Seizures in Critical Care

CURRENT CLINICAL NEUROLOGY

Daniel Tarsy, SERIES EDITOR

For other titles published in the series, go to
www.springer.com/series/7630

Seizures in Critical Care

A Guide to Diagnosis and Therapeutics

Second Edition

Edited by

Panayiotis Varelas, MD

Henry Ford Hospital
Detroit, MI
USA

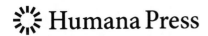 Humana Press

Editor
Panayiotis Varelas
Henry Ford Hospital
Detroit, MI
USA

ISBN 978-1-60327-531-6   e-ISBN 978-1-60327-532-3
DOI 10.1007/978-1-60327-532-3
Springer New York Dordrecht Heidelberg London

Library of Congress Control Number: 2009933998

Springer is part of Springer Science+Business Media (www.springer.com)

Preface to the Second Edition

Seizures in Critical Care: A Guide to Diagnosis and Therapeutics was published in the end of 2004. Based on the communication that my co-authors and I had with various health care providers, it was received very positively and was widely used as a reference book in many Intensive Care Units. It also received reviews in international journals and even from the World Federation of Neurology.

This positive attitude towards the book, and the fact that 5 years have passed since, made us entertain the idea of a second edition. My hope, as I have noted in the Preface of the first edition, was that " … it should constitute a testimony of the paucity of data in the field and become a starting point for well-organized research in the future." Although each one of us has a special interest in the field of seizures or ICU and follows closely the specific literature, it was the global curiosity to find what really happened during these 5 years—how much more the science has advanced and how much more we know now—that became the motive behind undertaking the daunting task of editing a specialized book like this.

There is new knowledge, indeed: several new studies, new antiepileptic medications, some of them available intravenously, and new published guidelines. This is not distributed evenly, however. Most chapters have undergone extensive revision due to an abundance of new data, few only moderately due to relative paucity of new information. Overall, the book looks fresh and new with the addition of a new chapter on neuromonitoring via continuous EEG in the ICU, complete re-writing of some chapters, addition of new cases with examples of EEGs and MRIs and new tables and figures. Authorities in their fields, Drs Dan Friedman and Larry Hirsch (continuous EEG monitoring), Denise Rhoney (neuropharmacology) and Paul Vespa (non-convulsive seizures in various brain injuries) joined the panel of previous authors to provide pertinent expertise to the readers.

Still a product of collaboration between various experts in the field of intensive care and epilepsy, this new edition is aimed at neurologists, general intensivists, neurosurgeons, and epileptologists. As with the first edition, our hope is that this new book will fulfill the need for more in-depth and specialized knowledge and will help provide specialized management in a very sick patient population.

Detroit, MI
May 2009

Panos Varelas, MD, PhD

Preface to the First Edition

Seizures are devastating events in one's life. Their very presence argues for something being wrong with the brain. In many places of the planet, they are still related to spirits or "sacred illness" and considered as either a curse or a reason for awe. Having been married to an epileptologist and been trained at Yale, one of the best Epilepsy centers in North America, I had a strong exposure and could not escape their spell. I became intrigued by the diversity of their presentation and fascinated by the possibility that various simple or complex behaviors, within the normal or abnormal range, could be explained by such an "obsolete" machine such as the electroencephalograph. Later on, after my training as a neuro-intensivist, my interest grew further while I was trying to find treatable causes in somnolent or comatose patients with various brain injuries in the ICU. This simplistic and mechanistic suspicion, that the patient's clinical status was due to an electrical discharge of the brain, led, I am sure, to several unnecessary requests for EEGs and trials of antiepileptics. Fortunately, I also had some unexpected successes.

Then, I started looking at the issue more closely and had revealing discussions with my peers, especially those who were not neuro-intensivists. To my surprise, two facts emerged: first, many in the ICU community, did not know what to seek, what to expect and how and when to treat; and second, while reviewing the literature, I could not find too much. Most of the articles were reporting small, uncontrolled series or personal experience. Few studies were conducted in the complex environment of an ICU. Very often, as with my personal experience, doubts regarding the epileptic nature of the phenomenon lingered. EEG, the gold-standard test, was difficult to interpret or inconsistently ordered. Seizures could be explained by more than one mechanism in many cases. In other cases, the response could be attributed not so much to the administration of the usual antiepileptics, but to the correction of more systemic derangements. Interaction between ICU medications and antiepileptics were frequent and puzzling to the treating physicians. Several of antiepileptics were either not available for parenteral administration or contraindicated due to specific organ failure. Finally, the newer antiepileptics were not well known and seldom used in the ICU.

Therefore, it did not take me too long to decide about the need for editing a book regarding seizures in the ICU. *Seizures in Critical Care: A Guide to Diagnosis and Therapeutics* is a collaborative effort. Experts in both the ICU and epilepsy fields mainly from North America but also from Europe contributed Chapters in this book. I tried to confine the content to the most common and interesting in the ICU, however. Norman Delanty's excellent book served as the starting point in many cases, but the scope was different. This book is much more balanced towards central nervous system insults, which can occur in the ICU. I encouraged reference to personal experience and included many real ICU cases with EEGs and neuroimages. Where data were lacking or information was contradictory, a very common situation indeed, the authors were advised to provide raw data and expert advice to the reader. Treatment of ICU seizures, most of the time uniform, is included in a separate Chapter. If more specific treatment is needed, for example pyridoxine for isoniazide-induced seizures, it is mentioned in the appropriate Chapter. Overall, our hope is that this book can serve as a useful aid in the everyday ICU and neurological practice for intensivists, neurologists, neurosurgeons, and any other health care professional or student in this expanding field. Most importantly in my mind, but less directly, it should constitute a testimony of the paucity of data in the field and become a starting point for well-organized research in the future.

Lastly, I would like to dedicate this effort to my parents, my grandfather (the shining star of my life) and all my teachers, who taught me the "ζείν"- living- and "ευ ζείν"- living well- of the ancients. I am also very grateful to all my co-authors, who did an excellent job and especially to my wife, Marianna, for her indirect contribution and support.

Detroit, MI   Panos Varelas, MD, PhD
February 2004

Series Editor's Introduction

The first edition of *Seizures in Critical Care: A Guide to Diagnosis and Therapeutics,* which appeared in 2005, filled an important need in the armamentarium of the neurological, neurosurgical, and medical intensivists who deal with seriously ill patients in the ICU setting. Unlike epilepsy, as it usually presents in the outpatient department, seizures in ICU patients are nearly always secondary phenomena that signify that something is seriously amiss in very ill patients with primary medical or surgical disease. The job of the intensivist is to identify the cause of the seizure or seizures, examine the myriad of potential contributing factors, and provide appropriate management and treatment that takes all aspects of the patient's illness into consideration. As in the first edition, Dr. Varelas and his associates recognize the extreme importance of prompt recognition, diagnosis, and sophisticated management of seizures in this group of seriously ill patients. Dr. Varelas has now recollected his group of contributors and produced a new and up to date compendium of what one needs to know in order to work effectively in this difficult and demanding area. A welcome addition to the new edition is the chapter by Friedman and Hirsch on the role of continuous monitoring in the ICU which is essential for the diagnosis and treatment of nonconvulsive seizures as these may be the most common form of seizures in this setting but are often missed in the evaluation of patients in stupor or coma. Recent technologic advances are described which allow for the simultaneous continuous monitoring of multiple ICU patients using new methods of data acquisition and analysis that allow for rapid and real-time transmission of information to the clinicians caring for the patient. The chapters on seizures due to metabolic causes and drug-induced seizures have new co-authors and have been revised and expanded while the other chapters have all been updated with new information and references. As in the first edition of this book, the issues discussed are all addressed with great common sense and sophistication by the very qualified contributors to this volume.

Daniel Tarsy MD
Professor in Neurology
Harvard Medical School
Beth Israel Deaconess Medical Center
Boston, MA

Contents

Contributors

Andrew Beaumont, MD, PhD
Department of Neurosurgery, Aspirus Spine and Neuroscience Institute,
Aspirus Wausau Hospital, Wausau, WI, USA

Lotfi Hacein Bey, MD
Interventional Neuro-Radiology, Radiological Associates of Sacramento
Medical Group Inc., Sacramento, CA, USA

Daniel Friedman, MD
Department of Neurology, Comprehensive Epilepsy Center,
Columbia University, New York, NY, USA

Romergyko Geocadin, MD
Associate Professor, Departments of Neurology, Anesthesiology-Critical
Care and Neurosurgery, Neurosciences Critical Care Division,
The Johns Hopkins Hospital, Baltimore, MD, USA

Errol Gordon, MD
Medical College of Wisconsin, Department of Neurology, Milwaukee,
WI, USA

Lawrence J. Hirsch, MD
Department of Neurology, Comprehensive Epilepsy Center,
Columbia University, New York, NY, USA

Matthew A. Koenig, MD
Assistant Professor, Departments of Neurology, Anesthesiology-Critical
Care and Neurosurgery, Neurosciences Critical Care Division,
The Johns Hopkins Hospital, Baltimore, MD, USA

Andreas R. Luft, MD
Department of Neurology, University of Tubingen, Tubingen, Germany

Marek A. Mirski, MD, PhD
Director, Neurosciences Critical Care Unit, Departments of Neurology,
Anesthesiology, & Critical Care Medicine and Neurosurgery, The Johns
Hopkins Hospital, Baltimore, MD, USA

Efstathios Papavassiliou, MD
Assistant Professor, Department of Neurosurgery, Beth Israel Deaconess
Medical Center, Harvard Medical School, Boston, MA, USA

Mohammed Rehman, DO
Fellow, Neurocritical Care, Henry Ford Hospital, Detroit, MI, USA

Denise Rhoney, PharmD, FCCP, FCCM
Associate Professor, Pharmacy Practice, Eugene Applebaum College of
Pharmacy & Health Sciences, Wayne State University, Detroit, MI, USA
Clinical Associate Professor, Department of Neurology, Wayne State
University School of Medicine, Detroit, MI, USA

Jenice Robinson, MD
Department of Neurology, Milton S Hershey Medical Center,
Penn State University College of Medicine, Hershey, PA, USA

Marianna V. Spanaki, MD, PhD, MBA
Director, Epilepsy Monitoring Unit, Senior Staff of Neurology,
Henry Ford Hospital, Detroit, MI, USA
Associate Professor of Neurology, Wayne State University, Detroit, MI, USA

Jose I Suarez, MD
Director, Vascular Neurology and Neurocritical Care, Associate Professor
of Neurology, Department of Neurology, Baylor College of Medicine,
Houston, TX, USA

Michel Torbey, MD, MPH, FAHA, FCCM
Director, Stroke Critical Care Program, Department of Neurology,
Medical College of Wisconsin, Milwaukee, WI, USA

Panayiotis N. Varelas, MD, PhD
Director, Neuro-Intensive Care Unit, Senior Staff Neurology &
Neurosurgery, Henry Ford Hospital, Detroit, MI, USA
Associate Professor of Neurology, Wayne State University, Detroit, MI, USA

Paul Vespa, MD, FCCM
Associate Professor of Neurosurgery and Neurology,
Director of Neurocritical Care, David Geffen School of Medicine,
University of California, Los Angeles, CA, USA

Zachary Webb, MD, DABPN, DABSM
Medical Director, Sleep Disorders Center, NorthStar Medical Specialists,
Bellingham, WA, USA

Eelco FM Wijdicks, MD, PhD, FACP
Professor of Neurology, Mayo Medical School, Medical Director,
Neurology–Neurosurgery Intensive Care Unit, Consultant,
Department of Neurology, Mayo Clinic, Rochester, MN, USA

Greg A. Worrell, MD
Division of Epilepsy, Department of Neurology, Mayo Clinic,
Rochester, MN, USA

Tarek Zakaria, MD
Division of Epilepsy, Department of Neurology, Mayo Clinic,
Rochester, MN, USA

Wendy C. Ziai, MD, MPH
Assistant Professor of Neurology, Anesthesia and Neurosurgery,
Neurosciences Critical Care Division, Departments of Neurology,
Neurosurgery, and Anesthesiology, Critical Care Medicine,
The Johns Hopkins Hospital, Baltimore, MD, USA

Chapter 1

Presentation and Pathophysiology of Seizures in the Critical Care Environment: An Overview

Marek A. Mirski

Abstract Seizures represent stereotypic electroencephalographic (EEG) and behavioral paroxysms as a consequence of electrical neurological derangement. Although seizures are often associated with stereotypic convulsive phenomena, in the ICU they are as likely to be subclinical as they are to express muscle contractions or behavioral symptoms. Hence, vigilance is required in the critical care setting. Due to the admission diagnoses and physiological derangements common to critically ill patients, the intensive care unit (ICU) hosts conditions appropriate for the manifestation of the entire spectrum of seizure disorders. Common etiologies of seizures in the ICU are due to primary neurological pathology or secondary to critical illness and clinical management. Alterations in neurotransmitter sensitivity via up- or down regulation of receptors, a decrease in inhibition, alterations in membrane pump functions, all may contribute to the high incidence of seizures in an ICU. Particularly prevalent as precipitants of seizures are hypoxia/ischemia, mass lesions, drug toxicity, and metabolic abnormalities. For optimal treatment, early diagnosis of the seizure type and its cause is important to ensure appropriate therapy. Most seizures and their recurrence are easily treated, and attention is focused on ascertaining the cause and correcting any medical abnormality. Convulsive status epilepticus represents the most feared seizure state, and requires emergent treatment before irreversible brain injury and severe metabolic disturbances occur. Treatment of seizures with anticonvulsants in an ICU is not without risks, and appropriate judgment and selection of therapeutic drugs are important.

Keywords Critical care, Seizures, Pathophysiology, GABA receptors, Nonconvulsive status, Convulsive status epilepticus

1.1. Introduction

Over the past several decades, a collective attempt has been made to define the precise circuitry of brain elements important in seizure expression, together with the physiological mechanisms that ignite these paroxysms. Such answers,

From: *Seizures in Critical Care: A Guide to Diagnosis and Therapeutics*: Current Clinical Neurology,
Second Edition, Edited by: P. Varelas, DOI 10.1007/978-1-60327-532-3_1,
© Humana Press, a part of Springer Science+Business Media, LLC 2005, 2010

in theory, would provide the necessary clues to successfully inhibit and prevent the ictal process. Nature, of course, thwarts our attempts to simplify the human condition, and perhaps the most unsettling physiological constraint is our inability to comprehend the intricacies of brain function. Seizures lie within that neurological realm.

In a comparative manner, the complex care environment of the intensive care unit (ICU) is to clinical management what the brain is to human physiology. We still remain appreciably uneducated as to the fundamental physiology that transitions normal brain excitation to ictal behavior. Seizures may occur in any individual, given the appropriate triggers. Our brains normally have a "cloak" of inhibition that aids in protecting us from paroxysmal excitation. Such protective measures become less effective when one is stricken with critical illness, and even less so given additional neurological injury, such as trauma, ischemia, or inflammation,. Coupled with the myriad of physiological derangements that commonly occur in the ICU setting, our risk for seizures becomes unsettlingly high. The ICU is, therefore, both the best environment to gain an understanding into the nature of seizures – based on the incidence, and the worst – because of the multiple and overlapping etiologic factors present. For intensivists, the complexities inherent in an ICU translate to the clinical truism that seizures may appear often and may manifest in severe form, with a few gross noncompliances to routine in-patient management.

As we have come to appreciate, seizures within the ICU are of many types, and the clinical characteristics of each are dependent on the region of brain involved. The term epilepsy, in fact, encompasses a wide variety of recurrent seizure disorders that have been classified in accordance with the location and extent of the seizure process within the brain. Fundamentally, seizures are of two types. They may be partial (focal) in nature or they may be generalized (Table 1-1). This distinction is appropriate for two reasons. First, the extent of cortical involvement differs between the groups. Second, and more important, each seizure type has a neuroanatomical mechanism that is fundamentally distinct. In the examination into their origin, many analytical tools and methods have been used. Surface and depth electroencephalographic recordings have provided the majority of evidence to date, although radiographic techniques such as radionuclide autoradiography, positron emission tomography, computed tomography (CT), and a variety of magnetic resonance (MR) sequence studies have proven to be of substantial value.

The greatest consideration in anatomical mapping has been given to focal epilepsies, in which structural disease is frequently apparent. These seizures display electroencephalographic and clinical manifestations consistent with the involvement of only a portion of the cortex and its corresponding functional systems (Fig. 1-1). Such events are precipitated by local excitatory aberrations of the corresponding cerebral mantle, with the spread typically to adjacent

Table 1-1. Common Presentation of Seizures in the ICU.

Seizure type	Clinical expression
Focal motor	Face or limb motor seizure, no alteration of sensorium
Generalized tonic-clonic	Loss of consciousness, generalized convulsions
Complex-partial	Disturbed sensorium, automatisms common
Non-convulsive status	Disturbed sensorium or loss of consciousness

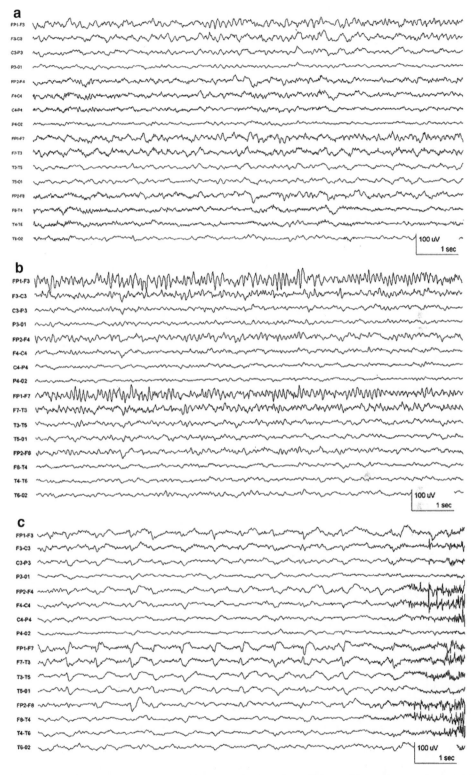

Fig. 1-1. Beginning of a partial (*left frontal temporal*) seizure in a 60-year-old man in complex partial status epilepticus due to vasculitis. (**b**) Thirty seconds after seizure onset. (**c**) The seizure ends with repetitive left frontal temporal sharp waves after 2 min and 7 s. Courtesy of Brenner RP (90)

cortical regions via local synaptic connections. Such ictal events are exemplified by the classic "Jacksonian march", a focal seizure that spreads along the cortical motor strip to progressively excite the neurons that control topographically associated limb musculature.

Other partial seizures, such as many of the temporal epilepsies, are formally described as partial complex because conscious contact with the environment is disturbed. The anatomy involved in this form of epilepsy is more complex than a simple partial seizure because of the recruitment of deeper brain elements that affect our conscious behavior. Most commonly, elements of the limbic brain, usually the hippocampus or amygdala and their connections, play a major role in the expression of these seizures. Automatisms frequent such ictal events – speech or behavioral mannerisms such as lip smacking, blinking, or repetitive hand movements. Such seizures that affect nonmotor regions of the cerebral cortex may be difficult to diagnose unless suspicion is high. Such patients may only appear noninteractive, or in a "fugue" state.

At the other end of the spectrum are the generalized seizures, where consciousness is affected and convulsions may occur throughout the face and extremities. Axial rigidity is not maintained, and the patient will fall if standing. Generalized seizures commonly begin with a focal cortical nidus, from which proceeds rapid spread of ictal activity. This "secondary" generalization may, in some circumstances, be too rapid for the electroencephalogram (EEG) to detect (Fig. 1-2). As a group, generalized seizures likely spread via cortical networks or cortical–subcortical circuits. The "primary" generalized seizures (example: absence epilepsy or primary tonic-clonic seizures) probably utilize brainstem/subcortical structures in the mediation and propagation of the paroxysmal activity (1–5).

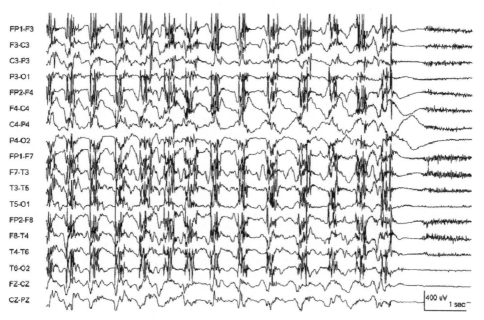

Fig. 1-2. Generalized spike and wave, best seen in the midline electrodes, with prominent superimposed repetitive muscle artifact during the clonic phase, followed by postictal suppression in a 22-year-old woman with a primary generalized tonic-clonic seizure. Courtesy of Brenner RP (90)

No cortical nidus is identified, and the deeper cerebral elements are the likely culprits in the initiation, or at least early propagation of these events (6–13). These primary generalized seizures are exemplified by bilaterally synchronous and symmetrical epileptiform discharges on EEG and clinical behavior typically characterized by loss of consciousness and generalized convulsive or paralytic motor phenomena. Although it is commonly stated that bilateral cortical involvement in a synchronized ictal EEG renders loss of consciousness, it has been demonstrated that there are exceptions (14, 15). Indeed, such descriptions support the fact that even during expression of "generalized seizures", there are brain regions seemingly uninvolved in the paroxysmal activity, and can maintain circuit integrity for a wakeful state. In the majority of instances of generalized seizures, no diffuse or focal brain disease or generalized metabolic disturbance can be convincingly demonstrated. Non-convulsive generalized seizures may also occur, and are more difficult to diagnose. As discussed later, such seizures often complicate the management of the comatose ICU patient.

In the intensive care unit (ICU) setting, seizures are a common neurological complication in both medical and post-surgical patients, and commonly arise from co-morbidities associated with the ICU experience (Table 1-2).

Table 1-2. Complications of Critical Illness – Seizure Predisposition.

Hypoxia/ischemia

Drug/substance toxicity

    Antibiotics

    Antidepressants

    Antipsychotics

    Bronchodilators

    Local anesthetics

    Immunosuppressives

    Cocaine

    Amphetamines

    Phencyclidine

Drug/substance withdrawal

    Barbiturates

    Benzodiazepines

    Opioids

    Alcohol

Infection & Fever

Metabolic abnormalities

    Hypophosphatemia

    Hypocalcemia

    Hypoglycemia

    Renal / hepatic dysfunction

Surgical injury (craniotomy)

Most ICU seizures occur in patients never having had a prior episode, or having neurological pathology as part of the primary admitting diagnosis. A review by Bleck et. al. noted that approximately 12% of patients admitted with nonneurological primary diagnoses incurred neurological events during their critical illness (16). Of these, seizures (28.1% incidence) closely followed metabolic encephalopathy (28.6%) as the leading neurological complication. Status epilepticus, the diagnosis most associated with seizures and the ICU is, in fact, a rare admission diagnosis (0.2%) as compared to the incidence of seizures as a complication (3.3%). Since seizures occur most often in non-primary neurological patients, it is important for the general clinician, intensivist, and consulting neurologist to be cognizant about the potential for seizures in the ICU and be aggressive in treating them.

Regardless of the seizure type, the medical management in an ICU and the environment itself unfortunately present unique challenges and difficulties with regards to the etiology, diagnosis, and treatment of seizures. Patients are critically ill, and the common scenario of multi-system organ dysfunction presents a variety of potential etiologies for cerebral disturbance, often predisposing to seizures. Also, treatment with sedatives, as a means to provide comfort to the patient, and paralytic agents to optimize therapy alike, hinder the neurological examination (17). Many pharmaceuticals used in an ICU, particularly the psychotropic medications, antibiotics, stimulants, and others may also lower seizure threshold (18, 19). Anticonvulsants and other medications may alternatively sedate the patient or enhance toxic responses, further delaying neurological recovery from the seizure episode (20). Such difficulties may lead to additional diagnostic studies and prolongation of ICU stay. Seizures may also accompany conditions that render the patient into a coma state – such as severe encephalopathy, trauma, or stroke (21–28), or following seemingly uncomplicated procedures in healthy patients. For example, of late, the phenomenon of Posterior Reversible Encephalopathy Syndrome (PRES) has been reported more frequently as a consequence of labor and delivery, and seizures can be one of its prominent manifestations (29). Recurrent or continuous seizure activity may prevent arousal, and requires EEG assessment for correct diagnosis. More seriously, recurrent seizures and status epilepticus (SE) are more difficult to suppress than simple focal or generalized convulsions and can be life-threatening when they occur as complications of primary neurological or other visceral organ disease. Finally, the ICU itself is an environment with considerable electrical field dispersion, often preventing optimal EEG recording.

The need to diagnose and effectively treat recurrent seizure activity is imperative. Multiple seizure events or convulsive SE may lead to acidosis, hyperthermia, rhabdomyolysis, and trauma with consequent higher morbidity and mortality (30, 31). Loss of protective airway reflexes is common in patients with prolonged or recurrent seizures, and promotes the likelihood of pulmonary aspiration. The duration of seizures of more than one hour is an independent predictor of poor outcome (odds ratio of almost 10) (31). Prolonged seizures increase the risk of cerebral damage due to excitotoxicity, intracellular Ca^{++} accumulation and apoptosis, epileptogenic synaptic reorganization and sprouting, and the depletion of energy stores with inhibition of protein and DNA synthesis (32).

1.2. Cellular Pathphysiology of ICU Seizures

Fundamentally, despite numerous phenotypic expressions of seizures and epilepsy syndromes, the manifestations of the ictal process emanate from a few common cellular mechanisms and brain loci. The cerebral cortex is the nidus for most clinically evident seizures; the hippocampus, the most rudimentary cortical element of the medial temporal lobe, also falls into that category. Regarding subcortical structures, it is well known that the thalamus plays a substantive role in mediating the paroxysms and supporting the hypersynchronous, rhythmic EEG activation. Specific research effort has prominently identified all three locations in seizure mechanisms, and implicated a variety of neuronal and glial functions (10, 33–36).

As evidenced by the cortical EEG, the fundamental marker for an epileptic paroxysm is the interictal spike, which is the electrical fingerprint of the intracellular paroxysmal depolarizing shift or PDS (Fig. 1-3). The interictal spike is generated by a synchronous firing of a network of local neurons, coupled

Abnormal Neuronal Firing

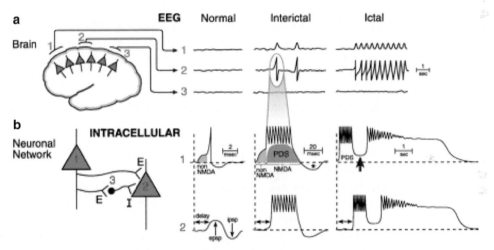

Fig. 1-3. Abnormal neuronal firing at the levels of (**a**) the brain and (**b**) a simplified neuronal network consisting of two excitatory neurons (90, 91) and an inhibitory interneuron (1). EEG (*top set of traces*) and intracellular recordings (*bottom set of traces*) are shown for the normal (*left column*), interictal (*middle column*), and ictal conditions (*right column*). Numbered traces refer to like-numbered recording sites. Note time scale differences in different traces. (**a**) Three EEG electrodes record activity from superficial neocortical neurons. In the normal case, activity is low voltage and "desynchronized" (neurons are not firing together in synchrony). In the interictal condition, large "spikes" are seen focally at electrode 2 (and to a lesser extent at electrode 1, where they might be termed "sharp waves"), representing synchronized firing of a large population of hyperexcitable neurons (expanded in time below). The ictal state is characterized by a long run of spikes. (**b**) At the neuronal network level, the intracellular correlate of the interictal EEG spike is called the "paroxysmal depolarization shift" (PDS). The PDS is initiated by a non-NMDA-mediated fast EPSP (*blue*) but is maintained by a longer, larger NMDA-mediated EPSP (*red*). The post-PDS hyperpolarization (*) temporarily stabilizes the neuron. If this post-PDS hyperpolarization fails (*right column, thick arrow*), ictal discharge can occur. The lowermost traces, recordings from neuron 2, show activity similar to that recorded in neuron 1, with some delay (double-headed arrow). Activation of inhibitory neuron 3 by firing of neuron 1 prevents neuron 2 from generating an action potential (the IPSP counters the depolarization caused by the EPSP). If it does reach firing threshold, neuron 2 then can recruit additional neurons, leading to an entire network firing in synchrony (seizure). Illustration by Marcia Smith and Alan Michaels. Courtesy Strafstrom (91)

with periods of inhibition via K^+ current-activated hyperpolarization. Neurons that are particularly readily disposed to such activity are the pyramidal cells of cortical layer V and the CA3 neurons within the hippocampus (37). These cells are synaptically linked to regional neurons that amplify the excitation within a synaptic network. The paroxysmal discharge may be induced by a local increase in excitation, a decrease inhibitory neurotransmission, or alteration in Na^+ or K^+ current conductance (38). Excitation is classically derived from direct stimulation of N-methyl,D-aspartate (NMDA) receptors or enhancement of synaptic transmission via reduction of K^+ current. Reduced inhibition may stem from antagonism of gamma-amino-butyric acid (GABA) activity at its receptor or decreasing GABA binding through chemical means, such as a reduction of local Mg^{++} (39–42).

The interictal spike may be effectively transitioned to an array of several spikes, or a "burst", by the presence of local burst-generating cells. These are made possible by persistent Na^+ and Ca^{++} slow action potential currents that function primarily in the dendritic formations, promoting prolonged depolarizations in the neuron soma (41, 43). The bursts appear to further manifest when there is alternating depolarization between the dendrites and soma (44). Network modeling of hippocampal cells has reproduced the EEG events of a tonic-clonic seizure (45, 46). The high frequency firing tonic component is triggered by prolonged somatic depolarizations, and the slower synchronous clonic seizure results from rhythmic bursting of slow-channel dendrite depolarizations. Continued depolarization of the neuronal membrane (contrast to the brief depolarization of a PDS), is responsible for the maintenance of successive rapid discharges inherent in a stereotypic seizure. Recurrent after discharges, as occur during a clonic seizure, are perpetuated by a reduction of the hyperpolarizations that occur following aberrant paroxysms such as the interictal spike.

Now that the susceptible tissue has undergone epileptiform transformation, the propagation to larger cortical terrain, or even to generalize, requires vital network pathways and connections (47, 48). On a regional scale, ictal events may spread by disruption of the local chemical environment, such as alterations in K^+ or Mg^{++}. Such spread is not very rapid, estimated at 50–200 mm/sec (49). Clinically important seizure propagation must clearly utilize synaptic transmission via networked connections. Even ectopic transmission has been proposed as a means to further enhance the spread or continuation of the ictal state (50). Such cortico-cortico or subcortico-cortico circuitry has only been occasionally identified (10, 35, 50–52) (example, Fig. 1-4).

We do know from clinical experience that there are many pathological conditions inherent in ICU patients – particularly those with primary cerebral disturbance, that predispose to seizures (Table 1-3). However, very little is known concerning the contribution of regional pathology on the predisposition to seizures, despite ready acknowledgement that injured regions of brain following a stroke or head injury appear more prone to paroxysms than native cortex (53). Similarly, brain tissue adjacent to "irritative elements" such as neoplasms with associated edema or vascular malformations has been associated with a high risk of manifesting seizures. The mechanisms leading to enhanced susceptibility have only recently been forthcoming (Table 1-4) (54, 55).

It is clear from work on cerebral neoplasia that tumors may have intrinsic cellular properties inciting an epileptogenic focus (56, 57). Other consequences of a mass lesion that impacts regional blood flow and supply (such as tumors

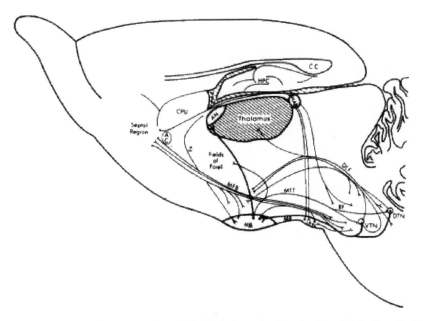

Fig. 1-4. Sagittal illustration of rat brain depicting one of the few identified subcortical pathways participating in the early propagation of experimental generalized seizures. In this case, the expression of seizures induced by the chemical convulsant pentylenetetrazol has been shown to be modulated by the perturbation of neuronal activity within the path from the brainstem (ventral & dorsal tegmental nuclei) synaptically linked to the hypothalamus, anterior thalamus (AN), and cingulate gyrus (31). Recent clinical trials of deep brain stimulation of AN for refractory epilepsy have been very promising (Medtronic-SANTE Trial). *MB* mammillary bodies, *MTT* mammillotegmental tracts, *VTN* ventral tegmental nuclei, *DTN* dorsal tegmental nuclei, *MFB*: median forebrain bundle; *CPU* caudate-putamen, *HPC* hippocampus, *DLF* dorsal longitudinal fasciculus; *MP* mammillary peduncle

Table 1-3. Common Etiologies of Seizures in the ICU.

Neurological pathology

    Neurovascular
     Stroke
     Arteriovenous malformations
     Hemorrhage
    Tumor
     Primary
     Metastatic
    CNS infection
     Abscess
     Meningitis
     Encephalitis
    Inflammatory disease
     Vasculitis
     Acute disseminated encephalomyelitis
    Traumatic head injury
     Contusion
     Hemorrhage
    Primary epilepsy
    Primary CNS metabolic disturbance (inherited)

Table 1-4. Pro-Convulsant Mechanisms Inherent in Cerebral Neoplastic and Vascular Malformations.

Intrinsic epileptogenic cellular properties (tumors)
Local impaired vascularization/ischemia
Denervation hypersensitivity
Axonal & synaptic plasticity
Decrease in regional GABA
Increase in local glutamate
Alteration of electrolyte ions – Mg^{++}
Increase in regional Fe^{++}

Adapted from Beaumont and Whittle (93).

Table 1-5. Intracranial Pathology and Relative Risk for Seizures.

Pathology	High risk
Stroke	Hemorrhagic
	Large cortical involvement
	Acute confusional state
Intracranial tumor	Cortical – primary
	Cortical – metastatic
Traumatic head injury	Cerebral contusion
	Acute subdural (SDH)
	Depressed skull fracture
	Penetrating missile injury
	Evacuation/chronic SDH

or AVMs) are the potential for local tissue ischemia, denervation hypersensitivity, alteration in neural plasticity, and disequilibrium of the local microchemistry – GABA, glutamate, Mg^{++}, etc (58–61). Some evidence also suggests alterations in intercellular iron ions (Fe^{++} or Fe^{+++}) may exist and predispose to seizures. Aside from the putative intrinsic epileptogenic characteristics of certain tumor types themselves, the pro-convulsant features listed above that have been associated with tumors and AVMs, may likely apply to cerebral tissue affected by head injury, stroke, and inflammatory conditions (Table 1-5). In the following chapters, there will be a detailed discussion relating to the specific etiologies and therapies for seizures occurring in the ICU arena.

1.3. Clinical Manifestations and Diagnosis

A focal or generalized seizure commonly lasts for several seconds or up to 1–2 min. During this period, alterations in hemodynamics and respiratory indices are typical in generalized convulsions, with increases usually recorded in heart rate and blood pressure. Ventilation may be impeded in the latter seizure type, with desaturation noted on pulse oximetry, often with excessive salivation. Interestingly, although grunting and gasping are encountered during a generalized tonic-clonic seizure, patients only rarely incur an aspiration event. If one should occur, it is almost always of the patient's oral secretions rather than gastric contents. Therefore, patient care during a violent convulsion is focused on protecting the patient from extremity injury, biting of the tongue, and maintenance of a clear airway during prolonged seizures. Brief desaturations are the rule, and require no special intervention. For the vast majority of simple convulsive episodes, protection of the airway beyond what is described above, or frank ventilatory support, is not indicated. A depressed sensorium is common following a generalized convulsion, requiring several additional minutes before baseline is re-established. Focal or generalized seizures may also lead to post-ictal focal deficits (Todd's paralysis), lasting up to several hours. These deficits are especially common in patients with pre-existing subtle weakness from a mass lesion or stroke, and seizures can accentuate these pre-convulsive neurological impairments. In contrast to generalized convulsive episodes, patients with focal seizures are fully cogent during their attack, and those with complex-partial seizures typically return rapidly to their baseline neurological state.

Most seizures that occur in an ICU setting, likely manifest as generalized tonic-clonic convulsions, including secondary generalization, with some reports observing approximately 90% of the presenting seizure as of this variety (16, 26). Focal seizures comprise the majority of remaining behaviorally disturbing seizure types. These data suggest that recognition of a seizure in the ICU is rarely a diagnostic dilemma. Although uncommon, patients who do present with complex-partial or other nonconvulsive seizures (9%) may be considerably more difficult to diagnose, especially in a critical care setting where sedative medication is often administered. That said, there is increasing concern that nonconvulsive SE (NCSE) may be much more prevalent in ICU patients. Recent data suggests that 5%–10% of ICU comatose patients were in NCSE (62). Other investigators have evidence to suggest that the incidence of non-convulsive seizures is alarmingly high, up to 34% of neurological ICU patients, and it is only for a lack of monitoring that these seizures are not detected (63, 64).

Specifically within the ICU setting, there have been reports of an interesting phenomenon known as "stimulus-induced seizures", whereby relatively minor tactile stimulation to the patient evokes a rhythmic, ictal EEG discharge and may be accompanied by overt motor clonic activity (65, 66). Hirsch et al have described these events as "stimulus-induced rhythmic, periodic, or ictal discharges" (SIRPIDs) (66). Such evoked responses are usually focal in nature. There are reports that focal stimulation may induce bilateral periodic discharges (PEDS) and a mild arousal response in comatose patients (67).

Besides overt behavioral manifestations, the scalp EEG is the diagnostic test of choice. Even when a seizure is noted by obvious clinical expression, evaluating the treatment success according to the presence or absence of motor paroxysms or level of consciousness may be occasionally misleading. Treatment of motor convulsions alone may be insufficient to prevent the continuation of seizure activity. The persistence of electrographic status without convulsions (NCSE) has been observed in 14% of patients treated for convulsive SE (68). Conversely, improvement in the neurological examination is often a poor clinical assessment tool, as 87% of patients successfully treated for convulsive SE and 100% of patients treated for NCSE remained comatose 12 h following the initiation of therapy (69). Therefore, it cannot be over emphasized that electrical monitoring of ICU patients is crucial in settings where seizures may be a complicating feature of critical illness. Unless a seizure fully resolves and the patient returns to an alert, cognitive baseline, an EEG is highly useful, if not mandatory to exclude ongoing ictal activity.

1.4. Overview of Status Epilepticus

Status epilepticus represents a distinct seizure phenomenon. Not simply a prolonged seizure, SE represents a reconfiguration of the excitatory and inhibitory network of normal brain (70). Most focal seizures do not secondarily spread to produce a generalized event because of local inhibitory circuitry (GABA-mediated) that prevents enlargement of the ictus. As seizures continue, it is known that a breakdown occurs within this cortical "inhibitory surround", thus making it easier for seizure activity to spread. In addition, the inhibitory events which assist in terminating the seizures also become disturbed. Thus, recurrent or prolonged seizures induce a positive feedback loop that help sustain, rather than inhibit further ictal activity. In essence, "seizures beget seizures" (70).

Exactly when a prolonged seizure or set of recurrent seizures is deemed to have become "SE" is a question that continues to evolve. Historically, since the 1960's, the minimum time of unremitting seizures before SE said to occur by experts in the field was arbitrarily assigned to 30 min. This included a single generalized seizure lasting greater than 30 min, or a group of repetitive seizures between which the patient had not fully recovered. Given the discussion regarding the risk of early neuronal injury, and a desire to adequately treat this disorder prior to irreversible cerebral insult, shorter seizure epochs have been more recently emphasized as SE. Based on the typical seizure duration of 1–2 min., it is reasonable to consider as SE any seizure events greater than 5–10 minutes in length. Such is now the tenet of the American Academy of Neurology and the American Epilepsy Society. There are several reports describing seizures of 10–29 min duration that have had spontaneous resolution without therapy, but consensus is that these represent a small population. It is strongly felt that a high risk-benefit ratio exists in not treating such patients as SE. If treatment was required to "stop" the clinically obvious seizure, EEG correlation again is advocated if the patient has not returned to their pre-ictal, alert condition.

There are three main subtypes of SE, two of which are prominent in the ICU. Generalized Convulsive SE (GCSE) represents the classic motor SE (Fig. 1-5). These seizures may be overt or have subtle motor manifestations, especially if the SE is prolonged. By far, GCSE is the most commonly reported SE subtype. Focal Motor SE (FMSE) or epilepsy partialis continuans, is relatively uncommon, and rare in the ICU. Continuous motor twitching of a single limb or a side of the face is most frequently observed. These seizures can be difficult to control with medications. It is not clear whether prolonged FMSE results in substantive injury to the cerebral cortex. Thus, reasonable attempts at control are advocated, but high-risk therapies such as induced pharmacological coma are rarely involved. Nonconvulsive SE (NCSE) is often used as an umbrella term incorporating a wide spectrum of continuous non-motor seizures. As a group, they may encompass primary generalized SE, such

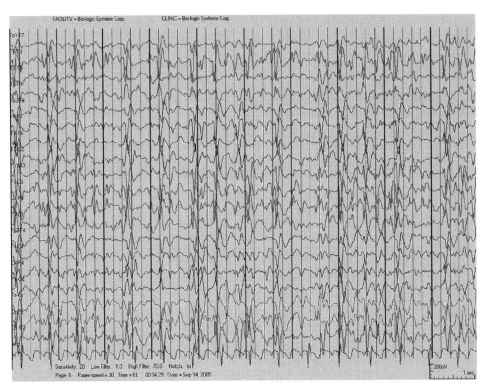

Fig. 1-5. This EEG shows diffuse multifocal or generalized spikes or spike waves that then pervade the recording during non-REM sleep, and 1.5–2.0 Hz generalized spike waves. Courtesy Kaplan (92)

as absence SE, which has a very stereotypic EEG, to secondary generalized seizures with variable EEG features (Fig. 1-6). Other terms within NCSE are complex-partial SE, subtle SE, nontonic-clonic SE, and subclinical SE. The hallmark is a diminishment of the neurological exam secondary to the seizure, but the patient may present clinically anywhere along the spectrum between being awake/ambulatory to coma. The true incidence of this subtype of SE is unknown and likely under recognized (64, 71). Pertinent to the ICU setting, a recent trend ascribes the label of NCSE to patients having suffered from severe anoxic/ischemic encephalopathy, when characteristic EEG spikes are present. When such EEG findings, consisting of bilateral periodic lateralizing epileptiform discharges (PLEDS), are present along with the appropriate clinical history, they portend a poor neurological outcome (72).

Although there is a strong consensus in aggressively treating GCSE (73–78), there is mixed opinion as to the proper management of NCSE (63, 68). These seizures are diagnosed by recurrent paroxysmal or epileptiform bursts on the cortical EEG. In the purest form, without prior evidence of cerebral injury or mass lesion, NCSE is typically benign. Apart from the altered cognition during the seizure that may be disabling, there is no evidence that permanent morbidity has been attributed to this form of SE. Thus, therapy should be directed towards chronic prevention of the attacks. In the ICU, however, most forms of NCSE are associated with a history of moderate to severe cerebral injury, as following an anoxic-ischemic event or trauma. Although associating the effects of NCSE on direct neuronal injury is difficult in this setting, most

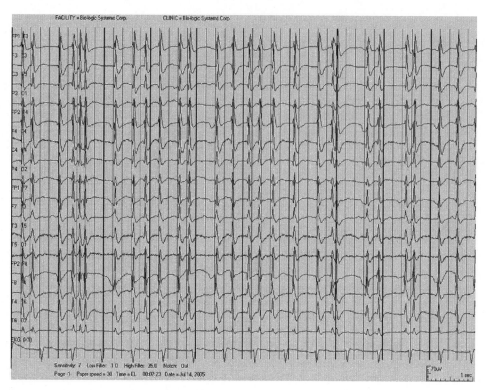

Fig. 1-6. This EEG shows generalized, but predominantly synchronous frontal epileptic discharges typical of GNSE. Courtesy Kaplan (92)

Table 1-6. Typical EEG Presentation of GCSE and NCSE SE.

Classic GCSE	Generalized spike or sharp wave pattern –begins from a normal background rhythm. SE is characterized by an unremitting spike activity or, more commonly, a crescendo-decrescendo pattern of major motor ictal periods interspersed with lower voltage paroxysmal activity. No abrupt termination or "postictal depression" is observed as following simple seizures.
NCSE	EEG is variable, with a number of EEG patterns being recognized. Generally, seizures such as complex-partial status resemble their non-SE counterparts.

epileptologists would agree that in such scenarios the presence of continuous paroxysmal activity may accentuate injury incurred by the primary insult. Therefore, it is felt prudent to attempt therapy as rapidly as is feasible. To what degree one should attempt to abolish the EEG paroxysms remains unclear, although even the induction of barbiturate coma has been performed.

As may be expected, monitoring by EEG is critical to the accurate diagnosis of SE, and for monitoring of the therapeutic response. This is especially true for both NCSE and prolonged convulsive SE, where there is a paucity of physical findings and the EEG may be the only effective tool for diagnosis (75–80). Table 1-6 lists common EEG features of GCSE and NCSE. For ongoing SE, EEG (preferably continuous) is mandatory to ensure effective treatment. Commonly, convulsive SE is incompletely treated with residual subtle EEG seizures or NCSE, despite cessation of motor ictal activity. Some clinical reports suggest residual electrographic seizures in almost 50% of patients with GCSE, and a 10–20% incidence of NCSE in those patients treated for GCSE with cessation of motor seizure activity (68).

1.5. Paroxysmal Lateralizing Epileptiform Discharges (PLEDS)

The significance of paroxysmal lateralizing epileptiform discharges (PLEDs) has been debated since their first designation in the early 1960's, but the fact not in dispute is their frequent attendance in ICU patients. Although not rigidly defined, PLEDs have been ascribed to the presence of spikes, sharp waves, or mix of sharp-spike waves that may have coincident slow waves that together appear on the EEG at regular, periodic intervals (Fig. 1-7) (81). Mostly described in patients with cortical injury, PLEDs have also been associated with patients with epilepsy syndromes and following bouts of severe seizures, such as SE. Ischemic stroke appears to be the most frequent etiology, but other brain conditions such as hemorrhage, neoplasms, cortical infection and inflammation, and even metabolic disturbances have been linked to this EEG phenomenon (82).

The underlying pathophysiological mechanisms remain unclear, but their similarity to the interictal spike suggests that similar chemical/membrane disturbances underlying the PDS may be fundamental. An interesting observation

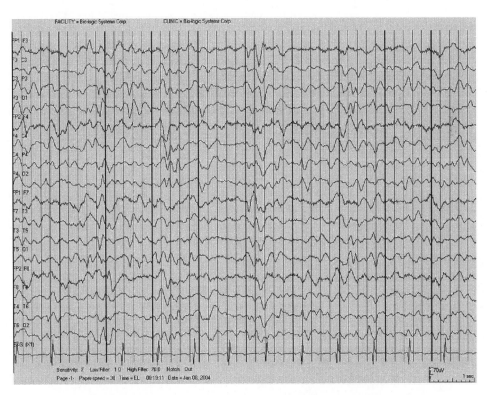

Fig. 1-7. This EEG shows bilateral, independent PLEDs occurring over the left and right frontal regions, without clinical correlate. Courtesy Kaplan (92)

has been made where clinically occurring PLEDs were linked to basal ganglia circuit function (83). This is of interest as it links subcortical activity with PLEDs, and thus connects this epileptiform phenotype with the basal ganglia association with seizures (84).

Many consider PLEDs a cerebral response to an acute focal process, although these paroxysms may last for several years if a stroke or mass lesion remains a physiological irritant. Although structural injury is the greatest stimulant for development of PLEDs, metabolic or diffuse alteration of cerebral function may be an etiologic factor in some patients (85). The presence or absence of coincident paroxysmal bursts leads to a subcategorization of "simple or proper PLEDs" or "PLEDs plus" (86). The disappearance of PLEDs either spontaneously or with anticonvulsant therapy has been well documented (87, 88).

Lacking consensus is the attribution of PLEDS to an active ictal state. It is clear that these discharges may come in the setting of a diagnosis of seizures, or simply with a structural lesion. Data does not appear to support definite conclusions that may be drawn from their presence, such as patient clinical outcome or as further risk for seizures (89). Some have observed that PLEDS may occur secondary to tactile stimulation in comatose patients associated with a clinical arousal response (67).

1.6. Conclusion

Seizures occurring in the ICU setting are more difficult to prevent, diagnose, and treat effectively than those manifesting outside the ICU or hospital. Particularly challenging is the diagnostic component of seizure management, especially when only subtle clinical evidence is present, and the EEG is not conclusive. The use of a variety of medications and the clinical management in an ICU all tend to lower, rather than elevate seizure threshold. A high index of suspicion is warranted by the intensivist, and early use of EEG surveillance can be vital in early detection. Treatment of seizures in an ICU setting can also be challenging, even when not dealing with SE. The ability to recognize and treat seizures is critical, however, as there exists clear evidence for potential grave neurological injury when seizures persist as SE. However, the treatment of seizures itself may impose new patient toxicity, and requires appropriate toxicity/benefit evaluation, as well as proper drug selection. Lastly, confronting the etiology of the seizures, assessing the risk for future episodes, and understanding treatment options can greatly assist in formulating their acute ICU and future therapeutic management.

References

1. Andy OJ, Mukawa J (1959) Brain stem lesion effects on electrically induced seizures (electroencephalographic and behavioral study). EEG Clin Neurophysiol 11:397
2. Bancaud J et al (1974) "Generalized" epileptic seizures elicited by electrical stimulation of the frontal lobe in man. EEG Clin Neurophysiol 37:275–282
3. Gloor P (1968) Generalized cortico-reticular epilepsies. Some considerations on the pathophysiology of generalized bilaterally synchronous spike and wave discharge. Epilepsia 9:249–263
4. Murphy JP, Gelhorn E (1945) Further investigations on diencephaliz-cortical relations and their significance for the problem of emotion. J Neurophys 8:431–455

5. Velasco F et al (1976) Specific and non-specific multiple unit activities during the onset of pentylenetetrazol seizures. II Acute lesions interruption non-specific system connections. Epilepsia 17:461–475

6. Green JD, Morin F (1953) Hypothalamic electrical activity and hypothalamo-cortical relationships. Am J Physiol 172:175–186

7. Jinnai D et al (1969) Effects of brain-stem lesions on metrazol-induced seizures in cats. Clin Neurophysiol 27:404–411

8. Kreindler A et al (1958) Electroclinical features of convulsions induced by stimulation of brain stem. J Neuro Phys 21:430–436

9. Mirski MA, Ferrendelli JA (1987) Interruption of the connections of the mamillary bodies protect against generalized pentylenetetrazol seizures in guinea pigs. J Neurosci 7:662–670

10. Mirski MA, Ferrendelli JA (1986) Anterior thalamic mediation of generalized pentylenetetrazol seizures. Brain Res 399:212–223

11. Mirski MA, Fisher RA (1993) Pharmacological inhibition of posterior hypothalamus raises seizure threshold in rats. Epilepsia 34(Suppl 6):12

12. Mirski MA, Ferrendelli JA (1986) Anterior thalamus and substantia nigra: two distinct structures mediating experimental generalized seizures. Brain Res 397:377–380

13. Mullen S et al (1967) Thalamic lesions for the control of epilepsy-a study of nine cases. Arch Neurol 16:277–285

14. Nogueira RG, Sheth KN, Duffy FH, Helmers SL, Bromfield EB (2008) Bilateral tonic-clonic seizures with temporal onset and preservation of consciousness. Neurology. 70(22 Pt 2), 2188–90. No abstract available

15. Bell WL, Walczak TS, Shin C, Radtke RA (1997) Painful generalised clonic and tonic-clonic seizures with retained consciousness. J Neurol Neurosurg Psychiatry 63:792–795

16. Bleck TP, Smith MC, Pierre-Louis SJC et al (1993) Neurologic complications of critical medical illness. Crit Care Med 21:98–103

17. Mirski MA, Muffelman B, Ulatowski JA, Hanley DF (1995) Sedation for the critically ill neurologic patient. Crit Care Med 23:2038–2053

18. Mirski MA, McPherson RW, Traystman RJ (1994) Dexmedetomidine lowers seizure threshold in a rat model of experimental generalized epilepsy. Anesthesiology 81:1422–1428

19. Wallace KL (1997) Antibiotic-induced convulsions. Crit Care Clinics 13:741–761

20. Dreifuss FE (1991) Toxic effects of drugs used in the ICU. Anticonvulsant agents. Crit Care Clin 7:521–532

21. Annegers JF, Hauser A, Coan SP, Rocca WA (1998) A population-based study of seizures after traumatic brain injuries. N Eng J Med 338:20–24

22. Arboix A, Garcia-Eroles L, Massons JB, Oliveres M, Comes E (1997) Predictive factors of early seizures after acute cerebrovascular disease. Stroke 28:1590–1594

23. Lee ST, Lui TN, Wong CW et al (1997) Early seizures after severe closed head injury. Can J Neurol Sci 24:40–43

24. Lee ST, Lui TN, Wong CW, Yeh YS, Tzaan WC (1995) Early seizures after moderate closed head injury. Acta-Neurochir-Wien 137:151–154

25. Sabo RA, Hanigan WC, Aldag JC (1995) Chronic subdural hematomas and seizures: the role of prophylactic anticonvulsive medication. Surg Neurol 43:579–582

26. Wijdicks EFM, Sharbrough FW (1993) New-onset seizures in critically ill patients. Neurology 43:1042–1044

27. Claassen J, Jetté N, Chum F et al (2007) Electrographic seizures and periodic discharges after intracerebral hemorrhage. Neurology 69:1356–1365

28. Yanagawa Y, Nishi K, Sakamoto T (2008) Hyperammonemia is associated with generalized convulsion. Intern Med 47:21–23

29. DeLorenzo RJ (1990) Status epilepticus: concepts in diagnosis and treatment. Semin Neurol 10:396–405

30. Striano P, Striano S, Tortora F, De Robertis E, Palumbo D, Elefante A, Servillo G (2005) Clinical spectrum and critical care management of Posterior Reversible Encephalopathy Syndrome (PRES). Med Sci Monit 11, CR549–53.

31. Towne AR, Pellock JM, Ko D, DeLorenzo RJ (1994) Determinants of mortality in status epilepticus. Epilepsia 35:27–34

32. Sloviter RS (1999) Status epilepticus-induced neuronal injury and network reorganization. Epilepsia 40:S34–S39 discussion S40-1

33. Clark S, Wilson WA (1999) Mechanisms of epileptogenesis. Adv Neurol 79: 607–630

34. Delgado-Escueta AV, Wilson WA, Olsen RW, and Porter eds. Advances in Neurology Vol 79. Jaspers Basic Mechanisms of the Epilepsies (1999) Lippincott. Wilkins and Williams, Philadelphia

35. McNamara JO (1999) Emerging insights into the genesis of epilepsy. Nature 399:A15–A22

36. Mirski MA et al (1997) Anticonvulsant effect of anterior thalamic high frequency electrical stimulation in the rat. Epilepsy Res 28:89–100

37. Connors BW (1984) Initiation of synchronized neuronal bursting in neocortex. Nature 310:685–687

38. Segal MM (2002) Sodium channels and epilepsy electrophysiology. Novartis Found Symp 241:173–180

39. Jeffreys JG (1994) Experimental neurobiology of the epilepsies. Curr Opin Neurol 7:113–122

40. Jeffreys JG (1995) Nonsynaptic modulation of neuronal activity in the brain: electric currents and extracellular ions. Physiol Rev 75:689–723

41. Le Beau FEN, Alger BE (1998) Transient suppression of $GABA_A$ – receptor-mediated IPSPs after epileptiform burst discharges in CA1 pyramidal cells. J Neurophysiol 79:659–669

42. Lopantsev V, Avioli M (1998) Laminar organization of epileptiform discharges in the rat entorhinal cortex in vitro. J Physiol 509:785–796

43. Traub RD, Jeffreys JG (1994) Are there unifying principles underlying the generation of epileptiform after-discharges in vitro? Prog Brain Res 102:383–394

44. Traub RD, Wong RK, Miles R, Michelson H (1991) A model of a CA3 hippocampal pyramidal neuron incorporating voltage-clamp data on intrinsic conductances. J Neurophysiol 66:635–660

45. Heinemann U, Lux HD, Gutnick MJ (1977) Extracellular free calcium and potassium during paroxysmal activity in the cerebral cortex of the cat. Exp Brain Res 27:237–243

46. Traynelis SF, Dingledine R (1988) Potassium-induced spontaneous electrographic seizures in the rat hippocampal slice. J Neurophysiol 59:259–276

47. Larkum ME, Zhu JJ, Sakmann B (1999) A new cellular mechanism for coupling inputs arriving at different cortical layers. Nature 398:338–341

48. McCormick DA, Contreras D (2001) On the cellular and network basis of epileptic seizures. Annual Rev Physiol 63:815–846

49. Traub RD, Jeffrey JG, Miles R (1993) Analysis of the propagation of disinhibition-induced afterdischarge along the guinea-pig hippocampal slice in vitro. J Physiol 472:267–287

50. Stasheff SF, Hines M, Wilson MA (1993) Axon terminal hyperexcitability associated with epileptogenesis in vitro I Orifin of ectopic spikes. J Neurophysiol 70:961–975

51. Mirski MA, Ferrendelli JA (1985) Selective metabolic activation of the mamillary bodies and their connections during ethosuximide-induced suppression of pentylenetetrazol seizures. Epilepsia 51:194–203

52. Mirski MA, Ferrendelli JA (1984) Interruption of the mammillothalamic tracts prevents seizures in guinea pigs. Science 226:72–74

53. Mirski MA, Varelos P (2001) Seizures in the ICU. J Neurosurg Anesthesiol 13:163–175

54. Gastaut JL, Sabet Hassan MS, Bianchi CL, Gastaut H (1979) Electroencephalography in brain edema (127 cases of brain tumour investigated by cranial computerized tomography). EEG Clin Electrophysiol 46:239–255

55. Williamson A, Patrylo PR, Lee S, Spencer DD (2003) Physiology of human cortical neurons adjacent to cavernous malformations and tumors. Epilepsia 44:1413–1419

56. Kim JH, Guimaraes PO, Shen MY, Masukawa LM, Spencer DD (1990) Hippocampal neuron density in temporal lobe epilepsy with and without glioma. Acta Neuropathol (Berlin) 80:41–45

57. Wolf HK, Wiestler OD (1993) Surgical pathology of chronic epileptic seizure disorders. Brain Pathol 3:371–380

58. Avoli M, Drapeau C, Pumain R, Olivier A, Villemure JG (1991) Epileptiform activity induced by low extracellular magnesium in the human cortex maintained in vitro. Ann Neurol 30:589–596

59. Gonzalez D, Elvidge AR (1962) On the occurrence of epilepsy caused by astrocytoma of the cerebral hemispheres. J Neurosurg 19:470–482

60. Sherwin A, Robitaille Y, Quesney F et al (1988) Excitatory amino acids are elevated in human epileptic cerebral cortex. Neurology 38:920–923

61. Singh R, Pathak DN (1990) Lipid peroxidation and glutathione peroxidase, glutathione reductase, superoxide dismutase, catalase and glucose-6-phosphate dehydrogenase activities in $FeCl_3$ induced epileptogenic foci in the rat brain. Epilepsia 31:15–26

62. Towne AR, Waterhouse EJ, Boggs JG et al (2000) Prevalence of nonconvulsive status epilepticus in comatose patients. Neurology 54:340–345

63. Jordan KG (1993) Continuous EEG and evoked potential monitoring in the neuroscience intensive care unit. J Clin Neurophysiol 10:445–475

64. Nuwer MR (2007) ICU EEG monitoring: nonconvulsive seizures, nomenclature, and pathophysiology. Clin Neurophysiol 118:1653–1654

65. Hirsch LJ, Pang T, Claassen J, Chang C, Khaled KA, Wittman J, Emerson RG (2008) Focal motor seizures induced by alerting stimuli in critically ill patients. Epilepsia 49:968–973

66. Hirsch LJ, Claassen J, Mayer SA, Emerson RG (2004) Stimulus-induced rhythmic, periodic, or ictal discharges (SIRPIDs): a common EEG phenomenon in the critically ill. Epilepsia 45:109–123

67. Koutroumanidis M, Tsatsou K, Bonakis A, Michael M, Tan SV. Stimulus-induced bilateral central periodic discharges, cortical myoclonus and arousal responses in mild reversible coma. Clin Neurophysiol 2008; e pub Sep 20

68. DeLorenzo RJ, Waterhouse EJ, Towne AR et al (1998) Persistent nonconvulsive status epilepticus after the control of convulsive status epilepticus. Epilepsia 39:833–840

69. Treiman DM, Meyers PD, Walton NY et al (1998) A comparison of four treatments for generalized convulsive status epilepticus. Veterans Affairs Status Epilepticus Cooperative Study Group. N Eng J Med 339:792–798

70. Fountain NB, Lothman EW (1995) Pathophysiology of status epilepticus. J Clin Neurophysiol 12:326–342

71. Abou Khaled KJ, Hirsch LJ (2008) Updates in the management of seizures and status epilepticus in critically ill patients. Neurol Clin 26:385–408

72. Garzon E, Fernandez RM, Sakamoto AC (2001) Serial EEG during human status epilepticus: evidence for PLED as an ictal pattern. Neurology 57:1175–1183

73. Mirski MA (1989) Rapid treatment of status epilepticus with low dose pentobarbital. Crit Care Report 1:150–156

74. Mirski MA, Williams MA, Hanley DF (1995) Prolonged pentobarbital and phenobarbital coma for refractory generalized status epilepticus. Crit Care Med 23:400–404

75. Drislane FW, Lopez MR, Blum AS, Schomer DL (2008) Detection and treatment of refractory status epilepticus in the intensive care unit. J Clin Neurophysiol 25(4):181–186

76. Legriel S, Mourvillier B, Bele N, Amaro J, Fouet P, Manet P, Hilpert F (2008) Outcomes in 140 critically ill patients with status epilepticus. Intensive Care Med 34(3):476–480

77. Minicucci F, Muscas G, Perucca E, Capovilla G, Vigevano F, Tinuper P (2006) Treatment of status epilepticus in adults: guidelines of the Italian League against Epilepsy. Epilepsia 47(Suppl 5):9–15

78. Slooter AJ, Vriens EM, Leijten FS, Spijkstra JJ, Girbes AR, van Huffelen AC, Stam CJ (2006) Seizure detection in adult ICU patients based on changes in EEG synchronization likelihood. Neurocrit Care 5:186–192

79. Trevathan E (2006) Ellen R. Grass Lecture: Rapid EEG analysis for intensive care decisions in status epilepticus. Am J Electroneurodiagnostic Technol 46:4–17

80. Rumbach L, Sablot D, Berger E, Tatu L, Vuillier F, Moulin T (2000) Status epilepticus in stroke: report on a hospital-based stroke cohort. Neurology 54:350–354

81. Young GB, Goodenough P, Jacono V, Schieven JR (1988) Periodic lateralized epileptiform discharges: electrographic and clinical features. Am J EEG Technol 28:1–13

82. Pohlman-Eden B, Hoch DB, Cochius JIU, Chiappa KH (1996) Periodic lateralized epileptiform discharges: a critical review. J Clin Neurophysiol 13:519–530

83. Gross DW, Quesney LF, Sadikot AF (1998) Chronic periodic lateralized epileptiform discharges during sleep in a patient with caudate nucleus atrophy: insights into the anatomical circuitry of PLEDs. EEG Clin Electrophysiol 107:434–438

84. Norden AD, Blumenfeld H (2002) The role of subcortical structures in human epilepsy. Epilepsy Behav 3:219–231

85. Raroque HG, Gonzales PCW, Jhaveri HS, Leroy RF, Allen EC (1993) Defining the role of structural lesions and metabolic abnormalities in periodic lateralized epileptiform discharges. Epilepsia 34:279–283

86. Reiher JR, Hollier LH, Sundt TM et al (1991) Periodic lateralized epileptiform discharges with transitional rhythmic discharges: association with seizures. EEG Clin Neurophysiol 78:12–17

87. Erkulvrawatr S (1977) Occurrence, evolution and prognosis of periodic lateralized epileptiform discharges in EEG. Clin Electroencephalogr 8:89–99

88. Markund ON, Daly DD (1971) Pseudoperiodic lateralized paroxysmal discharges in electroencephalogram. Neurology 21:975–981

89. Garcia-Morales I, Garcia MT, Galan-Davila L, Gomez-Escalonilla C, Saiz-Diaz R et al (2002) Periodic lateralized epileptiform discharges. J Clin Neurophysiol 19:172–177

90. Bremmer RP (2004) EEG in convulsive and nonconvulsive status epilepticus. J Clin Neurophysiol 21:319–331

91. Stafstrom CE (1998) Back to basics: the pathophysiology of epileptic seizures: a primer For pediatricians. Ped in Rev 19:342–351

92. Kaplan PW (2006) The EEG of status epilepticus. J Clin Neurophysiol 23:221–229

93. Beaumont A, Whittle IR (2000) The pathogenesis of tumour associated epilepsy. Acta Neurochir 142:1–15

Chapter 2

Diagnosing and Monitoring Seizures in the ICU: The Role of Continuous EEG for Detection and Management of Seizures in Critically Ill Patients

Daniel Friedman and Lawrence J. Hirsch

Abstract Recent advances in computer technology have made it possible to perform prolonged digital continuous video EEG monitoring of many critically ill patients simultaneously. Recent studies using continuous EEG monitoring (cEEG) have found that these patients, especially those with coma, acute brain injury, or prior clinical seizures, often have nonconvulsive seizures (NCSz), and that these may contribute to secondary brain injury. The majority of seizures in the critically ill are nonconvulsive and can only be identified with EEG recording. Rapidly improving quantitative EEG (qEEG) software speeds data review to allow screening of multiple prolonged recordings to detect NCSz and has the potential to provide continuous information about changes in brain function in real time at the bedside. Optimal sensitivity and specificity of qEEG tools are obtained with full electrode montages and careful maintenance of scalp electrodes. New electrode technologies, such as MRI-compatible electrodes, help reduce the burden on EEG technologists while limiting interruptions in recordings. In addition to detecting NCSz, cEEG can also be used for dynamic detection of other changes in brain function such as ischemia, and can be coupled with other modalities of monitoring brain physiology such as microdialysis, tissue oximetry, and intracranial electrophysiology. Together, these tools can allow early detection of brain at risk for injury and alert the physician to intervene before the damage becomes irreversible.

Keywords Continuous EEG monitoring, Intensive care unit, Neurotelemetry, Nonconvulsive seizures, Critical care, Status epilepticus

2.1. Introduction

Nonconvulsive seizures (NCSz) and nonconvulsive status epilepticus (NCSE) are increasingly recognized as common occurrences in the ICU where 8–48% of comatose patients undergoing continuous EEG monitoring (cEEG) may have

From: *Seizures in Critical Care*: *A Guide to Diagnosis and Therapeutics*: Current Clinical Neurology, Second Edition, Edited by: P. Varelas, DOI 10.1007/978-1-60327-532-3_2,
© Humana Press, a part of Springer Science+Business Media, LLC 2005, 2010

NCSz, depending on the study population (1–5) (Table 2-1). NCSz, as the term is used in this chapter, refers to electrographic seizures with little or no overt clinical manifestations. NCSE occurs when NCSz are prolonged; a common definition is continuous or near-continuous electrographic seizures lasting at least 30 min (2, 6, 7). Most patients with NCSz have purely electrographic seizures (1) (Table 2-1 and Fig. 2-1) but NCSz can be associated with other subtle signs such as face and limb twitching, nystagmus, eye deviation, pupillary abnormalities (including hippus), and autonomic instability (8–11). None of these signs is highly specific for NCSz and is often seen under other circumstances in the critically ill patient; thus, continuous EEG monitoring (cEEG) is necessary to diagnose NCSz. In this chapter, we will discuss the implementation of cEEG in the critically ill and how to review the data, including available quantitative EEG (qEEG) tools that enable efficient review of the vast amount of raw EEG generated by prolonged monitoring. We will also review which patients are appropriate candidates for cEEG, as well and the numerous EEG patterns that may be encountered. Finally, we will discuss future directions for cEEG and neurophysiological monitoring in the ICU.

2.2. How To Monitor

Obtaining high-quality cEEG recordings in the ICU is a challenge. Adequate technologist coverage is necessary to connect patients promptly, including on off-hours, and maintain those connections 24-h a day. Critically ill patients are frequently repositioned and transported to tests, which makes maintaining electrode integrity difficult. In our center, we employ collodion to secure disk electrodes, and check the electrodes twice daily, usually supplemented by keeping the live recordings visible remotely to see which patients require electrode maintenance. Newer electrodes, such as subdermal wires, which may be more secure and lead to less skin breakdown, may be appropriate for comatose patients who are expected to undergo cEEG for days to weeks (12). While these electrodes may take more time to apply, they require less maintenance and are MRI- and CT-compatible (both safe and not affecting image interpretation), thereby saving substantial technologist time. Concerns for image artifacts and patient safety make it necessary to remove and then reapply standard disk electrodes when patients undergo brain MRIs, but there has been some progress in creating practical MRI- and CT-compatible electrodes (13), including conductive plastic electrodes. These are now commercially available in the United States and have been safely used in MRI scanners with a field strength of up to 4 T (Fig. 2-2).

There are numerous sources of artifact in the ICU environment that make cEEG challenging. Some are easily identified and filtered out such as 60 Hz (or 50 Hz in Europe) line noise from nearby electrical equipment. Others, however, such as pacemaker artifact, chest percussion, vibrating beds, respirator activity, and intravenous drips, may be difficult to distinguish from seizures or other cerebral activity (14, 15) (Fig. 2-3). Simultaneous digital video recording is useful for distinguishing brain signals from artifacts, especially rhythmic patterns such as those seen with chest percussion. In addition, video recording helps correlate EEG patterns with patient behaviors. In some cases, periodic EEG patterns can be determined to be ictal if they are time-locked to subtle patient movements (16). In addition, some significant

Table 2-1. Summary of Studies Using EEG Monitoring to Detect Nonconvulsive Seizures in Critically Ill Patients.

Study	Study population	EEG type	Design	N	Percentage of patients with any seizures	Percentage of seizure patients who had NCSz only
Privitera et al.(5)	Patients with altered level of consciousness or suspected subclinical seizures anywhere in medical center.	Routine EEG[1]	Prospective	198	37	100 (32% had no subtle clinical signs)
Jordan (104)	Patients admitted to neuro-ICU undergoing cEEG.	cEEG	Retrospective	124	35	74
DeLorenzo et al. (35)	All patients with prior convulsive SE and altered level of consciousness without clinical seizure activity.	cEEG	Prospective	164	48	100 (29% NCSE)
Vespa et al. (105)	All patients with moderate to severe traumatic brain injury admitted to the neuro-ICU.	cEEG	Retrospective	94	22	52
Towne et al. (4)	ICU patients in coma without clinical seizure activity.	Routine EEG	Retrospective	236	8	100 (NCSE)
Vespa et al. (78)	Patients admitted to neuro-ICU with stroke or intracerebral hemorrhage.	cEEG	Prospective	109	19	79
Claassen et al. (1)	Patients of all ages with unexplained decreased level of consciousness or suspected subclinical seizures	cEEG	Retrospective	570	19	92
Pandian et al. (3)	Neuro-ICU patients undergoing cEEG for diagnostic purposes or for titration of intravenous therapy for SE	cEEG	Retrospective	105	68	27 (NCSE)
Jette et al. (33)	Patients <18 years admitted to ICU with unexplained decreased level of consciousness or suspected subclinical seizures.	cEEG	Retrospective	117	44	75
Claassen et al. (51)	Patients with intracerebral hemorrhage with unexplained decreased level of consciousness or suspected subclinical seizures	cEEG	Retrospective	102	31	58
Oddo et al. (36)	Medical ICU patients without known brain injury undergoing with unexplained decreased level of consciousness or suspected subclinical seizures	cEEG	Retrospective	201	10 (additional 17% with PEDs)	67

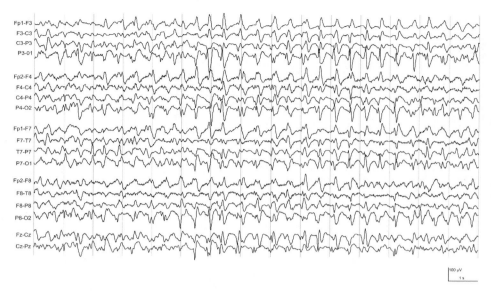

Fig. 2-1. Nonconvulsive status epilepticus (SE). This is the EEG from a 29-year-old man with a history of liver transplantation and chronic immunosupression who presented with convulsive SE due to encephalitis. He was treated with intravenous anticonvulsants, and movements ceased, but he remained comatose. His EEG demonstrated electrographic seizure activity without clinical correlate

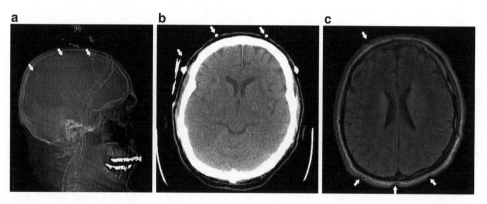

Fig. 2-2. CT- and MRI-compatible EEG electrodes. (**a**) A CT "scout" image demonstrating the placement of a full montage of conductive plastic electrodes (*white arrows*) on the scalp of a patient undergoing cEEG monitoring. (**b**) An axial image from the CT scan from the same patient demonstrating minimal artifact due to the electrodes (*white arrows*). Note there is no evidence of "streaking" common to head CT with conventional electrodes. (**c**) Axial FLAIR MRI performed 3 days later with electrodes in place. Note only minimal image artifact near the scalp (*white arrows*)

EEG patterns in the critically ill appear after the patient is stimulated, which is easily determined by reviewing the video (17, 18).

The number of electrodes used in cEEG studies varies considerably. In our center, we typically perform "full electrode" recordings using 16 or more active electrodes in addition to 1 or 2 reference electrodes and cardiac leads. Other authors have used reduced electrode configurations (19). The advantage of a reduced electrode system is that it is faster to apply and easier to maintain. It is also easier to work around other neuro-monitoring devices, surgical wounds, or ventricular drains common in NICU patients.

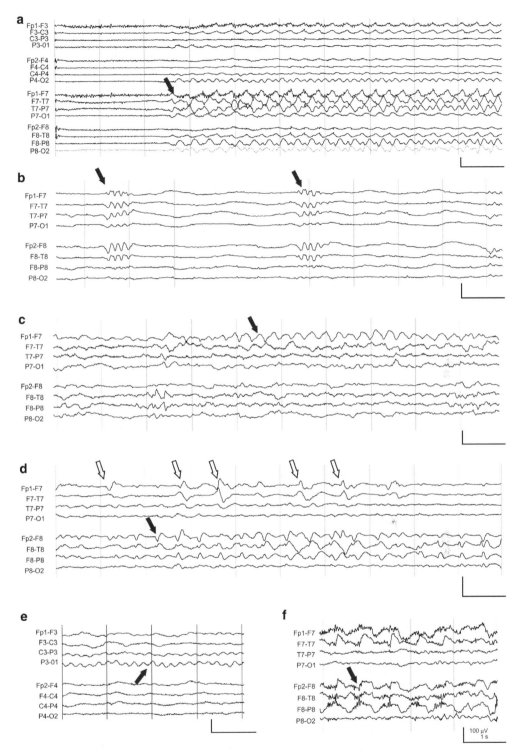

Fig. 2-3. Common ICU EEG artifacts. (**a**), Rhythmic bitemporal artifact due to chest compression in a medical ICU patient (*arrow*). (**b**) Respirator artifact due to fluid collecting in the tubing (*arrow*). These patterns are easily recognized on simultaneous video recording, as they are synchronized with respirations. (**c**) Left temporal rhythmic waveforms (*arrow*) due to patting in an infant. This pattern is sometimes easy to confuse with seizures without video, as it often shows a physiological field with evolution in frequency and amplitude. (**d**) Semirhythmic right temporal artifact (*black arrow*) due to chest percussion mimicking right PLEDs or potentially ictal activity in a patient with true left hemisphere PLEDs (*white arrows*). (**e**) Right occipital 5-Hz rhythmic artifact (*arrow*) due to percussion bed activity (**f**) Rhythmic 1–1.5-Hz artifact (*arrow*) due to chewing in an edentulous patient

However, a full electrode configuration improves the ability to distinguish brain signals from artifacts, aids in spatial localization of pathological activity, and provides a safety factor in case one or more leads fail, including allowing qEEG calculations and alarms to continue to function adequately (20). In addition, reduced electrode methods, especially when coupled to qEEG tools, may miss clinically significant events. For instance, Shellhaas et al. (21) found that neonatologists evaluating amplitude-integrated EEG using only two electrodes for seizure detection, a technique employed in purpose-built devices common in neonatal ICUs, detected only 12–38% of seizures identified using conventional electrode arrangements. Although emergent below-the-hairline EEG recordings have only moderate sensitivities and specificities (22), they are almost certainly better than no EEG at all; a full EEG should be done when possible to confirm or refute the results.

2.3. Data Analysis

Several days of cEEG generates gigabytes of data that, in its raw form, are time-consuming for a neurophysiologist to review, especially if many patients are being monitored simultaneously. Furthermore, the raw EEG may be difficult for nonexperts, such as ICU physicians and nurses, to interpret at the bedside. Therefore, concerning electrographic events may not be noticed until several hours later, when the file is reviewed by the neurophysiologist. Computing advances have enabled the use of qEEG algorithms to reduce the data and provide graphical representation of significant patterns and trends to speed up review. Some of the commonly employed qEEG methods are discussed below (see (23) for a detailed review).

Many qEEG data reduction and trending tools are based on transforming the raw cEEG into a time–frequency series using algorithms such as short time Fourier transform or continuous wavelet transform. Several hours of cEEG recordings can be reduced to a single screen of time–frequency values using a compressed spectral array or density spectral array. The time–frequency data can be averaged over scalp regions or hemispheres to further reduce the data. Using these techniques, the abrupt changes in cEEG spectral power in a relatively narrow frequency range during seizures are highlighted, allowing quick assessment of seizure frequency and duration (Fig. 2-4). Time–frequency transformation of the cEEG can be further manipulated to provide a single scalar value for each epoch of time. For instance, Claassen et al. (24) showed that the ratio of total hemispheric power in the alpha frequency band (8–13 Hz) to the total power in the delta frequency band (1–4 Hz) after maximal alerting, or post-stimulation alpha–delta ratio (ADR), was the most useful qEEG parameter for detecting delayed cerebral ischemia in patients with high-grade subarachnoid hemorrhage (SAH). Hemispheric asymmetries in spectral power, computed as ratio of left and right total power for all EEG frequencies or as relative differences at each frequency, can be used to quickly identify focal seizures (e.g., Fig. 2-4). The greatest utility of reducing the cEEG to single scalar values is that these values can easily be displayed and interpreted on bedside monitors like heart rate and blood pressure. This could allow early identification of neurophysiological events by the ICU staff and alarms to trigger patient examination and could lead to more responsive treatment.

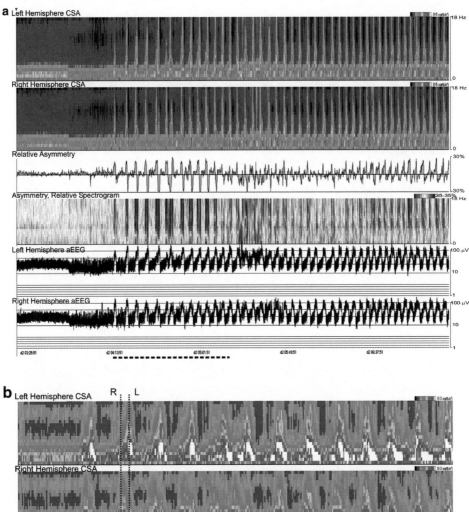

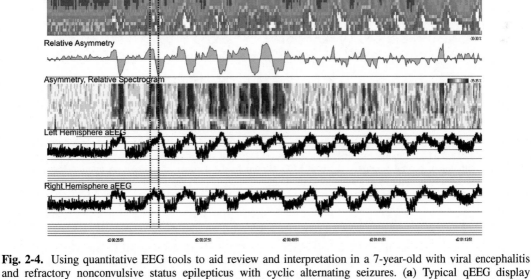

Fig. 2-4. Using quantitative EEG tools to aid review and interpretation in a 7-year-old with viral encephalitis and refractory nonconvulsive status epilepticus with cyclic alternating seizures. (**a**) Typical qEEG display showing long-term trends in spectral power between 0 and 18 Hz for both hemispheres (*top two panels*), relative interhemispheric asymmetry index (middle; up=right on relative asymmetry tracing, and red=more power on right on asymmetry spectrogram), and hemispheric amplitude-integrated EEG (*bottom two panels*) for five hours of recoding. (**b**) enlargement of the region in **a** marked by the *dash line*. There is an alternating pattern of increased spectral power at all frequencies on the right (R), and then the left (L) hemispheres.

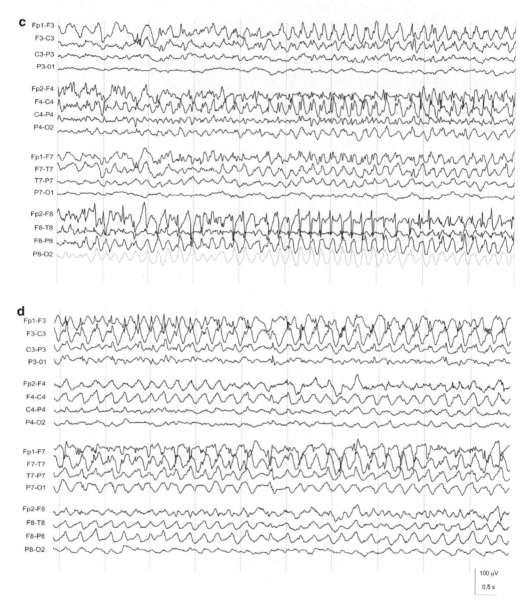

Fig. 2-4. (continued) This also corresponds to fluctuating asymmetry index between hemispheres and increased hemispheric aEEG. These changes in qEEG measures reflect right-maximal seizures (R; raw EEG shown in c), alternating with left-maximal seizures, (L; raw EEG shown in d), a form of alternating cyclic electrographic seizures (106), which we refer to as "ping-pong seizures"

Other trending algorithms highlight amplitude measures, which can also be used to detect seizures. Amplitude-integrated EEG (aEEG) computes statistical measures such as mean, maximum, minimum, and percentiles of the smoothed and full-wave-rectified EEG signal (Figs. 2-4 and 2-5). These tools are commonly used in commercial devices in neonatal ICUs (25) to assess the background EEG and occasionally to detect seizures, although these qEEG-based devices may be insensitive for detecting seizures (21). Reliance on qEEG tools without the ability to review the raw EEG

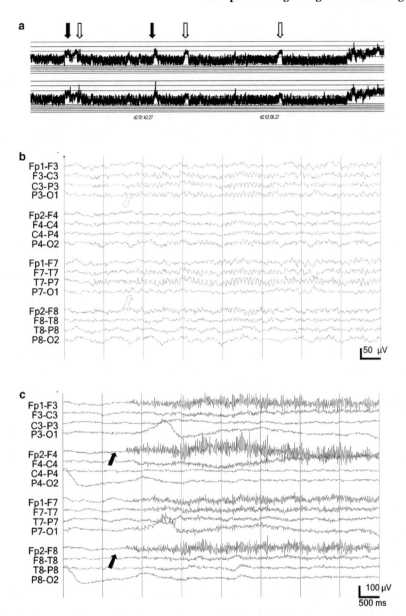

Fig. 2-5. Limits of seizure detection using amplitude-integrated EEG in a 64-year-old man with central nervous system lymphoma and altered mental status. (**a**) A plot of the average amplitude-integrated EEG (aEEG) for the left (*top*) and right (*bottom*) hemispheres demonstrates frequent transient elevations in the EEG amplitude (*open arrows*) that correspond to left temporal electrographic seizures. A typical seizure is shown in (**b**) with the onset indicated by the arrows. At times, similarly shaped peaks in the aEEG trend (*solid arrows*) occurred that correspond to movement/muscle artifact such as that seen in (**c**). It is not possible to differentiate seizures from artifact by the aEEG tracing alone

for noncerebral signals can also lead to false positive seizure detections (Fig. 2-5); thus, qEEG should only be interpreted in conjunction with the raw EEG wave forms and confirmed by electroencephalographers whenever possible.

Quantitative EEG tools can also calculate the degree of burst-suppression of the EEG background to allow for easy titration of medication to induce coma, a common treatment of status epilepticus (SE), or refractory elevated intracranial pressure (ICP) (26). EEG-based monitors such as bispectral index (27), patient state index (28), and Narcotrend (29) have been in use in operating rooms and ICUs for over a decade to monitor depth of sedation. While these single-purpose devices use proprietary algorithms, evaluation of the raw cEEG or qEEG measures can also provide information about arousal in the paralyzed patient (30). Unlike cEEG, these devices cannot detect seizures, and their performance has not been tested adequately in brain-injured patients.

In our experience, no one qEEG tool is appropriate for all patients or even for the same patient at all times. Situations may occur where one tool is more susceptible to certain artifacts or is less sensitive to the seizures the individual patient may have. Instead, we employ multiple tools simultaneously to screen the initial cEEG record and focus particularly on reviewing the raw EEG data at times where there appear to be clear changes in the qEEG measures from baseline (Fig. 2-4). Once the patient's seizure pattern is identified, the parameters of the qEEG tools can be further refined to highlight this pattern and improve the recognition of subsequent seizures.

With Internet-based networking, it is now practical to monitor dozens of patients in multiple ICUs. If there is sufficient network capability in the hospital, cEEG can be streamed live over the network and can be interpreted in real time if needed (and personnel are available). In addition, cEEG can be reviewed remotely from home or from a distant hospital site using virtual private networks and virtual network computing (20). However, in current practice, cEEG is not yet a truly real-time technology at most centers. In our center, records are routinely reviewed by neurophysiologists or technologists three times daily. Records can be reviewed more frequently if there are suspicious clinical events or medications are being titrated. However, as most NCSz have little or no detectable clinical correlate, they may go unrecognized for several hours with only intermittent review. It is clear that we need to move towards continuous real-time monitoring via use of quantitative EEG alarms and around-the-clock "neurotelemetrists" to respond to the alarms and review the long-term trends.

2.4. Who To Monitor

Recent studies using routine and cEEG monitoring have helped to identify which patients are at risk for NCSz and, therefore, may benefit from cEEG. The causes of NCSz and NCSE in ICU patients are similar to the causes of convulsive seizures in these patients. These include acute structural lesions, infections, metabolic derangements, toxins, withdrawal, and epilepsy, all common diagnoses in the critically ill patient (31). However, NCSz are the more common ictal manifestation (or lack thereof) in ICU patients (1–5). NCSz are even more common in the pediatric population, especially in infants (1, 20, 32, 33). Recent prospective studies using cEEG have indentified the incidence of NCSz and NCSE in various patient populations. These studies are summarized in Table 2-1.

While it may not be surprising that patients with acute brain injuries (1, 34) and recent convulsive SE (35) have a high risk of NCSz, NCSz also occur in medical or surgical ICU patients, including in those without known structural brain injury. Critically ill medical and surgical patients are susceptible to many toxic, electrolyte, and metabolic abnormalities that may cause both mental status changes and seizures. In the Columbia series, 21% of patients monitored with cEEG with toxic-metabolic encephalopathy as their primary neurologic diagnosis had NCSz. In other series, 5–25% of patients with acute NCSz had metabolic derangements as the likely etiology of their seizures (4, 6). In a recent study of 201 medical ICU patients without known brain injury that underwent cEEG monitoring, 22% of patients had periodic epileptiform discharges (PEDs) or seizures; sepsis and acute renal failure were significantly associated with both PEDs and seizures (36).

2.5. What To Look For

The background, interictal, and ictal EEG patterns of the critically ill patient are significantly different from those encountered in ambulatory patients (37, 38). Ictal patterns may include rhythmic epileptiform discharges or rhythmic waves at greater than 3 Hz. However, in critically ill patients, rhythmic or periodic patterns occurring at a rate of less than 3 per second can be ictal as well. One set of criteria for defining NCSz is shown in Table 2-2. It should be noted that these criteria reflect expert consensus and there are periodic patterns common to critically ill patients where the relationship to seizures is unknown (39). In practice, it is often difficult to determine whether periodic activity in a comatose patient reflects seizure activity, a brain at risk for seizures, or, perhaps, has no relationship to seizures (as is widely thought to be the case with triphasic waves seen in metabolic encephalopathy).

Table 2-2. Criteria for Diagnosing Nonconvulsive Seizures (adapted from (39), Who Modified the Criteria of (6)).

Any pattern lasting at least 10 s satisfying any one of the following three primary criteria

Primary criteria

- Repetitive generalized or focal spikes, sharp-waves, spike-and-wave complexes at $\geq$ 3/s

- Repetitive generalized or focal spikes, sharp-waves, spike-and-wave, or sharp-and-slow wave complexes at < 3/s and the secondary criterion

- Sequential rhythmic, periodic, or quasi-periodic waves at $\geq$1/s and unequivocal evolution in frequency (gradually increasing or decreasing by at least 1/s, e.g., 2–3/s), morphology, or location (gradual spread into or out of a region involving at least two electrodes). Evolution in amplitude alone is not sufficient. Change in sharpness without other change in morphology is not enough to satisfy evolution in morphology

Secondary criterion

Significant improvement in clinical state or appearance of previously absent normal EEG patterns (such as posterior-dominant "alpha" rhythm) temporally coupled to acute administration of a rapidly acting antiepileptic drug. Resolution of the "epileptiform" discharges leaving diffuse slowing without clinical improvement and without appearance of previously absent normal EEG patterns would not satisfy the secondary criterion.

While certain periodic discharges may be more closely related with systemic metabolic abnormalities, such as triphasic waves in hepatic encephalopathy, others may reflect injured tissue at risk for seizures such as periodic lateralized epileptiform discharges (PLEDs) and generalized periodic epileptiform discharges (GPEDs) (40–42) (Fig. 2-6). There is convincing evidence to suggest that PLEDs are sometimes ictal. For instance, PLEDs can be time-locked to focal clonic movements in some patients with focal motor SE (16). Positron emission tomography in a patient with frequent PLEDs demonstrated increased regional glucose metabolism similar to what is seen with focal seizures (43). Single-photon emission CT (SPECT) imaging in patients with PLEDs demonstrated increased regional cerebral perfusion that normalized when the PLEDs resolved (44, 45). In addition, frequent PLEDs in elderly patients have been associated with a confusional state that resolves spontaneously or with diazepam treatment (46). However, other studies have described cases where PLEDs are clearly non-ictal such as in some epilepsy patients with chronic interictal PLEDs (47). In addition, when some patients with PLEDs and acute brain injury demonstrate seizures, the EEG pattern is often faster and with different morphology (48). Given the close association with seizures and the fact they are at times clearly associated with behavioral changes, some authors view PLEDs as an unstable state in an "irritable" brain, lying along an ictal–interictal continuum (39, 42).

A common practice used to distinguish ictal from non-ictal periodic EEG patterns in the critically ill is to see whether they are abolished by a trial of short-acting benzodiazepines (Table 2-3 and Fig. 2-7). However, almost all periodic discharges, including triphasic waves seen in metabolic encephalopathy and the discharges of Creutzfeldt-Jakob Disease, are attenuated by benzodiazepines (49). Thus, unless there is clinical improvement accompanying the EEG change, the test is not helpful. Unfortunately, improvement can take substantial time even if the activity represents NCSE and is aborted with benzodiazepines. However, a substantial portion of ICU patients with nonconvulsive seizures or NCSE will improve neurologically, and usually within a day of treatment. For example, Drislane et al. (50) showed that 56% of critically ill patients without anoxic injury treated for NCSzs demonstrated mental status improvement. Although noncomatose patients were more likely to improve (81%), 48% of comatose patients improved as well. Our protocol for attempting to prove the presence of NCSE is shown in Table 2-3. It is important to recognize that lack of clinical improvement does not exclude NCSE – it simply does not help determine its presence or absence.

While there is consistent evidence that the presence of PEDs (and nonconvulsive seizures) are an independent risk factor for worse prognosis in intracerebral hemorrhage (ICH) (51), SAH, (52), sepsis(36), and after GCSE (35, 53), it is unclear whether these and other periodic discharges require treatment and how aggressive this treatment should be. Laboratory studies and computer modeling are beginning to probe the network mechanisms that mediate periodic discharges in the injured brain (54).

Another common pattern in encephalopathic ICU patients is epileptiform activity triggered by stimulation or arousals. The evoked activity may be anywhere on the interictal to ictal spectrum and we have termed it "stimulus-induced rhythmic, periodic, or ictal discharges" (17) (SIRPIDs). There is usually no clinical correlate, as with most ICU seizures, but a small number of patients will have

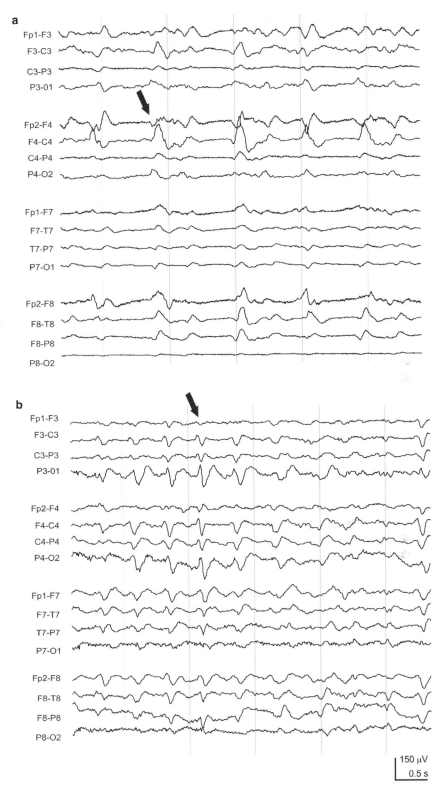

Fig. 2-6. Periodic discharges in critically ill patients. (**a**) Right frontal PLEDs occurring at 1 Hz (*arrow*) in an 82-year-old man after resection of a bifrontal meningioma. The patient subsequently developed right frontal electrographic seizures. (**b**) Generalized periodic discharges at 1–2 Hz in a 79-year-old patient with dementia, renal disease, and altered mental status. Although these waveforms have a triphasic morphology at times, the pattern subsequently evolved to 2.5–3 Hz GPEDs consistent with NCSz and was associated with modest elevations in neuron-specific enolase, a marker of neuronal injury, to 14 (reference range 3.7–8.9)

Table 2-3. Benzodiazepine Trial for the Diagnosis of Nonconvulsive Status Epilepticus (adapted from Jirsch and Hirsch (11)).

Appropriate patients have rhythmic or periodic focal or generalized epileptiform
  discharges on EEG with altered level of consciousness

Need to monitor EEG, pulse oximetry, blood pressure, ECG, and respiratory rate with dedicated nurse

Antiepileptic drug trial

- Sequential small doses of rapidly acting short-duration benzodiazepine such as midazolam at 1 mg/dose
- Between doses, repeated clinical and EEG assessment
- Trial is stopped after any of the following

  1. Persistent resolution of the EEG pattern (and exam repeated)

  2. Definite clinical improvement

  3. Respiratory depression, hypotension, or other adverse effect

  4. A maximum dose is reached (such as 0.2 mg/kg midazolam, though higher may be needed if the patient is
    on chronic benzodiazepines)

Test is considered positive if there is resolution of the potentially ictal EEG pattern AND either an improvement in the clinical state or the appearance of previously absent normal EEG patterns (e.g., posterior-dominant "alpha" rhythm). If EEG improves but patient does not, the result is equivocal.

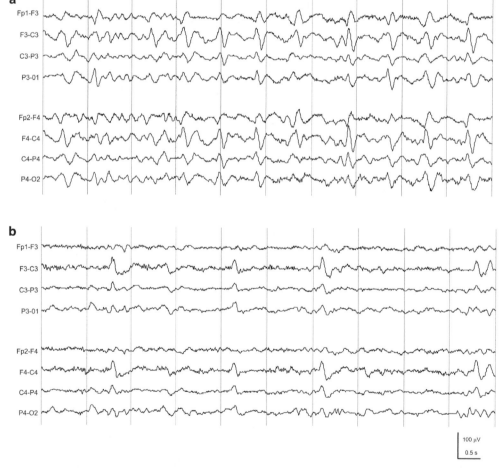

Fig. 2-7. Benzodiazepine trial in a 51-year-old man with multiple medical problems including chronic liver disease and HIV who was admitted to the medical ICU with sepsis. Despite treatment, he continued to have poor mental status. (**a**) Initial cEEG monitoring showed GPEDs at 1–2 Hz. (**b**) Following the administration of lorezapam 1 mg IV, the GPEDs became less frequent and the patient became responsive and followed commands, strongly suggesting that the initial pattern was ictal

focal motor seizures consistently elicited by alerting stimuli (18). This is most likely a result of hyperexcitable cortex that is activated by the usual arousal pathways, which involve the upper brainstem, thalamus, and widespread thalamo-cortical projections. This epileptiform activity may become clinically apparent if it causes synchronous activation of motor pathways. At our center, technologists stimulate patients twice daily to assess for the presence of SIRPIDs

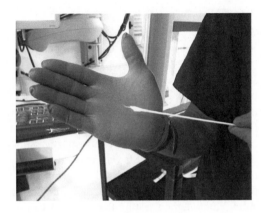

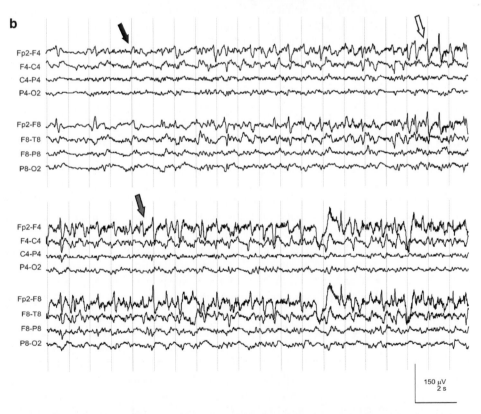

Fig. 2-8. Testing for stimulus induced rhythmic, periodic, or ictal discharges in critically ill patients. (**a**) EEG technologist demonstrating the cotton applicator used to provide nasal noxious stimulation to comatose patients undergoing cEEG twice daily. (**b**) SIRPIDs induced following noxious stimulation (*black arrow*) in an 84-year-old woman who was comatose following evacuation of a large right subdural hematoma. Shortly after stimulation, right frontal periodic discharges are seen. After several seconds, repetitive left hand movements emerge (*red arrow*) that are time-locked to the discharges. She subsequently became more responsive following treatment with anticonvulsants

(Fig. 2-8). The treatment and prognostic implications of SIRPIDs are currently unknown, but the relationship between ictal discharges and arousals raises the possibility that limiting unnecessary stimulation in patients with SIRPIDs may be beneficial. This can be studied fairly easily, particularly when cerebral micro-dialysis is being utilized.

2.6. Why Monitor

While NCSz are common in the critically ill, the evidence that they worsen outcomes and require prompt identification and treatment is mixed (55, 56). In several studies, the presence of NCSE and delay to diagnosis and treatment were each associated with significantly higher mortality (6, 57), though mortality in patients with NCSE may be most related to the underlying cause (58). In addition, while NCSE may be associated with poor prognosis in the critically ill elderly (59), one retrospective study showed that aggressive treatment of NCSz and NCSE was associated with worse outcomes in this population (60). Because of the conflicting outcome data, much of the justification for identifying and treating NCSz in the critically ill comes from human and animal data demonstrating that seizures can lead to neuronal injury. To date, there has not been a prospective controlled trial to determine whether treating NCSz or NCSE improves neurologic outcomes.

There is a large body of evidence that prolonged seizures, even if non-convulsive, can lead to neuronal damage in several animal models. In a seminal study, Meldrum et al. (61) found that paralyzed and artificially ventilated baboons had hippocampal cell loss after treatment with a convulsant. Cell death occurred after 60 min of continuous electrographic seizures despite careful control of oxygenation, temperature, and metabolic status. In rodent models, electrical and chemoconvulsant-induced SE is associated with cell loss, free-radical production, inflammation, gliosis, and synaptic reorganization (62). Pathological changes can be seen in the absence of overt convulsions and can have profound long-term effects such as impaired performance on cognitive tasks (63) and the development of epilepsy (64). There is also some evidence from animal models that even single or multiple brief seizures may lead to cell death and cognitive impairment (65, 66). Even in the absence of cell death, brief seizures in certain animal models can lead to alterations in gene expression (67), impaired long-term potentiation which is related to memory (68), and reduced threshold for subsequent seizures (69). SE in humans has also been associated with hippocampal cell loss in postmortem studies (70). In hospitalized patients, SE is associated with neuronal injury as demonstrated by elevated levels of serum neuron-specific enolase (NSE), including in patients without detectable acute brain injury (e.g., from seizure activity alone) (71, 72). In fact, even complex partial seizures in ambulatory patients with epilepsy can lead to elevated NSE (73). While the sequelae of NCSz and NCSE are not as well understood, evidence suggests that they can lead to neuronal damage in humans. DeGiorgio et al. (74) showed that NSE levels, though elevated after all seizures, were especially high following NCSz and seizures of partial onset even in absence of acute brain injury.

In addition to direct pathological effects of seizures themselves, seizure may also worsen the extent of injury from the inciting neurological injury. Seizures can place increased metabolic, excitotoxic, and oxidative stress on at-risk brain leading to irreversible injury. For instance, microdialysis studies in patients with TBI demonstrated increases of extracellular glutamate to excitotoxic levels following NCSz (75) as well as associated elevated lactate/pyruvate ratios and ICP (76). Glycerol, a marker of cellular breakdown, has also been found to be elevated in the microdialysate after NCSz in TBI patients (77). Compared to patients without NCSz who had similar injuries, impaired brain metabolism and increased ICP could be seen up to 100 h after injury (76). As mentioned above, NCSz in ICH were associated with increased mass effect on serial imaging, as well as worse NIHSS (National Institutes of Health Stroke Scale) scores in one study (78) and expansion of hematoma size in another (51); there was a trend towards worse outcomes in those with NCSzs in both studies. Seizures are also associated with increased metabolic demand, which may worsen injury to ischemic brain, particularly the penumbra. NCSz were associated with increased infarct volumes and higher mortality rates following middle cerebral artery occlusion in rats, (79) and treatment resulted in reduced volumes (80). In addition, even brief seizures can lead to hemodynamic changes, such as increased cerebral blood flow (CBF) (81), which may lead to transient and potentially injurious elevations in ICP even in the absence of tonic-clonic activity (82, 83). Finally, seizures are associated with peri-injury depolarizations, a process related to cortical spreading depression and which seems to be very common and to contribute to secondary neuronal injury itself (84, 85)

2.7. How Long To Monitor

Several recent studies have address the duration of cEEG monitoring required to diagnose NCSz in critically ill patients. In their study of NICU patients, Pandian et al. (3) found that routine EEGs (30 min) detected seizures in only 11% of patients, while subsequent cEEG (mean duration of 2.9 days) detected seizures in 28%. In 110 critically ill patients with seizures detected by cEEG (92% of patients had purely nonconvulsive seizures), Claassen et al. (1) found that only half of patients had their first seizure within the first hour of monitoring. Although 95% of noncomatose patients had their first seizure within 24 h, only 80% of comatose patients had a seizure by this time (Fig. 2-9). After 48 h of monitoring, the first seizure had occurred in 98% of noncomatose versus 87% of comatose patients. Coma and the presence of PEDs predicted a delay in the time to first seizure (>24 h). Similarly, Jette et al. (33) found that 50% of 51 children with nonconvulsive seizures had their first seizure within 1 h, and 80% within 24 h. Therefore, we feel monitoring for 24 h is probably sufficient to rule out NCSz in noncomatose patients without PEDs, but longer periods may be required for comatose patients or those with epileptiform discharges.

2.8. Future Directions

In addition to detecting seizures, cEEG can be used to identify other changes in brain physiology. In recent years, there has been renewed interest in using cEEG for the detection of brain ischemia. It has been known for some time that EEG changes occur within seconds of reduction in CBF (86, 87), which is the basis for intraoperative EEG monitoring of ischemia during carotid

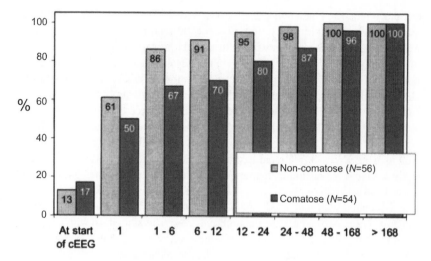

Duration of cEEG monitoring to record first seizure (hr)

Fig. 2-9. Summary plot of time to detect first seizure in 110 critically ill patients undergoing continuous EEG monitoring who had convulsive or nonconvulsive seizures (>90% were nonconvulsive). (Reproduced with permission from Claassen et al. 2004)

endarterectomy (88–90). In these patients, as CBF falls below 25–30 mL/100 g/min, there is a progressive loss of higher frequencies and prominent slowing of background EEG activity. When CBF falls below 8–10 mL/100 g/min, which is low enough to cause irreversible cell death, all EEG frequencies are suppressed (91, 92). Therefore, cEEG can detect a window where intervention can potentially prevent permanent brain injury.

Recent advances in computing have allowed for the real-time application of qEEG tools for extracting time–frequency data to measure changes in the background EEG rhythms. The ability to reduce EEG patterns usually identified by visual review to scalar values allows for prolonged use of cEEG monitoring in the ICU to detect cerebral hypoperfusion or other acute processes, especially in comatose or sedated patients where clinical examination is limited. In a study of 32 primarily good-grade SAH patients, Vespa et al. (19) found that a reduction in the variability of relative alpha frequency (a visual scoring of a tracing displaying 6–14 Hz expressed as a percentage of total power between 1–20 Hz) was 100% sensitive and 50% specific for vasospasm as detected by transcranial Doppler (TCD) or angiography. In the majority of patients, qEEG changes preceded the diagnosis of vasospasm by over 2 days. In a study of 34 poor-grade SAH patients (Hunt–Hess grade 4 and 5), Claassen et al. (93) found that the post-stimulation alpha/delta ratio was the most useful qEEG parameter for detection of delayed cerebral ischemia: a reduction in the post-stimulation ratio of alpha to delta frequency power of >10% relative to baseline in six consecutive epochs of cEEG was 100% sensitive and 76% specific for delayed cerebral ischemia. A reduction of >50% in a single epoch was 89% sensitive and 84% specific. However, these studies examined the use of qEEG for ischemia detection in a retrospective manner, and the performance of these tools in patient management has yet to be tested rigorously; this is largely due to the lack of practical software to detect these changes in an automated fashion and alert ICU staff in a timely manner. In addition to ischemia, cEEG monitoring can be used to detect evolving intracranial hemorrhages or masses (94) and systemic metabolic changes.

Real-time application of cEEG monitoring – neurotelemetry – including using automated alarm systems at the bedside, as exists with cardiac telemetry in almost all hospitals today, is becoming an approachable goal. Reducing the raw cEEG to a few displayed variables using qEEG tools will make it a practical tool that can be interpreted by nurses and intensivists or by neurotelemetry technicians. In addition, trend and critical value alarms can be used to alert staff to changes in neurological status (23). Computer algorithms have been successfully used to detect ongoing seizures in patients in epilepsy monitoring units (95). Because seizure patterns in the critically ill are different from ambulatory patients, new algorithms must be designed to detect seizures in this patient population (23). Refining techniques to help identify patterns of interest is an area of active research (96, 97). Improvement is needed, as many qEEG and data reduction tools are not sufficiently specific (98) and are susceptible to contamination by artifacts (Fig. 2-5). While ICU staff can be easily trained to review raw cEEG traces for obvious artifacts and even pathological patterns (94), a neurophysiologist must still be available to verify the interpretation.

In parallel with these technical advancements, continued research is needed to confirm that real-time monitoring is a necessary goal. Further studies need to be performed in both laboratory models and in prospective clinical trials to examine whether identifying and treating NCSz early improves outcomes, though this is already known for ischemia and is likely to be the case for other acute brain processes such as elevated ICP. It is also necessary to determine the relationship of the different periodic and rhythmic EEG patterns in the critically ill to ongoing brain injury to identify targets for intervention (39). Studies are also needed to determine whether using cEEG to detect ischemia improves patient outcomes and to identify the time window for intervention after a change is detected by cEEG.

Continuous EEG monitoring is just one of the modalities available to evaluate brain physiology in the ICU. ICP monitoring using intraventricular catheters or intraparenchymal probes, brain tissue oxygenation monitors, CBF monitoring and brain metabolism monitoring using microdialysis probes (99), all provide critical data about brain physiology. The use of these methods in combination with cEEG may help further understanding of the complex relationships between CBF, tissue oxygenation, cerebral metabolism, and neuronal activity in the injured brain (Fig. 2-10). In addition, the combined use of these methods may be able to compensate for some of the shortcomings of the individual methods. For instance, microdialysis and tissue oxygenation probes sample only the immediate area of brain into which they are inserted and can miss new injury to a remote area of the brain that may be detected by cEEG because of the wide spatial coverage. Conversely, there are situations, such as barbiturate coma, where the relationship between EEG activity and tissue ischemia is limited and other methods may be necessary to detect new ischemic injury (90).

Finally, new research is examining the utility of electrophysiological monitoring beyond conventional scalp EEG. Recent studies in patients with severe trauma brain injury (TBI) using subdural electrodes found episodes of cortical spreading depression, i.e., slow and prolonged peri-injury depolarizations lasting several minutes or longer, near injured brain (84). Similar types of cortical depolarizations have been observed in animal models of stroke where they are associated with infarct enlargement due to NMDA (N-methyl D-aspartate)-receptor-mediated injury (100). Recently, these events have also been demonstrated in patients with large middle cerebral artery strokes (101) and in patients with SAH (102), where they have been associated with delayed cerebral ischemia. Preliminary studies at our center (103) demonstrated that a small depth electrode inserted near injured cortex in severely brain injured patients was able to detect seizures and other epileptiform activity (Fig. 2-10) as well as changes in background activity from ischemia or hemorrhage that was not apparent on scalp EEG. It is possible that many focal seizures occurring across the cerebral cortex, but not synchronized sufficiently to generate scalp EEG changes, may contribute to impaired consciousness in some comatose patients without evidence of seizures on cEEG. Whether targeting these events for therapy improves patient outcomes needs to be determined. When possible, we use individualized, physiology-driven data (such as the lactate/pyruvate ratio and glutamate on microdialysis) to decide which EEG patterns require additional treatment and which do not.

2.9. Summary

Nonconvulsive seizures are common in brain injured patients with altered mental status and even in critically ill patients without structural brain injury. Seizures can contribute to depressed level of consciousness and cause secondary neuronal injury. Therefore, in our center, we recommend cEEG for all critically ill patients with acute brain injury and altered mental status and for patients with fluctuating or unexplained impaired mental status. Patients who are encephalopathic but not comatose are typically monitored for 24 h to exclude NCSz. However, patients who are comatose, who have PEDs, or who are having sedation/antiepileptic drugs withdrawn should undergo at least 48 h of cEEG. Once NCSz or equivocal periodic patterns are identified, monitoring can continue for several days. If NCSz are identified, cEEG is necessary to monitor the response to treatment and, more importantly, correlate improvement in the cEEG findings with improvement in the patient's clinical status. If the cEEG demonstrates periodic activity that is suspicious for, but not definitively, seizure activity, further monitoring can help the neurophysiologist gather additional evidence for or against the ictal nature of the pattern (e.g., to see whether there are unequivocal seizures). This monitoring requires 24-h technician coverage to connect patients and perform maintenance; appropriate information technology infrastructure; neurophysiologists available to review the data; and tools to speed up data review. While this requires a substantial amount of resources, it is feasible,

Fig. 2-10. (continued) glutamate and lactate and decrease in pyruvate. The lactate/pyruvate ratio increased dramatically to greater that 700 (normal <30; >40 associated with neuronal injury) suggesting significantly increased brain metabolic stress. (**b**) Scalp (*black traces*) and miniature depth electrode (*blue traces*) recording prior to meperidine (*open arrow*) demonstrates diffuse attenuation and slowing over the scalp and at the depth electrode. (**c**) During the period after meperidine administration when lactate/pyruvate ratio peaked (*closed arrow*), the scalp EEG was obscured by artifact. However, depth electrode recordings demonstrated periodic discharges and rhythmic delta activity at some of the leads (*red arrow*)

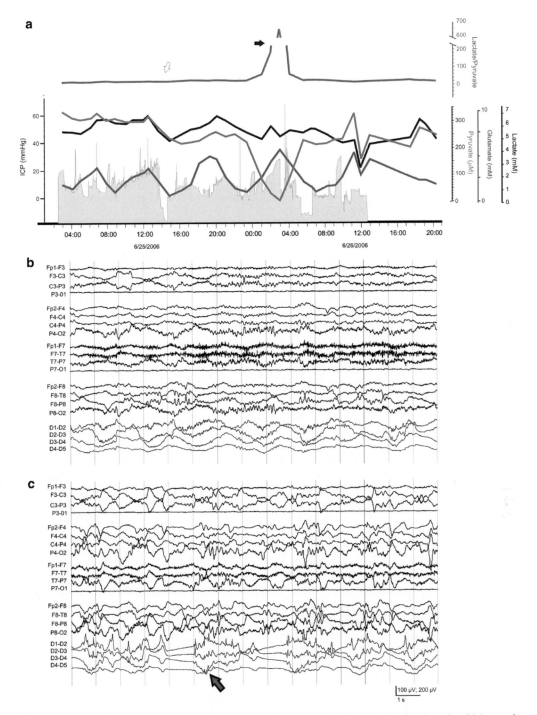

Fig. 2-10. Multimodality monitoring in a 61-year-old with a Hunt–Hess grade 5 subarachnoid hemorrhage due to a ruptured right anterior communicating artery aneurysm, vasospasm, and coma. A "bundle" consisting of a microdialysis probe, brain tissue oximetry monitor, intracerebral pressure transducer, and an eight-contact miniature depth electrode was placed in the right frontal lobe at the bedside. Continuous EEG was recorded simultaneously. (**a**) Levels of major cerebral metabolites in the microdialysate over time including lactate (*black line*), pyruvate (*blue line*), glutamate (*green line*), and the lactate/pyruvatre ratio (*red line*; note broken *y*-axis for clarity) as well as ICP (*blue bars* with area under the curve shaded *gray*). At approximately 1 a.m. on 6/26, the patient was given a bolus of meperidine for shivering, which was followed by a rapid increase in brain tissue

and cEEG is routinely employed in many neuroscience ICUs around the world. In addition, cEEG has applications outside of NCSz detection, which can expand the number of patients who may benefit from monitoring. Advances in the use of cEEG for ischemia detection and general brain function monitoring can make it a widely applicable tool for dynamic assessment of neurological function, in combination with other monitoring modalities, with the potential to detect brain injury moments after it occurs.

References

1. Claassen J, Mayer SA, Kowalski RG, Emerson RG, Hirsch LJ (2004) Detection of electrographic seizures with continuous EEG monitoring in critically ill patients. Neurology 62(10):1743–8
2. Jordan K (1999) Nonconvulsive status epilepticus in acute brain injury. J Clin Neurophysiol 16(4):332–40
3. Pandian JD, Cascino GD, So EL, Manno E, Fulgham JR (2004) Digital video-electroencephalographic monitoring in the neurological-neurosurgical intensive care unit: clinical features and outcome. Arch Neurol 61(7):1090–4
4. Towne AR, Waterhouse EJ, Boggs JG et al (2000) Prevalence of nonconvulsive status epilepticus in comatose patients. Neurology 54(2):340–5
5. Privitera M, Hoffman M, Moore JL, Jester D (1994) EEG detection of nontonic-clonic status epilepticus in patients with altered consciousness. Epilepsy Res 18(2):155–66
6. Young GB, Jordan KG, Doig GS (1996) An assessment of nonconvulsive seizures in the intensive care unit using continuous EEG monitoring: an investigation of variables associated with mortality. Neurology 47(1):83–9
7. Walker M, Cross H, Smith S et al (2005) Nonconvulsive status epilepticus: Epilepsy Research Foundation Workshop Reports. Epileptic Disord 7(3):253–96
8. Lowenstein DH, Aminoff MJ (1992) Clinical and EEG features of status epilepticus in comatose patients. Neurology 42(1):100–4
9. Kaplan PW (2002) Behavioral Manifestations of Nonconvulsive Status Epilepticus. Epilepsy Behav 3(2):122–39
10. Husain AM, Horn GJ, Jacobson MP (2003) Non-convulsive status epilepticus: usefulness of clinical features in selecting patients for urgent EEG. J Neurol Neurosurg Psychiatry 74(2):189–91
11. Jirsch J, Hirsch LJ (2007) Nonconvulsive seizures: developing a rational approach to the diagnosis and management in the critically ill population. Clin Neurophysiol 118(8):1660–70
12. Young GB, Ives JR, Chapman MG, Mirsattari SM (2006) A comparison of sub-dermal wire electrodes with collodion-applied disk electrodes in long-term EEG recordings in ICU. Clin Neurophysiol 117(6):1376–9
13. Mirsattari SM, Lee DH, Jones D, Bihari F, Ives JR (2004) MRI compatible EEG electrode system for routine use in the epilepsy monitoring unit and intensive care unit. Clin Neurophysiol 115(9):2175–80
14. Young GB, Campbell VC (1999) EEG monitoring in the intensive care unit: pitfalls and caveats. J Clin Neurophysiol 16(1):40
15. Hirsch LJ (2004) Continuous EEG monitoring in the intensive care unit: an overview. J Clin Neurophysiol 21(5):332–40
16. Snodgrass SM, Tsuburaya K, Ajmone-Marsan C (1989) Clinical significance of periodic lateralized epileptiform discharges: relationship with status epilepticus. J Clin Neurophysiol 6(2):159–72
17. Hirsch LJ, Claassen J, Mayer SA, Emerson RG (2004) Stimulus-induced rhythmic, periodic, or ictal discharges (SIRPIDs): a common EEG phenomenon in the critically ill. Epilepsia 45(2):109–23

18. Hirsch LJ, Pang T, Claassen J et al (2008) Focal motor seizures induced by alerting stimuli in critically ill patients. Epilepsia 49(6):968–73

19. Vespa PM, Nuwer MR, Juhász C et al (1997) Early detection of vasospasm after acute subarachnoid hemorrhage using continuous EEG ICU monitoring. Electroencephalogr Clin Neurophysiol 103(6):607–15

20. Kull LL, Emerson RG (2005) Continuous EEG monitoring in the intensive care unit: technical and staffing considerations. J Clin Neurophysiol 22(2):107

21. Shellhaas RA, Soaita AI, Clancy RR (2007) Sensitivity of amplitude-integrated electroencephalography for neonatal seizure detection. Pediatrics 120(4):770–7

22. Kolls BJ, Husain AM (2007) Assessment of hairline EEG as a screening tool for nonconvulsive status epilepticus. Epilepsia 48(5):959–65

23. Scheuer ML, Wilson SB (2004) Data analysis for continuous EEG monitoring in the ICU: seeing the forest and the trees. J Clin Neurophysiol 21(5):353–78

24. Claassen J, Hirsch LJ, Kreiter KT et al (2004) Quantitative continuous EEG for detecting delayed cerebral ischemia in patients with poor-grade subarachnoid hemorrhage. Clin Neurophysiol 115(12):2699–710

25. Toet MC, van der Meij W, de Vries LS, Uiterwaal CS, van Huffelen KC (2002) Comparison between simultaneously recorded amplitude integrated electroencephalogram (cerebral function monitor) and standard electroencephalogram in neonates. Pediatrics 109(5):772–9

26. Eisenberg HM, Frankowski RF, Contant CF, Marshall LF, Walker MD (1988) High-dose barbiturate control of elevated intracranial pressure in patients with severe head injury. J Neurosurg 69(1):15–23

27. Simmons LE, Riker RR, Prato BS, Fraser GL (1999) Assessing sedation during intensive care unit mechanical ventilation with the Bispectral Index and the Sedation-Agitation Scale. Crit Care Med 27(8):1499–504

28. Prichep LS, Gugino LD, John ER et al (2004) The Patient State Index as an indicator of the level of hypnosis under general anaesthesia. Br J Anaesth 92(3):393–9

29. Bauerle K, Greim CA, Schroth M, Geisselbrecht M, Kobler A, Roewer N (2004) Prediction of depth of sedation and anaesthesia by the NarcotrendTM EEG monitor. Br J Anaesth 92(6):841–5

30. Roustan JP, Valette S, Aubas P, Rondouin G, Capdevila X (2005) Can electroencephalographic analysis be used to determine sedation levels in critically ill patients? In: IARS: 1141–1151

31. Abou Khaled KJ, Hirsch LJ (2006) Advances in the management of seizures and status epilepticus in critically ill patients. Crit Care Clin 22(4):637–59

32. Clancy RR, Legido A, Lewis D (1988) Occult neonatal seizures. Epilepsia 29(3):256–61

33. Jette N, Claassen J, Emerson RG, Hirsch LJ (2006) Frequency and predictors of nonconvulsive seizures during continuous electroencephalographic monitoring in critically ill children. Arch Neurol 63(12):1750–5

34. Vespa P (2005) Continuous EEG monitoring for the detection of seizures in traumatic brain injury, infarction, and intracerebral hemorrhage: "to detect and protect". J Clin Neurophysiol 22(2):99–106

35. DeLorenzo RJ, Waterhouse EJ, Towne AR et al (1998) Persistent nonconvulsive status epilepticus after the control of convulsive status epilepticus. Epilepsia 39(8):833–40

36. Oddo M, Carrera E, Claassen J, Mayer SA, Hirsch LJ. (2009) Continuous Electroencephalography in the Medical Intensive Care Unit. Crit Care Medicine 37(6): 2051–2056

37. Young GB (2000) The EEG in Coma. J Clin Neurophysiol 17(5):473

38. Kaplan PW (2004) The EEG in metabolic encephalopathy and coma. J Clin Neurophysiol 21(5):307–18

39. Chong DJ, Hirsch LJ (2005) Which EEG patterns warrant treatment in the critically ill? Reviewing the evidence for treatment of periodic epileptiform discharges and related patterns. J Clin Neurophysiol 22(2):79–91

40. Reiher J, Rivest J, Grand'Maison F, Leduc CP (1991) Periodic lateralized epileptiform discharges with transitional rhythmic discharges: association with seizures. Electroencephalogr Clin Neurophysiol 78(1):12–7

41. Husain AM, Mebust KA, Radtke RA (1999) Generalized periodic epileptiform discharges: etiologies, relationship to status epilepticus, and prognosis. J Clin Neurophysiol 16(1):51–8

42. Pohlmann-Eden B, Hoch DB, Cochius JI, Chiappa KH (1996) Periodic lateralized epileptiform discharges–a critical review. J Clin Neurophysiol 13(6):519–30

43. Handforth A, Cheng JT, Mandelkern MA, Treiman DM (1994) Markedly increased mesiotemporal lobe metabolism in a case with PLEDs: further evidence that PLEDs are a manifestation of partial status epilepticus. Epilepsia 35(4):876–81

44. Assal F, Papazyan JP, Slosman DO, Jallon P, Goerres GW (2001) SPECT in periodic lateralized epileptiform discharges (PLEDs): a form of partial status epilepticus? Seizure 10(4):260–5

45. Bozkurt MF, Saygi S, Erbas B (2002) SPECT in a patient with postictal PLEDs: is hyperperfusion evidence of electrical seizure? Clin Electroencephalogr 33(4):171–3

46. Terzano MG, Parrino L, Mazzucchi A, Moretti G (1986) Confusional states with periodic lateralized epileptiform discharges (PLEDs): a peculiar epileptic syndrome in the elderly. Epilepsia 27(4):446–57

47. Westmoreland BF, Klass DW, Sharbrough FW (1986) Chronic periodic lateralized epileptiform discharges. Arch Neurol 43(5):494–6

48. Brenner RP (2002) Is it status? Epilepsia 43(Suppl 3):103–13

49. Fountain NB, Waldman WA (2001) Effects of benzodiazepines on triphasic waves: implications for nonconvulsive status epilepticus. J Clin Neurophysiol 18(4):345–52

50. Drislane FW, Lopez MR, Blum AS, Schomer DL (2008) Detection and treatment of refractory status epilepticus in the intensive care unit. J Clin Neurophysiol 25(4):181–6

51. Claassen J, Jette N, Chum F et al (2007) Electrographic seizures and periodic discharges after intracerebral hemorrhage. Neurology 69(13):1356–65

52. Claassen J, Hirsch LJ, Frontera JA et al (2006) Prognostic significance of continuous EEG monitoring in patients with poor-grade subarachnoid hemorrhage. Neurocrit Care 4(2):103–12

53. Jaitly R, Sgro JA, Towne AR, Ko D, DeLorenzo RJ (1997) Prognostic value of EEG monitoring after status epilepticus: a prospective adult study. J Clin Neurophysiol 14(4):326–34

54. Frohlich F, Bazhenov M, Sejnowski TJ (2008) Pathological effect of homeostatic synaptic scaling on network dynamics in diseases of the cortex. J Neurosci 28(7):1709

55. Aminoff MJ (1998) Do nonconvulsive seizures damage the brain?–No. Arch Neurol 55(1):119–20

56. Young GB, Jordan KG (1998) Do Nonconvulsive seizures damage the brain?–Yes. Arch Neurol 55(1):117–9

57. Vespa PM, Nuwer MR, Nenov V et al (1999) Increased incidence and impact of nonconvulsive and convulsive seizures after traumatic brain injury as detected by continuous electroencephalographic monitoring. J Neurosurg 91(5):750–60

58. Shneker BF, Fountain NB (2003) Assessment of acute morbidity and mortality in nonconvulsive status epilepticus. Neurology 61(8):1066–73

59. Bottaro FJ, Martinez OA, Pardal MM, Bruetman JE, Reisin RC (2007) Nonconvulsive status epilepticus in the elderly: a case-control study. Epilepsia 48(5):966–72

60. Litt B, Wityk RJ, Hertz SH et al (1998) Nonconvulsive status epilepticus in the critically ill elderly. Epilepsia 39(11):1194–202

61. Meldrum BS, Vigouroux RA, Brierley JB (1973) Systemic factors and epileptic brain damage Prolonged seizures in paralyzed, artificially ventilated baboons. Arch Neurol 29(2):82–7

62. Holmes GL (2002) Seizure-induced neuronal injury: animal data. Neurology 59(9 Suppl 5):S3–6

63. Krsek P, Mikulecka A, Druga R et al (2004) Long-term behavioral and morphological consequences of nonconvulsive status epilepticus in rats. Epilepsy Behav 5(2):180–91

64. Lothman EW, Bertram EH, Bekenstein JW, Perlin JB (1989) Self-sustaining limbic status epilepticus induced by 'continuous' hippocampal stimulation: electrographic and behavioral characteristics. Epilepsy Res 3(2):107–19

65. Cavazos JE, Das I, Sutula TP (1994) Neuronal loss induced in limbic pathways by kindling: evidence for induction of hippocampal sclerosis by repeated brief seizures. J Neurosci 14(5 Pt 2):3106–21

66. Kotloski R, Lynch M, Lauersdorf S, Sutula T (2002) Repeated brief seizures induce progressive hippocampal neuron loss and memory deficits. Prog Brain Res 135:95–110

67. Saffen DW, Cole AJ, Worley PF, Christy BA, Ryder K, Baraban JM (1988) Convulsant-induced increase in transcription factor messenger RNAs in rat brain. Proc Natl Acad Sci U S A 85(20):7795–9

68. Zhou JL, Shatskikh TN, Liu X, Holmes GL (2007) Impaired single cell firing and long-term potentiation parallels memory impairment following recurrent seizures. Eur J NeuroSci 25(12):3667–77

69. Dube C, Chen K, Eghbal-Ahmadi M, Brunson K, Soltesz I, Baram TZ (2000) Prolonged febrile seizures in the immature rat model enhance hippocampal excitability long term. Ann Neurol 47(3):336–44

70. DeGiorgio CM, Tomiyasu U, Gott PS, Treiman DM (1992) Hippocampal pyramidal cell loss in human status epilepticus. Epilepsia 33(1):23–7

71. Rabinowicz AL, Correale J, Boutros RB, Couldwell WT, Henderson CW, DeGiorgio CM (1996) Neuron-specific enolase is increased after single seizures during inpatient video/EEG monitoring. Epilepsia 37(2):122–5

72. DeGiorgio CM, Gott PS, Rabinowicz AL, Heck CN, Smith TD, Correale JD (1996) Neuron-specific enolase, a marker of acute neuronal injury, is increased in complex partial status epilepticus. Epilepsia 37(7):606–9

73. Palmio J, Keranen T, Alapirtti T et al (2008) Elevated serum neuron-specific enolase in patients with temporal lobe epilepsy: A video-EEG study. Epilepsy Res 81(2–3):155–60

74. DeGiorgio CM, Heck CN, Rabinowicz AL, Gott PS, Smith T, Correale J (1999) Serum neuron-specific enolase in the major subtypes of status epilepticus. Neurology 52(4):746–9

75. Vespa P, Prins M, Ronne-Engstrom E et al (1998) Increase in extracellular glutamate caused by reduced cerebral perfusion pressure and seizures after human traumatic brain injury: a microdialysis study. J Neurosurg 89(6):971–82

76. Vespa PM, Miller C, McArthur D, et al. Nonconvulsive electrographic seizures after traumatic brain injury result in a delayed, prolonged increase in intracranial pressure and metabolic crisis. Critical care medicine 2007

77. Vespa P, Martin NA, Nenov V et al (2002) Delayed increase in extracellular glycerol with post-traumatic electrographic epileptic activity: support for the theory that seizures induce secondary injury. Acta Neurochir Suppl 81:355–7

78. Vespa PM, O'Phelan K, Shah M et al (2003) Acute seizures after intracerebral hemorrhage: a factor in progressive midline shift and outcome. Neurology 60(9):1441–6

79. Hartings JA, Williams AJ, Tortella FC (2003) Occurrence of nonconvulsive seizures, periodic epileptiform discharges, and intermittent rhythmic delta activity in rat focal ischemia. Exp Neurol 179(2):139–49

80. Williams AJ, Tortella FC, Lu XM, Moreton JE, Hartings JA (2004) Antiepileptic drug treatment of nonconvulsive seizures induced by experimental focal brain ischemia. J Pharmacol Exp Ther 311(1):220–7

81. Johnson DW, Hogg JP, Dasheiff R, Yonas H, Pentheny S, Jumao-as A (1993) Xenon/CT cerebral blood flow studies during continuous depth electrode monitoring in epilepsy patients. AJNR 14(1):245–52

82. Gabor AJ, Brooks AG, Scobey RP, Parsons GH (1984) Intracranial pressure during epileptic seizures. Electroencephalogr Clin Neurophysiol 57(6):497–506

83. Marienne JP, Robert G, Bagnat E (1979) Post-traumatic acute rise of ICP related to subclinical epileptic seizures. Acta Neurochir Suppl (Wien) 28(1):89–92

84. Fabricius M, Fuhr S, Bhatia R et al (2006) Cortical spreading depression and peri-infarct depolarization in acutely injured human cerebral cortex. Brain 129(Pt 3):778–90

85. Fabricius M, Fuhr S, Willumsen L et al (2008) Association of seizures with cortical spreading depression and peri-infarct depolarisations in the acutely injured human brain. Clin Neurophysiol 119(9):1973–84

86. Sundt TM Jr, Sharbrough FW, Anderson RE, Michenfelder JD (1974) Cerebral blood flow measurements and electroencephalograms during carotid endarterectomy. J Neurosurg 41(3):310–20

87. Sundt TM Jr, Sharbrough FW, Piepgras DG, Kearns TP, Messick JM Jr, O'Fallon WM (1981) Correlation of cerebral blood flow and electroencephalographic changes during carotid endarterectomy: with results of surgery and hemodynamics of cerebral ischemia. Mayo Clin Proc 56(9):533–43

88. Sharbrough FW, Messick JM Jr, Sundt TM Jr (1973) Correlation of continuous electroencephalograms with cerebral blood flow measurements during carotid endarterectomy. Stroke; a journal of cerebral circulation 4(4):674–83

89. Zampella E, Morawetz RB, McDowell HA et al (1991) The importance of cerebral ischemia during carotid endarterectomy. Neurosurgery 29(5):727–30 discussion 30–31

90. Arnold M, Sturzenegger M, Schaffler L, Seiler RW (1997) Continuous intraoperative monitoring of middle cerebral artery blood flow velocities and electroencephalography during carotid endarterectomy. A comparison of the two methods to detect cerebral ischemia. Stroke; a journal of cerebral circulation 28(7):1345–50

91. Astrup J, Siesjo BK, Symon L (1981) Thresholds in cerebral ischemia – the ischemic penumbra. Stroke; a journal of cerebral circulation 12(6):723–5

92. Jordan KG (2004) Emergency EEG and continuous EEG monitoring in acute ischemic stroke. J Clin Neurophysiol 21(5):341–52

93. Claassen J, Hirsch LJ, Emerson RG, Mayer SA (2002) Treatment of refractory status epilepticus with pentobarbital, propofol, or midazolam: a systematic review. Epilepsia 43(2):146–53

94. Jordan KG (1999) Continuous EEG monitoring in the neuroscience intensive care unit and emergency department. J Clin Neurophysiol 16(1):14

95. Gotman J (1999) Automatic detection of seizures and spikes. J Clin Neurophysiol 16(2):130

96. Agarwal R, Gotman J, Flanagan D, Rosenblatt B (1998) Automatic EEG analysis during long-term monitoring in the ICU. Electroencephalogr Clin Neurophysiol 107(1):44–58

97. Shah AK, Agarwal R, Carhuapoma JR, Loeb JA (2006) Compressed EEG pattern analysis for critically ill neurological-neurosurgical patients. Neurocrit Care 5(2):124–33

98. Adams DC, Heyer EJ, Emerson RG et al (1995) The reliability of quantitative electroencephalography as an indicator of cerebral ischemia. Anesth Analg 81(1):80–3

99. Wartenberg KE, Schmidt JM, Mayer SA (2007) Multimodality monitoring in neurocritical care. Crit Care Clin 23(3):507–38

100. Hartings JA, Rolli ML, Lu XC, Tortella FC (2003) Delayed secondary phase of peri-infarct depolarizations after focal cerebral ischemia: relation to infarct growth and neuroprotection. J Neurosci 23(37):11602–10

101. Dohmen C, Sakowitz OW, Fabricius M et al (2008) Spreading depolarizations occur in human ischemic stroke with high incidence. Ann Neurol 63:720–728

102. Dreier JP, Woitzik J, Fabricius M et al (2006) Delayed ischaemic neurological deficits after subarachnoid haemorrhage are associated with clusters of spreading depolarizations. Brain 129(12):3224

103. Waziri AE, Arif H, Oddo M et al (2007) Early experience with a cortical depth electrode for ICU neurophysiological monitoring in patients with acute brain injury. Epilepsia 48(s6):125

104. Jordan KG (1995) Neurophysiologic monitoring in the neuroscience intensive care unit. Neurol Clin 13(3):579–626

105. Vespa PM, Nenov V, Nuwer MR (1999) Continuous EEG Monitoring in the Intensive Care Unit: Early Findings and Clinical Efficacy. J Clin Neurophysiol 16(1):1

106. Friedman DE, Schevon C, Emerson RG, Hirsch LJ (2008) Cyclic electrographic seizures in critically ill patients. Epilepsia 49(2):281–7

Chapter 3

Stroke and Critical Care Seizures

Panayiotis N. Varelas and Lotfi Hacein-Bey

Abstract Patients with hemorrhagic stroke are usually admitted for observation to an intensive care unit (ICU). A smaller percentage of patients with ischemic stroke are also admitted, as well as those patients with cerebral venous thrombosis or those who have undergone carotid endarterectomy. All these patients are at risk for seizures. Those with hemorrhagic stroke are usually at two to three times higher risk than those with ischemic stroke, but several characteristics of the stroke modify the risk of having a seizure. In most cases, an early seizure within the first few days after the ictus has a different significance from a late seizure after the patient has been discharged from the ICU or the hospital. In addition, a significant role is played by the type of treatment offered to these patients – medical, surgical, or endovascular. Despite an abundance of studies examining the incidence and characteristics of poststroke seizures, there are several questions still to be answered regarding appropriate treatment institution and duration.

Keywords Ischemic, Hemorrhagic stroke, Subarachnoid hemorrhage, Arteriovenous malformation, Carotid endarterectomy, Hyperperfusion syndrome, Cerebral sinus thrombosis

3.1. Introduction

Seizures following stroke have been reported since the nineteenth century. In 1864, Hughlings Jackson reported convulsions in the paralyzed side after a middle cerebral artery (MCA) embolism (1), and a few years later, in 1885 William Gowers introduced the term "post-hemiplegic epilepsy" (2).

Seizures can occur early following a stroke (within the first 2 weeks) or start at later stages. They can occur >24 h before clinical evidence of stroke ("antecedent" seizures) or within the 24 h period before or after the initial neurologic deficit ("at onset" or "acute phase" seizures)(3, 4). Early seizures may be seen during the index admission in the intensive care unit (ICU) for stroke, or may occur later in the course of the event, justifying admission or

From: *Seizures in Critical Care: A Guide to Diagnosis and Therapeutics*: Current Clinical Neurology, Second Edition, Edited by: P. Varelas, DOI 10.1007/978-1-60327-532-3_3,
© Humana Press, a part of Springer Science+Business Media, LLC 2005, 2010

readmission to the unit. Three major questions arise in the ICU when a patient with stroke develops one or more seizures: (1) How do the seizures impact on the stroke? (2) Are the fits, especially the early ones, a mode of entrance into epilepsy? (3) When is antiepileptic treatment appropriate. One may encounter several difficulties while reviewing the literature in an attempt to address the importance of the problem: Many studies are old, from the precomputed tomography (CT) era, retrospective, are based on small numbers of patients, do not include all types of stroke, or consider the timing (not differentiating between early or late seizures). It is important, however, to differentiate between early and late poststroke seizures because there are several clinical, etiological, and prognostic differences, justifying a separate analysis (5). Moreover, in several studies, the time between stroke onset and admission is unclear, making it uncertain whether the seizures occurred before a healthcare personnel encountered the patient; this is an important detail since many seizures occur during the very first hours after the onset of a stroke. Finally, many studies do not control effectively for the presence of antiepileptic medications when the seizures occur, potentially underestimating the natural history of poststroke seizures.

3.2. Seizures After Ischemic Stroke

3.2.1. Clinical Studies

The reported incidence of poststroke seizures varies between 4.4% and 13.8% depending on the subgroups included in the analysis, the methods used to evaluate the stroke and the follow-up period (5–13). A male preponderance has been reported in two studies (5, 14). Early seizures (definition varying from the first 24 h to the first 4 weeks post stroke) usually occur at the stroke onset in 1.8–33% of patients and constitute most poststroke seizures (5, 6, 8, 9, 11, 12, 15–19). Most early seizures occur immediately poststroke, and the majority of those are inaugural of stroke (12). Late poststroke seizure occurrence also depends on the definition and the duration of follow-up, with a reported incidence of 2.5–67% of cases (6, 10, 12, 19–23). Recurrent seizures (epilepsy) can occur after stroke in 4–9% of patients (24, 25). Although some studies have reported that early seizures did not lead to the development of late seizures (26, 27), the cumulative risk for epilepsy may reach 19% in 6 years, a figure 22 times higher than the expected age-specific incidence of epilepsy in the general population (16). Loiseau et al., in a large epidemiological study from southwestern France, found that cerebrovascular disease was the most frequently recognized etiology of seizures in the aging population: it was the underlying cause in 36.6% of patients with spontaneous seizures and in 53.9% of the patients with confirmed epilepsy (14). Therefore, although only 5% of epilepsy is due to cerebrovascular disease (pre-CT data from Rochester, Minnesota) (16), because stroke incidence is high in the elderly, it may account for 25–50% of new epilepsy cases in this population segment (14, 28–32).

Most of the seizures after stroke have a focal onset and are of the simple partial type (9–11, 33, 34). Almost half of them show secondary generalization, making it difficult in the ICU to differentiate between the two types, unless the onset was witnessed or there is continuous video-electroencephalography (EEG) monitoring.

Complex partial seizures are less frequent, although in one retrospective study, their incidence reached 24% of all poststroke seizures (34). The incidence of primary generalized seizure lies between the two, although this may be an overestimate, most authorities agreeing that a major portion of them are secondary generalized (35).

There have been very few studies conducted in a stroke unit or other ICU, since most stroke patients are managed in an acute floor setting and get admitted to an ICU environment only if they have significant comorbidities or they deteriorate. In this chapter, we provide a review of all currently available data, so that the reader may form his own opinion.

Several studies were conducted in the pre-CT era, the most notable being that by Louis and McDowell who reviewed the records of 1,000 patients with presumed thrombotic infarction based on clinical criteria (10). The incidence of seizures was 7.7%. Early seizures were reported in 55% and late seizures in 45% of 60 patients. Epilepsy developed in 3% of patients with early seizures and 81% of patients with late seizures during an average follow-up period of 27 months.

Another early report of a large stroke population admitted to an Acute Stroke Unit in Toronto found 83/827 (10%) patients to have seizures during the first admission or during the 2–5-year follow-up (36). Seizures occurred only in patients with hemispheric lesions and were equally represented in those with infarcts and hemorrhages. Early seizures (within 1 week) occurred in 57% of those patients (39% within the first day). By the first year, 88% of those 83 patients had seizures. Mortality during the first week was not different in patients with and without seizures.

In a retrospective analysis of 90 patients with post-ischemic stroke seizures, immediate seizures (defined as occurring within 24 h) were observed in 30% and early seizures (within 2 weeks) in 33% (33). Overall, 98% of the initial poststroke seizures were observed within 2 years. The authors could identify the precipitating factors for initial seizures in four patients (one with hypoglycemia, one with hyponatremia and two with fever due to pneumonia). Early seizures were more likely partial, and late seizures generalized. Recurrent seizures occurred in 35/90 (39%) patients, with a mean follow-up of 30 months. Eighty six percent of patients with recurrent seizures had identifiable precipitating factors, the major being noncompliance with the antiepileptic medications. There was no difference in the recurrence rate between patients with early (40%) and late seizures (38%).

In a retrospective analysis of medical records from Taiwan, approximately 2,000 patients were admitted with presumed cerebral infarction, and 118 of them had seizures (34). A bimodal distribution of post-thrombotic stroke seizures was found, with an early peak within 2 weeks (early seizures) and a late one between 6 months and 1 year (34). Early seizures were reported in 13/118 (11%) patients with seizures and late seizures in 66/118 (66%). However, this study has several limitations, because 42/118 patients were with unknown interval between seizure and stroke onset. Twenty three out of 118 patients (19.5%) with a first seizure had silent infarcts proven by CT of the head and no history of previous stroke. In patients with a single infarct (excluding lacunes and border zone infarcts), the frontal and the temporal lobes were the most commonly involved lobes, either solely or partially (58% each), followed by the parietal lobe (43%) and the occipital lobe (20%). Most of the seizures were simple partial (58%) or complex partial (24%) with or without secondary generalization. Status epilepticus (SE) occurred in 15% of the patients. For patients with ischemic stroke, epilepsy developed in 35% of patients after early seizures and in 90% of patients with late seizures.

In another hospital-based study from Buenos Aires, Argentina, 22 (10%) of 230 patients with stroke developed seizures, including 7.1% with ischemic stroke and 25% with intracerebral hemorrhage (ICH) (6). The risk for seizures was higher in those patients with ICH, cortical involvement, and large stroke (defined as a lesion involving more than one lobe). Early onset seizures (within the first month) occurred in 54.5% and seizure recurrence in 6/22 (27%) of patients with seizures. There was no difference in the type, location, and size of stroke between those patients with early and late seizures.

In a prospective study conducted in Birmingham, UK, 230 patients were followed for at least 27 months after acute stroke (11). Early seizures at the onset of stroke (defined as within a 24-h period before or after the initial neurological deficit onset) occurred in 13 (5.7%) patients, all with strokes in the internal carotid artery distribution. In the ischemic stroke subgroup, the percentage was 4.3%; in the ICH, 10.7%; and in the subarachnoid hemorrhage group (SAH), 11.1%. Mortality in patients with seizures was significantly higher than for the whole stroke group only during the first 48 h after admission. This study has several limitations. Only 86% of patients were admitted to the hospital within the first 48 h of stroke onset, and only 20% had confirmation of the stroke type by CT, angiogram, or necropsy. Six out of 13 patients with seizures had epilepsy or were taking antiepileptic medications before the onset of the stroke. None of the remaining patients with poststroke seizures who survived their stroke (5/7) had further seizures during a minimum follow-up of 30 months. The authors concluded that antiepileptics failed to control seizures in these patients.

A large prospective study was conducted in Australia, following 1,000 patients admitted for stroke (9). The incidence of early seizures (within 2 weeks) was 4.4% (44 patients) and in 43/44 (97%) occurred within the first 48 h. Four patients had SE (0.4%), and 18 (1.8%) had multiple seizures. All patients who received antiepileptic treatment (77%) had readily controlled seizures. The highest incidence of early seizures (15.4%) was found in patients with supratentorial lobar or extensive (lobar and deep) ICH, followed by 8.5% in patients with SAH, 6.5% in patients with carotid territory infarcts and 3.7% in patients with hemispheric transient ischemic attacks (TIAs). No early seizures were found in any patients with subcortical, lacunar, or vertebrobasilar distribution infarcts or deep cerebral or infratentorial ICHs. There was no difference in the incidence of seizures after cardioembolic infarct compared to large-vessel extracranial disease. In the ICH subgroup, arteriovenous malformation as a cause of lobar ICH was found to have a strong association with early seizures ($p = 0.001$).

As a follow-up to the previous study from Australia, the same authors reported the incidence of late seizures (defined as seizures occurring after discharge) in 31/44 patients with early seizures without TIA, who survived (37). Late seizures occurred in 32% of these patients, compared to 10% of patients matched for age, sex, and type of stroke without early seizures, from the same cohort. In patients with ischemic stroke, late seizures occurred in 26% and 0%, respectively, and in patients with ICH in 62.5% and 25%, respectively.

The mean time from early to late seizure was 12 months (3 months to 2.5 years), and the type of seizure was not associated with seizure recurrence. Twenty one patients were on antiepileptic treatment at discharge, but the authors could not conclude about their usefulness in preventing late seizures because of the small numbers.

Early seizures (within 2 weeks) occurred in 2.5% of 1,200 patients admitted for acute stroke in a large retrospective study from China (15). The incidence of early seizures was 2.3% in infarction, 2.8% in ICH and 2.7% in SAH. There was no association between the stroke subtype and early seizure occurrence. Carotid artery territory cortical infarctions had a 10-fold increased incidence of seizures compared to non-cortical infarctions and lobar ICH had a 20-fold increased incidence compared to non-lobar ICH ($p < 0.001$). Two-thirds of early seizures were partial, 24% generalized, and 10% SE.

Another large retrospective hospital-based study was conducted in Marseille, France (12). Seventy eight patients out of 2016 (3.9%) developed seizures after acute stroke and were followed for an average of 30.2 months. The authors observed a biphasic chronological distribution of seizures: early seizures (within the first month) were observed in 28/78 (36%) of patients with seizures and late seizures (after the 3d month) in 64%. Among those with early seizures, two-thirds of the seizures occurred within the first 24 h (23% of all seizures), and among those with the late ones, two-thirds occurred between the 3rd and 12th months (42% of all seizures). Compared to ischemic strokes, ICH was followed more frequently by early seizures ($p = 0.05$). The proportion of seizures following cardioembolic stroke was similar to that from other causes. Simple partial seizures (with or without secondary generalization) were observed in 64%, primary generalized in 32%, and complex partial in 4% of patients. SE presenting as first seizure occurred in 14% of cases. EEG was performed in 97% of patients with seizures and showed focal slowing abnormalities in 63% and focal irritative abnormalities in 37% of cases. The earlier it was performed after the stroke (within the first 48 h or not), the higher was the percentage of irritative abnormalities found. Recurrent seizures occurred in 51% of 70 patients with seizures that survived the stroke, and no difference was found between those with early or late seizure onset.

In a retrospective, hospital-based study from Palermo, Italy, 217 out of 4,425 (4.7%) patients with acute stroke had one or more seizures (38). Seizures after ischemic stroke occurred in 4.7% of patients and after ICH, in 5.7%. In the ischemic group, seizures heralded the stroke in 10.7% of patients with seizures, were early (within 2 weeks) in 44.3% and late in 44.9% of patients with seizures. The location of ischemic stroke was cortical in 45.5% of cases, subcortical in 32.6%, and mixed in 21.9%.

In a prospective hospital-based registry of 1,099 patients with stroke conducted in Barcelona, Spain, 27 (2.5%) had early (within the first 48 h) seizures (17). Younger age, confusional syndrome, hemorrhagic stroke, large lesion size, and involvement of parietal and temporal lobes were more frequently found in patients who developed early seizures. There was no increased frequency of early seizures in patients with TIAs, embolic infarcts, and lacunar strokes. Patients with seizures had 33.3% mortality (vs. 14.2% for those without seizures, $p = 0.02$). Presence of early seizures after stroke was an independent predictor of in-hospital mortality (odds ratio (OR), 95%CI 6.17, 2.13–17.93). In a subsequent article, with one more year of data included, the authors reported similar findings regarding early seizures: In the multivariate analysis only cortical involvement (6, 2.5–14) and acute agitated confusional state (4.4, 1.4–13.8) were independent predictors for early poststroke seizures (39).

In a prospective multicenter international study (Seizures after Stroke Study Group, SASS), 1897 patients with acute stroke were admitted to teaching hospitals (7). Seizures were present in 8.6% of patients with ischemic stroke and 10.6% of patients with ICH. Early onset seizures (within 2 weeks) occurred in 4.8% of patients with ischemic stroke. Forty percent of all seizures (3.4% of patients with ischemic stroke) occurred within the first 24 h. Recurrent seizures (epilepsy) occurred in 2.5% of all patients (28% of patients who had seizures) or 2.1% of patients with ischemic stroke (55% of patients with late onset seizures). Partial seizures accounted for 52% of all seizures. The 1-year actuarial risk for seizures was 20% for patients with ICH and 14% for patients with ischemic stroke. Using a Cox proportional hazards model, late onset seizures conveyed in the total cohort an almost 24-fold increased risk for epilepsy. In the ischemic stroke group, cortical involvement and stroke disability (as measured by the modified Canadian Neurological score) were independent factors for the development of seizures and late onset seizures for the development of epilepsy (a 12-fold increased risk).

In a retrospective study from Hong Kong, 34/994 patients (3.4%) with stroke developed poststroke seizures. No patient with subarachnoid hemorrhage or posterior circulation infarct developed seizures. Male sex and cortical stroke location were the only independent factors associated with seizures (ORs 3.2, 95%CI 1.45–7.08, and 3.83, 1.05–14, respectively). Early seizures (within 30 days from onset of stroke) occurred in 1.6% (47% of patients with poststroke seizures) and epilepsy in 0.7% (40).

In a prospective study from Norway, 484 patients were followed for 7–8 years after ischemic stroke. Poststroke epilepsy (defined as ≥2 seizures ≥1 week after the stroke) developed in 5.7% of patients, and in all of them it was partial epilepsy. Scandinavian Stroke Scale (SSS) score <30 on admission was a significant independent predictor for developing poststroke epilepsy (OR 4.9) (41).

More recently, a large study from Turkey evaluated 1,428 patients admitted to a stroke unit for developing epilepsy over a mean follow-up period of 5.5 years. Although details regarding the timing of seizure presentation are not provided, 3.6% of patients developed epilepsy (2.7% with ischemic and 12.8% with hemorrhagic stroke and 26.6% with venous infarction). Using Trial of Org 10172 in Acute Stroke Treatment (TOAST) classification criteria (42), the authors reported poststroke epilepsy in 2.7% of patients with atherothrombotic stroke, in 2.6% with cardioembolic stroke, and in 1.3% with lacunar stroke (43).

Another retrospective study from Turkey evaluated 1,880 patients with stroke and found 200 (10.6%) of them having seizures. These patients with seizures were compared with 400 control patients, but there was no matching between the groups. Instead, the controls were matched to the rest of the patients without seizures (i.e., they were a good random sample). This study is unique because it reported similar incidence of seizures between ischemic (10.6%) and hemorrhagic (10.7%) strokes. Early seizures (within 2 weeks) occurred in 38.5% of patients with seizures and late seizures in 61.5% (44).

Lastly, a large retrospective study from Croatia evaluated 3,542 patients with stroke and seizures, defined as convulsions immediately before or within 24 h from the onset of neurological deficits. Seizures were observed in 1.43% of patients with ischemic stroke and in 3.76% of patients with hemorrhagic stroke. Total inpatient mortality was 21.4% in the group without seizures, and significantly more (30.8%) in the group with seizures (45).

The only prospective hospital-based study conducted in the ICU examining the incidence of poststroke seizures was conducted at UCLA, Los Angeles, CA, using continuous EEG (CEEG) monitoring (46). None of the ischemic stroke patients received prophylactic antiepileptic treatment. All patients with ICH were covered with such a regimen. Despite the prophylaxis difference, seizures occurred in 18/63 (28%) of patients with ICH and 3/46 (6%) patients with ischemic stroke (OR 5.7, 95%CI 1.4–26.5, $p < 0.004$). Most seizures (89%) occurred within the first 72 h after the insult and most of them (76%) were nonconvulsive (unresponsive patients with absence of overt convulsions).

Most of the aforementioned studies are hospital-based studies, introducing a potential bias for more severe stroke admissions. Such bias can be avoided by studying population-based cohorts. These studies give information for both acute onset seizures after stroke (usually hospitalized patients) and for the long-term risk (and thus influence the decision about prophylactic antiepileptic management).

The oldest population-based study was conducted in Rochester, Minnesota and included 535 patients with first ischemic stroke (47). Onset seizures (within 24 h) occurred in 4.8% of these patients and early seizures (within 1 week) in 6%. The cumulative probability of developing late seizures (after the first week) within the first year was 3% (a risk 23-fold higher than for the general population); by 5 years, 7.4%: and by 10 years, 8.9%. In the multivariate analysis, anterior hemisphere location of the infarct was a strong predictor of early seizures (OR 4, 95%CI 1.2–13.7). Early seizures and stroke recurrence were independent predictors for late seizures and recurrent seizures (epilepsy). A criticism of these results may be based on the fact that several patients had their first stroke in the 1960s, when computed tomography was not available and might have had hemorrhagic instead of ischemic strokes.

Another large prospective population-based study was performed in France between 1985 and 1992 (5). Using the Stroke Registry of Dijon, the authors reported 90 (5.4%) patients with early seizures (within the first 15 days) out of 1,640 patients with acute stroke, with an understudy population of 150,000. All patients had CT of the head, and all patients with seizures underwent an EEG evaluation. Patients with cerebral infarct due to atheroma had seizures in 4.4%, those with cardiogenic embolus in 16.6%, those with lacunes in 1%, and those with TIAs in 1.9%. An interesting observation in this study is the high incidence of seizures with infarcts of the occipital lobe (11.3%). There were no seizures in patients with brainstem, thalamic, cerebellar, or retinal infarcts. The authors reported higher incidence of seizures after cardioembolic infarction (20.8%) compared to infarction from atheroma (5%, $p = 0.01$) in the anterior circulation distribution. There was no such difference in the vertebrobasilar distribution. This study is also interesting because it reports male predominance as an independent factor for early seizures after stroke and also EEG findings. All patients with seizures had abnormal EEGs: nonspecific focal slow waves in 43 patients, bilateral slow waves in 18, periodic lateralized epileptiform discharges (PLEDs) in 15, paroxysmal features in 10, and electrical partial SE in 4.

A second large, prospective, population-based study was conducted in Besancon, France (22). Out of 3,205 patients with first-time ischemic or hemorrhagic stroke, 159 (5%) had first-time seizures. Early onset seizures occurred in 57 (1.8%) patients, and late ones in 102 (3.2%) patients. During a mean follow-up period of 47 months, 68/135 (50%) patients with a first post-stroke seizure had seizure recurrence. A second seizure occurred more often in patients with late as opposed to early seizures ($p < 0.01$). Occipital involvement and late onset first seizure were independent predictors of multiple seizure recurrences.

A large European population study was conducted in the Oxfordshire community, UK (8). Over 4 years, 675 patients with first stroke were registered from a study population of about 105,000. Onset seizures (within the first 24 h) occurred in 14 (2%) of acute stroke patients and were generalized in 7, simple partial in 6, and complex partial in 1. The risk for onset seizures was higher in patients with SAH (6%) and ICH (3%) than in patients with ischemic stroke (2%). Onset seizures conveyed a 7.5 times higher risk (95%CI 2.5–23) for subsequent seizures in comparison to patients with acute stroke but no onset seizures. In the actuarial analysis, the cumulative risk for seizures after ischemic stroke was 4.2% (2.2–6.2%) within the first year and 9.7% (3.7–15.7%) within 5 years. The risks for seizures from ICH were 19.9% (1.5–38.3%) and 26.1% (0–54.8%) and from SAH 22% (2.6–41.8%) and 34.3% (0–100%), respectively. Survivors of total anterior circulation infarction had a 34% (12–57%) risk for post-stroke seizures within 2 years, a risk much higher than in those with other stroke subtypes. On the other hand, the lowest risk for seizures was found in those patients with lacunar strokes (only 3% developed seizures) and in those who were independent at 1 month post stroke (actuarial risk at 5 years 4.2% (0.1–8.3%)). Compared to the general population, ischemic stroke conveyed a 29-fold increased risk for seizures within the first year and a 21-fold increased risk within the second year. This difference was accentuated in the age group < 65 years, where the risk for seizures within the first year was 76-fold increased compared to the general population without stroke. Interestingly, in this age group and during the second year, the risk for seizures, although still higher than for the general population, was lower than for the other age groups (17.2-fold increase vs. 18.5–23.2-fold increase in patients > 65 years old). Thus, younger patients were noted to have a dramatically increased risk for seizures during the first year after stroke, which dropped during the second year.

Another population-based study was conducted in Copenhagen, where 1,195 patients with acute stroke out of a population of 240,000 inhabitants were followed for 3 years (18). Early seizures (within the first 14 days after stroke) occurred in 4.2% of patients, most within the first 72 h (86%). Early seizures were only related to the severity of stroke, as estimated by the Scandinavian Stroke Scale (SSS). For each 10-point increase in the SSS, the risk for early seizures increased by a factor of 1.65 (95%CI 1.4–1.9). This study did not include patients with SAH. Although ICH was more frequent in patients with early seizures than without (17% vs. 7%), in the multivariate analysis it dropped as a predictor of seizures. Mortality in patients with early seizures was 50% compared with 20% in patients without seizures, but seizures did not stand as an independent predictor of mortality in the multivariate analysis (only stroke severity predicted mortality). Indeed, this study found that, in survivors, early seizures were associated with a better outcome. The authors explained this finding by suggesting that seizures were emanating from a larger ischemic penumbra, which represents salvageable brain tissue. Interestingly, in a subsequent analysis of this cohort, followed for 7 years, the authors reported that 3.2% of patients developed poststroke epilepsy, which was independently associated with younger age, higher onset stroke severity, larger lesion size, intracerebral hemorrhage or presence of early seizures (48).

In another population-based study (Northern Manhatan Stroke Study – NOMASS), seizures within the first 7 days of the stroke onset occurred in 4.1% of all 904 patients enrolled and in 3.1% of 704 patients with ischemic strokes (49). The most common type of seizures was complex partial seizures (48.7%), followed by primary generalized (24.3%), simple partial (10.8%) and undetermined (16.2%) seizures. Compared to ischemic infarcts, seizures post ICH conferred a 2.4-times increased risk for subsequent seizures (95%CI, 1.2–5.2). Compared to deep infarcts, lobar infarcts conferred an 11 times increased risk for seizures (95%CI 2.6–47.6). Deep and lobar ICH, as well as SAH, also correlated with a significantly higher risk for seizures than deep ischemic infarcts (7.9, 1.4–43.6; 25.3, 5.1–125.2; and 13.2, 2.7–86.4, respectively). In a subgroup with recorded National Institutes of Health Stroke Scale (NIHSS) scores, seizures were more commonly associated with NIHSS >15 on admission. Early seizures post ischemic stroke were not independently predictive of 30-day case fatality, a finding that was in conflict with earlier studies (17).

A large prospective study from Lausanne, Switzerland, using the Lausanne Stroke Registry, reported 43/3,628 (1.2%) patients with seizures (50). Those patients with seizures were matched for age, sex, and location-type of lesion with two controls without seizures, from the same cohort. Early seizures (within the first 24 h) occurred in 23/3,270 (0.7%) patients with ischemic stroke and 14/352 (3.97%) patients with ICH. Patients with infarcts were statistically fewer than those with ICH to develop seizures. Hemorrhagic infarcts were associated with seizures, but embolic infarcts were not. All lesions in patients with seizures involved the cortex, except for three (one deep posterior circulation infarct and two striatocapsular ICH). In the multivariate analysis, a high blood cholesterol level was an independent predictor for decreased risk for early seizures (OR 0.18, 95%CI 0.06–0.54).

More recently, a large population-based study from Cincinnati, Ohio, evaluated 6044 patients with acute stroke and reported 190 (3.1%) of them having acute onset seizures (within the first 24 h). No difference was found between first-ever versus recurrent strokes on the incidence of seizures. Ischemic strokes and TIAs had an overall 2.4% incidence of these early seizures, in contrast with 7.9% for ICH and 10.1% for SAH. Of the patients with ischemic stroke, there was higher incidence of seizures in cardioembolic (3%) versus small- or large-vessel ischemic strokes (1.7%). Independent risk factors for seizure development included hemorrhagic stroke, younger age, and pre-stroke Rankin score of ≥1 (51). Table 3-1 summarizes the aforementioned studies of stroke and seizures, as well as percentages of early, late, recurrent (epilepsy), or total seizures.

Table 3-1. Studies With Reported Seizure Incidence After a Stroke.

Study	Type of study	No of patients	Type of stroke	Total seizures	Early seizures	Late seizures	Epilepsy
Louis and McDowell (10)	R	1,000	Isc	7.7%	3.3%	2.7%	3% early, 81% late
Black et al. (36)	R	827	Isc, hem	10%	57%*	43%*	
Gupta et al. (33)	R	90	Isc		33%*	1 year 40%* 2 years 24%*	39%*
Sung et al. (34)	R	118	Isc	5.9%	11%8	66%*	35% early* 90% late*
Lancman et al. (6)	R	230	Isc, ICH	10%	5.4%	2.7%	
Shinton et al. (11)	P	230	Isc, ICH, SAH		5.7%		
Kilpatrick et al. (9)	P	1,000	Isc, ICH, SAH		4.4%	32% early* 10% without early*	
Lo et al. (15)	R	1,200	Isc, ICH, SAH		2.5%		
Milandre et al. (12)	R	2,016	Isc, ICH	3.9%	1.4%	2.5%	1.7%
Daniele et al. (38)	R	4,425	Isc, ICH	Isc 4.7% ICH 5.7%	Isc 2.6% ICH 3.6%	Isc 2.1% ICH 2.1%	
Arboix et al. (39)	P	1,099	Isc, ICH, SAH		2.5%		
Bladin et al. (7)	P	1,897	Isc, ICH	Isc 8.6% ICH 10.6%	Isc 4.8% ICH 7.9%	Isc 3.8% ICH 2.6%	Isc 2.1% ICH 2.6%
Vespa et al. (46)	P	109	Isc, ICH	Isc 6% ICH 28%	6%		
So et al. (47)	R	535	Isc		6%	1 year 3% 5 year 7.4% 10 year 8.9%	
Giroud et al. (5)	P	1,640	Isc, ICH, SAH	Ath 4% Card 16.6% Lac 1% TIA 1.7%	5.4%		
Berges et al. (22)	P	3,205	Isc, hem	5%	1.8%	3.2%	50%**
Burn et al. (8)	P	675	Isc, ICH, SAH	Isc 4.2%/9.7% ICH 19.9%/26.1% SAH 22%/34.3%	2%		

Reith et al. (18, 48)	P	1,195	Isc, ICH	4.1%	Isc 3% ICH 8%	3.2%
Labovitz et al. (49)	P	904	Isc, ICH, SAH		Isc 3.1% ICH 7.3% SAH 8%	
Devuyst et al. (50)	P	3,628	Isc, ICH	1.02%	Isc 0.7%*** ICH 3.97%***	
Neau et al. (94) +	R	65	Isc	10.8%		
Lamy et al. (20)++	P	581	Isc		2.4%	1 year 3.1% 3 years 5.5%	2.3%
Cheung et al. (40)	R	994	Isc, ICH, SAH	3.4%	Isc 3.3% ICH 4.1% SAH 0%	0.7%
Cordonnier et al. (97)	P	202	Isc, ICH		5.4% Isc 4.5% ICH 12%	6.9% Isc 6.8% ICH 8%
Lossius et al. (41)	P	484	ICH			5.7%
Benbir et al. (43)	P	1,428	Isc, ICH, CVT	3.6%		Isc 2.7% ICH 12.8% CVT 26.6%
Misirli et al., (44)	R	1,880	Isc, ICH	10.6%	4.1%	6.5%
Szaflarski et al. (51)	P	6,044	Isc, ICH, SAH	3.1%	Isc 2.4% ICH 7.9% SAH 10.1%	
Basic-Baronica et al. (45)	R	3,542	Isc, ICH	1.8%	Isc 1.43% ICH 3.76%	

P prospective, *R* retrospective, *Isc* ischemic, *ICH* intracerebral hemorrhage, *hem* hemorrhage, *SAH* subarachnoid hemorrhage, *Ath* atheroma, *Card* cardioembolic, *CVT* cerebral venous thrombosis, *Lac* lacunar, *TIA* transient ischemic attack, * = % of patients with seizures, ** = of survivors with first seizure, *** excluding 6 pts with prodromal seizures, + = age group 15–45 years, ++ = age group 18–55 years.

3.2.2. Status Epilepticus

SE is defined as a seizure or a series of repetitive seizures without recovery between episodes that lasts more than 30 min (52, 53). SE may be an additional risk factor for increased mortality and morbidity after stroke, through systemic metabolic changes, increased risk for herniation secondary to elevated intracranial pressure, cardiac arrhythmias leading to sudden death, or increased risk of aspiration pneumonia (49). Thus SE is an unquestionable reason for ICU admission.

Acute stroke is the third most common cause for SE (53), accounting for approximately 20% of all SE cases (54–56). In a retrospective study, 8% of all initial poststroke seizures presented as SE (6% focal and 2% generalized) (33). SE was more common with early (14%) than late (5%) onset seizures, but did not occur as recurrent seizures. This was demonstrated in the largest pre-CT retrospective study of seizures following non-embolic cerebral infarction, which found most SE attacks to occur in the acute poststroke phase (10). In another retrospective study, SE occurred in 13% of 118 patients with thrombotic stroke and was generalized tonic-clonic (GTC) in 60%. This latter study reported only one patient with SE as the initial stroke manifestation and another three with SE in the acute stroke phase: 60% of patients had SE as late seizure manifestation post infarction (34). Milandre et al. found that 14% of their patients with initial poststroke seizures were in SE (12), and Lo et al. that 10% of early seizure patients were in SE (15). Within the first 7 days following an ischemic stroke, SE occurs in 0.9% of patients (NOMASS population-based study) and represents 15.8–27% of all seizures after stroke (49, 57).

A large, prospective, population-based study was conducted in Besançon, France (57). Out of 3,205 patients with first-time strokes, 159 (5%) had first-time seizures. SE occurred in 31/159 (19%) patients with poststroke seizures. Partial SE occurred in 12 patients, nonconvulsive SE (NCSE) in 10, generalized in 6, and unclassifiable in 3. SE occurred in 22/2742 (0.8%) patients with ischemic stroke and 22/116 (19%) patients with ischemic stroke who had poststroke seizures. SE occurred in 9/463 (1.9%) patients with ICH and 9/43 (21%) patients with ICH and poststroke seizures. There was no significant difference between the two etiologies of stroke (ischemic stroke or ICH) regarding the occurrence of poststroke SE. In 4/3,205 (0.12%) patients stroke initially manifested as SE and in 17/159 (11%) SE occurred as the first poststroke epileptic symptom. In patients with SE, it manifested as the first epileptic syndrome in 17/31 (55%) patients (in 7 as "early" SE within the first 2 weeks and in 10 as "late" SE), and in 14 patients it followed another seizure after the stroke (in 2 patients it was "early" SE and in 12 patients it was "late" SE). In an average 47 month follow-up of the 16/17 surviving patients with SE as the first epileptic symptom, only 3 (19%) developed additional episodes of SE and 50% were SE or seizure free. By contrast, all 14 patients with SE after one or more seizures had recurrences: 5 with SE (36%) and 9 (64%) with only seizures. Thus, SE as the first epileptic symptom was associated with a lower risk for subsequent seizures ($p < 0.01$). Such favorable association was not noted with early or late occurrence of SE. Fifteen out of 31 (48%) patients with poststroke SE died. In five of them (16%, all with infarction), SE was considered the direct cause of death. There was no significant difference in mortality for patients with poststroke seizures and poststroke SE.

Permanent neurologic deterioration after SE occurred in two patients only, and transient deterioration in 13 patients. However, there was no radiological change in these 15 patients. In another large multicenter study of 346 patients with generalized convulsive SE, mortality reached 11% in those patients with stroke as the precipitating cause (54).

Another large, retrospective, hospital-based study was reported from Turkey (58). Out of 1,174 patients with first-time stroke, 180 (15.3%) developed poststroke seizures, of which 17 (9% or 1.45% of the whole cohort) developed SE. Twelve patients manifested SE after ischemic stroke and five after ICH. There was no difference between the group with SE and the group with poststroke seizures regarding sex, age, stroke risk factors, seizure types, EEG findings, stroke type (ischemic or hemorrhagic), topography or cortical involvement, or size of the lesion. However, SE occurred more frequently among more disabled patients (Rankin scale >3, $p=0.002$). Early onset (within the first week) SE was found in 7/17 patients, of whom SE occurred as the first epileptic symptom in 6 (stroke begun as SE in 2 patients) and as SE after at least one seizure in one patient. Late onset SE was found in 10/17 patients, of whom SE occurred as the first epileptic symptom in 3. Five of seven patients with early onset SE compared to none of those patients with late onset SE experienced recurrence of SE ($p=0.003$). Mortality was not different among patients with SE (53%) compared to those with poststroke seizures (50%). However, it was higher in those patients with early onset SE, than in those with late onset seizures ($p=0.049$). Death was the direct consequence of SE in two patients (12%). Poor functional disability was the only independent clinical factor for developing poststroke SE, and age for mortality after poststroke SE.

More recently, in the large prospective study from Lausanne, Switzerland, SE was reported in 3/37 (8%) patients with early seizures after stroke, but in only 0.08% of all patients with ischemic infarction or ICH in this cohort (50).

Lastly, a prospective study from Turkey evaluated 121 patients with SE and reported that 30 (24.8%) were associated with stroke. This study does not report incidence of poststroke SE. All stroke types were evenly distributed within the early onset group (within 2 weeks), whereas only ischemic stroke was found in the late onset group (after 2 weeks). Posterior cerebral artery (PCA) infarcts were significantly more common within the late onset group. NCSE was more frequent than convulsive SE in the early onset group (59). Table 3-2 is a summary of the aforementioned studies reporting SE incidence after stroke.

3.2.3. Pathophysiology

Although the vast majority of seizures follow stroke, they can also precede it. Many studies excluded epileptic patients from the analysis if they suffered a stroke and had concurrent seizures. Others, however, reported the outcomes in these patients with "vascular precursor epilepsy" (10, 34). In one particular study from the UK, 46% of patients who developed seizures after acute stroke were epilepsy patients, raising the possibility that patients with epilepsy may have more frequent seizures after a stroke than patients without epilepsy (11). This could be explained either through recurrent or continuous focal ischemia capable of inducing an epileptogenic cortical focus or the activation

Table 3-2. Studies With Reported Status Epilepticus (SE) Incidence After a Stroke.

Study	Type of study	No of pts	SE	Comments
Sung et al. (34)	R	118	15%	0.8% initial stroke manifestation
Kilpatrick et al. (9)	P	1000	0.4%	Pts with early seizures
Lo et al. (15)	R	1,200	0.25%	Pts with early seizures
Milandre et al. (12)	R	2,016	0.5%	
Gupta et al. (33)	R	90	8%	14% of pts with early seizures
				5% of pts with late seizures
Labovitz et al. (49)	P	904	0.9%	
Rumbach et al. (57)	P	3,205	Isc 0.9%	0.12% initial stroke manifestation
			ICH 1.9%	19% pts with SE had recurrent SE, when first epileptic symptom
				36% pts with SE had recurrent SE, when SE followed seizures
Velioglu et al. (58)	R	1,174	1.45%	0.17% initial stroke manifestation
			Isc 1%	71% pts with SE had recurrence, when early onset SE
			ICH 0.45%	0% pts with SE had recurrence, when late onset SE
Devuyst et al. (50)	P	3,628	0.08%	Excluding 6 pts with prodromal seizures
Lamy et al. (20)	P	581	0.34%	age group 18–55 years

P prospective, *R* retrospective, *Isc* ischemic, *ICH* intracerebral hemorrhage.

of epileptiform discharges by regional hypoxia in patients with partial or primary generalized epilepsy, a mechanism not yet demonstrated in non-epileptic patients (3). In another study from Taiwan, four patients had seizures preceding the thrombotic stroke onset from a few hours to 2–3 days (34). In the Oxfordshire study, 2% of patients had a seizure in the year before the stroke, a threefold increase compared to the general population (8). Another case–control study of 230 patients showed an eightfold increased risk of epilepsy before stroke (60). A more recent population-based study from the UK matched 4709 patients who had seizures beginning at or after the age of 60 with controls and followed them for 5–7 years. In the group with seizures, 10% of patients developed strokes while in the control group only 4.4% did. In a Cox model, the estimated relative hazard of stroke at any point for patients with seizures compared with the control group was 2.89 (61). In addition, the previously cited large prospective study from Switzerland reported 6/3628 (0.16%) patients with seizures within the week preceding the stroke onset (50). Three patients had infarcts and three, ICH. The authors suggest that these pre-stroke seizures are caused by an initially preclinical lesion, which, because of rebleeding, developing edema, or extension or dysfunction of adjacent or remote structures (diaschisis), evolves into a clinical stroke syndrome. Because up to 11% of patients with first clinical strokes have asymptomatic cerebral infarctions on computed tomography (half of which involve the cortex) (62), it is conceivable that the preceding seizures arise from these asymptomatic lesions (34). Two studies support this theory: In the first study, 15/132 (11.4%) patients with late age onset seizures and no history of stroke had infarcts on CT of the head versus 2 of age- and sex-matched controls ($p=0.003$). However, 60% of these infarcts were lacunes (63). In another study, 75/387 (19%) of patients older than 50 years with new-onset seizures had ischemic lesions on CT of the head, making cerebral vascular disease the most frequently identified cause of late-in-life onset epilepsy (32).

Onset seizures after acute stroke have common features with acute seizures after traumatic brain injury and imply a common pathogenesis (7, 8). Since there may be a free time interval between the development of late seizures after early poststroke seizures, the pathophysiologic mechanisms may differ between early and late seizures or be evolving in time (12). Early seizures are thought to emanate from electrically irritable tissue in the penumbra of the lesion (64, 65) due to regional metabolic dysfunction and excitotoxic neurotransmitter release, such as glutamate (66). Dysfunction of inhibitory GABAergic circuits is another possibility. Accumulation of Ca^{2+} and Na^+ inside the cell results in depolarization of the cellular membrane and the activation of several intracellular cascades. This has been shown in animal models of stroke (67), where cortical neurons in the neocortex and hippocampus had altered membrane potentials and increased excitability (68, 69), as well as in vitro models of hippocampal neuron cultures, where a single 30-min 5-μM glutamate exposure produced dead cells or cells manifesting recurrent epileptiform discharges and with increased intracellular calcium levels (66). In a rat model, Nedergaard and Hansen showed that the penumbral depolarization after MCA occlusion either spreads depression waves (from K^+ or glutamate release from the core of the infarct) or ischemic depolarizations (due to blood flow fluctuations around the threshold of anoxic membrane failure) (70). These derangements do not remain stationary but constitute an evolving process. In a rat model of forebrain ischemia, there was a differential seizure threshold to infused pro-epileptic agents, which changed over time (71). Therefore, it is suggested that after an initial critical period, estimated around 3 h, the progression of the penumbra tissue towards necrosis leads to lessened epileptogenic activity, which accounts for the decrease in seizure frequency between 3 and 24 h after stroke (50). These findings are supported by another neurophysiological study using transcranial magnetic stimulation, where 6 out 84 patients with stroke showed a decrease in duration of the silent period in either the arm or leg of the affected side compared to the unaffected limb (72). Five of these six patients had early or late poststroke focal seizures and no interictal epileptiform activity on the EEG. The authors suggested that this finding was due to decreased cortical inhibitory activity related to functional or structural impairment of GABAergic interneurons.

The potential role that hypoxemia may play, in addition to the presence of a penumbra, is exemplified in a large retrospective study from Belgium. Two hundred and thirty-seven patients with poststroke seizures were compared with 939 stroke patients without seizures. The interesting finding from this study was that the only independent factors associated with poststroke seizures were partial anterior circulation syndrome/infarct and presence of chronic obstructive pulmonary disease (COPD). The authors suggested that nocturnal desaturations in patients with COPD play an additional role to stroke (73).

Late seizures probably are due to gliosis and the development of meningocerebral cicatrix, leading to persistent hypoperfusion and anoxia, dendritic deformation, and hypersensitivity or denervation supersensitivity (3, 33, 65).

A summary of possible mechanisms for seizures in varying temporal relationships to stroke can be found in the articles by Armon et al. (3) and Solverman et al. (65). Poststroke seizures are associated with more severe brain ischemia as shown by positron emission tomography (74). Seizures associated with migraine may be warning signs of an underlying cerebral infarction (75). A causal relationship between TIAs and seizures has been difficult to establish. Repetitive involuntary movements in association with TIAs have been reported. EEG in these patients did not show epileptiform activity and the movements did not respond to phenytoin (3, 76)

Although the involvement of the cerebral cortex after ischemic stroke is thought to be necessary for the occurrence of seizures, there have been several reports of seizures associated with lesions involving subcortical structures. For instance, lacunar infarcts have been implicated in the development of seizures, either through more widespread cerebrovascular disease and involvement of adjacent cortex not apparent on the CT of the head or because subcortical lesions, such as those in the caudate head, which may induce seizures (5, 27). Four out of 13 patients with seizures after acute stroke had subcortical lesions in a prospective study from Birmingham, UK (11). Only 3 out of 273 (1%) patients with lacunar infarcts had seizures in the previously quoted large prospective study from Dijon, France (5). In the same population, the authors reported in a different study, that 11/13 (85%) patients with seizures and CT-proven lenticulostriate strokes had an associated ipsilateral posterofrontal or anterotemporal cortical ischemic lesion demonstrated by magnetic resonance imaging (MRI). On single photoemission computed tomography (SPECT), 13/13 (100%) patients had decreased cerebral blood flow (CBF) in the ipsilateral frontal area. Also, in patients with a lenticulostriate stroke, a larger size of both the subcortical and ipsilateral cortical ischemic lesions is predictive of seizures (77). Five patients (3%) in the Oxfordshire study with lacunes had seizures (8) and another 5 patients with lacunes and grand mal seizures have been reported in a case series from Israel (78). In the multicenter, prospective SASS study, 2.6% of patients with lacunes developed seizures, but 7/8 had also other identifiable reasons (7). In a prospective hospital-based registry, 113 patients with non-lacunar subcortical infarcts were studied. Seizures occurred in four (3.5%) of these patients, all with striatocapsular infarcts: two within the first 24 h, one within the first month, and one within the first year. Cardioembolic strokes were more common in patients with seizures (79). In the Hong Kong study, 1.5% of patients with lacunar strokes developed seizures, contrasting with the 8.8% of those with total anterior circulation infarcts, and 7% of those with partial anterior circulation infarcts (40). In the recent Turkish study, epilepsy developed in 1.3% of patients with lacunar strokes (43). Other large studies have not found an association between lacunes and seizures (9).

Seizures associated with embolic infarcts may be due to commonly seen hemorrhagic conversion, since iron deposition in rat brain tissue is known to be epileptogenic (80). The same way, iron deposition may play a significant role in seizure development after ICH, although this mechanism does not adequately explain the early onset frequently seen. In addition, thrombin is thought to play a significant role in seizures after ICH. In a rat model of ICH, thrombin injected into the brain at concentrations found in hematomas produced brain edema and immediate focal motor and electrographic seizures in all animals. When a-NAPAP, a thrombin inhibitor, was added to the thrombin injection, none of the animals had clinical or EEG seizure activity and brain edema was reduced (81).

How much do seizures affect the evolution of the triggering stroke? The effect of seizures on the infarcted area, through hypoxia, lactic acidosis, ionic changes, and a higher metabolic demand of the brain is thought to lead to persistent worsening of the neurologic deficits (17, 82). In one particular study, persistent partial motor poststroke seizures led to persistent worsening of the prior neurologic deficit in 10/48 patients, without new CT or MRI findings (82). However, several other studies have failed to demonstrate worsening of prognosis after poststroke seizures (9, 11, 18, 49).

Another interesting recent finding was the association of poststroke seizures with subsequent development of dementia. In the Lille, France, large prospective stroke/dementia cohort, cognitive function before and after a stroke was evaluated longitudinally with a battery of tests. Early poststroke seizures (within 1 week from stroke onset) were independently predicting new-onset dementia within 3 years (hazard ratio 3.81, 95%CI 1.13–12.8). The authors suggested that seizures were a marker of an underlying condition associated with an increased risk for dementia, such as more severe vascular pathology, an underlying preclinical degenerative disease such as Altheimer's, or poststroke complications (83).

3.2.4. EEG Findings

Occasionally, EEG may be helpful in the ICU in the evaluation of poorly defined poststroke neurological symptoms (65), such as focal weakness (Todd's paralysis) or coma (due to NCSE) (84). Conventional analog EEG, computer-assisted digitized EEG, and continuous EEG recordings have all been used in the ICU (84, 85). Normal EEG after poststroke seizures has been reported in 4–15% of cases (9, 12, 15, 33). Using CEEG monitoring in the ICU, Vespa et al., concluded that electrographic poststroke seizures are 4 times more frequently detected than clinical poststroke seizures (46). A more recent study from Switzerland evaluated 100 patients admitted to a stroke unit with acute stroke (ischemic in 91 and hemorrhagic in 9 patients). CEEG was performed for a mean duration of 17 h 34 min. Epileptic activity occurred in 17 patients and consisted of repetitive focal sharp waves in 7, repetitive focal spikes in 7, and PLEDs in 3. Although clinical seizures occurred in three patients before CEEG (only one had repetitive focal spikes on CEEG), electrical seizures were recorded only in two patients without clinical seizures. On multivariate analysis, stroke severity (higher NIHSS) was the only independent predictor (86).

Abnormalities on the EEG may have a differential predictive value regarding the development of seizures after cerebral infarction. Holmes found that 98% of poststroke patients with sharp waves, spikes, and PLEDs on the EEG developed seizures, but did not correlate these findings with seizure recurrence (13). Twenty six percent of patients who developed poststroke seizures had PLEDs in this study, compared to only 2% of those who never had one. The prognostic significance of poststroke PLEDs has also been emphasized in another retrospective study, which noted that all four patients with PLEDs on the initial EEG had recurrent seizures (33). Conversely, in patients with poststroke seizures focal irritative abnormalities (electrographic seizures, epileptiform abnormalities, PLEDs) can be found on the average in one-fourth of cases and focal slowing in two-thirds (12, 15, 33). Epileptiform abnormalities on EEG performed within the first 24 h ("unless the patient was critically ill") were found in 14% of patients with peristroke seizures in a large recent prospective study (50). The specificity of the test is poor, since similar findings are not uncommon in patients with stroke without seizures (12). The frequency of irritative abnormalities can be influenced by the timing and the repetition rate of the test. This may explain why in a prospective study from Denmark, epileptiform abnormalities were reported in only 2/77 (2.6%) patients with supratentorial strokes (24). EEGs were obtained in all patients within the first week after the stroke and repeated at 3 and 6 months. All seven patients who developed epilepsy in this series had focal delta and theta activity on the EEG. One patient had epileptiform activity at 3 months poststroke before he developed epilepsy and another on the first EEG recorded 6 days after stroke and 5 days after the first seizure. The authors conclude that EEG was not helpful in determining the risk for developing epilepsy. Fig. 3-1 shows a patient who was in SE after an old ischemic stroke. Fig. 3-2 shows another patient who developed a stroke followed by seizures while driving.

3.2.5. Neuroimaging

Diffusion-weighted MRI (DWI) and apparent diffusion coefficient (ADC) changes have been well described during acute ischemic stroke. In the acute phase, because of energy substrate depletion and Na^+/K^+ – ATPase pump failure, ionic changes lead to cytotoxic edema and decreased diffusion of water. On DWI, ischemic brain appears brighter (high signal) than normal brain, while it is darker on ADC maps (low ADC=decreased signal). Later, when the cells die and cellular membranes are disrupted, these changes reverse (decreased DWI signal and increased ADC signal). However, neuroimaging changes have also been reported after repetitive seizures or SE or NCSE (87), making interpretation more difficult when these conditions coexist. Low density changes on CT and high signals on T2-weighted MRI (that do not respect vascular territories), leptomeningeal contrast enhancement (indicative of alteration of the blood–brain barrier and vasogenic edema), local hyperperfusion on magnetic resonance angiography (MRA), and cerebral activation on functional MRI, all reversible, have been well associated with partial epilepsy and could help differentiate between ischemic stroke and seizure activity (88, 89). Senn et al. reported a patient with partial status that had high DWI and ADC

Fig. 3-1. An 81-year-old African American woman with history of old stroke and left side residual hemiplegia was admitted to the neuro-ICU for altered mental status. Continuous EEG exhibited 162 electrographic seizures during the first day of recording, emanating from the right hemisphere. She was treated with IV valproic acid and IV phenytoin. Two days later, the EEG showed only interictal activity and after an additional two days only mild to moderate encephalopathy, while her mental status was improving. (**a**). CT of the head showing an encephalomalacic area on the right frontoparietal area from the old ischemic stroke (*white arrow*). (**b**) Continuous EEG showing the beginning (**b**.1), evolution (**b**.2), and end (**b**.3) of a single electrographic seizure (without clinical correlate other than diminished mental status). The rhythmic, high amplitude theta/delta activity starts over P4, P8, and O2, but later spreads to the whole right hemisphere

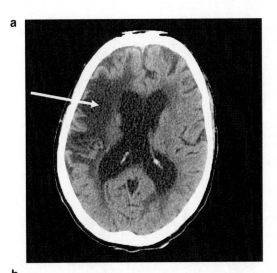

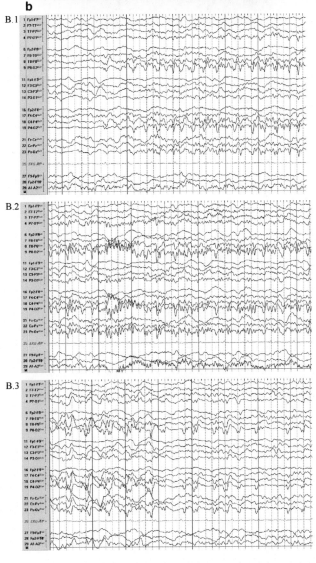

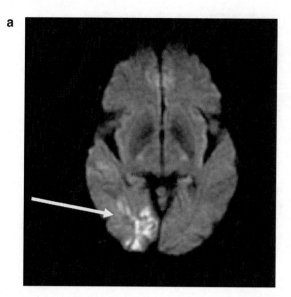

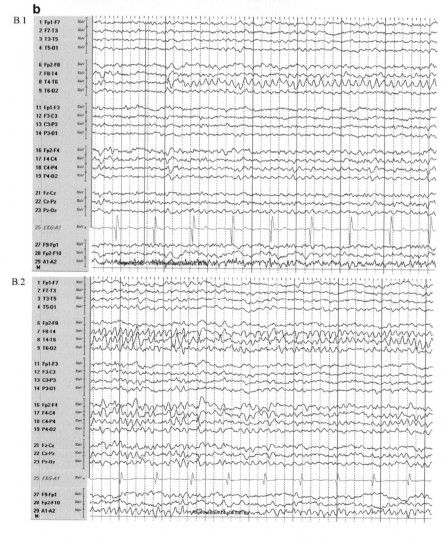

signal in the affected areas at the onset of seizures. Seven days later, DWI signal had regressed and ADC had further increased, and 10 days later there was marked regression of all signals and signs of focal atrophy (88). These findings contrast with those of Lansberg et al., who reported three patients with complex partial SE and decrease in ADC on the first day (89). These differences may be due to timing of the MRI during SE. So far, to our knowledge, no data exist regarding neuroimaging findings of poststroke seizures, except for one patient with mitochondrial encephalomyopathy (MELAS) and recurrent SE (90).

3.2.6. Seizures Post Stroke in the Young and the Elderly

Non-hemorrhagic stroke in young patients (before 45) accounts for 3–10% of all infarctions and has low mortality (1.5–8%) (91–93). Very few studies have examined the incidence of poststroke seizures in this younger population.

In a retrospective analysis of 65 young patients (aged 15–45) with stroke, who were followed for an average of 32 months (range 12–59), the incidence of seizures was 10.8% and all of them occurred in patients with carotid artery territory infarction (94).

In a prospective, multicenter European study (the PFO-ASA study), 581 patients with cryptogenic ischemic stroke, aged 18–55 years, were followed for an average of 38 months for seizures (20). None of the six deaths was related to the occurrence of a seizure. Early seizures (within 1 week post-stroke) occurred in 14/581 (2.4%) of patients, 71% of them within the first 24 h. Two patients developed SE, one as an inaugural event. Rankin scale ≥ 3 (OR, 95%CI, 3.9, 1.2–12.7) and cortical involvement (7.7, 1–61.1) were the only clinical and radiologic independent variables associated with early seizures. Late seizures occurred in 20/581 (3.4%) with a mean delay of 12.9 months post stroke. Six of these patients had early seizures, and 4/6 were on antiepileptic treatment when the first late seizure occurred. Early seizures (5.1, 1.8–14.8), cortical signs (4.5, 1.6–13.1), and size of infarct larger than one-half hemisphere (9.7, 3.1–30.8) were independent predictors for late seizure development. Recurrent, unprovoked late seizures were found in 11/20 (55%) patients with late seizures, and the risk for epilepsy was 2.3% within 3 years in this patient population.

The incidence of seizures in the elderly is close to that in the first decade of life. With increasing age, more patients have an identifiable cause for their seizures and thus more seizures may have a focal onset (95). Luhdorf et al. followed all patients within a definite area who developed seizures after the age of 60. The dominant cause of seizures was previous stroke in 32% of cases (30). In a retrospective population-based study from Saskatchewan, Canada, 46/84 (55%) of patients 60 years and older with new onset seizures had acute

---

Fig. 3-2. An 84-year old African American woman with diabetes was admitted to the neuro-ICU after a motor vehicle accident (she was the driver) without head trauma or loss of consciousness. During her transfer, she was found hypoglycemic and developed generalized tonic-clonic seizures. An MRI showed a right occipital stroke and an EEG revealed several seizures emanating from the right temporal-occipital areas. She was loaded with phenytoin and levetiracetam IV and the seizures stopped. (**a**) Diffusion-weighted imaging of the MRI showing the R inferior tempo-occipital stroke (white arrow). (**b**) EEG showing the beginning from T4–T6 of a seizure (**b**.1). This seizure evolved over the entire right hemisphere (**b**.2)

or remote cause identified (symptomatic). Of those, 22/46 (48% or 26% of all patients with new seizures) were due to acute or old stroke. All patients with non-life-threatening strokes had excellent prognosis, with seizures resolving in all but one patient. No information is provided about the number of elderly patients admitted to an ICU in these studies (96).

Similar findings were noted in a large, prospective epidemiological study conducted in Southwest France (14). The annual incidence of seizures in patients older than 60 years was 127/100,000. Cerebrovascular disease was the most frequently recognized cause in this age group and represented 36.6% of patients with spontaneous seizures and 54% of patients with confirmed epilepsy.

More recently, a prospective study from Lille, France, evaluated 202 patients with acute stroke (median age 76 years) for the presence of pre-existing dementia. Early seizures developed in 5.4% of patients in this cohort. Stroke patients with pre-existing dementia had an increased risk of late seizures, but not for early seizures. Any factor increasing the risk of seizures (drugs, metabolic changes), the authors concluded, should be avoided in these patients (97).

3.2.7. Treatment of Post-Ischemic Stroke Seizures

Seizures at the onset of an ischemic stroke were considered a contraindication for IV tissue plasminogen activator (t-PA) (98), although data addressing this issue are missing. In a prospective study from Calgary, Canada, 230 patients were eligible for IV t-PA (admission within the 3-h window), but did not receive the treatment for various reasons (99). Seizures at the stroke onset were the reason for the exclusion in 2/230 (0.9%) of these patients. In a recent large prospective study, 60% of peristroke seizures occurred between the stroke onset and 3 h (during the IV t-PA treatment window) and only 26% between 3 and 24 h (50). Interestingly, seizures occurring during the period of thrombolysis with IV t-PA may represent a sign of reperfusion or hyperperfusion and may enhance the thrombolytic process (100–102). Although in these small case series these seizures were associated with a dramatic recovery, they may also herald hemorrhagic conversion, and an urgent CT of the head should be considered if clinically the patient deteriorates.

The most recent guidelines from the Stroke Council of the American Stroke Association include a change in the recommendations regarding withholding thrombolysis in the presence of seizures at the onset of stroke. If the physician is convinced that the residual impairments are due to the stroke and are not post-ictal phenomena, due to the presence of a seizure at the time of the stroke onset, the patient may still be eligible for t-PA thrombolysis (103). This change was based on newer but poor evidence-based data. In a case report, a patient who presented with seizures, in whom the combination of DWI/PWI MRI and MRA confirmed the diagnosis of an embolic ischemic stroke, was treated with IV t-PA with clinical and radiological improvement (104). In another study, 9/116 (7.7%) patients who presented within 3 h from symptom onset and were eligible for thrombolysis had a concern of seizure at stroke onset. The median age was 73 years and the median NIHSS score was 12. CT angiography showed proximal MCA occlusion in two and distal MCA occlusion in three patients. All five patients had evidence of infarction on follow-up. Three of these patients received IV t-PA because they were deemed to have "ischemic tissue at risk". Four patients had normal CT and CT angiography studies and recovered completely in 24 h. The authors concluded that CT angiography was a useful modality in differentiating Todd's paralysis from early seizure and ischemia by detection of intracranial occlusion and may contribute to decision making for thrombolysis (105).

The same recent guidelines from the Stroke Council of the American Stroke Association did not change compared to the previous ones regarding the utility of prophylactic antiepileptic drug (AED) administration, and prophylactic treatment was not recommended (Class III, Level of Evidence C) (103). They also recognized that there are only few data concerning the efficacy of these drugs in the treatment of poststroke patients who have experienced seizures. Their recommendation was to base the treatment on the established management of recurrent seizures complicating any acute neurological illness (Class I, Level of Evidence B) (103). In the following paragraphs we will try to summarize the data available and have an in-depth look at the problem an intensivist faces.

As mentioned before, there are no randomized, controlled trials evaluating specific treatment options in poststroke seizures. Bladin et al. argue that such a trial would pose extensive logistic challenges and would likely be unethical (7). Prophylactic treatment for seizures after ischemic stroke is controversial. The duration of treatment is also unknown. Should these patients be admitted to an ICU when they present with a seizure in the context of an acute or subacute stroke? Armon et al. have summarized the rationale for treating seizures at the onset of a stroke, as follows: (a) control of persistent or recurrent seizures (SE) (b) prevention of seizures within the first day of stroke (c) prevention within the first 2 weeks post stroke, and (d) prevention of recurrence of seizures after the first 2 weeks or the appearance of late seizures (3). We suggest adapting the same rationale to the ICU setting by tailoring it to the following issues: (a) whether or not to treat a seizure that accompanies a stroke, (b) whether to treat recurrent seizures or SE, (c) whether to treat preventively poststroke seizures, (d) whether to prevent late seizures from occurring after an early seizure, or (e) whether to prevent epilepsy from developing after early or late seizures.

The current consensus in ischemic stroke management is to not treat patients unless they present with a first seizure or they have known preexisting epilepsy (106). If a patient had prestroke seizures, the rationale for covering him/her with antiepileptics is based on the prevention of preexisting epilepsy to manifest in its usual form post stroke or as SE (3). However, even before the occurrence of the first seizure, some subgroups of non-epileptic patients may be at higher risk for seizure development. Large infarct size, cortical involvement hemorrhagic stroke, and severe stroke (5–7, 15, 18, 20, 33, 37, 39, 47, 49, 107) are typical situations where a physician could consider covering the patient with antiepileptic treatment to prevent early seizures, especially if other comorbidities make a seizure manifestation an unacceptably high risk for complications.

The occurrence of one or more seizures may trigger the decision to use antiepileptics, although that decision may also depend on the type and location of stroke. Because of the risk of progression to SE, further damage to the ischemic penumbra leading to deterioration of the stroke or aspirating oral secretions or vomitus, we believe these patients should be admitted and treated in a neonatal (NICU) or a stroke unit. Are there any data that support this approach? In the series of Milandre et al. 51% of patients with seizures developed recurrent seizures, multiple in two-thirds of them (12). In the series by Gupta et al., 39% of patients had recurrent seizures, multiple in 57% of them (33). In neither study was there any difference in the recurrence rate, whether the seizures occurred early or late post-stroke. In the Oxfordshire study, 3% of patients with cerebral infarction developed a single post stroke seizure and another 3% recurrent seizures, which overall occurred infrequently. The percentages for those with total anterior circulation infarction were 5% and 11% and in those with lacunes 2% and 1%, respectively. However, 40% of patients with seizures within the first 24 h post ischemic stroke and 50% post ICH developed later seizures, although the numbers are very small (8). Patients with lobar ICH or SAH had 14% and 8% incidence of early seizures in the Manhattan population study, and the authors suggested prophylaxis for these subgroups for the first 24 h only, since almost 90% of seizures occurred within that time frame (49).

Usually late poststroke seizures are not encountered in the ICU, unless one is dealing with SE. Occasionally, however, a patient who is admitted for another medical reason to the ICU develops seizures that cannot be related to a drug or a metabolic derangement. Or the patient may develop seizures in the context of a recurrent stroke and it may be difficult (if there is no clear focality in the seizure onset or in the EEG) to associate the seizure with the new or the old stroke. As with early seizures, there are data supporting the use of antiepileptic coverage for these late seizures. From the SASS study, although late onset seizures (after the first 2 weeks) occurred in only 3.8% of all patients with ischemic stroke, they led to epilepsy in 55% of these patients, and their presence was the only independent predictor for the development of epilepsy (7). This has also been noted in other studies (34, 47) and in younger patient populations (20).

The role played by antiepileptic medications in preventing early or late poststroke seizures is also unclear (9, 11). In a retrospective study, 88% of patients with post-infarction seizures were controlled with monotherapy, mostly phenytoin, whereas another smaller percentage was initially started on multidrug regimen (33). An Israeli group retrospectively compared 35 patients with post-ischemic stroke treated immediately with antiepileptic medications for 2 years after their first early seizure, with 26 patients who were untreated until they developed a second seizure (108). The assignment was made on the basis of on the admission service that had accepted the patients. The mean time for the development of a first seizure post stroke was 5.7 days and for the second 15.2 months. During the initial 2-year post event period, the group that was treated immediately had lower relapse (14.3% vs. 38.5%, $p=0.03$) and higher seizure-free rates (85% vs. 61%, $p=0.042$). However, the treated group after discontinuing the antiepileptic treatment had the same seizure risk than the untreated group during the period between the first and the second seizure (4.8% vs. 6.2%, $p=0.6$). This protective role of antiepileptic medications was not confirmed in other larger studies. In a recent multicenter prospective European study of younger patients (<55 years old) with cryptogenic ischemic stroke, antiepileptic treatment did not prevent late seizures in patients with early seizures (20).

Which antiepileptic agents are most effective in preventing poststroke seizures is also unknown. Overall, poststroke seizures seem easily controlled, and monotherapy usually suffices. Because the majority of seizures have a focal onset, first-line drugs in the ICU are parenteral agents, such as phenytoin or fosphenytoin (65). However, if the patient's mental status and swallowing ability allows oral administration of other agents, such as carbamazepine or oxcarbamazepine, those should be considered.

The potential effect that antiepileptic medications may have on ischemia or rehabilitation should also been considered. Some antiepileptics, such as carbamazepine, topiramate, or sodium valproate, have additional neuroprotective properties against cerebral ischemia (109, 110). On the other hand, other studies also suggest that pheny-toin, barbiturates, and benzodiazepines may have a negative effect on recovery from stroke (111). These older agents also have interactions with common drugs used for treatment or secondary prevention of stroke, such as warfarin or salicylic acid (106).

Because of more favorable side-effect profile and tolerability, newer agents such as lamotrigine should be also considered as monotherapy. Other oral agents, that are approved only for adjunctive treatment and are commonly used as monotherapy, such as topiramate, leviracetam, zonisamide, and tiagabine, could also be used in individual cases. Age may also be another important factor for a decision which agent to use, since most stroke patients are elderly (106). The International League Against Epilepsy has concluded that only lamotrigine and gabapentin have level A evidence to allow recommendation as first-line monotherapy for elderly adults with partial-onset seizures (112). Gabapentin has been used as monotherapy in 71 patients with late poststroke seizures in an uncontrolled study from Barcelona, Spain (113). The initial dose of gabapentin was established on the basis of weight: 900 mg/d for patients weighing under 75 kg and 1,200 mg/d for patients weighing over 75 kg. If seizures recurred, the dose was increased by 300 mg/d. Seizures were observed in 18.2% of patients during an average follow-up period of 30 months. Overall, these patients achieved better control than patients with newly diagnosed nonvascular partial epilepsy (114). Another monotherapy used in 25 elderly patients with late poststroke seizures was levetiracetam. After 6 months, 76% of patients were still receiving the drug (at a median dose of 1,052 mg/day (range 1–2 g/day) and 89.5% of them were seizure-free (115).

The duration of the antiepileptic treatment is also unknown. Most experts use the EEG together with the clinical picture and stroke type to decide about the length of treatment. Armon et al. suggested a 12-month seizure-free interval and an EEG without epileptiform activity to consider withdrawing the treatment for cortical ICH and seizures. For non-hemorrhagic stroke and one or more GTC seizures (at the onset or early on), they suggested a 1–2 week course with phenytoin, then tapering if the EEG does not show an epileptogenic focus. If such a focus is present they suggested a longer treatment. The same approach was used for epilepsia partialis continua, with the objective of minimizing the likelihood of secondary generalization (3). Table 3-3 represents a suggested algorithm for the treatment of poststroke seizures.

3.3. Intracerebral Hemorrhage (ICH)

3.3.1. Clinical Studies

Although there are no widely accepted guidelines for ICH admission to an ICU, most physicians prefer to admit patients with moderate to large size (> 30 cc) hematomas to the stroke unit or ICU for initial observation. One of

Table 3-3. Treatment with AntiEpileptic Medications After Ischemic Stroke.

1. Infarct and pre-existing seizures: continue or restart antiepileptic regimen, keep therapeutic levels.

2. Infarct and no seizures:

   Observe.

   Consider Rx if large, cortical infarct, with hemorrhagic component or significant co-morbidities (lung, heart, presence of aneurysm, etc.) for at least 2 weeks

3. Infarct and early first seizure:

   Start monotherapy. If subcortical or lacune, continue for 2 weeks. If anterior circulation cortical infarct, continue for 1–2 years (seizure-free interval). Assess with EEG before discontinuation?

4. Infarct and SE:

   Treat according to SE protocol in the NICU. Continue Rx for at least 4 years (seizure-free interval) if SE was the first epileptic symptom. Assess with EEG before discontinuation and individualize. Treat indefinitely, if SE followed early or late seizures.

5. Infarct and late first seizure:

   Treat with monotherapy for at least 2 years (seizure-free interval). Assess with EEG before discontinuation and individualize.

the signs of ICH that would make an admission to the ICU particularly likely is early seizures, although there are no data supporting that approach. Seizures post ICH can develop with the same crude incidence rate in the ICU and in other non-ICU services (116), but probably could be recognized earlier and managed more safely in a unit environment if they recur.

Several studies have reported the incidence of post-ICH seizures ranging between 0% and 31% (5, 7, 27, 38, 46, 116–124), with the highest incidence reported from the NICU, where patients were monitored with CEEG (46, 124). No particular sex association with seizures has been reported (46, 122). At least one study has reported lower frequency of post-ICH seizures in black patients (122). Most studies have found that post-hemorrhagic stroke seizures occur more frequently than post-ischemic stroke seizures (5–7, 9), although there are a few that did not find this association (11, 36). Cortical involvement has been postulated to be more common in patients who develop seizures, since one of the earliest studies by Richardson and Dodge (125). As with ischemic stroke, most of post-ICH seizures are of the partial type with or without secondary generalization in 67–71% of cases (27, 46, 119, 123). Only one study found seizures to be more often generalized (122). Most of the studies providing information about the natural history of ICH have limitations.

Using the Besançon Stroke Registry, Tatu et al. identified 350 patients with primary ICH (120). Seizures occurred in 39/350 (11.1%) patients and were the presenting symptom of ICH in 20/350 (5.7%) patients, although their incidence varied with the location of the hematoma: 22.7% with lobar, 8% with putaminal, 1.8% with thalamic, and none with cerebellar ICH. Among 191 patients admitted within 12 h of onset, 51 (26.7%) experienced an early clinical worsening, but no data are presented about the subgroup with seizures. In another study, however, seizures were not found to be associated with neurological deterioration in non-comatose patients with ICH (126). The vast majority of studies after CT became available are hospital based and retrospective.

An interesting study with clinical and radiological details (through medical record review) was conducted in the Bronx, NY (122). Seizures occurred in 19/112 (17%) patients with supratentorial ICH, all within 24 h from the ICH onset. A major limitation of this study is that, in all but one patient, seizures manifested before arriving to the emergency room. This may account for a possible overrepresentation of generalized (68%) versus focal (32%) seizures. Another limitation is the short median follow-up period of 60 days. Patients with bleeding diatheses (anticoagulant- or alcohol-induced thrombocytopenia) and cortical extension of the hemorrhage were more likely to have seizures. No association was found between seizure occurrence and level of consciousness or Glasgow coma score (GCS) on admission, hemorrhage size, presence of midline shift, or subarachnoid or intraventricular extension.

Another large chart review study from Taipei, Taiwan, reported 126 patients with seizures out of 1,402 patients with ICH (9%) (119). The authors, however, excluded from their analysis those patients who had any type of surgery post ICH. In those medically treated patients who were followed for an average of slightly less than 2 years, seizures occurred in 4.6%. More than half were early seizures (within 2 weeks) and in 30% they were the first manifestation of ICH. Overall, 90% of seizures occurred within the first year post ICH. The incidence of epilepsy after ICH was 2.5%. Twenty nine percent of patients with early seizures developed epilepsy compared to 93% of those with late seizures (we calculated the OR for seizure recurrence for late compared to early seizures at 29.4, 95%CI 5.9–146.4, $p < 0.001$). More patients with lobar compared to deep-seated hematomas developed early or late seizures, SE, or epilepsy.

One retrospective study from New Orleans, LA, examined the incidence of seizures after primary or secondary (neoplasms or vascular lesions) ICH (121). Thirty three out of 222 patients (15%) had seizures within 12 months of follow-up. Hematoma location played a role: 32% of frontal ICH had seizures, 36% with parietal, 37% with temporal, and only 6% with occipital. None of the patients with caudate head involvement or IVH had seizures. Of those patients with immediate or early seizures (up to 72 h after onset of ICH), 70% had recurrent seizures. All patients with seizures after the first 72 h had recurrences, but no patient had seizures while on antiepileptic treatment after the first 4 months.

In a retrospective, hospital-based study from Palermo, Italy, 217 out of 4,425 (4.9%) patients with acute stroke had one or more seizures (38). Seizures after ischemic stroke occurred in 4.7% of patients and after ICH in 5.7%. In the ICH group, seizures heralded stroke in 3.3%, were early (within 2 weeks) in 60%, and late in 36.7% of cases. Lobar ICH and seizures was found in 67% of cases, subcortical in 20%, and massive in 13%.

In another retrospective study from Rome, Italy, the authors reported seizures in 55/298 (18%) patients with primary ICH (123). A limitation of this study is that almost 40% of ICH was diagnosed before the CT era. In 42% of patients with seizures, these were the inaugural symptom of ICH, in 18% they were early (within 2 weeks), and in 25% they were late. Seizures were seen in 35% of lobar ICH and only 8% of deep-seated hematomas. Epilepsy developed in 9% of patients with inaugural seizures, in 29% with early seizures, and in 93% of patients with late seizures.

In a series of 123 patients with primary ICH, from Birmingham, AL, followed for an average of 4.6 years or until death, 31 (25%) patients had seizures according to retrospective chart review (27). In 50% of patients with seizures, these occurred within 24 h of the ICH and in 13%, seizures were the inaugural symptom. Overall, two-thirds of seizures occurred within the first 48 h. Cumulative seizure incidence was 50% within 5 years. Seizure incidence was highest with bleeding into lobar cortical structures (54%), low with basal ganglionic hemorrhages (19%), and zero with thalamic hemorrhages. Within the basal ganglia, caudate involvement predicted seizures, and within the cortex temporal or parietal involvement also predicted seizures. Although cumulative seizure incidence was high (50%) by year 5, prevalence of recurrent seizures (epilepsy) was much lower: 13% in 30-day to 2-year survivors and 6.5% in 2- to 5-year survivors. The authors estimated the incidence of post-ICH seizures compared to the general population to be15 times higher within the first 2 years and 8 times higher within the third through the fifth year. Hematoma size in this (27) and other studies (7) was not found to be associated with seizures.

In the prospective study from Dijon, France, the authors reported a 16.2% incidence of seizures in patients with supratentorial ICH and none in those with infratentorial ICH (5). Seizures were more frequent in patients with lobar ICH and cortical involvement (22.7%) than those with deep ICH (2.5%) or those with cortical infarction (6.8%, $p=0.001$).

In a prospective multicenter international study, 1,897 patients with acute stroke were admitted to teaching hospitals and followed for an average of 9 months (7). Seizures were present in 10.6% of patients with ICH. Early onset seizures (within 2 weeks) occurred in 7.9% of patients, 57% of which occurred during the first 24 h. The 1-year actuarial risk for seizures was 20% for patients with ICH. Recurrent seizures occurred in all patients with late seizures (after the first 2 weeks). Using a Cox proportional hazards model, ICH conveyed an almost twofold increased risk for seizures (hazard ratio 1.85; (95%CI, 1.3–2.7, $p=0.002$). The only independent predictor for seizures was cortical involvement by the ICH. According to the authors, the sudden development of a space-occupying lesion with mass effect, focal ischemia, and blood products are all variables thought to play a role in the development of early seizures after ICH (7).

A prospective hospital-based study from Siena, Italy, found that 57/761 (7.5%) patients had seizures post spontaneous supratentorial ICH (116). The crude incidence rate of seizures in the intensive care was 5.1%, not different from other services admitting ICH patients. An interesting finding was that those patients with previous stroke did not have a higher incidence of immediate (within 24 h) or early (within 30 days) seizures after the index ICH compared to those without previous strokes. Thirty-two (4.2%) patients had immediate seizures, the majority (62.5%) being simple partial ones. In a multivariate analysis, lobar location of ICH and smaller volume of ICH (≤18 cc) were independent predictors of immediate seizures (OR, 95%CI were 4, 3.45–4.65, $p<0.001$ and 1.6, 1.02–4.5, respectively). Only one patient with immediate seizures had recurrent seizures. Twenty-five out of 650 patients who survived the first ICH day (3.8%) had early seizures, the majority (52%) generalized ones. Lobar location (2.8, 1.6–4.8, $p=0.0002$), neurologic complications (2.2, 1.5–3.3), and prophylactic antiepileptic treatment (in this study, phenobarbital, which reduces the risk of early seizures, 0.58, 0.39–0.87) were the only independent predictors for early seizures. Immediate early seizures or SE were not independent predictors of in-hospital mortality. The cumulative actuarial risk for seizures within 5 days of the ICH onset was 7.2%, and within 30 days 8.1%. For those with seizures and a mean follow-up of 59 months, the risk was 27% for relapse within 5 years and was associated with clinical events such as infarct, hematoma enlargement, and discontinuation of medications. Prophylactic antiepileptic treatment was given in 65.1% of patients on the basis of the judgment of the responsible physician. Younger patients with larger hematomas and midline shift were more likely to be treated. The risk for early seizures was reduced with prophylactic treatment only in patients with lobar ICH (0.62, 0.4–0.96, $p=0.033$). The authors reach the interesting conclusion that the likelihood of immediate seizures is influenced by predisposing factors that are inherent to the ICH.

Another large prospective study from Barcelona, Spain, evaluated all patients admitted with ICH within a 10-year period (1986–1995). Seizures occurred in 11/229 patients (4.8%). After adjusting for covariates, seizures were associated only with lobar ICH (OR 11.2, 95%CI 2.2–56.8) (127).

In a large retrospective study of Chinese patients from Hong Kong, 9/222 (4.1%) patients developed post-ICH seizures. Cortical location of ICH was as significant risk factor for seizure occurrence in ICH patients. There was no difference of poststroke seizure incidence in this study between patients with ischemic stroke (3.3%) and ICH (4.1%) (40).

In a large recent prospective study from Turkey, epilepsy developed almost 5 times more frequently in patients admitted to a stroke unit with ICH compared to ischemic stroke 12.8% vs. 2.7%) (43).

Lastly, the large population-based study from Cincinnati, OH, showed a 7.9% incidence of early seizures (within 24 h) after ICH/IVH, which is contrasting with the mere 2.4% after acute ischemic stroke. Hemorrhagic stroke, younger age, and pre-stroke Rankin ≥1 were independent predictors of these early seizures (51).

Three studies, conducted in NICUs, examined the incidence of post-ICH seizures. Two of them used CEEG monitoring and are important because they reported the highest incidence of seizures post ICH. In a prospective ICU study, Vespa et al. examined the incidence of poststroke seizures using CEEG monitoring (46). All patients with ICH were preventively covered with antiepileptic treatment (phenytoin, with therapeutic levels 14–18 mg/dL). None of the ischemic stroke patients received such prophylaxis, unless they had surgery, ventriculostomy, or seizures. Seizures occurred in 18/63 (28%) of patients with ICH and 3/46 (6%) patients with ischemic stroke (OR 5.7, 95%CI 1.4–26.5). Most seizures (89%) occurred within the first 72 h after the insult and most of them (76%) were nonconvulsive (unresponsive patients with absence of overt convulsions). In the ICH subgroup, where there was a trend of more arteriovenous malformation (AVM) representation in the seizures subgroup ($p=0.07$), seizures occurred more frequently with intraventricular extension of blood and with lobar rather than subcortical location of the hematoma (2, 0.59–7). More than one-third of post ICH seizures (38.9%), however, developed with subcortical ICH locations. The NIHSS score increased more in the seizure group than in the group of ICH without seizures, and the same was true for the midline shift at the level of the septum pellucidum.

There was a weak tendency towards larger ICH volume during repeat CT in those patients with seizures compared to those without ($p<0.16$). By the same token, a nonsignificant correlation with higher mortality was found in the group of ICH patients with seizures (27.8%) compared to those with ICH without seizures (15%). In the multivariate analysis, seizures were independently predicted by age, location of ICH, presence of IVH, and initial volume tercile (<30 cc, 30–60 cc, or >60 cc), but not by the initial NIHSS score. Outcome in those patients with ICH was predicted by the initial NIHSS score and age. Seizures had only a trend effect ($p<0.06$) on outcome as measured by GOS.

More recently, Claassen et al. retrospectively examined all patients with ICH admitted at Columbia Presbyterian hospital in New York and monitored by CEEG. The vast majority of these 102 patients (96%) was admitted to the neurological ICU. Impaired mental status was found in 57% of patients on admission and in 76% at the time of EEG initiation. Seizures occurred in 31% of these patients. In 19 patients, the clinical seizures occurred before hook-up to the EEG. Eighteen percent of patients had electrographic seizures. Importantly, only 1 of these 18 patients also had clinical seizures while on CEEG. Therefore, the vast majority of these seizures were subclinical and would not have been detected without CEEG. In the 18 patients with EEG seizures, 56% had the first seizure recorded within 1 h, 72% within 24 h, and 94% within 48 h of CEEG initiation. Electrographic seizures occurred in 29% of patients with a superficial ICH (within 1 mm of the cortex), in 23% of patients with lobar ICH, and in 11% with deep hemorrhages. NCSE occurred in seven patients (i.e., in 7%, or in 39% of those with electrographic seizure activity). Only an increase in ICH volume of ≥30% between admission and 24-h follow-up CT scan was independently associated with electrographic seizures (OR 9.5, 95%CI 1.7 to 53.8). Periodic epileptiform discharges were less frequently seen in those with ICH located at least 1 mm from the cortex (OR 0.2, 0.1 to 0.7) and were independently associated with poor outcome (OR 7.6, 2.1 to 27.3). Focal stimulus-induced rhythmic, periodic, or ictal discharges (SIRPIDS) were also independently associated with poor outcome (OR 15.6, 2.7–90.5), but electro-graphic seizures, which were significantly more present in patients with poor outcome than in those with better outcome (44% vs. 21%), lost their predictive significance when adjusted for other covariates (124).

The third study conducted at the Neurocritical Care Unit at Johns Hopkins Hospital differs from the other two, because it evaluated seizures on presentation (witnessed by family, emergency medical service (EMS), or the emergency department, before the admission to the unit) and obviously did not use any EEG confirmation. All the 125 patients with ICH, however, were managed in the NICU. Seizures on presentation occurred in 17% of patients. After adjusting for covariates, seizures on presentation had no significant impact on 30-day mortality or outcomes at discharge in this cohort (128).

3.3.2. SE Following ICH

SE occurs in 0.8 to 1.9% of patients with ICH. This incidence, however, is higher in studies using CEEG monitoring for detection and can reach 7% (124). In those patients with ICH who develop seizures, SE occurs in 14–21% (12, 116, 119).

The incidence of SE after ICH was specifically addressed in the large prospective, population study from Besançon, France (57). ICH triggered

SE in nine patients or SE occurred in 9/463 (1.9%) of patients with ICH. Among patients with first-time poststroke seizures, 9/43 (21%) had ICH and SE. Although SE followed ICH more than twice as frequently compared to ischemic stroke, etiology did not reach significance for SE in this cohort. ICH was more common among patients with SE as the first poststroke seizure symptom (6/17, 35.3%) than among those with SE occurring after one or more seizures (3/14, 21.4%). In another study from Taiwan, SE was found in 11/1402 (0.8%) patients with ICH. Among those patients who developed seizures, SE occurred in 11/64 (17%). SE was the first ever seizure type post ICH in nine patients and the first manifestation of ICH in six patients. Mortality in this series reached 36% for patients with seizures and SE, while it was 24% in those with seizures without SE (119). In a recent study from Italy, SE occurred in 1.1% of patients with ICH and in 14% of those who developed seizures post ICH (116). SE occurred exclusively in patients with lobar ICH, but in the multivariate analysis alcohol abuse was the only independent predictor for SE (OR 3.4, 95%CI 1.2–9.6).

In a recent retrospective study, Bateman et al. used the Nationwide Inpatient Sample for the years 1994–2002 to derive data about GCSE after ICH. Two hundred and sixty-six patients (0.3%) out of 102,763 admitted with ICH developed GCSE. Using multivariate analysis, higher rate of GCSE was associated with African American and Hispanic race, renal disease, coagulopathy, brain tumor, alcohol abuse, and sodium imbalance, while increasing age and hypertension were associated with lower rates of GCSE (129).

3.3.3. Pathophysiology of Seizures Post ICH

As mentioned above in the pathophysiology of ischemic stroke, the theory of seizure development after ICH is based on the fact that iron contained in the hemoglobin residing in the clot is a known trigger for cellular depolarization in animal models (80). This mechanism does not adequately explain the early onset of seizures frequently seen after ICH. Another factor thought to play a significant role in seizure generation after ICH is thrombin. When thrombin was injected into a rat brain at concentrations found in hematomas, it produced brain edema and immediate focal motor and electrographic seizures in all animals. When a-NAPAP, a thrombin inhibitor, was added to the thrombin injection, none of the animals had clinical or EEG seizure activity, and brain edema was reduced (81).

ICH may also influence gene expression. In a recent adult rat model, gene expression was assessed using Affymetrix microarrays in the striatum and the overlying cortex at 24 h after intracranial infusions of blood into the striatum. ICH upregulated 108 and downregulated 126 genes in the striatum, and upregulated 170 and downregulated 69 genes in the cortex. These results suggest that ICH-related downregulation of GABA-related genes and potassium channels might contribute to perihematoma cellular excitability and increased risk of post-ICH seizures (130).

3.3.4. Treatment of Seizures Post ICH

The appropriateness of treating seizures that follow ICH has not been addressed specifically in the literature: neither has the usefulness of prophylactic treatment, knowledge about which is only inferred from observational studies, as randomized trials are lacking. The guidelines published by the Stroke Council of the American Heart Association emphasize this lack of evidence currently available, but suggest antiepileptic treatment for 1 month and then tapering and discontinuation of the treatment if no seizures occur (131).

Immediate, early seizures or even SE do not appear to increase mortality after ICH (116), but their effect on morbidity post ICH is not known. In one retrospective study, which also included ICH from underlying vascular or neoplastic lesions, patients were followed for 1 year (121). All patients with ICH from an underlying lesion that was previously causing seizures were noted to have seizure recurrences, despite antiepileptic treatment, but none after the first 4 months.

The only currently available study of ICU stroke patients, evaluated with CEEG monitoring, found a higher incidence of seizures post ICH than post-ischemic stroke, despite the fact that all ICH patients were systematically covered with antiepileptic medications upon admission and none of the ischemic stroke patients was on prophylactic treatment (46). The results of this study make us and others (116, 122, 132) believe that antiepileptic treatment should be given prophylactically to all patients with lobar supratentorial ICH or with cortical ICH involvement. Among lobar ICH patients, the temporoparietal location appears to confer a higher seizure risk (27, 118). Other high risk subgroups include the elderly and those with high-initial ICH volume (> 60 cc) (46). If neurological complications (such as brain ischemia or rebleeding) occur after the ICH, early seizures may occur more often and prophylactic antiepileptic treatment may indeed be effective (116). If the seizures occur after the first two weeks, most authorities recommend long-term antiepileptic treatment (123, 133), because late seizures are strongly associated with epilepsy development (119).

The effect of surgery on occurrence of seizures is also unknown. The study by Faught et al. did not find any increase in the incidence of seizures: in their series, 22/31 patients with post ICH seizures were symptomatic before any surgery and 9 only after a surgical procedure (27). In one retrospective study, patients who had surgical clot removal had a higher incidence of late than early seizures (43% compared to 33%), but only 1 out of 15 patients eventually developed epilepsy (123). Prophylactic treatment aimed at preventing postoperative seizures does not seem to be effective: 5/27 (18.5%) patients in a chart review analysis had seizures while still on antiepileptics after surgery compared to 3/17 (17.6%) who were never treated (27). A recent study agreed with these findings: the rate of surgery was not different in those patients with immediate or early seizures and those without seizures (116). Thus, we do not recommend prophylactic treatment in the ICU just because the patient underwent a surgical procedure, if there are no other high-risk factors present.

Since alcoholic patients post ICH have more than threefold increased risk for SE (116), we recommend antiepileptic treatment in this patient subgroup in the ICU with agents that increase GABAergic inhibition (benzodiazepines or phenobarbital).

Table 3-4 represents a suggested algorithm for the treatment of ICH-related seizures.

Table 3-4. Treatment with AntiEpileptic Medications After ICH.

1. ICH and pre-existing seizures: Continue or restart antiepileptic regimen, keep therapeutic levels.

2. ICH and no seizures:

   Observe.

   Consider Rx for 1 month, if the patient is older or has lobar ICH (especially temporal-parietal) or ICH with cortical involvement.

   Treat if there is an underlying structural lesion (AVM or other lesion) or history of alcohol abuse.

3. ICH and early seizure:

   Treat for at least 2 years (seizure-free interval). Assess with EEG before discontinuation?

4. ICH and SE:

   Treat according to SE protocol in the NICU. Continue long-term Rx. Consider discontinuing Rx after at least 2 years (seizure-free interval) if there were concurrent etiologic factors, such as alcohol abuse, that are not present at time of discontinuation. Assess with EEG before discontinuation.

5. ICH and late seizures:

   Treat indefinitely.

3.4. Subarachnoid Hemorrhage

3.4.1. Clinical Studies

All patients with spontaneous SAH should be admitted to the NICU; most of them have longer length of stay compared to other types of stroke. It is not unusual to witness abnormal motor activity and loss of consciousness at the onset of SAH, usually preceding the ICU admission. Many patients have opisthotonos or tonic extension posturing of the arms and legs. Studies examining the incidence of seizures published in the pre-CT era had several limitations. The clinical phenomena that were witnessed were seldom described, and most of the articles were not focused on this subject, but rather on other aspects of SAH. In addition, several changes took place in the management of SAH in the 1990s. The most important are early angiography and surgery, endovascular treatment and modern management in the NICU, leading to a decrease in mortality from 49% to between 20% and 30% (134). As result of the improvements in diagnosis and treatment, the earlier and more recent cohorts may have different characteristics. Early seizures after SAH have been reported in 1.1–16% of patients (135–141) and late seizures in 5.1–14% (136, 138, 140–144), depending on the definition used and inherent biases to the sampling of patients. In studies with aneurysmal SAH, anterior cerebral or communicating artery aneurysms had the highest incidence of seizures, followed by middle cerebral artery aneurysms (138, 145).

The evolution in our diagnostic capabilities in the NICU and the spectrum of clinical presentation of seizures is nicely illustrated in a case report of a patient with tonic-clonic movements, unresponsiveness, and profound bradycardia after coiling of a giant left ICA aneurysm abutting the left temporal lobe. By using video-EEG monitoring, the authors discovered that the bradycardia spell was preceded by an ictal discharge over the left frontotemporal region. This patient was successfully treated with valproate and was advised to have a cardiac pacemaker implanted (146).

Seizures or epilepsy as a result of an unruptured cerebral aneurysm are rare. In a literature review, until 2003, Kamali et al. found only 14 epilepsy patients in whom intracranial aneurysm was found (and described another 5 patients). They noted that the majority of epileptic patients had giant, usually middle cerebral artery, aneurysms. The mechanisms implicated were calcification of the aneurismal wall with compression or ischemia in the adjacent tissue or distal emboli emanating from the aneurysm sac (147). After the aneurysm bleeds, the pathophysiology may not be the same, however. Although several pathophysiologic mechanisms for seizure development after SAH have been considered in early studies, such as intracranial pressure (ICP) elevation, intracerebral hematoma, infarction, or vasospasm, most experts now agree that the majority of the previously described seizures were indeed non-epileptic phenomena, consistent with either acutely released brainstem reflexes or preterminal events secondary to decreased cerebral perfusion or brain herniation (139, 148). The pathogenesis of post-SAH seizures remains speculative and most likely multifactorial. For early seizures, direct irritation of the cerebral cortex by blood seems a more plausible mechanism than vasospasm that usually develops 4–7 days later. An association of onset seizures to brain ischemia from an "ultra-early arterial vasospasm" described by Qureshi et al. (149), however, remains a possibility (140). For late seizures, factors such as cerebral infarction or operative trauma may play a more important role (136). Hyponatremia maybe another etiology for seizures after SAH, but the cutoff level of sodium that may provoke seizures is unknown. In a recent study, 179/316 patients with SAH (56.6%) developed hyponatremia (Na^+ <135 mmol/L). In the majority, hyponatremia was due to SIADH (syndrome of inappropriate antidiuretic hormone) (69%) in these series. Seizures developed in 14.5% of patients with Na^+ <130, but there was no difference in the incidence of seizures between patients with plasma Na^+ <125 mmol/L and patients with Na^+ between 125 and 130 mmol/L (150).

One of the first systematic approaches to evaluate the incidence of seizures after SAH was the retrospective study by Hart et al. from the pre-CT era (139). They evaluated 100 patients with SAH and based their results on clinical data and in the majority of cases on unwitnessed seizures. There were 30 episodes of seizure activity in 26 patients. Nineteen percent of patients experienced seizures at the onset or within the first 12 h after SAH, most during the first few minutes. There was no correlation between those seizures and the incidence of rebleeding or the prognosis. Late seizures (after the first 12 h) occurred in 11/93 (12%) patients who survived. In 73% of these, seizures manifested during acute rebleeding. Patients with acute rebleeding had a 20% incidence of seizures, almost the same as those who experienced seizures at the onset of the initial bleeding (19%). Overall, 90% of all post-SAH seizures were temporally related to acute hemorrhage. The mortality of those patients with late seizures was 64% and the mortality of those who survived the first 12 h after the initial SAH without late seizures 38%, but the difference did not reach significance. Neither the authors did find any difference in the rebleeding rate or mortality between those patients treated with antiepileptic medications and those who never received any.

In a chart review study from Saskatoon, Canada, seizures were observed in 31/131 (24%) patients with spontaneous SAH not related to AVMs (136). Early seizures (within 2 weeks) were found in 20% and late seizures (with a mean follow-up of 23 months) in 4%. Nineteen out of 26 (73%) early seizures occurred during the first 24 h post SAH, and only 2 (7.7%) patients with early seizures developed late seizures beyond 4 weeks. There was no difference in mortality between patients with or without early seizures. Neither a difference was found in the incidence of intracerebral hematoma or rebleeding. No specific predilection for seizures in relation to the location of supratentorial aneurysms was reported, but no seizures occurred with infratentorial ones. The authors question the need for routine prophylactic long-term antiepileptic treatment for patients with early seizures.

Another study from Detroit, MI, that randomly selected 100 charts for review, reported pre-hospital seizures in 17.9% of patients post SAH, with an additional 7.4% having questionable seizures (145). In-hospital seizures developed in 4.1% of patients, a mean 14.5 days from ictus, and in 8% of discharged patients (all of them with pre-hospital and none with in-hospital seizures). This study is interesting because it reports length of stay in ICU, which was longer for patients with seizures (median 15 days vs. 10 for those without seizures, $p=0.06$). Seizures were more frequent in men than in women. There were no other clinical or radiologic predictors of seizures, although there was a trend for higher Fisher scores and Graeb IVH scores to be associated with a seizure. Intracerebral hematomas induced by SAH were not associated with seizures regardless of size. No difference between groups with or without seizures regarding mortality or discharge disposition was found. A limitation of this study is the absence of multivariate analysis.

Other studies, however, have found an association between post-SAH seizures and increased mortality and disability. In a prospective hospital-based study from Lisboa, Portugal, onset seizures (within the first 12 h) occurred in 16/ 253 (6.3%) patients with SAH (137). Rebleeding (OR 8.4, 95%CI 2.8–25.1), severe disability at discharge, or death (4.1, 1.4–11.6) were significantly more frequent in the univariate analysis in patients with seizures. Rebleeding, however, did not happen on the same day as the seizure; so, it was difficult to establish a cause and effect relationship. Only one patient in that series developed epilepsy 1 year later.

A retrospective series from Melbourne, Australia, reported on SAH patients with seizures who were age- and sex-matched with two control patients who did not have seizures (140). Thirty-two out of 412 (7.8%) patients had onset seizures. Late seizures occurred in 17/412 (4.1%) patients. All patients with late seizures, except one, were on antiepileptic treatment. Onset seizures were independently predicted by the total score of blood on the initial CT described by Hijdra et al. (151). Disability 6 weeks after admission was predicted by onset seizures (OR 7.8, 95%CI 1.1–13.9), initial GCS <6 (13.7, 2.2–228) and cisternal blood score (1.1, 1.08–1.18). The proportion of patients with onset seizures declined with increasing age (23% in those <31 years old and 4% in those >50 years). Remarkably, 71% of patients ≤31 years old with fatal outcome had onset seizures, compared to only 4% in those >50 years old. Late seizures were independently predicted by onset seizures (27.4, 2.3–330) and rebleeding (94.4, 4.1–186), but not by aneurysmal etiology, initial GCS, amount of blood on CT, vasospasm, or hydrocephalus.

Several studies have reported on the incidence of seizures in a stroke population, including, but not specifically focusing on, SAH. In a large prospective study from Victoria, Australia, Kilpatrick et al. reported 6/71

(8.5%) patients with post-SAH seizures (9). None of the patients with early seizures had late seizures after discharge (37). In a prospective study from Dijon, France, the authors reported seizures in 4/24 (16.4%) patients with SAH (5). In another prospective study from Birmingham, UK, seizures at the onset of SAH (24 h before or after the development of the neurologic deficit) occurred in 1/9 (11.1%) patients (11). In another large study from Barcelona, Spain, 1/28 (3.6%) patients with first ever SAH developed early seizures (39). Finally, two population-based studies reported on the incidence of seizures after SAH: one from Oxfordshire, UK, where 6/33 (18%) patients had either single or recurrent seizures [2 (6%) patients with seizure at the onset] (8) and one from Manhattan, NY, where 4/50 (8%) patients had early seizures and 1/50 (2%) SE (49). Lastly, in the study from Hong Kong, no seizure was observed in the 20 Chinese patients with SAH (out of 994 patients with stroke included) (40).

The issue of long-term development of epilepsy after SAH has been examined in several studies. In the only population-based study on this topic, patients treated between 1958 and 1968 for aneurysmal SAH were compared to the general population of Iceland (152). Eleven out of 44 (25%) patients with SAH developed epileptic seizures, 70% being the same patients who had a seizure within the first 2 weeks following SAH (relative risk 7, 95%CI 2.3–21.6). In this study, which predates modern neuroimaging, neurosurgical and NICU care, the patients with the more severe neurologic residuals had also a higher risk for developing epilepsy.

In a retrospective study of 177 patients with aneurysmal SAH, from Kuopio, Finland, early seizures occurred in only 2 (1.13%) patients, late seizures in 25 (14%) and recurrent seizures in 21 (12%) (141). Most seizures were partial or secondary generalized, with a mean latency of 8.4 months after the operation. Pre-operative Hunt & Hess grade was a significant factor for epilepsy (33% of grade III–IV patients developed epilepsy) and middle cerebral artery aneurysm location, complications of SAH (hematoma, vasospasm with infarction, shunt-dependent hydrocephalus), or persistent neurological deficits (hemiparesis, dysphasia, visual field defects) for late seizure occurrence.

In another retrospective hospital-based study from Rotterdam, The Netherlands, 35/381 (9%) patients were noted to have one or more epileptic seizures 12 h to 1,761 days (median 18 days) after the initial bleed (138). In this study, patients with SAH were observed in the ICU for 28 days or until death or surgery (usually on day 12), and seizures that occurred within the first 12 h following either the initial or subsequent hemorrhage, surgery, or hyponatremia were excluded from the analysis. In the multivariate analysis, a high cisternal blood score (graded semiquantitatively 0–30 points) and rebleeding were independent predictors of epilepsy (hazards ratios 2.06, 95%CI 1.03–4 and 3.02, 1.23–7.43, respectively) even after exclusion of those patients who received peri-operative antiepileptic treatment.

In a prospective study from Auckland, New Zealand, 24/123 (20%) patients followed 4 to 7 years after SAH had seizures: 2 had a seizure at the onset, 9 within the first 2 postoperative weeks, 10 after discharge within the first year, and 3 after the first year (153). Seizures were related to aneurysmal SAH. Age was an independent predictor of seizures (the younger the patient, the more likely the seizure) and so was the GOS score at 10 weeks (the worse the score, the higher the likelihood to experience a seizure).

More recently, two studies from Taiwan examined the incidence and outcomes of seizures after SAH. The first was a large retrospective study which followed 217 patients with SAH treated with clipping of cerebral aneurysm for an average of 78.7 months (range 24–157 months) (154). Forty-six patients (21.2%) had at least one seizure post SAH. Seventeen patients (7.8%) had onset seizures, 5 (2.3%) had preoperative seizures, 4 (1.8%) had postoperative seizures and no recurrence, 21 (9.7%) had at least one seizure episode after the first week postoperatively, and 15 (6.9%) developed late epilepsy . Unadjusted variables associated with onset seizures were younger age (< 40 years old), loss of consciousness of more than 1 h at ictus, and Fisher Grade ≥3. Onset seizure was also a significant predictor of persistent neurological deficits (Glasgow Outcome Scale Scores 2–4, OR 4.2, 95%CI 1.4–12.3) at follow-up. Factors associated with the development of late epilepsy were loss of consciousness of more than 1 h at ictus and persistent postoperative neurological deficit.

The second retrospective study from Taiwan followed 137 patients with SAH admitted in 2004–2005 for a mean 14 months. Seizures occurred in 21 patients who had SAH, including acute symptomatic seizures in 11.7% and unprovoked seizures (in the absence of precipitating factors) in 3.6%. No patient developed SE. No prophylactic AEDs were administered. Patients with seizures, however, received AEDs which were later discontinued if no recurrence ensued. After a minimum of 1-year follow-up, the mean GOS was not different between patients with seizures and those without. Higher mean World Federation of Neurological Surgeons (WFNS) grade on presentation was predictive of seizure in a Cox's proportional hazards model (155).

The incidence of seizures may also depend on the detection method. Using CEEG monitoring for all patients with SAH admitted to the NICU at Columbia Presbyterian Hospital, NY, who developed unexplained coma or neurological deterioration, Dennis et al. found that 8/26 (31%) were in NCSE, an average of 18 days (range, 5–38 d) after SAH onset. All eight patients were receiving prophylactic AEDs. Four patients were persistently comatose and four demonstrated deterioration to stupor or coma; only one exhibited overt GTC seizures before entering into coma; two patients had subtle eye blinking and facial twitching. A worst Hunt and Hess grade of IV or V, older age, ventricular drainage, and cerebral edema on CT were identified as unadjusted risk factors for NCSE. NCSE was successfully terminated for five patients (63%), but only one experienced clinical improvement, which was transient. All eight patients eventually died after a period of prolonged coma (156).

A subsequent analysis from the same group was published by Claassen et al (157). All patients were initially managed in an NICU and had received a loading dose of fosphenytoin. Antiepileptic treatment was discontinued after discharge from the hospital, unless the patients had a seizure. Thirty-one out of 431 (7%) patients had in-hospital seizures and an additional 9 (2%) had NCSE evaluated with CEEG monitoring. Seizures were more common in patients with prior epilepsy (33%). In those patients without a prior history of epilepsy, seizures were associated with a higher mortality rate at 12 months (65% compared to 23% in patients without seizures, $p < 0.001$) and a higher incidence of epilepsy (17% compared to 7% in patients without seizures, $p = 0.36$). Most (8/9, 89%) patients with NCSE were dead by 12 months. New onset epilepsy, defined as ≥2 unprovoked seizures after discharge, occurred in 7% of patients with SAH (an additional 4% had only one seizure after discharge) and was

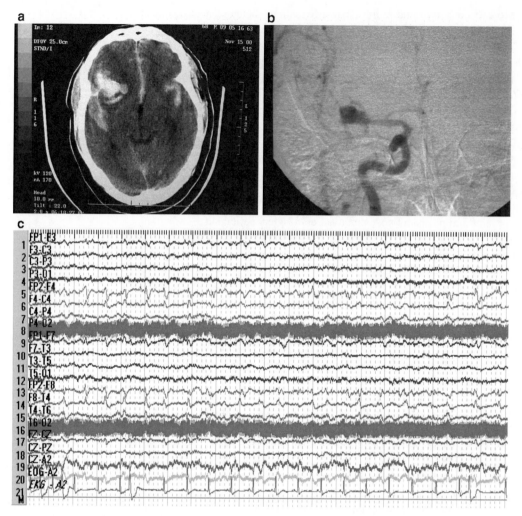

Fig. 3-3. An 68-year-old African American male was admitted with SAH and found to host a right MCA aneurysm, which was clipped on day 1. Six days later, the patient developed two episodes of left upper extremity shaking. (**a**) CT of the head demonstrating the SAH with a right frontotemporal large clot. (**b**) Cerebral angiogram revealing the right MCA aneurysm. (**c**) EEG recording obtained 1 h after the seizures demonstrating semi-periodic sharp waves over the right frontal area and phase reversal over F8 on a theta-delta background. This interictal activity was partially affected by the administration of 2 mg IV lorazepam. The patient was loaded with phenytoin and never experienced another seizure activity during the in-hospital period

independently predicted by the presence of subdural hematoma (SDH) or cerebral infarction at any time point. Most seizures were secondary generalized (76%). Patients who developed epilepsy at 12 months were more severely disabled, had a reduced quality of life, and had increased anxiety, as measured by various scales. Fig. 3-3 presents an ICU patient who developed focal seizures probably due to a combination of contralateral hematoma and surgical treatment of the aneurysm.

3.4.2. Treatment of Seizures after SAH

The main reason to use prophylactic antiepileptic treatment after SAH in the ICU is to decrease the likelihood of aneurysm re-rupture, which usually has catastrophic consequences. Another reason is to avoid changes in the ICP and

CBF, which could further compromise brain tissue perfusion in case of cerebral edema or vasospasm. Drugs that potentially reduce the seizure threshold, such as ε-aminocaproic acid (158), may be another reason of concern. Finally, the prevention of kindling effect of early seizures upon the development of epilepsy may be another reason for prophylaxis, although recent data suggest that antiepileptics may only mask or suppress seizures and not prevent epilepsy from developing. It is unclear whether antiepileptics can really do the job, since there are no prospective, randomized trials.

A chart review study from Detroit, MI, revealed that 4/95 (4%) patients had an in-hospital seizure (145). Three out of four patients were on antiepileptic medications (two on phenytoin and one on carbamazepine) with therapeutic levels at the time of seizure. Seventy-three percent of the total cohort received a loading dose of antiepileptic medication and 99% of those, a maintenance dose with phenytoin. Therapy was initiated within 24 h of hospitalization. The duration of therapy was not related to the occurrence of seizures. Antiepileptic therapy was prescribed at the time of discharge for 41% of patients with pre-hospital seizures and for all patients with in-hospital seizures. None of the patients with in-hospital seizures had recurrent seizures after discharge, but 8/56 (14%) patients, all with pre-hospital seizures, had seizures after discharge (50% of them on treatment, with higher than therapeutic levels when the seizure occurred). The median time to discontinuation of antiepileptic treatment was 40 days (range 12–730). Thus, most seizures in this study would be considered unpreventable since they occurred before admission to the ICU, and those that occurred after admission to the ICU were, in three-fourths, not prevented with antiepileptics. The authors also suggest that, because the incidence of in-hospital seizures (4%) was lower than the incidence of adverse effects from the antiepileptics (7%), long-term treatment may not be beneficial.

In a prospective hospital-based study from Portugal, onset seizures were more common in patients with hemiparesis (OR 5.2, 95%CI 1.6–16.6), Hunt & Hess grade 4 or 5 (5.3, 1.5–18.6), Fisher grade 3 or 4 (4.8, 1.3–17.4), and when an aneurysm was found in angiography (8.6, 1.1–68.1) (137). All patients with onset seizures were prescribed phenytoin 300 mg/day and 4/16 of those had recurrent seizures between 12 and 24 h after SAH onset, but only one of the survivors had recurrent and difficult-to-control seizures at 1 year of follow-up. Based on a 25% early seizure recurrence rate, the authors find it reasonable to prescribe antiepileptic treatment during hospitalization to patients with onset seizures. Long-term prophylactic treatment did not seem successful to the authors, although the numbers in the study were too small to allow confident statements.

In the recently quoted prospective study from Columbia-Presbyterian Hospital, NY, 9% of patients had in-hospital seizures or NCSE after SAH (157). At 12 months, 4% had one seizure and another 7% two or more seizures after discharge. Interestingly, 18% of the patients who developed epilepsy were on antiepileptic treatment at the time their first post-hospital seizure occurred and 94% were treated at 12 months. In the same study, in-hospital seizures after SAH were not identified as predictors of epilepsy. The authors mention the unpublished results of an American Association of Neurological Surgeons survey, where 24% of participants routinely treat patients with SAH with antiepileptics for 3 months, whether in-hospital seizures occur or not, and suggest that prophylactic treatment after discharge is not warranted if there is neither cerebral infarction nor SDH, two independent variables predictive of epilepsy in this study.

This statement was partially triggered by data supporting a negative influence of antiepileptic drugs, such as phenytoin, on motor and cognitive recovery after stroke (111) or head trauma (159).

In a study from Australia, onset seizures post SAH correlated with a large amount of blood on CT of the head and were independent predictors for both late seizures and disability at 6 weeks (140). Based on these results, the authors recommend early antiepileptic treatment in patients with a large amount of blood on CT and long-term treatment for those with onset seizures.

In addition to the direct effect of SAH on seizure incidence, surgical or endovascular treatment of an aneurysm may also contribute to early post-procedure seizures or epilepsy. Earlier studies reported a 10–25% incidence of epilepsy after aneurysm surgery (141). More recent studies report a lower rate of early seizures of 1.9–5% (141, 144, 160–162). The efficacy of antiepileptics in this patient population is also unknown. Postoperative phenytoin administration in mixed craniotomy patients at high risk for seizures was ineffective and associated with toxicity (163, 164), and prophylactic antiepileptic administration after supratentorial craniotomy is not routinely recommended (165).

A retrospective study of 177 patients surgically treated for ruptured aneurysms, was reported from Kuopio, Finland (141). All patients were started on phenytoin treatment during surgery and maintained for 2–3 months or longer (if they developed seizures). The authors conclude that low preoperative grade patients have a very low risk for epilepsy and that treatment with phenytoin can be discontinued by 3 months after the operation, if no high risk factors are present, such as high pre-operative Hunt & Hess grade, middle cerebral artery aneurysm location, complications of SAH (hematoma, vasospasm with infarction, shunt-dependent hydrocephalus) or persistent neurological deficits (hemiparesis, dysphasia, visual field defects).

Sheib et al. did not find any need for prophylactic phenytoin in a prospective study of 100 consecutive patients who survived aneurysm surgery and were followed for 4 years (161). In this series only, 3% of patients developed post-operative epilepsy and there was no difference in seizure incidence between the groups with or without antiepileptic prophylaxis.

Bidzinski et al. reported a 7% risk for two or more seizures (epilepsy) in a prospective study of 121 patients operated for cerebral aneurysms (only 3 with unruptured aneurysms) and followed for 12 months after discharge (143). Another three patients had a single seizure during the observation period. No prophylactic perioperative antiepileptic treatment was administered in this series, unless epilepsy developed. Another eight patients had seizures during the perioperative period, but only one developed epilepsy during the follow-up period. None of these patients was treated with antiepileptic medications. Although a total of 18/121 (15%) patients had seizures during the perioperative or follow-up period, the authors concluded that prophylactic antiepileptic treatment is not justified after aneurysmal surgery.

A large retrospective study of perioperative short-term antiepileptic prophylaxis was conducted at Columbia Presbyterian Hospital in NY, NY (162). Patients at high risk for seizures (previous history of epilepsy, perioperative hematomas or infarction, concomitant AVMs) were excluded from the analysis. All patients with SAH were admitted to the NICU. and those with unruptured aneurysms to the neurosurgical floor. All were loaded with antiepileptics and were maintained on a daily dose. Medications were then stopped within 7 days of surgery, on average after 3.1 days (or after 5.3 days of average total treatment duration). Postoperative seizures occurred in 5.4% of patients (4.5% for those with ruptured and 6.9% for those with unruptured aneurysms). Early postoperative seizures (within 14 days from surgery) occurred in 1.9% of patients (1.5% of ruptured and 2.6% of unruptured aneurysms) and late postoperative seizures in 3.5% (3% of ruptured and 4.4% of unruptured aneurysms). Two-thirds of early postoperative seizures occurred in patients with significant intracranial complications, such as hematomas or infarcts. Only 2/6 patients had therapeutic antiepileptic levels when the early seizures occurred, but all were reloaded and maintained on treatment for 1 year without any further seizures. Late seizures developed in 8/11 patients within 3 months of surgery and were easily controlled with antiepileptic medications. In the multivariate analysis there was no association between total or postoperative duration of treatment and risk of early or late seizures. The authors concluded that early postoperative seizures should always be evaluated for ongoing intracranial pathology. They also recommend loading the patients the day before surgery, but not using antiepileptics after surgery for more than seven days if the patients are at low perioperative risk for seizures.

This "short" prophylactic treatment with AEDs may be important in the context of few new studies challenging the safety of older-generation drugs in patients with SAH. A recent study from Columbia Presbyterian hospital in NY studied 527 SAH patients and calculated a "phenytoin burden" for each by multiplying the average serum level of phenytoin by the time in days between the first and last measurements, up to a maximum of 14 days from ictus. Phenytoin burden was associated with poor functional outcome at 14 days (OR, 1.5 per quartile, 95%CI, 1.3–1.8), but not at 3 months. This effect remained significant after correction for admission GCS, fever, stroke, age, NIHSS $\geq$10, hydrocephalus, clinical vasospasm, and aneurysm rebleeding. Higher quartiles of phenytoin burden were associated with worse telephone interview for cognitive status scores at hospital discharge and at 3 months. The authors warned that burden of exposure to phenytoin may predict poor neurologic and cognitive outcome after SAH (166).

More recently, Rosengart et al. examined data collected in 3552 patients with SAH who were entered into four prospective, randomized, double-blind, placebo-controlled international trials conducted between 1991 and 1997 (167). In these older studies, 90% of patients had the aneurysms treated surgically. AEDs were used in 65.1% of patients (53% phenytoin, 19% Phenobarbital and 2% carbamazepine) and the prescribing pattern was mainly dependent on the treating physicians: the prevalence of AED use varied dramatically across study country and center. Australia, Canada, Italy and the US prescribed AEDs in >50% of cases. After adjustment, patients treated with AEDs had ORs of 1.56 (95%CI 1.16–2.10) for worse outcome at 3 months based on the GOS. Unfortunately, the adjustment covariates for outcome, in addition to AED use, included only study center, WFNS grade, age, and admission systolic BP only, but no incidence of seizures or study drug treatment arm, which reflects the limitations of compiling data from various studies. Treatment with AEDs also conferred higher in-hospital complications than no treatment: 1.87 (95%CI 1.43–2.44) for cerebral vasospasm, 1.61 (95%CI 1.25–2.06) for neurological deterioration, 1.33 (95%CI 1.01–1.74) for cerebral infarction, and 1.36 (95%CI 1.03–1.80) for elevated temperature during hospitalization.

Echoing these three aforementioned studies, Chumnanvej et al. retrospectively compared two regimens of prophylactic AEDs after SAH: long term (from admission to discharge) and short term (for only 3 days post admission) (168). More than 95% of patients had the aneurysm secured within 3 days from admission, approximately 80% by clipping. The 3-day phenytoin regimen produced a statistically significant reduction in the rate of phenytoin complications (hypersensitivity reactions). Additionally, several patients were switched from phenytoin to another AED for, presumably, drug fever. On the other hand, the percentage of patients who had seizures, early on or later, was not different between the two regimens. The authors concluded that a 3-day regimen of phenytoin prophylaxis is adequate to prevent seizures in SAH patients.

Lastly, an argument against phenytoin use is that it may interfere with the metabolism of commonly used medications after SAH. One of them is nimodipine, a calcium channel antagonist administered for 21 days after SAH, which has been found to improve outcomes. This drug is hepatically metabolized by the P450 3A4 cytochrome, which can be induced by phenytoin (and hence reduce the bioavailability of nimodipine, with unknown consequences) (169). An alternative AED, such as sodium valproate (169), could be administered instead in a parenteral formulation in the ICU. The same may be true for levetiracetam, a renally excreted, last-generation AED, which in animal models of SAH has been shown to improve functional outcomes and reduce vasospasm (170).

One would expect aneurysms treated with endovascular approaches to have a lower risk for seizures for lack of additional injury from a craniotomy. A large study conducted in Oxford, England, examined the risk for seizures after endovascular treatment of cerebral aneurysms (171). The authors prospectively followed 243 patients treated with Gugliemi Detachable Coils (GDC) for up to 7.7 years. Only 3 patients had epilepsy and were already on antiepileptic regimen when they developed SAH and 33 other patients (12%) received prophylactic treatment after they bled. Ictal seizures (within 24 h from ictus) occurred in 26/243 (11%) patients and were independently predicted by loss of consciousness, MCA location of the aneurysm, and antiepileptic treatment. However, no distinction was made between loss of consciousness from SAH and seizure causing loss of consciousness. Moreover, antiepileptic treatment might have been prescribed because an individual patient experienced an ictal seizure. Seven out of 233 (3%) patients developed late seizures, but 3 already had epilepsy and only 4 (1.7%) had de novo seizures. None of the patients with late seizures presented during the peri-procedural period (i.e., within 30 days) and none with ictal seizures experienced late seizures. Only half of them (0.85%) had recurrent seizures and required long-term antiepileptic treatment. Late seizures were independently predicted by a history of epilepsy before SAH, cerebrospinal fluid (CSF) shunting or drainage procedure and antiepileptic medications. This latter finding could probably be explained by the fact that patients who experienced ictal seizures were covered with antiepileptic medications before referral. The authors concluded that there is no need for peri-procedural seizure prophylaxis with antiepileptics and that the low incidence of de novo late seizures is also a reason for not prophylactically using long-term treatment.

The large International Subarachnoid Aneurysm Trial (ISAT) provided important data regarding incidence of seizures after coiling or clipping.

Table 3-5. Treatment with AntiEpileptic Medications After SAH.

1. SAH and pre-existing seizures: continue or restart antiepileptic regimen, keep therapeutic levels.

2. SAH and no seizures:

   Low risk patients: Rx until aneurysm is secured

   High-risk patients (high H&H grade, high Fisher grade, aneurysm found, hemiparesis): Rx during hospitalization. Long-term Rx if SDH (before or after surgery) or infarct.

   Post craniotomy-clipping: Rx for 7 days. Rx for at least 1–2 years (seizure-free interval) if high H&H grade, MCA aneurysm, hematoma, infarct, shunt-dependent hydrocephalus or persistent neurological deficits. Assess with EEG before discontinuation?

   Post GDC: No Rx. Consider Rx for at least 1–2 years (seizure-free interval) if patients were on antiepileptic medications before or have shunt-dependent hydrocephalus. Assess with EEG before discontinuation?

3. SAH and onset or early seizures:

   Rx during hospitalization.

   Consider long-term Rx after discharge, for at least 1–2 years (seizure-free interval), if large amount of blood on CT, infarct, hematoma, SDH or hemiparesis. Assess with EEG before discontinuation?

   Post-craniotomy clipping: Rx during hospitalization. Rx for at least 1–2 years (seizure-free interval) if high H&H grade, MCA aneurysm, hematoma, infarct, shunt-dependent hydrocephalus or persistent neurological deficits. Assess with EEG before discontinuation?

   Post GDC: Rx during hospitalization. Consider Rx for at least 1–2 years (seizure-free interval) if patients were on antiepileptic medications before or have shunt-dependent hydrocephalus. Assess with EEG before discontinuation?

In this randomized, multicenter trial comparing these two treatment options in patients who were suitable for either treatment, 2143 patients were randomly assigned to neurosurgical clipping ($n = 1070$) or endovascular coiling ($n = 1073$) arm. The risk for seizures was included in the secondary outcomes. The mean follow-up was 4 years at the time the study was published. There was a highly significant reduction of seizures in the endovascular compared to the surgical group: at 1 year after the SAH, 46 seizures were recorded in the endovascular group and 88 in the surgical group. After the first year, another 14 and 24 seizures were recorded, respectively. Overall, the endovascular arm exhibited relative risk for seizures of 0.52, 0.37–0.74 compared to the neurosurgical arm of treatment (172). In summary, a tentative algorithm for treating seizures after SAH is presented in Table 3-5.

3.5. Arteriovenous Malformations

3.5.1. Clinical Studies

AVM are abnormal fistulae between arteries and veins in the brain without an intervening capillary bed. They occur in 0.1% of the population and typically present before the age of 40, equally among men and women (173). Although their etiology is unknown, they are thought to arise from developmental derangements of cerebral vessels and thus have to be differentiated from arteriovenous fistulae caused by trauma or occlusion of branch arteries or venous sinuses. The most common presentation is intracranial hemorrhage (30–82%), which is also the most common reason for ICU admission, other than AVM treatment (surgical, endovascular, or multidisciplinary) or seizures (multiple or in succession). Seizures are the initial symptoms in 16–53% of AVM cases. Most seizures are simple partial or partial complex. Although focal seizure onset may be an indicator of the location of the lesion, in upto 62% seizures can be GTC. Headache, learning disabilities, and focal neurologic deficits unrelated to hemorrhage are less common (174–181).

Seizures that occur in the ICU in a patient with an AVM are either related to the AVM itself (with or without a hemorrhage) or may develop as a complication following surgical, endovascular, or radiosurgical treatment of the AVM. Factors associated with the development of pre-treatment seizures were recently reported in a large series of AVMs from the Massachussets General Hospital. Seizures were statistically associated with male sex, age of less than 65 years, AVM size of more than 3 cm, and temporal lobe AVM location. Posterior fossa and deep locations were statistically associated with the absence of seizures (182). Mechanisms thought to play a role in the pathogenesis of epilepsy in patients with AVMs include secondary epileptogenesis in the ipsilateral temporal cortex, gliosis from previous hemorrhage and hemosiderin deposition into the cortex, focal cerebral ischemia from a steal syndrome, and neurochemical changes on or around the lesion (183–185).

A more recent prospective study from Columbia Presbyterian Hospital in New York, which reported data from the time of diagnosis to the time of treatment, showed that 183/622 (29%) of patients with AVMs presented with seizures unrelated to hemorrhage. Although this important study reported an annual hemorrhage rate of 1.3% for unruptured and 5.9% for ruptured AVMs, seizure presentation was not included in the analysis of risks for hemorrhage (186).

Because of a higher incidence of re-hemorrhage after the initial one (18% compared to 2% for those without hemorrhage, (177)), aggressive treatment of AVMs is advocated to avoid hemorrhage rather than to control seizures (187). This has also led to limited data regarding the natural history of seizures in these patients. In 138 conservatively managed patients with AVMs, Crawford et al. found a 19% risk of seizures at 20 years using a life survival analysis, compared to 57% in 96 patients treated surgically (176). Older studies showed poor control of seizures after surgical AVM removal, development of new seizures (188, 189) or no difference (178).

More recent studies, however, indicate a lower risk of postoperative seizures, which may depend on the history of seizures before the surgical intervention: <40% in patients with pre-operative seizures and <10% in those without such history (187, 190, 191). Factors that increase the incidence of postoperative seizures in AVM patients include age <30 years at seizure onset, preoperative seizure duration >12 months, AVM size >3 cm, location in the medial temporal or peri-Rolandic cortex, previous hemorrhage, or hemosiderin deposition (184, 185, 187, 190). The effect of intracerebral hematomas on the incidence of poststroke seizures was examined in a prospective ICU study using CEEG monitoring (46). Seizures occurred in 18/63 (28%) of patients with ICH and 3/46 (6%) patients with ischemic stroke (ORs 5.7, 95%CI 1.4–26.5, $p < 0.004$). In patients with ICH, there was a trend toward increased AVM representation in the seizures subgroup ($p = 0.07$).

3.5.2. Treatment of AVM-Related Seizures

Although there is a broad consensus to treat AVM-related epilepsy with antiepileptic medications (usually with a good response), many would also argue for a prophylactic approach. More controversial is the need, timing, and duration of antiepileptic treatment after surgery, embolization, or radiotherapy, and there are no studies from which solid recommendations may be drawn (174). Overall, there are data supporting a better prognosis with early seizures (within 30 days post ICH or surgery) (178, 187), but most studies do not report details about the antiepileptic treatment used.

Piepgras et al. reported a series of 280 patients with surgically treated AVMs, and mean follow-up of 7.5 years. Sixteen out of 163 patients (10%) without preoperative seizures had perioperative seizures and 6/117 patients (5%) with preoperative seizures had worsening of their seizures during hospitalization. At the last follow-up, 87.5% and 83%, respectively, of patients with early seizures were noted to be seizure free (187).

In a large, prospective study from Australia, 114 postoperative patients with AVMs were followed for a mean of 48 months (22 months–8.5 years) (192). Preoperative seizures were present in 53 patients (46%). Only 15 (13%) had seizures associated with an acute and newly diagnosed ICH. Neither AVM size nor AVM localization to temporal cortex or other eloquent brain areas was related to pre- or postoperative seizures. A total of 24 patients (21%) had post-operative seizures, including 14 of 53 (26%) of those with pre-operative and 10 of 61 (16%) of those without preoperative seizures. Preoperative seizures were not associated with the development of postoperative seizures. All patients were put on antiepileptic medications (those patients with preoperative seizures were maintained on their previous regimen) for at least 12 months post resection. The majority of postoperative seizures in those 24 patients occurred during the first 12 months while on antiepileptic treatment. In only 6/24 patients (25%) did the post-operative seizures appear after the first 12 months. In four of these patients, the seizures developed after withdrawal of the antiepileptic regimen. Poor neurologic outcome at 12 months was an independent predictor of postoperative seizures (OR, 95%CI 1.5, 1.01–2.3). Fig. 3-4 presents a patient who continued to have complex partial seizures even after resection of a frontal cavernous angioma.

The effect of radiosurgery on seizures has also been studied. Because of the delayed effect of this treatment, patients can be encountered in the ICU in the immediate posttreatment period or later, if admitted because of a seizure. A small risk for seizures as a complication of radiosurgery was reported in a large international study (10/1255 (0.8%) of patients with new-onset seizures and 12/1255 (1%) of patients with seizures in addition to other symptoms) (193). It seems likely that the time of AVM obliteration does not correlate well with seizure control. In fact, seizures can be controlled faster, before confirmation of complete AVM obliteration (194–196). The predominant theory suggests an independent effect of irradiation on epileptogenesis of cerebral tissue surrounding the AVM (due to an effect on AVM thrombosis and reduction of a steal phenomenon from the surrounding ischemic areas) (193, 195). In a study from Finland, 129 patients with inoperable cerebral AVMs were treated by stereotactic proton beam irradiation (linear accelerator, LINAC) (195). Symptomatic epilepsy was present in 29 patients (22.5%) and was markedly relieved by radiosurgery leading to cessation of the seizures in 16 (55.2%)

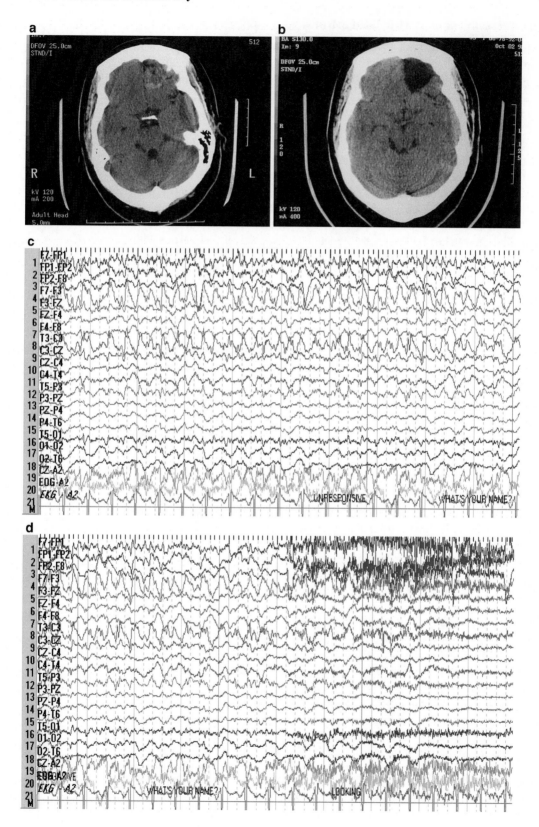

patients, with a mean follow-up period 4.5 years. In another retrospective study, Kurita et al. reported the results of gamma knife radiosurgery in 35 patients with unruptured epileptogenic AVMs (followed for a mean of 43 months) and in another 22 patients with non-epileptogenic AVMs (followed for a mean of 30 months). He found an association between the number and duration of pre-treatment seizures and posttreatment seizure outcome: 92% of patients with ≤5 seizures before radiosurgery were seizure-free after the treatment (vs 50% with >5 seizures, OR 2.8, 95%CI 0.09–0.7). Also 94% of patients with seizures for ≤ 6 months before radiosurgery were seizure free after treatment (vs. 64% with >6 months of seizures, 2.2, 0.046–0.58)(196).

The largest series reporting seizure control after gamma knife radiosurgery also comes from Japan (194). Epilepsy presented in 79/462 (17.1%) patients. Fifty-eight cases presented with seizures as the initial symptoms (group A) and the other 21 cases mostly had seizures following intracranial haemorrhage (group B). Seizures decreased in most of the cases (mean follow-up 24 months) in relation to nidus obliteration: good seizure control was achieved in 94.7% of completely obliterated and 77.1% of incompletely obliterated AVMs. Initial seizures were also more easily controlled than subsequent or secondary ones: seizures either decreased or disappeared in 91.6% of group A and 62.5% of group B patients. The overall results of this study indicated that seizures improved in 85.5%, were unchanged in 11.6%, and deteriorated in 2.9% of patients.

Two recent studies followed patients with seizures due to AVMs and treated with radiosurgery. In the first study from the Mayo Clinic in Rochester, MN, 70/285 (24.6%) of patients had seizures before the treatment. The authors report on 65 patients with seizures before the gamma knife treatment, who were followed for a median 48 months (range 12–144). Using the Engel Seizure Frequency Scoring System (range: 0=seizure-free, no antiepileptics to 12=status epilepticus), 26 patients (51%) were seizure-free and overall 40 patients (78%) had an excellent outcome (nondisabling simple partial seizures only) at 3-year follow-up after radiosurgery. Factors associated with seizure-free or excellent outcomes included a low seizure frequency score (<4) before radiosurgery and AVM of smaller size and diameter. Interestingly, although all patients were on antiepileptic drugs before radiosurgery, only four of them were off drugs 3 years after the treatment and the remainder had no significant change in their regimen. Twenty-three patients had intractable partial epilepsy prior to treatment. Twelve (52%) of 23 and 11 of 18 (61%) patients with medically intractable partial epilepsy had excellent outcomes at years 1 and 3, respectively (197).

The most recent study regarding gamma knife treatment comes out of Seoul, South Korea. Lim et al. followed 246 patients, 60 of which (24%) had seizures before the treatment. The authors however, focused on 43 of these patients with seizures as the initial symptom (i.e., without hemorrhage) and followed

---

Fig. 3-4. An 32-year-old African American female with CPS seizures since age 17. (**a**) CT of the head before and (**b**) CT of the head after resection of a left frontal cavernous angioma. (**c**) EEG 3 months after the resection showing an electrographic seizure over the left frontotemporal area. The patient had staring episodes and mouth automatisms during the event, while on therapeutic carbamazepine (**d**). The same seizure activity later stopping abruptly (right side of the epoque)

them for a median 46 months (range 8 months to 12 years). The type of seizures was general tonic-clonic in 28, focal motor or sensory in 7, and partial complex in 8. During follow-up after radiosurgical treatment, 23/43 (53.5%) were seizure-free (20 patients still on antiepileptic drugs, which they were slowly tapering after being 2 years seizure-free for 2 years), 10 (23.3%) had significant improvement, 8 (18.6%) were unchanged, and 2 (4.6%) patients had aggravated seizures. Twenty-six patients had angiographic follow-up for over 2 years. Significantly more patients with angiographic obliteration were seizure-free: 11/13 (84.6%) patients with complete obliteration were seizure-free versus only 4/13 (36.3%) with partial obliteration. Fifteen patients had experienced intractable seizure before radiosurgery, despite antiepileptic drugs. After radiosurgery, seizures disappeared in eight (53%) patients. Seizure frequently decreased in another five (33%) and two patients (14%) were unchanged but none was aggravated. Five (71%) of seven patients with complete obliteration, and two (40%) of five patients with partial obliteration were seizure-free (181).

It is evident from the above studies that no details of antiepileptic treatment are provided, and so it is difficult for the intensivist to draw safe conclusions regarding when and how long to cover the patients.

There are not many data about embolization, because it is usually considered an adjunctive treatment for AVMs. In an older study reporting data from the 1980s, 33/49 patients received only embolization and the rest additional surgery or radiosurgery (198). Four patients developed early focal seizures hours after treatment, which were easily controlled. Long-term follow-up revealed that 9/21 (43%) patients, who presented with seizures, experienced either a significant reduction in the frequency of their attacks or an easier control of the seizures with medications.

Although most previous reports were about single modality treatments, now there are emerging data on multimodality approaches. The intensivist may encounter patients at various stages of treatment and should be aware of factors that may alter the risk for seizures or specific antiepileptic treatment needs. However, only scant data are available. A study from Stanford, CA, reported on 33 patients who underwent radiosurgery followed by microsurgical resection 1–11 years later. Embolization was also offered to 25 patients prior to surgery. Out of nine patients who already had seizures at the time the AVM was diagnosed, three improved, and four became seizure-free, and three developed new onset seizures after the combination of treatments (199).

In the aforementioned retrospective study from the Massachusetts General Hospital, a multidisciplinary neurovascular team treated 424 patients with cerebral AVMs with surgical resection, radiosurgery, or embolization, either alone or in combination (182). One hundred and forty-one patients (33%) experienced seizures before treatment. Follow-up data were available in 110 (78%) of these patients for a mean period of 2.9 years after treatment. Using the Engel Seizure Outcome Scale, there were 73 (66%) Class I (free of disabling seizures), 11 (10%) Class II (rare disabling seizures), 1 (0.9%) Class III (worthwhile improvement), and 22 (20%) Class IV (no worthwhile improvement) outcomes. Sixteen (5.7%) patients experienced new-onset seizures after treatment. A limited seizure history (<5 seizures before treatment), association of seizures with intracranial hemorrhage, GTC seizure type, deep and posterior fossa AVM locations, surgical resection, and complete AVM obliteration were

Table 3-6. Treatment with AntiEpileptic Medications in Case of an AVM.

1. AVM and pre-existing seizures – no AVM treatment:

   Treat indefinitely or according to post-AVM Rx.

2. AVM and no seizures:

   Observe

   Consider Rx if patient is male, < 65 years old, has > 3 cm AVM or an AVM in the temporal lobe.

3. AVM and surgical Rx:

   Treat independently of presence of preoperative seizures for at least 2 years (seizure-free interval) or indefinitely if poor neurologic outcome at 12 months

4. AVM and radiosurgery:

   Treat for 1–2 weeks, if no history of seizures

   If AVM presented with seizures, treat up to 2 years (seizure-free interval) if seizures were the initial symptom, or up to 4 years (seizure-free interval) if seizures were secondary symptoms (e.g., after ICH). Assess with EEG before discontinuation?

   Treat indefinitely if patient had pre-radiosurgery Rx > 5 seizures or the duration of seizures was > 6 months.

5. AVM and embolization:

   Treat for 1–2 weeks if no pre-existing seizures

   Continue Rx if pre-existing seizures or post-procedural seizures for at least 1–2 years (seizure-free interval). Assess with EEG before discontinuation?

6. AVM and multi-modality Rx:

   Treat for 1–2 weeks if no pre-existing seizures

   If pre-existing seizures, continue antiepileptic Rx for 1 year (seizure-free interval) if low risk factors for seizures are present: patient had < 5 seizures before multimodality Rx, seizures were associated with ICH, they were generalized tonic-clonic type, the AVM was in the posterior fossa, it was surgically resected, or there was complete AVM obliteration. Assess with EEG before discontinuation? Continue antiepileptic Rx for at least 2 years (seizure-free interval), if low risk for seizures factors are not present. Assess with EEG before discontinuation?

statistically associated with Class I outcomes. In the whole cohort, surgery resulted in seizure elimination in 81%, radiosurgery in 43%, and embolization in 50% of patients treated. When only completely obliterated AVMs were considered, there were no statistically significant differences between surgery, radiosurgery, and embolization. Table 3-6 represents a suggested algorithm for the treatment of AVM-related seizures.

3.6. Reperfusion–Hyperperfusion Syndrome

First described by Sundt et al. (200), the reperfusion syndrome is an uncommon constellation of symptoms usually encountered following carotid endarterectomy [0.4–2% of cases (201, 202)] or other revascularization procedures, such as percutaneous transluminal angioplasty (PTA) (203, 204), extracranial–intracranial arterial bypass (205), or innominate endarterectomy (206). It comprises transient focal seizures (always emanating from the vascular territory ipsilateral to the treated artery), ipsilateral headache with atypical migrainous features, and intracerebral hemorrhage or brain edema, usually a few days to up to 3 weeks after revascularization (207). The syndrome should not be related to thromboembolism, and no new infarct should be demonstrated on neuroimaging (208). Occasionally, SE ensues (65). Severe ICA stenosis with preoperative internal carotid artery/common carotid artery (ICA/CCA) pressure ratio <0.7 leads to significant increase of CBF in both hemispheres after CEA, more pronounced ipsilaterally (209). In many centers, these patients are monitored in the ICU for the first few postoperative days (210).

Seizures are thought to result from cerebral embolization from the operative site [although some authors require a stricter definition of the syndrome and exclude thromboembolism (208)], hemorrhage secondary to the lack of autoregulation, or simply the reperfusion syndrome effect. If they occur during or early after surgery, they are more likely caused by intraoperative or immediate postoperative embolization or inadequate perfusion during clamping of the carotid. The predisposing role of preoperative strokes towards seizures in symptomatic patients is unclear. If seizures occur late during the postoperative course, especially when there is severe carotid stenosis and if preceded by headache, they are most likely caused by the hyperperfusion syndrome (207). The syndrome is thought to be due to impaired cerebral autoregulation, as a result of chronic cerebral hypoperfusion distal to high-grade carotid stenosis (211). The intracranial distal arterioles are maximally and chronically dilated and do not respond to the flush of blood by vasoconstriction after correction of the stenosis. Carotid baroreceptor insensitivity and the secondary hypertensive response after CEA are additional factors (203), as most patients have uncontrolled hypertensive blood pressure levels both before and after surgery (207). The role played by volatile anesthetics that produce cerebral vasodilation, such as isoflurane (202), various vasoactive peptides secreted from perivascular sensory nerves (212), and oxidants that develop before (213) or inflammatory cytokines (and the no-reflow phenomenon) after (213) revascularization is still unclear. Pathological findings in the hyperperfusion syndrome resemble the findings in hypertensive encephalopathy and the reperfusion syndrome after cerebral AVM resection (207).

Sundt et al. reported a 11/1,145 (0.9%) incidence of seizures after CEA (200). A total of 20 (1.8%) patients in their series displayed the characteristic constellation of symptoms, which was given the name "hyperperfusion syndrome." Seizures presented between the fifth and seventh postoperative day. Five patients had a history of preoperative strokes and two developed postoperative ICH. Riegel et al. reported the lowest incidence of seizures so far in their large series from the Mayo Clinic (10/2,439, 0.4%), which included some patients from Sundt's series (214). Four patients had a history of preoperative strokes, and seven had a Xenon CBF study during surgery, which demonstrated an increase in CBF ipsilaterally to the CEA. Nine of 10 patients had initial focal onset of seizures, which then generalized. Although all patients had PLEDs on EEG, all had complete resolution of their neurologic deficits. The authors suggested that patients with preoperative hypertension and high-grade bilateral carotid stenoses were at the greatest risk for developing seizures post CEA. They recommended caution with anticoagulant or antiplatelet agents in these patients and prompt treatment of blood pressure and seizures.

Kieburtz et al. described 8 patients with focal and generalized seizures following 650 CEAs (1.2%) (215). Six patients had pre-CEA TIAs, while two were asymptomatic. Seizures occurred with a mean of 7.6 (range 6–13) days after CEA. All patients initially had focal motor seizures contralateral to the side of the CEA, but six patients had seizures that became generalized.

All patients had post-ictal hemiparesis. Lorazepam given initially and phenytoin/phenobarbital sodium for maintenance resulted in control of the seizures. CT showed old strokes in two patients (one ipsilateral to the CEA and the other contralaterally), diffuse cerebral edema ipsilateral to the CEA in another two, ICH in one, and no abnormalities in three. Five patients without CT evidence of stroke were normal at follow-up and had no further seizures. The other three patients had mild deficits. One developed a chronic seizure disorder.

Reversible cerebral edema was reported in 5/184 (2.7%) patients with severe carotid stenosis or occlusion who underwent CEA or bypass (207). Headache, focal neurologic deficits, and white matter edema on CT developed after discharge from the hospital. Focal seizures occurred in four and generalized seizures in three of these patients, and the EEG showed PLEDs in two and ipsilateral slowing in another two of them. The authors suggested that hyperperfusion syndrome has been underreported and that many cases of cerebral edema, especially in older series, were misinterpreted as cerebral infarction.

In a large prospective study from the UK, Naylor et al. identified 8/949 (0.8%) patients who developed seizures after CEA (216). Seven were treated hypertensives but four patients had labile blood pressure (BP) preoperatively. Five had severe bilateral carotid disease and four had vertebral/subclavian stenoses. Five required treatment for postoperative hypertension. Two suffered seizures <36 h of CEA, the remainder at 3–8 days. All eight had significantly elevated blood pressure at onset of seizures. CT scanning/autopsy showed normal scans in three patients, white matter edema in four, and petechial or diffuse ICH in two . Seven developed a post-ictal neurological deficit (stroke in five, TIA in two). In this case series, post-CEA seizure was associated with adverse outcomes (one patient died, one had a disabling stroke, and four had non-fatal strokes). Interestingly, the authors report that clinicians treating these patients in acute medical units were generally unaware of the "post-CEA hyperperfusion syndrome" and tended to treat the hypertension less aggressively.

In a retrospective study of CEAs from Brooklyn, NY, 9/404 (2%) patients developed hyperperfusion syndrome and 3 of them seizures (201). One of these patients had intraoperative mean ICA volume flow by carotid artery duplex scanning of 178 ml/min, which during seizures 1 week postoperatively increased to 632 ml/min and subsequently decreased to 141 ml/min after symptoms subsided. This study suggested that contralateral CEA within 3 months from the index CEA may be a predictive factor for hyperperfusion syndrome.

In a retrospective study from India, 6/87 (7%) patients developed hyperperfusion syndrome after stenting (47 cases) or CEA (40 cases) (210). Two patients were the presenting symptom in 2 patients and occurred 5 h and 1 day after the intervention. Both patients had either high-degree stenosis in one side or occlusion and occlusion on the opposite side. Although only the second patient had an ICH, they both died.

In another large retrospective study from Los Angeles, CA, 6/1602 (0.4%) developed hyperperfusion syndrome, and only one developed seizures 8 days after the surgery (202). This patient was treated for 3 months with phenytoin, without recurrence.

Percutaneous transluminal angioplasty (PTA) and stenting is gaining acceptance as a safe alternative to CEA in some patient subgroups. Two patients who developed seizures secondary to hyperperfusion syndrome have also been reported by Schoser et al. 16 h and 3 days after PTA and stenting of the ICA (203, 204). Although the management of seizures is not discussed in the article, marked increase of cerebral blood flow velocity (CBFV) was demonstrated by transcranial Doppler (TCD). Two patients reported by Ho et al. with high-grade bilateral ICA stenoses and pre-existing hypertension developed recurrent seizures with focal onset and secondary generalization 7 h and 14 days, respectively, after successful endovascular treatment (204). Seizures were controlled by intravenous diazepam and phenytoin, and by lowering the blood pressure during the events. CT of the head did not reveal new infarcts, and follow-up angiograms showed widely patent ICAs. In a retrospective study from Canada, 129 patients underwent reperfusion procedures (208). Hyperperfusion syndrome developed in 4/129 (3.1%) patients with CEA and 3/44 (6.8%) patients with ICA stenting. Two patients developed delayed seizures. In a large retrospective study from the Cleveland Clinic, OH, 5/450 (1.1%) patients post carotid artery stenting developed hyperprfusion syndrome within a median of 10 h (range 6 h to 4 days) (217). One patient developed a seizure on the fifth postoperative day. The authors concluded that similar to patients after CEA, patients after ICA stenting may be at higher risk for hyperperfusion syndrome, if they have a critical ICA stenosis of ≥90%, severe contralateral ICA disease, poor collateral flow, hypertension, and recent stroke or ischemia.

TCD can be used in the ICU to evaluate patients with a suspicion of hyperperfusion syndrome. Thirty-six high-grade stenosis patients (> 90% stenosis of ICA) were evaluated with TCD before and after IV infusion of 1 g acetazolamide (218). Thirty-three patients showed increased MCA CBFVs after the challenge (preserved reserve capacity) and three decreased (loss of reserve capacity). After CEA, those three patients developed unilateral headache and an increase of mean MCA CBFVs, while the other 33 patients showed little difference. None of these patients developed seizures, suggesting a mild hyperperfusion syndrome.

In a landmark paper, Jorgensen and Schroeder evaluated 95 patients with TCD before and after symptomatic CEA (211). Hyperperfusion syndrome developed in 18/95 (19%) and two separate groups were identified: in nine patients symptoms lasted for a mean of 3 h and in the other nine for a mean of 12 days. The longer the duration of the symptoms of hyperperfusion, the more likely the preoperative finding of increased mean blood pressure gradient across the stenosis, and the lower the CO_2 reactivity index on both sides of the brain and the absence of decrease of the pulsatility index during CO_2 inhalation. Following surgery in patients with symptoms of hyperperfusion, MCA CBFVs were shown to decrease significantly with labetalol from a mean high of 104 cm/sec to 68 cm/sec on the side of CEA, a reaction not seen on the contralateral side. This asymmetric response diminished over time as the episodes of hyperperfusion subsided. At discharge, cerebral CO_2 reactivity improved bilaterally in these patients, a change not seen in patients without the hyperperfusion syndrome. Interestingly, 2/9 (22%) patients with longer lasting hyperperfusion symptoms developed seizures on the fifth–sixth postoperative day. MCA CBFVs on the side of the CEA in these two patients during seizures were 104 and 120 cm/s with MAP 130 and 120 mmHg, respectively. After labetalol was administered, mean arterial pressure (MAP) dropped to 100 and 67 mmHg and CBFVs to 38 and 60 cm/s, respectively, and the seizures stopped.

Table 3-7. Treatment with AntiEpileptic Medications After Revascularization.

1. Revascularization and pre-existing seizures: Continue Rx.
2. Revascularization and immediate or early (< day 5) seizure:

   Neuroimaging to rule out ICH or artery to artery embolization

   Treat seizures as after stroke
3. Revascularization and late seizure (fifth day–3d week), with focal onset contralateral to procedure side:

   Neuroimaging to rule out ICH

   If pre-existing high-grade stenosis and history of severe hypertension plus headache now: Treat hyperperfusion syndrome with lorazepam and phenytoin or phenobarbital or valproic acid IV and hypertension with IV labetalol or enalaprilat or clonidine to reduce SBP to a level where CBFVs by TCD are symmetrical. Continue Rx for at least 3 weeks and discontinue if neuroimaging negative

In both patients, MCA CBFVs contralateral to the CEA remained unchanged, implying a defective cerebral autoregulation only present on the side ipsilateral to the CEA. Both patients who developed seizures had contralateral ICA occlusions, consistent with previous observations (210, 214). None had postoperative infarcts on CT of the head, although they demonstrated patchy edema. These results prompted the authors to suggest that post-CEA patients should have their blood pressure meticulously controlled and that TCD may help identify patients at high risk for developing the hyperperfusion syndrome and seizures. If anticipated, a baseline study before or another immediately after surgery may be helpful (207, 211, 219).

Another monitor used in neuro-ICUs is transcranial near-infrared spectroscopy. Using this method to monitor regional cerebral oxygen saturation (rSO_2), Ogasawara examined 50 patients with CEA (220). Post-CEA hyperperfusion (CBF increase of ≥100%, compared with preoperative values) was observed for six patients, one of which developed hyperperfusion syndrome with seizures on the sixth postoperative day.

All this strongly suggests that high-risk patients (history of hypertension, bilateral high grade stenoses, low CBFVs or CO_2 reactivity by TCD, previous contralateral CEA within 3 months) should be monitored in the ICU for symptoms of hyperperfusion syndrome after revascularization of the cerebral vessels (210). The blood pressure should be tightly controlled and, if symptoms develop, the first step of treatment should include further lowering of BP (to a level of equalization of ipsilateral and contralateral CBFVs (211)). The ICU staff should be alerted to the possibility of seizures. Neuroimaging to exclude a new ICH or infarct should be considered if there is new change in the neurological exam. Table 3-7 represents a suggested algorithm for the treatment of reperfusion–hyperperfusion syndrome -related seizures.

3.7. Cerebral Vein and Dural Sinus Thrombosis

3.7.1. Clinical Studies

Several medical or surgical complications have been associated with the development of cerebral venous thrombosis (CVT). Also, CVT is somewhat frequently encountered in ICU patients with the following conditions: various infectious processes (local or systemic), hematologic disorders (genetic prothrombotic conditions [such as antithrombin III or protein C or S deficiencies, hyperhomocysteinemia, Factor V Leiden mutation, prothrombin gene mutation, Factor VIII excess, leukemia, thrombocytemia, paroxysmal nocturnal hemoglobinuria), cancer, non-infectious inflammatory disease, Behçet disease, nephrotic syndrome, dehydration and congestive heart failure, complications of pregnancy and the puerperium, and mechanical causes, such as lumbar puncture (LP) alone or associated with the diagnosis of multiple sclerosis, and high doses of corticosteroids (221–226). Patients with CVT are also frequently admitted to the ICU for cerebral edema, signs of increased intracranial pressure (headache, papilledema), focal neurologic deficits, or seizures.

Outcomes after CVT in recent years have improved, with mortality in the 5–10% range and independent life in almost 80–86% of patients (227–231). The outcome may be less favorable in hospitals without stroke units or early accessibility to MRI (227).

Seizures occur frequently after CVT, and in several cases they are the presenting sign. Indeed, seizures were present in the first clinical description of CVT in 1825 by Ribes (232). In the angiographically proven cases reported by Bousser et al., Jacksonian or grand mal seizures occurred in 11/38 (29%) patients and were the fourth most common symptom, following headache (74%), papilledema (45%), and hemiplegia (34%) (233). In more recent studies, however, seizures have been recorded as one of the two most common signs of CVT (227, 230, 234).

It is interesting to note that several of the causative factors for CVT can also independently cause seizures (head trauma, intracranial surgery, central nervous system (CNS) infection, primary or secondary brain tumors, vasculitis), although no attempt has been made to differentiate the relative roles of each (233, 235). Other common etiologies for CVT include the aforementioned conditions, but in up to a quarter of cases the etiology remains unknown. Since lumbar punctures (LPs) are commonly performed in the ICUs, the reported association between CVT and LP is of special interest to the intensivist. All five patients reported by Wilder-Smith et al. developed a characteristic pattern of headache (initially postural, then continuous) and seizures after LP or complicated peridural anesthesia and were found to have CVT (223). Three out of the four tested had Factor V Leiden deficiency. Other similar cases of CVT after LP complicated by seizure onset have also been reported (236–238).

Several studies report on the incidence of early or late seizures.

In a retrospective study of 78 patients with CVT, generalized seizures occurred in 24 (31%) patients and were the presenting symptom in 13 (17%, seven with partial motor and six with generalized seizures) (239). Seizures were associated with a poor outcome in the univariate analysis and were included in a prognostic scale (0–11 points) developed by the authors, with 0.98 positive prognostic value for good and 0.96 positive prognostic value for poor prognosis.

In another retrospective study from the Bronx, NY, seizures were observed in 35/112 (31%) patients with acute CVT. Only 5% of patients had epilepsy after a mean follow-up period of 77.8 months (229). Among those patients with early seizures and follow-up records, 4/28 (14%) had epilepsy, all with focal signs in the acute stage of CVT. Those seizures manifested in three of four patients during the first year and in one patient 2 years after CVT.

The authors concluded that because of the low risk of recurrent seizures and of late recurrences, antiepileptic treatment seems appropriate only for 1-year post CVT, after which it can be tapered off gradually, unless seizures recur.

In the prospective, randomized, placebo-controlled Dutch-European Cerebral Sinus Thrombosis Trial, low molecular weight heparin (nadroparin 180 anti-factor Xa units/kg/day for 3 weeks, followed by oral anticoagulation with a target international normalized ratio (INR) 2.5–3.5 for 10 weeks) was compared to placebo (240). Seizures were reported in 28/59 (47%) patients, but the study did not comment on their relationship with outcomes at 12 weeks (228).

In a prospective French study from Lille, seizures were the most common symptom overall, occurred in 28/55 (50.9%) patients with CVT and were the presenting symptom in 1 (1.8%) patient (227). There is no mention of antiepileptic treatment in this series. With a median follow-up of 36 months, recurrent seizures developed in 7/28 (25%) patients with seizures in the acute stage (i.e., 14.5% of all 3-year survivors from CVT). Focal or generalized seizures were not associated with outcome as measured with the modified Rankin disability score.

In another prospective study from Portugal (VENOPORT study), data were collected retrospectively for 51 patients and prospectively in another 91 patients (who were followed for an average of one year) with CVT (235, 241). Early seizures (within the first 2 weeks after the diagnosis) were observed in 31/91 (34%) patients. In 29 (31.9%) patients, early seizures were the presenting feature of CVT (in one patient seizures evolved to grand mal SE). The frequency of seizures was the same whether the superior sagital sinus (33%) or the lateral/sigmoid sinus (25%) was thrombosed, but no seizures were observed in the seven patients with involvement of the deep venous system. Early seizures were independently predicted by sensory deficits (OR 7.8, 95%CI 0.8–74.8) and the presence of a parenchymal lesion on admission, including focal edema, ischemic infarct, or hemorrhage (3.7, 1.4–9.4). Late seizures were found in 6/43 (14%) of survivors in the retrospective arm of the study (241) and in 8/84 (9.5%) of survivors in the prospective arm (235), who were followed up to 10 months from the onset of the CVT. Epilepsy developed in 4/84 (4.8%) patients. Seven out of eight (87.5%) patients with late seizures were on antiepileptic treatment when the seizures occurred. Late seizures were generalized in almost two-thirds of patients and were independently predicted by the presence of hemorrhage on the neuroimaging study performed upon admission. Only in the univariate analysis, late seizures were more common in patients with early seizures (19% vs. 5% in those patients without early seizures). In the multivariate analysis, early or late seizures were not independent predictors of increased mortality or dependency, although early seizures directly contributed to death in two patients (intractable SE and cardiorespiratory arrest after grand mal seizure). The authors concluded that prophylactic AEDs during the first year after CVT is justified only in those patients with hemorrhage on CT/MRI or early symptomatic seizures, but could probably be avoided in patients without such high risk factors.

Another small prospective study from Lyon, France, reported a high percentage of pro-thrombotic states in patients with CVT admitted in a stroke unit (242). Seizures were observed in 8/16 (50%), 5 of whom had a hemorrhagic infarct.

A prothrombotic state was detected in 6/8 (75%, a high factor VIII level in four patients), the same percentage as in patients without seizures.

In a prospective study (with a retrospective arm) from Germany, 79 patients with CVT were followed for an average of 52 months (231). Twenty-two patients required NICU admission and mechanical ventilation. Thirty-one (39.2%) patients developed seizures and all were treated with AEDs (phenytoin IV in 20, barbiturates IV in 4, and oral AEDs in 7 patients). More than two seizures despite antiepileptic treatment was among other factors (age, the NIHSS on admission, venous infarct, and hemorrhagic transformation of the venous infarct) significantly related to acute death (15% of patients). Epilepsy developed in 9/58 (16%) of surviving patients during the long-term follow-up and was associated with more than two seizures despite antiepileptic treatment during hospitalization.

In a retrospective multicenter study from Italy, focal deficits and/or seizures were recorded in 19/35 (54.3%) patients with cortical and 4/13 (30.8%) patients with deep CVT (234). EEG was performed in 18 patients, and in two-thirds, revealed diffuse abnormalities. Only 2/18 (11%) of EEGs showed epileptic focal abnormalities. All patients with seizures, except one, were treated with AEDs.

Another large prospective study from Turkey included 1,428 patients with stroke, among which 15 had CVT. Four of these patients developed seizures (26.6%), a significantly higher percentage than ICH (12.7%) or ischemic stroke (2.7%) (43).

In a large prospective study from Germany, 194 patients with CVT were admitted in two hospitals over a period of 28 years (243). Early seizures (within the first 14 days) occurred in 86 (44.3%) patients, the majority of which had focal onset and subsequent Todd's paralysis. SE occurred in 11 (12.8%) patients. Patients with early seizures were more likely to be admitted to the NICU than patients without seizures. Among patients with seizures, mortality was 3 times higher in those with SE than in those without SE (36.4% and 12%, respectively). Motor deficit (OR 5.8, 95%CI 2.98–11.42), ICH (2.8, 1.46–5.56), and cortical vein thrombosis (2.9, 1.43–5.96) were independent predictors of early seizures. The authors concluded that prophylactic antiepileptic treatment may be an option for patients with these predictor variables.

Most recently, results of the International Study on Cerebral Vein and Dural Sinus Thrombosis (ISCVT) have been published (230, 244). This prospective, multicenter study included 624 patients. Most patients were treated with heparin (83%), and only 13.4% had a poor outcome (death or dependency). Prognostic factors for poor outcome were age >37 years, male sex, coma, mental status disorder, hemorrhage on admission CT scan, thrombosis of the deep cerebral venous system, CNS infection, and cancer. Presenting seizures occurred in 245 (39.3%, the second most common symptom after headache), and early seizures (within 2 weeks) in 43 (6.9%) patients with CVT. Sixty percent of early seizures were in reality recurrent, because they occurred in patients with presenting seizures. Supratentorial lesion (4.05, 2.74–5.95), cortical vein thrombosis (2.31, 1.44–3.73), sagittal sinus thrombosis (2.18, 1.50–3.18), and puerperal CVT (2.06, 1.19–3.55) were associated with presenting seizures, whereas supratentorial lesion (3.09, 1.56–9.62) and presenting seizures (1.74, 0.90–3.37) predicted early seizures.

3.7.2. Treatment of Seizures Related to CVT

The treatment of seizures that follow CVT obeys the same principles as the treatment of seizures not related to this condition (see Chapter 11). If onset or presenting seizures occur, they should be treated with AEDs, because presenting seizures are predictive of early seizures based on the International study on Cerebral Vein and Dural Sinus Thrombosis (ISCVT) results (244). In this large study, the risk of early seizures in patients with supratentorial lesions and presenting seizures was significantly lower when AED prophylaxis was used (1 patient with seizures out of 148 patients with AEDs vs. 25 out of 47 patients without AEDs, OR 0.006, 95%CI 0.001–0.05).

Should every patient with CVT be treated prophylactically with AEDs? In a recent Cochrane Review, Kwan et al. did not find any randomized and quasi-randomized controlled trial for treatment of seizures after CVT. Based on that, the authors concluded that there is no evidence to support or refute the use of antiepileptic drugs for the primary or secondary prevention of seizures related to CVT (245). However, other studies have reported factors associated with seizure incidence, such as supratentotial lesions, motor or sensory deficits, ICH, or isolated cortical vein thrombosis (235, 243, 244). These patients should probably be started on AEDs, because early seizures can lead to neurologic or systemic deterioration, SE, or death (244). In the ISCVT study, however, seizures were not an independent predictor of death and/or dependency (230). Moreover, the duration of treatment is unclear. Prolonged treatment for 1 year should be considered in patients with CVT who developed early seizures and ICH, because late seizures may occur within the first 12 months (227, 229, 235, 243).

How does treatment, which is aimed at recanalizing the thrombosed venous channel using various available options, affect the incidence or severity of seizures? Few data are currently available to help answer that question. In the Dutch–European prospective study, seizures occurred in 16/30 (53%) patients on the nadroparin arm and in 12/29 (41%) patients on the controls arm ($p > 0.05$). In the most recent prospective Dutch study, 20 patients with severe CVT (i.e., selected for thrombolysis if they had an altered mental status, coma, straight sinus thrombosis, or large space-occupying lesions) were treated with urokinase infused into the sinuses (246). Some patients received thrombosuction with a rheolytic catheter, combined with thrombectomy via a Fogerty catheter. Six patients died in these case series by transtentorial herniation. Interestingly, seizures occurred less frequently in the fatal cases (1/6) than in the surviving patients (10/14). Even the single patient with SE had an excellent outcome. Although no specific mention about AEDs was found in this study, the explanation provided for the better outcomes in patients with seizures was that some of these patients might have been enrolled in the study with decreased mental status or coma due to seizures (and not due to severe infarcts or ICHs) and quickly recovered with antiepileptic treatment.

Are seizures in patients with CVT treated with IV heparin more likely to lead to fatal complications? One retrospective study from Freiburg, Germany, analyzed 79 patients with CVT (247). All patients received a 5,000 IU IV bolus of heparin and a subsequent infusion with target aPTT of 80–90 s. There was no difference in fatal compared to nonfatal outcome in those patients with seizures (58% of all patients) or those patients with series of seizures or status (28% of patients with seizures).

Table 3-8. Treatment with AntiEpileptic Medications After CVT.

1. CVT and no seizures:
Observe.
Consider Rx if there are supratentorial lesions or parenchymal lesion (focal edema, infarct, or hemorrhage), focal motor or sensory deficits, or cortical vein thrombosis on the admission CT/MRI. Continue Rx for at least 1 year (seizure-free interval). Assess with EEG before discontinuation?
2. CVT and onset or early seizures:
Treat with monotherapy first for 1 year (seizure-free interval). Assess with EEG before discontinuation?

Other studies evaluating novel treatments for CVT usually do not report data regarding seizures, either because the numbers are too small to draw meaningful conclusions or because they have a different focus. Niwa et al. reported treating a woman in her 10th month of pregnancy and with superior sagittal sinus thrombosis with direct t-PA instillation (248). The patient presented with generalized seizure and tetraparesis, but was discharged without neurologic deficit. Another interesting and informative case was reported by Gerszten et al., who treated an 18-year-old man with deep cerebral venous system thrombosis secondary to antithrombin III deficiency (249). The patient, who presented with a focal motor seizure, was started on antiepileptics and became comatose with fixed pupils before he received the endovascular treatment. He was treated with urokinase delivered in the straight sinus and the vein of Galen 27 h after the onset and despite the presence of edema in both basal ganglia and thalami bilaterally and a hemorrhage in the left thalamus. The procedure resulted in deep system recanalization, and subsequently continuous infusion of heparin was given. The patient remained in the ICU on pentobarbital coma for 20 days for ICP control, but eventually improved to the point of living independently and was able to graduate from high school on time. Table 3-8 represents a suggested algorithm for the treatment of CVT-related seizures.

References

1. Jackson J. On the scientific and empirical investigation of epilepsies. In: Taylor J, (ed) Selected writtings of John Hughlings Jackson. London: Hodder and Stoughton, 1931; 233
2. Gowers W (1964) Epilepsy and other chronic convulsive disorders. Dover, New York, p 106
3. Armon C, Radtke RA, Massey EW (1991) Therapy of seizures associated with stroke. Clin Neuropharmacol 14:17–27
4. Barolin GS (1982) The cerebrovascular epilepsies. Electroencephalogr Clin Neurophysiol Suppl, 287–295
5. Giroud M, Gras P, Fayolle H, Andre N, Soichot P, Dumas R (1994) Early seizures after acute stroke: a study of 1, 640 cases. Epilepsia 35:959–964
6. Lancman ME, Golimstok A, Norscini J, Granillo R (1993) Risk factors for developing seizures after a stroke. Epilepsia 34:141–143
7. Bladin CF, Alexandrov AV, Bellavance A, Bornstein N, Chambers B, Cote R et al (2000) Seizures after stroke: a prospective multicenter study. Arch Neurol 57:1617–1622
8. Burn J, Dennis M, Bamford J, Sandercock P, Wade D, Warlow C (1997) Epileptic seizures after a first stroke: the Oxfordshire Community Stroke Project. BMJ 315:1582–1587

9. Kilpatrick CJ, Davis SM, Tress BM, Rossiter SC, Hopper JL, Vandendriesen ML (1990) Epileptic seizures in acute stroke. Arch Neurol 47:157–160
10. Louis S, McDowell F (1967) Epileptic seizures in nonembolic cerebral infarction. Arch Neurol 17:414–418
11. Shinton RA, Gill JS, Melnick SC, Gupta AK, Beevers DG (1988) The frequency, characteristics and prognosis of epileptic seizures at the onset of stroke. J Neurol Neurosurg Psychiatry 51:273–276
12. Milandre L, Broca P, Sambuc R, Khalil R (1992) [Epileptic crisis during and after cerebrovascular diseases. A clinical analysis of 78 cases]. Rev Neurol 148:767–772
13. Holmes GL (1980) The electroencephalogram as a predictor of seizures following cerebral infarction. Clin Electroencephalogr 11:83–86
14. Loiseau J, Loiseau P, Duche B, Guyot M, Dartigues JF, Aublet B (1990) A survey of epileptic disorders in southwest France: seizures in elderly patients. Ann Neurol 27:232–237
15. Lo YK, Yiu CH, Hu HH, Su MS, Laeuchli SC (1994) Frequency and characteristics of early seizures in Chinese acute stroke. Acta Neurol Scand 90:83–85
16. Hauser WA, Kurland LT (1975) The epidemiology of epilepsy in Rochester, Minnesota, 1935 through 1967. Epilepsia 16:1–66
17. Arboix A, Comes E, Massons J, Garcia L, Oliveres M (1996) Relevance of early seizures for in-hospital mortality in acute cerebrovascular disease. Neurology 47:1429–1435
18. Reith J, Jorgensen HS, Nakayama H, Raaschou HO, Olsen TS (1997) Seizures in acute stroke: predictors and prognostic significance. The Copenhagen Stroke Study. Stroke 28:1585–1589
19. Camilo O, Goldstein LB (2004) Seizures and epilepsy after ischemic stroke. Stroke 35:1769–1775
20. Lamy C, Domigo V, Semah F, Arquizan C, Trystram D, Coste J et al (2003) Early and late seizures after cryptogenic ischemic stroke in young adults. Neurology 60:400–404
21. Paolucci S, Silvestri G, Lubich S, Pratesi L, Traballesi M, Gigli GL (1997) Poststroke late seizures and their role in rehabilitation of inpatients. Epilepsia 38:266–270
22. Berges S, Moulin T, Berger E, Tatu L, Sablot D, Challier B et al (2000) Seizures and epilepsy following strokes: recurrence factors. Eur Neurol 43:3–8
23. De Carolis P, D'Alessandro R, Ferrara R, Andreoli A, Sacquegna T, Lugaresi E (1984) Late seizures in patients with internal carotid and middle cerebral artery occlusive disease following ischaemic events. J Neurol Neurosurg Psychiatry 47:1345–1347
24. Olsen TS, Hogenhaven H, Thage O (1987) Epilepsy after stroke. Neurology 37:1209–1211
25. Viitanen M, Eriksson S, Asplund K (1988) Risk of recurrent stroke, myocardial infarction and epilepsy during long-term follow-up after stroke. Eur Neurol 28:227–231
26. Fish DR, Miller DH, Roberts RC, Blackie JD, Gilliatt RW (1989) The natural history of late-onset epilepsy secondary to vascular disease. Acta Neurol Scand 80:524–526
27. Faught E, Peters D, Bartolucci A, Moore L, Miller PC (1989) Seizures after primary intracerebral hemorrhage. Neurology 39:1089–1093
28. Sundaram MB (1989) Etiology and patterns of seizures in the elderly. Neuroepidemiology 8:234–238
29. Mahler ME (1987) Seizures: common causes and treatment in the elderly. Geriatrics 42:73–78
30. Luhdorf K, Jensen LK, Plesner AM (1986) Etiology of seizures in the elderly. Epilepsia 27:458–463

31. Dam AM, Fuglsang-Frederiksen A, Svarre-Olsen U, Dam M (1985) Late-onset epilepsy: etiologies, types of seizure, and value of clinical investigation, EEG, and computerized tomography scan. Epilepsia 26:227–231
32. de la Sayette V, Cosgrove R, Melanson D, Ethier R (1987) CT findings in late-onset epilepsy. Can J Neurol Sci 14:286–289
33. Gupta SR, Naheedy MH, Elias D, Rubino FA (1988) Postinfarction seizures. A clinical study. Stroke 19:1477–1481
34. Sung CY, Chu NS (1990) Epileptic seizures in thrombotic stroke. J Neurol 237:166–170
35. Pohlman-Eden B, Hoch D, Cochius J, Hennerici M (1996) Stroke and epilepsy: critical review of the literature. Cerebrovasc Dis 6:332–338
36. Black SE, Norris JW, Hachinski V (1983) Post-stroke seizures. Stroke 14:134
37. Kilpatrick CJ, Davis SM, Hopper JL, Rossiter SC (1992) Early seizures after acute stroke. Risk of late seizures. Arch Neurol 49:509–511
38. Daniele O, Caravaglios G, Ferraro G, Mattaliano A, Tassinari C, Natale E (1996) Stroke-related seizures and the role of cortical and subcortical structures. J Epilepsy 9:184–188
39. Arboix A, Garcia-Eroles L, Massons JB, Oliveres M, Comes E (1997) Predictive factors of early seizures after acute cerebrovascular disease. Stroke 28:1590–1594
40. Cheung CM, Tsoi TH, Au-Yeung M, Tang AS (2003) Epileptic seizure after stroke in Chinese patients. J Neurol 250:839–843
41. Lossius MI, Ronning OM, Slapo GD, Mowinckel P, Gjerstad L (2005) Poststroke epilepsy: occurrence and predictors–a long-term prospective controlled study (Akershus Stroke Study). Epilepsia 46:1246–1251
42. Adams HP Jr, Woolson RF, Biller J, Clarke W (1992) Studies of Org 10172 in patients with acute ischemic stroke. TOAST Study Group. Haemostasis 22:99–103
43. Benbir G, Ince B, Bozluolcay M (2006) The epidemiology of post-stroke epilepsy according to stroke subtypes. Acta Neurol Scand 114:8–12
44. Misirli H, Ozge A, Somay G, Erdogan N, Erkal H, Erenoglu NY (2006) Seizure development after stroke. Int J Clin Pract 60:1536–1541
45. Basic Baronica K, Sruk A, Planjar-Prvan M, Bielen I (2008) Seizures in the peracute stage of stroke: incidence and effect on inpatient mortality. Acta Med Croatica 62:29–32
46. Vespa PM, O'Phelan K, Shah M, Mirabelli J, Starkman S, Kidwell C et al (2003) Acute seizures after intracerebral hemorrhage: a factor in progressive midline shift and outcome. Neurology 60:1441–1446
47. So EL, Annegers JF, Hauser WA, O'Brien PC, Whisnant JP (1996) Population-based study of seizure disorders after cerebral infarction. Neurology 46:350–355
48. Kammersgaard LP, Olsen TS (2005) Poststroke epilepsy in the Copenhagen stroke study: incidence and predictors. J Stroke Cerebrovasc dis 14:210–214
49. Labovitz DL, Hauser WA, Sacco RL (2001) Prevalence and predictors of early seizure and status epilepticus after first stroke. Neurology 57:200–206
50. Devuyst G, Karapanayiotides T, Hottinger I, Van Melle G, Bogousslavsky J (2003) Prodromal and early epileptic seizures in acute stroke: does higher serum cholesterol protect? Neurology 61:249–252
51. Szaflarski JP, Rackley AY, Kleindorfer DO, Khoury J, Woo D, Miller R et al (2008) Incidence of seizures in the acute phase of stroke: A population-based study. Epilepsia 49:974–981
52. Celesia GG (1976) Modern concepts of status epilepticus. JAMA 235:1571–1574
53. DeLorenzo RJ, Hauser WA, Towne AR, Boggs JG, Pellock JM, Penberthy L et al (1996) A prospective, population-based epidemiologic study of status epilepticus in Richmond, Virginia. Neurology 46:1029–1035
54. Scholtes FB, Renier WO, Meinardi H (1994) Generalized convulsive status epilepticus: causes, therapy, and outcome in 346 patients. Epilepsia 35:1104–1112

55. Towne AR, Pellock JM, Ko D, DeLorenzo RJ (1994) Determinants of mortality in status epilepticus. Epilepsia 35:27–34

56. Barry E, Hauser WA (1993) Status epilepticus: the interaction of epilepsy and acute brain disease. Neurology 43:1473–1478

57. Rumbach L, Sablot D, Berger E, Tatu L, Vuillier F, Moulin T (2000) Status epilepticus in stroke: report on a hospital-based stroke cohort. Neurology 54:350–354

58. Velioglu SK, Ozmenoglu M, Boz C, Alioglu Z (2001) Status epilepticus after stroke. Stroke 32:1169–1172

59. Afsar N, Kaya D, Aktan S, Sykut-Bingol C (2003) Stroke and status epilepticus: stroke type, type of status epilepticus, and prognosis. Seizure 12:23–27

60. Shinton RA, Gill JS, Zezulka AV, Beevers DG (1987) The frequency of epilepsy preceding stroke Case-control study in 230 patients. Lancet 1:11–13

61. Cleary P, Shorvon S, Tallis R (2004) Late-onset seizures as a predictor of subsequent stroke. Lancet 363:1184–1186

62. Kase CS, Wolf PA, Chodosh EH, Zacker HB, Kelly-Hayes M, Kannel WB et al (1989) Prevalence of silent stroke in patients presenting with initial stroke: the Framingham Study. Stroke 20:850–852

63. Roberts RC, Shorvon SD, Cox TC, Gilliatt RW (1988) Clinically unsuspected cerebral infarction revealed by computed tomography scanning in late onset epilepsy. Epilepsia 29:190–194

64. Heiss WD, Huber M, Fink GR, Herholz K, Pietrzyk U, Wagner R et al (1992) Progressive derangement of periinfarct viable tissue in ischemic stroke. J Cereb Blood Flow Metab 12:193–203

65. Silverman IE, Restrepo L, Mathews GC (2002) Poststroke seizures. Arch Neurol 59:195–201

66. DeLorenzo RJ, Sun DA, Blair RE, Sombati S (2007) An in vitro model of stroke-induced epilepsy: elucidation of the roles of glutamate and calcium in the induction and maintenance of stroke-induced epileptogenesis. Int Rev Neurobiol 81:59–84

67. Comi AM, Weisz CJ, Highet BH, Johnston MV, Wilson MA (2004) A new model of stroke and ischemic seizures in the immature mouse. Pediatr Neurol 31: 254–257

68. Buchkremer-Ratzmann I, August M, Hagemann G, Witte OW (1998) Epileptiform discharges to extracellular stimuli in rat neocortical slices after photothrombotic infarction. J Neurol Sci 156:133–137

69. Congar P, Gaiarsa JL, Popovici T, Ben-Ari Y, Crepel V (2000) Permanent reduction of seizure threshold in post-ischemic CA3 pyramidal neurons. J Neurophysiol 83:2040–2046

70. Nedergaard M, Hansen AJ (1993) Characterization of cortical depolarizations evoked in focal cerebral ischemia. J Cereb Blood Flow Metab 13:568–574

71. Kim DC, Todd MM (1999) Forebrain ischemia: effect on pharmacologically induced seizure thresholds in the rat. Brain Res 831:131–139

72. Kessler KR, Schnitzler A, Classen J, Benecke R (2002) Reduced inhibition within primary motor cortex in patients with poststroke focal motor seizures. Neurology 59:1028–1033

73. De Reuck J, Proot P, Van Maele G (2007) Chronic obstructive pulmonary disease as a risk factor for stroke-related seizures. Eur J Neurol 14:989–992

74. De Reuck J, Decoo D, Algoed L et al (1995) Epileptic seizures after thromboembolic cerebral infarcts: a positron emission tomographic study. Cerebrovasc Dis 5:328–333

75. Shuaib A, Lee MA (1987) Seizures in migraine: warning of an underlying cerebral infarction? Headache 27:500–502

76. Yanagihara T, Piepgras DG, Klass DW (1985) Repetitive involuntary movement associated with episodic cerebral ischemia. Ann Neurol 18:244–250

77. Giroud M, Dumas R (1995) Role of associated cortical lesions in motor partial seizures and lenticulostriate infarcts. Epilepsia 36:465–470

78. Avrahami E, Drory VE, Rabey MJ, Cohn DF (1988) Generalized epileptic seizures as the presenting symptom of lacunar infarction in the brain. J Neurol 235:472–474

79. Bentes C, Pimentel J, Ferro JM (2001) Epileptic seizures following subcortical infarcts. Cerebrovasc Dis 12:331–334

80. Willmore LJ, Sypert GW, Munson JB (1978) Recurrent seizures induced by cortical iron injection: a model of posttraumatic epilepsy. Ann Neurol 4:329–336

81. Lee KR, Drury I, Vitarbo E, Hoff JT (1997) Seizures induced by intracerebral injection of thrombin: a model of intracerebral hemorrhage. J Neurosurg 87:73–78

82. Bogousslavsky J, Martin R, Regli F, Despland PA, Bolyn S (1992) Persistent worsening of stroke sequelae after delayed seizures. Arch Neurol 49:385–388

83. Cordonnier C, Henon H, Derambure P, Pasquier F, Leys D (2007) Early epileptic seizures after stroke are associated with increased risk of new-onset dementia. J Neurol Neurosurg Psychiatry 78:514–516

84. Jordan KG (1999) Continuous EEG monitoring in the neuroscience intensive care unit and emergency department. J Clin Neurophysiol 16:14–39

85. Pohlmann-Eden B, Cochius J, Hoch D, Hennerici M (1997) Stroke and Epilepsy: critical review of the literature. Part II. Cerebrovasc Dis 7:2–9

86. Carrera E, Michel P, Despland PA, Maeder-Ingvar M, Ruffieux C, Debatisse D et al (2006) Continuous assessment of electrical epileptic activity in acute stroke. Neurology 67:99–104

87. Chu K, Kang DW, Kim JY, Chang KH, Lee SK (2001) Diffusion-weighted magnetic resonance imaging in nonconvulsive status epilepticus. Arch Neurol 58:993–998

88. Senn P, Lovblad KO, Zutter D, Bassetti C, Zeller O, Donati F et al (2003) Changes on diffusion-weighted MRI with focal motor status epilepticus: case report. Neuroradiology 45:246–249

89. Lansberg MG, O'Brien MW, Norbash AM, Moseley ME, Morrell M, Albers GW (1999) MRI abnormalities associated with partial status epilepticus. Neurology 52:1021–1027

90. Kim HS, Kim DI, Lee BI, Jeong EK, Choi C, Lee JD et al (2001) Diffusion-weighted image and MR spectroscopic analysis of a case of MELAS with repeated attacks. Yonsei Med J 42:128–133

91. Kappelle LJ, Adams HP Jr, Heffner ML, Torner JC, Gomez F, Biller J (1994) Prognosis of young adults with ischemic stroke A long-term follow-up study assessing recurrent vascular events and functional outcome in the Iowa Registry of Stroke in Young Adults. Stroke 25:1360–1365

92. Kristensen B, Malm J, Carlberg B, Stegmayr B, Backman C, Fagerlund M et al (1997) Epidemiology and etiology of ischemic stroke in young adults aged 18 to 44 years in northern Sweden. Stroke 28:1702–1709

93. Rozenthul-Sorokin N, Ronen R, Tamir A, Geva H, Eldar R (1996) Stroke in the young in Israel. Incidence and outcomes. Stroke 27:838–841

94. Neau JP, Ingrand P, Mouille-Brachet C, Rosier MP, Couderq C, Alvarez A et al (1998) Functional recovery and social outcome after cerebral infarction in young adults. Cerebrovasc Dis 8:296–302

95. Hauser WA (1992) Seizure disorders: the changes with age. Epilepsia 33(Suppl 4):S6–S14

96. Holt-Seitz A, Wirrell EC, Sundaram MB (1999) Seizures in the elderly: etiology and prognosis. Can J Neurol Sci 26:110–114

97. Cordonnier C, Henon H, Derambure P, Pasquier F, Leys D (2005) Influence of pre-existing dementia on the risk of post-stroke epileptic seizures. J Neurol Neurosurg Psychiatry 76:1649–1653

98. Tissue plasminogen activator for acute ischemic stroke (1995) The National Institute of Neurological Disorders and Stroke rt-PA Stroke Study Group. N Engl J Med 333:1581–1587

99. Barber PA, Zhang J, Demchuk AM, Hill MD, Buchan AM (2001) Why are stroke patients excluded from TPA therapy? An analysis of patient eligibility. Neurology 56:1015–1020

100. Rodan LH, Aviv RI, Sahlas DJ, Murray BJ, Gladstone JP, Gladstone DJ (2006) Seizures during stroke thrombolysis heralding dramatic neurologic recovery. Neurology 67:2048–2049

101. Hafeez F, Razzaq MA, Levine RL, Ramirez MA (2007) Reperfusion seizures: a manifestation of cerebral reperfusion injury after administration of recombinant tissue plasminogen activator for acute ischemic stroke. J Stroke Cerebrovasc Dis 16:273–277

102. Seeck M, Vulliemoz S (2007) Seizures during stroke thrombolysis heralding dramatic neurologic recovery. Neurology 69:409–410

103. Adams HP Jr, del Zoppo G, Alberts MJ, Bhatt DL, Brass L, Furlan A et al (2007) Guidelines for the early management of adults with ischemic stroke: a guideline from the American Heart Association/American Stroke Association Stroke Council, Clinical Cardiology Council, Cardiovascular Radiology and Intervention Council, and the Atherosclerotic Peripheral Vascular Disease and Quality of Care Outcomes in Research Interdisciplinary Working Groups: the American Academy of Neurology affirms the value of this guideline as an educational tool for neurologists. Stroke 38:1655–1711

104. Selim M, Kumar S, Fink J, Schlaug G, Caplan LR, Linfante I (2002) Seizure at stroke onset: should it be an absolute contraindication to thrombolysis? Cerebrovasc Dis 14:54–57

105. Sylaja PN, Dzialowski I, Krol A, Roy J, Federico P, Demchuk AM (2006) Role of CT angiography in thrombolysis decision-making for patients with presumed seizure at stroke onset. Stroke 37:915–917

106. Ryvlin P, Montavont A, Nighoghossian N (2006) Optimizing therapy of seizures in stroke patients. Neurology 67:S3–S9

107. Davalos A, Cendra E, Genis D, Lopez-Pousa S (1988) The frequency, characteristics and prognosis of epileptic seizures at the onset of stroke. J Neurol Neurosurg Psychiatry 51:1464

108. Gilad R, Lampl Y, Eschel Y, Sadeh M (2001) Antiepileptic treatment in patients with early postischemic stroke seizures: a retrospective study. Cerebrovasc Dis 12:39–43

109. Leker RR, Neufeld MY (2003) Anti-epileptic drugs as possible neuroprotectants in cerebral ischemia. Brain Res 42:187–203

110. Costa C, Martella G, Picconi B, Prosperetti C, Pisani A, Di Filippo M et al (2006) Multiple mechanisms underlying the neuroprotective effects of antiepileptic drugs against in vitro ischemia. Stroke 37:1319–1326

111. Goldstein LB (1998) Potential effects of common drugs on stroke recovery. Arch Neurol 55:454–456

112. Glauser T, Ben-Menachem E, Bourgeois B, Cnaan A, Chadwick D, Guerreiro C et al (2006) ILAE treatment guidelines: evidence-based analysis of antiepileptic drug efficacy and effectiveness as initial monotherapy for epileptic seizures and syndromes. Epilepsia 47:1094–1120

113. Alvarez-Sabin J, Montaner J, Padro L, Molina CA, Rovira R, Codina A et al (2002) Gabapentin in late-onset poststroke seizures. Neurology 59:1991–1993

114. Chadwick DW, Anhut H, Greiner MJ, Alexander J, Murray GH, Garofalo EA et al (1998) A double-blind trial of gabapentin monotherapy for newly diagnosed partial seizures. International Gabapentin Monotherapy Study Group 945–77. Neurology 51:1282–1288

115. Garcia-Escriva A, Lopez-Hernandez N (2007) The use of levetiracetam in monotherapy in post-stroke seizures in the elderly population. Revista de neurologia 45:523–525

116. Passero S, Rocchi R, Rossi S, Ulivelli M, Vatti G (2002) Seizures after spontaneous supratentorial intracerebral hemorrhage. Epilepsia 43:1175–1180

117. Ropper AH, Davis KR (1980) Lobar cerebral hemorrhages: acute clinical syndromes in 26 cases. Ann Neurol 8:141–147

118. Kase CS, Williams JP, Wyatt DA, Mohr JP (1982) Lobar intracerebral hematomas: clinical and CT analysis of 22 cases. Neurology 32:1146–1150

119. Sung CY, Chu NS (1989) Epileptic seizures in intracerebral haemorrhage. J Neurol Neurosurg Psychiatry 52:1273–1276

120. Tatu L, Moulin T, El Mohamad R, Vuillier F, Rumbach L, Czorny A (2000) Primary intracerebral hemorrhages in the Besancon stroke registry. Initial clinical and CT findings, early course and 30-day outcome in 350 patients. Eur Neurol 43:209–214

121. Weisberg LA, Shamsnia M, Elliott D (1991) Seizures caused by nontraumatic parenchymal brain hemorrhages. Neurology 41:1197–1199

122. Berger AR, Lipton RB, Lesser ML, Lantos G, Portenoy RK (1988) Early seizures following intracerebral hemorrhage: implications for therapy. Neurology 38:1363–1365

123. Cervoni L, Artico M, Salvati M, Bristot R, Franco C, Delfini R (1994) Epileptic seizures in intracerebral hemorrhage: a clinical and prognostic study of 55 cases. Neurosurg Rev 17:185–188

124. Claassen J, Jette N, Chum F, Green R, Schmidt M, Choi H et al (2007) Electrographic seizures and periodic discharges after intracerebral hemorrhage. Neurology 69:1356–1365

125. Richardson E, Dodge P (1954) Epilepsy in cerebral vascular disease: a study of the incidence and nature of seizures in 104 consecutive autopsy proven cases of cerebral infarction and hemorrhage. Epilepsia 3:49–74

126. Mayer SA, Sacco RL, Shi T, Mohr JP (1994) Neurologic deterioration in noncomatose patients with supratentorial intracerebral hemorrhage. Neurology 44:1379–1384

127. Arboix A, Comes E, Garcia-Eroles L, Massons J, Oliveres M, Balcells M et al (2002) Site of bleeding and early outcome in primary intracerebral hemorrhage. Acta Neurol Scand 105:282–288

128. Naval NS, Abdelhak TA, Zeballos P, Urrunaga N, Mirski MA, Carhuapoma JR (2008) Prior statin use reduces mortality in intracerebral hemorrhage. Neurocrit Care 8:6–12

129. Bateman BT, Claassen J, Willey JZ, Hirsch LJ, Mayer SA, Sacco RL et al (2007) Convulsive status epilepticus after ischemic stroke and intracerebral hemorrhage: frequency, predictors, and impact on outcome in a large administrative dataset. Neurocrit Care 7:187–193

130. Lu A, Tang Y, Ran R, Ardizzone TL, Wagner KR, Sharp FR (2006) Brain genomics of intracerebral hemorrhage. J Cereb Blood Flow Metab 26:230–252

131. Broderick JP, Adams HP Jr, Barsan W, Feinberg W, Feldmann E, Grotta J et al (1999) Guidelines for the management of spontaneous intracerebral hemorrhage: A statement for healthcare professionals from a special writing group of the Stroke Council, American Heart Association. Stroke 30:905–915

132. Diringer MN (1993) Intracerebral hemorrhage: pathophysiology and management. Crit Care Med 21:1591–1603

133. Qureshi AI, Tuhrim S, Broderick JP, Batjer HH, Hondo H, Hanley DF (2001) Spontaneous intracerebral hemorrhage. N Engl J Med 344:1450–1460

134. Mayberg MR, Batjer HH, Dacey R, Diringer M, Haley EC, Heros RC et al (1994) Guidelines for the management of aneurysmal subarachnoid hemorrhage. A statement for healthcare professionals from a special writing group of the Stroke Council, American Heart Association. Stroke 25:2315–2328

135. Zondra B, Buresova J (1994) Epileptic seizures following subarachnoideal haemorrhage. Acta Univ Palacki Olomuc Fac Med 137:61–63

136. Sundaram MB, Chow F (1986) Seizures associated with spontaneous subarachnoid hemorrhage. Can J Neurol Sci 13:229–231

137. Pinto AN, Canhao P, Ferro JM (1996) Seizures at the onset of subarachnoid haemorrhage. J Neurol 243:161–164

138. Hasan D, Schonck RS, Avezaat CJ, Tanghe HL, van Gijn J, van der Lugt PJ (1993) Epileptic seizures after subarachnoid hemorrhage. Ann Neurol 33:286–291

139. Hart RG, Byer JA, Slaughter JR, Hewett JE, Easton JD (1981) Occurrence and implications of seizures in subarachnoid hemorrhage due to ruptured intracranial aneurysms. Neurosurgery 8:417–421

140. Butzkueven H, Evans AH, Pitman A, Leopold C, Jolley DJ, Kaye AH et al (2000) Onset seizures independently predict poor outcome after subarachnoid hemorrhage. Neurology 55:1315–1320

141. Keranen T, Tapaninaho A, Hernesniemi J, Vapalahti M (1985) Late epilepsy after aneurysm operations. Neurosurgery 17:897–900

142. Ukkola V, Heikkinen ER (1990) Epilepsy after operative treatment of ruptured cerebral aneurysms. Acta Neurochir (Wien) 106:115–118

143. Bidzinski J, Marchel A, Sherif A (1992) Risk of epilepsy after aneurysm operations. Acta Neurochir (Wien) 119:49–52

144. Ohman J (1990) Hypertension as a risk factor for epilepsy after aneurysmal subarachnoid hemorrhage and surgery. Neurosurgery 27:578–581

145. Rhoney DH, Tipps LB, Murry KR, Basham MC, Michael DB, Coplin WM (2000) Anticonvulsant prophylaxis and timing of seizures after aneurysmal subarachnoid hemorrhage. Neurology 55:258–265

146. Maramattom BV, Britton JW, Ghearing GR, Wijdicks EF (2004) Ictal bradycardia after endovascular treatment of an aneurysm. Case illustration. J Neurosurg 101:546

147. Kamali AW, Cockerell OC, Butlar P (2004) Aneurysms and epilepsy: an increasingly recognised cause. Seizure 13:40–44

148. Haines SJ (1988) Decerebrate posturing misinterpreted as seizure activity. Am J Emerg Med 6:173–177

149. Qureshi AI, Sung GY, Suri MA, Straw RN, Guterman LR, Hopkins LN (1999) Prognostic value and determinants of ultraearly angiographic vasospasm after aneurysmal subarachnoid hemorrhage. Neurosurgery 44:967–973 discussion 973–964

150. Sherlock M, O'Sullivan E, Agha A, Behan LA, Rawluk D, Brennan P et al (2006) The incidence and pathophysiology of hyponatraemia after subarachnoid haemorrhage. Clin Endocrinol (Oxf) 64:250–254

151. Hijdra A, Brouwers PJ, Vermeulen M, van Gijn J (1990) Grading the amount of blood on computed tomograms after subarachnoid hemorrhage. Stroke 21:1156–1161

152. Olafsson E, Gudmundsson G, Hauser WA (2000) Risk of epilepsy in long-term survivors of surgery for aneurysmal subarachnoid hemorrhage: a population-based study in Iceland. Epilepsia 41:1201–1205

153. Ogden JA, Utley T, Mee EW (1997) Neurological and psychosocial outcome 4 to 7 years after subarachnoid hemorrhage. Neurosurgery 41:25–34

154. Lin CL, Dumont AS, Lieu AS, Yen CP, Hwang SL, Kwan AL et al (2003) Characterization of perioperative seizures and epilepsy following aneurysmal subarachnoid hemorrhage. J Neurosurg 99:978–985

155. Lin YJ, Chang WN, Chang HW, Ho JT, Lee TC, Wang HC et al (2008) Risk factors and outcome of seizures after spontaneous aneurysmal subarachnoid hemorrhage. Eur J Neurol 15:451–457

156. Dennis LJ, Claassen J, Hirsch LJ, Emerson RG, Connolly ES, Mayer SA (2002) Nonconvulsive status epilepticus after subarachnoid hemorrhage. Neurosurgery 51:1136–1143 discussion 1144

157. Claassen J, Peery S, Kreiter KT, Hirsch LJ, Du EY, Connolly ES et al (2003) Predictors and clinical impact of epilepsy after subarachnoid hemorrhage. Neurology 60:208–214

158. Feffer SE, Parray HR, Westring DW (1978) Seizure after infusion of aminocaproic acid. JAMA 240:2468

159. Dikmen SS, Temkin NR, Miller B, Machamer J, Winn HR (1991) Neurobehavioral effects of phenytoin prophylaxis of posttraumatic seizures. JAMA 265:1271–1277

160. Fabinyi GC, Artiola-Fortuny L (1980) Epilepsy after craniotomy for intracranial aneurysm. Lancet 1:1299–1300

161. Sbeih I, Tamas LB, O'Laoire SA (1986) Epilepsy after operation for aneurysms. Neurosurgery 19:784–788

162. Baker CJ, Prestigiacomo CJ, Solomon RA (1995) Short-term perioperative anticonvulsant prophylaxis for the surgical treatment of low-risk patients with intracranial aneurysms. Neurosurgery 37:863–870 discussion 870–861

163. Shaw MD (1990) Post-operative epilepsy and the efficacy of anticonvulsant therapy. Acta Neurochir Suppl (Wien) 50:55–57

164. North JB, Penhall RK, Hanieh A, Frewin DB, Taylor WB (1983) Phenytoin and postoperative epilepsy. A double-blind study. J Neurosurg 58:672–677

165. Foy PM, Chadwick DW, Rajgopalan N, Johnson AL, Shaw MD (1992) Do prophylactic anticonvulsant drugs alter the pattern of seizures after craniotomy? J Neurol Neurosurg Psychiatry 55:753–757

166. Naidech AM, Kreiter KT, Janjua N, Ostapkovich N, Parra A, Commichau C et al (2005) Phenytoin exposure is associated with functional and cognitive disability after subarachnoid hemorrhage. Stroke 36:583–587

167. Rosengart AJ, Huo JD, Tolentino J, Novakovic RL, Frank JI, Goldenberg FD et al (2007) Outcome in patients with subarachnoid hemorrhage treated with antiepileptic drugs. J Neurosurg 107:253–260

168. Chumnanvej S, Dunn IF, Kim DH (2007) Three-day phenytoin prophylaxis is adequate after subarachnoid hemorrhage. Neurosurgery 60:99–102 discussion 102–103

169. Wong GK, Poon WS (2005) Use of phenytoin and other anticonvulsant prophylaxis in patients with aneurysmal subarachnoid hemorrhage. Stroke 36:2532 author reply 2532

170. Wang H, Gao J, Lassiter TF, McDonagh DL, Sheng H, Warner DS et al (2006) Levetiracetam is neuroprotective in murine models of closed head injury and subarachnoid hemorrhage. Neurocrit Care 5:71–78

171. Byrne JV, Boardman P, Ioannidis I, Adcock J, Traill Z (2003) Seizures after aneurysmal subarachnoid hemorrhage treated with coil embolization. Neurosurgery 52:545–552 discussion 550–542

172. Molyneux AJ, Kerr RS, Yu LM, Clarke M, Sneade M, Yarnold JA et al (2005) International subarachnoid aneurysm trial (ISAT) of neurosurgical clipping versus endovascular coiling in 2143 patients with ruptured intracranial aneurysms: a randomised comparison of effects on survival, dependency, seizures, rebleeding, subgroups, and aneurysm occlusion. Lancet 366:809–817

173. Brown RD Jr, Wiebers DO, Torner JC, O'Fallon WM (1996) Frequency of intracranial hemorrhage as a presenting symptom and subtype analysis: a population-based study of intracranial vascular malformations in Olmsted Country, Minnesota. J Neurosurg 85:29–32

174. Ogilvy CS, Stieg PE, Awad I, Brown RD Jr, Kondziolka D, Rosenwasser R et al (2001) AHA Scientific Statement: Recommendations for the management of intracranial arteriovenous malformations: a statement for healthcare professionals from a special writing group of the Stroke Council, American Stroke Association. Stroke 32:1458–1471

175. Lazar RM, Connaire K, Marshall RS, Pile-Spellman J, Hacein-Bey L, Solomon RA et al (1999) Developmental deficits in adult patients with arteriovenous malformations. Arch Neurol 56:103–106

176. Crawford PM, West CR, Shaw MD, Chadwick DW (1986) Cerebral arteriovenous malformations and epilepsy: factors in the development of epilepsy. Epilepsia 27:270–275

177. Mast H, Mohr JP, Osipov A, Pile-Spellman J, Marshall RS, Lazar RM et al (1995) "Steal" is an unestablished mechanism for the clinical presentation of cerebral arteriovenous malformations. Stroke 26:1215–1220

178. Murphy MJ (1985) Long-term follow-up of seizures associated with cerebral arteriovenous malformations. Results of therapy. Arch Neurol 42:477–479

179. Osipov A, Koennecke HC, Hartmann A (1997) Seizures in cerebral arteriovenous malformations: type, clinical course, and medical management. Interventional Neuroradiol 3:37–41

180. Turjman F, Massoud TF, Sayre JW, Vinuela F, Guglielmi G, Duckwiler G (1995) Epilepsy associated with cerebral arteriovenous malformations: a multivariate analysis of angioarchitectural characteristics. AJNR Am J Neuroradiol 16:345–350

181. Lim YJ, Lee CY, Koh JS, Kim TS, Kim GK, Rhee BA (2006) Seizure control of Gamma Knife radiosurgery for non-hemorrhagic arteriovenous malformations. Acta Neurochir 99:97–101

182. Hoh BL, Chapman PH, Loeffler JS, Carter BS, Ogilvy CS (2002) Results of multimodality treatment for 141 patients with brain arteriovenous malformations and seizures: factors associated with seizure incidence and seizure outcomes. Neurosurgery 51:303–309 discussion 309–311

183. Wolf HK, Roos D, Blumcke I, Pietsch T, Wiestler OD (1996) Perilesional neurochemical changes in focal epilepsies. Acta Neuropathol (Berl) 91:376–384

184. Yeh HS, Privitera MD (1991) Secondary epileptogenesis in cerebral arteriovenous malformations. Arch Neurol 48:1122–1124

185. Kraemer DL, Awad IA (1994) Vascular malformations and epilepsy: clinical considerations and basic mechanisms. Epilepsia 35(Suppl 6):S30–S43

186. Stapf C, Mast H, Sciacca RR, Choi JH, Khaw AV, Connolly ES et al (2006) Predictors of hemorrhage in patients with untreated brain arteriovenous malformation. Neurology 66:1350–1355

187. Piepgras DG, Sundt TM Jr, Ragoowansi AT, Stevens L (1993) Seizure outcome in patients with surgically treated cerebral arteriovenous malformations. J Neurosurg 78:5–11

188. Foy PM, Copeland GP, Shaw MD (1981) The incidence of postoperative seizures. Acta Neurochir (Wien) 55:253–264

189. Forster DM, Steiner L, Hakanson S (1972) Arteriovenous malformations of the brain. A long-term clinical study. J Neurosurg 37:562–570

190. Yeh HS, Tew JM Jr, Gartner M (1993) Seizure control after surgery on cerebral arteriovenous malformations. J Neurosurg 78:12–18

191. Falkson CB, Chakrabarti KB, Doughty D, Plowman PN (1997) Stereotactic multiple arc radiotherapy. III–Influence of treatment of arteriovenous malformations on associated epilepsy. Br J Neurosurg 11:12–15

192. Thorpe ML, Cordato DJ, Morgan MK, Herkes GK (2000) Postoperative seizure outcome in a series of 114 patients with supratentorial arteriovenous malformations. J Clin Neurosci 7:107–111

193. Flickinger JC, Kondziolka D, Lunsford LD, Pollock BE, Yamamoto M, Gorman DA et al (1999) A multi-institutional analysis of complication outcomes after arteriovenous malformation radiosurgery. Int J Radiat Oncol Biol Phys 44:67–74

194. Kida Y, Kobayashi T, Tanaka T, Mori Y, Hasegawa T, Kondoh T (2000) Seizure control after radiosurgery on cerebral arteriovenous malformations. J Clin Neurosci 7(Suppl 1):6–9

195. Heikkinen ER, Konnov B, Melnikov L, Yalynych N, Zubkov Yu N, Garmashov Yu A et al (1989) Relief of epilepsy by radiosurgery of cerebral arteriovenous malformations. Stereotact Funct Neurosurg 53:157–166

196. Kurita H, Kawamoto S, Suzuki I, Sasaki T, Tago M, Terahara A et al (1998) Control of epilepsy associated with cerebral arteriovenous malformations after radiosurgery. J Neurol Neurosurg Psychiatry 65:648–655

197. Schauble B, Cascino GD, Pollock BE, Gorman DA, Weigand S, Cohen-Gadol AA et al (2004) Seizure outcomes after stereotactic radiosurgery for cerebral arteriovenous malformations. Neurology 63:683–687

198. Fournier D, TerBrugge KG, Willinsky R, Lasjaunias P, Montanera W (1991) Endovascular treatment of intracerebral arteriovenous malformations: experience in 49 cases. J Neurosurg 75:228–233

199. Steinberg GK, Chang SD, Levy RP, Marks MP, Frankel K, Marcellus M (1996) Surgical resection of large incompletely treated intracranial arteriovenous malformations following stereotactic radiosurgery. J Neurosurg 84:920–928

200. Sundt TM Jr, Sharbrough FW, Piepgras DG, Kearns TP, Messick JM Jr, O'Fallon WM (1981) Correlation of cerebral blood flow and electroencephalographic changes during carotid endarterectomy: with results of surgery and hemodynamics of cerebral ischemia. Mayo Clin Proc 56:533–543

201. Ascher E, Markevich N, Schutzer RW, Kallakuri S, Jacob T, Hingorani AP (2003) Cerebral hyperperfusion syndrome after carotid endarterectomy: predictive factors and hemodynamic changes. J Vasc Surg 37:769–777

202. Wagner WH, Cossman DV, Farber A, Levin PM, Cohen JL (2005) Hyperperfusion syndrome after carotid endarterectomy. Ann Vasc Surg 19:479–486

203. Schoser BG, Heesen C, Eckert B, Thie A (1997) Cerebral hyperperfusion injury after percutaneous transluminal angioplasty of extracranial arteries. J Neurol 244:101–104

204. Ho DS, Wang Y, Chui M, Ho SL, Cheung RT (2000) Epileptic seizures attributed to cerebral hyperperfusion after percutaneous transluminal angioplasty and stenting of the internal carotid artery. Cerebrovasc Dis 10:374–379

205. Stiver SI, Ogilvy CS (2002) Acute hyperperfusion syndrome complicating EC-IC bypass. J Neurol Neurosurg Psychiatry 73:88–89

206. MacGillivray DC, Valentine RJ, Rob CG (1987) Reperfusion seizures after innominate endarterectomy. J Vasc Surg 6:521–523

207. Breen JC, Caplan LR, DeWitt LD, Belkin M, Mackey WC, O'Donnell TP (1996) Brain edema after carotid surgery. Neurology 46:175–181

208. Coutts SB, Hill MD, Hu WY (2003) Hyperperfusion syndrome: toward a stricter definition. Neurosurgery 53:1053–1058 discussion 1058–1060

209. Schroeder T, Sillesen H, Sorensen O, Engell HC (1987) Cerebral hyperperfusion following carotid endarterectomy. J Neurosurg 66:824–829

210. Gupta AK, Purkayastha S, Unnikrishnan M, Vattoth S, Krishnamoorthy T, Kesavadas C (2005) Hyperperfusion syndrome after supraaortic vessel interventions and bypass surgery. J Neuroradiol 32:352–358

211. Jorgensen LG, Schroeder TV (1993) Defective cerebrovascular autoregulation after carotid endarterectomy. Eur J Vasc Surg 7:370–379

212. Macfarlane R, Moskowitz MA, Sakas DE, Tasdemiroglu E, Wei EP, Kontos HA (1991) The role of neuroeffector mechanisms in cerebral hyperperfusion syndromes. J Neurosurg 75:845–855

213. Bacon PJ, Love SA, Gupta AK, Kirkpatrick PJ, Menon DK (1996) Plasma antioxidant consumption associated with ischemia/reperfusion during carotid endarterectomy. Stroke 27:1808–1811

214. Reigel MM, Hollier LH, Sundt TM Jr, Piepgras DG, Sharbrough FW, Cherry KJ (1987) Cerebral hyperperfusion syndrome: a cause of neurologic dysfunction after carotid endarterectomy. J Vasc Surg 5:628–634

215. Kieburtz K, Ricotta JJ, Moxley RT III (1990) Seizures following carotid endarterectomy. Arch Neurol 47:568–570

216. Naylor AR, Evans J, Thompson MM, London NJ, Abbott RJ, Cherryman G et al (2003) Seizures after carotid endarterectomy: hyperperfusion, dysautoregulation or hypertensive encephalopathy? Eur J Vasc Endovasc Surg 26:39–44

217. Abou-Chebl A, Yadav JS, Reginelli JP, Bajzer C, Bhatt D, Krieger DW (2004) Intracranial hemorrhage and hyperperfusion syndrome following carotid artery stenting: risk factors, prevention, and treatment. J Am Coll Cardiol 43:1596–1601

218. Sbarigia E, Speziale F, Giannoni MF, Colonna M, Panico MA, Fiorani P (1993) Post-carotid endarterectomy hyperperfusion syndrome: preliminary observations for identifying at risk patients by transcranial Doppler sonography and the acetazolamide test. Eur J Vasc Surg 7:252–256

219. Powers AD, Smith RR (1990) Hyperperfusion syndrome after carotid endarterectomy: a transcranial Doppler evaluation. Neurosurgery 26:56–59 discussion 59–60

220. Ogasawara K, Konno H, Yukawa H, Endo H, Inoue T, Ogawa A (2003) Transcranial regional cerebral oxygen saturation monitoring during carotid endarterectomy as a predictor of postoperative hyperperfusion. Neurosurgery 53:309–314 discussion 314–305

221. Aidi S, Chaunu MP, Biousse V, Bousser MG (1999) Changing pattern of headache pointing to cerebral venous thrombosis after lumbar puncture and intravenous high-dose corticosteroids. Headache 39:559–564

222. Stam J (2003) Cerebral venous and sinus thrombosis: incidence and causes. Adv Neurol 92:225–232

223. Wilder-Smith E, Kothbauer-Margreiter I, Lammle B, Sturzenegger M, Ozdoba C, Hauser SP (1997) Dural puncture and activated protein C resistance: risk factors for cerebral venous sinus thrombosis. J Neurol Neurosurg Psychiatry 63:351–356

224. Ehtisham A, Stern BJ (2006) Cerebral venous thrombosis: a review. The Neurologist 12:32–38

225. Ferro JM, Canhao P (2008) Acute treatment of cerebral venous and dural sinus thrombosis. Curr treat options neurol 10:126–137

226. Kurkowska-Jastrzebska I, Wicha W, Dowzenko A, Vertun-Baranowska B, Pytlewski A, Boguslawska R et al (2003) Concomitant heterozygous factor V Leiden mutation and homozygous prothrombin gene variant (G20210A) in patient with cerebral venous thrombosis. Med Sci Monit 9:CS41–CS45

227. Breteau G, Mounier-Vehier F, Godefroy O, Gauvrit JY, Mackowiak-Cordoliani MA, Girot M et al (2003) Cerebral venous thrombosis 3-year clinical outcome in 55 consecutive patients. J Neurol 250:29–35

228. de Bruijn SF, de Haan RJ, Stam J (2001) Clinical features and prognostic factors of cerebral venous sinus thrombosis in a prospective series of 59 patients. For The Cerebral Venous Sinus Thrombosis Study Group. J Neurol Neurosurg Psychiatry 70:105–108

229. Preter M, Tzourio C, Ameri A, Bousser MG (1996) Long-term prognosis in cerebral venous thrombosis. Follow-up of 77 patients. Stroke 27:243–246

230. Ferro JM, Canhao P, Stam J, Bousser MG, Barinagarrementeria F (2004) Prognosis of cerebral vein and dural sinus thrombosis: results of the International Study on Cerebral Vein and Dural Sinus Thrombosis (ISCVT). Stroke 35:664–670

231. Stolz E, Rahimi A, Gerriets T, Kraus J, Kaps M (2005) Cerebral venous thrombosis: an all or nothing disease? Prognostic factors and long-term outcome. Clin Neurol Neurosurg 107:99–107

232. Ribes M (1825) Des recherches faites sur la phlebite. Revue Medicale Francaise et Etrangere et Journal de clinique de l' Hotel-Dieu et de la Charite de Paris 3:5–41

233. Bousser MG, Chiras J, Bories J, Castaigne P (1985) Cerebral venous thrombosis–a review of 38 cases. Stroke 16:199–213

234. Terazzi E, Mittino D, Ruda R, Cerrato P, Monaco F, Sciolla R et al (2005) Cerebral venous thrombosis: a retrospective multicentre study of 48 patients. Neurological Sciences 25:311–315

235. Ferro JM, Correia M, Rosas MJ, Pinto AN, Neves G (2003) Seizures in cerebral vein and dural sinus thrombosis. Cerebrovasc Dis 15:78–83

236. Hubbert CH (1987) Dural puncture headache suspected, cortical vein thrombosis diagnosed. Anesth Analg 66:285

237. Ravindran RS, Zandstra GC, Viegas OJ (1989) Postpartum headache following regional analgesia; a symptom of cerebral venous thrombosis. Can J Anaesth 36:705–707

238. Schou J, Scherb M (1986) Postoperative sagittal sinus thrombosis after spinal anesthesia. Anesth Analg 65:541–542

239. Barinagarrementeria F, Cantu C, Arredondo H (1992) Aseptic cerebral venous thrombosis proposed prognostic scale. J Stroke Cerebrovasc Dis 1:34–39

240. de Bruijn SF, Stam J (1999) Randomized, placebo-controlled trial of anticoagulant treatment with low-molecular-weight heparin for cerebral sinus thrombosis. Stroke 30:484–488

241. Ferro JM, Lopes MG, Rosas MJ, Ferro MA, Fontes J (2002) Long-term prognosis of cerebral vein and dural sinus thrombosis. results of the VENOPORT study. Cerebrovasc Dis 13:272–278

242. Cakmak S, Derex L, Berruyer M, Nighoghossian N, Philippeau F, Adeleine P et al (2003) Cerebral venous thrombosis: clinical outcome and systematic screening of prothrombotic factors. Neurology 60:1175–1178

243. Masuhr F, Busch M, Amberger N, Ortwein H, Weih M, Neumann K et al (2006) Risk and predictors of early epileptic seizures in acute cerebral venous and sinus thrombosis. Eur J Neurol 13:852–856

244. Ferro JM, Canhao P, Bousser MG, Stam J, Barinagarrementeria F (2008) Early seizures in cerebral vein and dural sinus thrombosis: risk factors and role of antiepileptics. Stroke 39:1152–1158

245. Kwan J, Guenther A (2006) Antiepileptic drugs for the primary and secondary prevention of seizures after intracranial venous thrombosis. Cochrane Database Syst Rev 3: CD005501.

246. Stam J, Majoie CB, van Delden OM, van Lienden KP, Reekers JA (2008) Endovascular thrombectomy and thrombolysis for severe cerebral sinus thrombosis: a prospective study. Stroke 39:1487–1490

247. Mehraein S, Schmidtke K, Villringer A, Valdueza JM, Masuhr F (2003) Heparin treatment in cerebral sinus and venous thrombosis: patients at risk of fatal outcome. Cerebrovasc Dis 15:17–21

248. Niwa J, Ohyama H, Matumura S, Maeda Y, Shimizu T (1998) Treatment of acute superior sagittal sinus thrombosis by t-PA infusion via venography–direct thrombolytic therapy in the acute phase. Surg Neurol 49:425–429

249. Gerszten PC, Welch WC, Spearman MP, Jungreis CA, Redner RL (1997) Isolated deep cerebral venous thrombosis treated by direct endovascular thrombolysis. Surg Neurol 48:261–266

Chapter 4

Traumatic Brain Injury and Seizures in the ICU

Andrew Beaumont

Abstract Seizures may occur in up to 22% of ICU patients with severe traumatic brain injury. There is a relatively high risk of nonconvulsive seizures in this population. Seizures may exacerbate the injury process and disrupt both patient care and family coping. Therefore, seizures should be recognized quickly and treated promptly. The clinician should have a high index of suspicion for seizures, especially in patients with clearly defined risk factors for seizure development. Continuous EEG monitoring should be considered in those patients who are considered to be at high risk of clinical or subclinical seizures. Seizure prophylaxis with antiepileptics is supported by the literature for the prevention of early seizures (defined as <7 days post-injury) but not for late seizures. Phenytoin and carbamazepine have been used in this setting, and both have been found to be efficacious in preventing early seizures. Phenytoin has several features that make it the best first line agent. Anticonvulsants have not been found to reduce the incidence of developing late posttraumatic seizures and therefore, prolonged prophylaxis with antiepileptics is not currently supported.

Keywords Traumatic brain injury, Nonconvulsive seizures, Seizure prophylaxis

4.1. Introduction

Traumatic brain injury (TBI) is an important health problem. In the US, an estimated 1.5–2.0 million people experience traumatic brain injury each year (1). Nearly a quarter of a million of these patients require hospitalization (2), and about 52,000 of these events result in death (3). This incidence equates to one hospitalization per 1,000 people each year (2). Many of these patients are admitted to the intensive care unit for initial stabilization and monitoring. The lifetime medical care costs of head injuries occurring in the US in 1985 were estimated to total $4.5 billion, including $3.5 billion for hospital costs. Seizures are a well known complication of traumatic brain injury with reported incidences ranging from 2 to 12% (4–14). The incidence of seizures is higher in severe TBI and also with penetrating injury (5, 15). Posttraumatic seizures are classified into immediate (<24 h), early, and late, on the basis of the relationship

From: *Seizures in Critical Care: A Guide to Diagnosis and Therapeutics*: Current Clinical Neurology, Second Edition, Edited by: P. Varelas, DOI 10.1007/978-1-60327-532-3_4,
© Humana Press, a part of Springer Science+Business Media, LLC 2005, 2010

between the time of injury and the time of seizure onset. The mechanisms that generate posttraumatic seizures are not known, and there may be differences in the pathophysiology of early and late seizures. Posttraumatic epilepsy is defined as two or more unprovoked seizures following injury, and must be viewed from a different perspective as a single post-TBI seizure (16).

One of the main goals of ICU care in TBI should be the prevention of physiological stresses that can worsen the injury. These secondary insults include hypoxia, hypotension, hyper/hypoglycemia, hypo/hyperperfusion, and neurotoxicity. Seizures are known to cause intense metabolic stress and also release significant quantities of neurotransmitters. Vespa et al. (2007) examined continuous EEG and microdialysis from ten patients with severe TBI and seizures with a matched cohort of ten patients without seizures (17). Seizures were associated with a higher mean intracranial pressure and a high mean lactate/pyruvate ratio.

Seizures, therefore, represent a potential for secondary insult, and some studies have demonstrated that they are associated with a worse outcome in TBI (18). It is, therefore, important to recognize seizures in patients with TBI and to treat them aggressively; care must also be given to diagnose nonconvulsive seizures promptly. Their significance in affecting outcome post-TBI is unknown, but they may be a potential risk factor. In addition, patients with recognized risk factors for post-traumatic seizures should receive anticonvulsant prophylaxis.

This chapter will review data regarding the incidence of posttraumatic seizures, particularly in the ICU population. Methods for diagnosing posttraumatic seizures will be reviewed, along with experimental data and current hypotheses regarding their pathophysiology. Methods of treating seizures in TBI and current recommendations for seizure prophylaxis will be discussed.

4.2. Incidence of Seizures in Traumatic Brain Injury

Estimates of the incidence of posttraumatic seizures have varied widely, ranging from 2 to 12% (6, 10, 14, 19). Most of these studies have been based on the civilian population and may be quite different from studies that addressed the problem in military populations. In the Vietnam Head Injury Study, 53% of veterans who had penetrating head injuries developed posttraumatic epilepsy, and half of those patients had seizures even 15 years after injury. However, the relative risk of developing epilepsy in these patients dropped from 580 times higher than the general age-matched population in the first year after TBI to 25 times higher, after 10 years (7). These studies used clinical evidence of seizure activity for establishing the diagnosis. A more recent prospective, nonrandomized, nonblinded study using continuous EEG monitoring in the ICU found that 22% of moderately to severely injured TBI patients experienced seizures (20). This study by Vespa et al. (1999) examined 94 patients with moderate to severe TBI for up to 14 days postinjury. Of the 22% patients with seizures, 52% had nonconvulsive or clinically silent seizures, and one-third of the group had status epilepticus. Interestingly, except for one patient without any clinical seizure activity, the patients in status had minimal clinical signs, including rhythmic facial twitching, eyelid fluttering, and irregular myoclonus that could easily be missed. All patients with status epilepticus died, compared with a 24% mortality rate in the non-seizure group. Other studies have indicated that seizures and nonconvulsive status epilepticus may occur more commonly than thought in the ICU. Young et al. (21) found that 43 of 127 (34%) critically ill, non-TBI patients had seizures in the ICU, on the basis of continuous EEG monitoring. Seventeen out of 43 (39.5%) were found to be in nonconvulsive status. Ronne-Engstrom and Winkler (2006) used continuous EEG in 70 patients with TBI and found a 33% incidence of seizures with onset 1–5 days after injury (22). Older age and low energy trauma were risk factors for developing seizures.

The incidence of late seizures is reported to vary according to injury severity. Annegers et al. (4) followed 4,541 cases of traumatic brain injury in Olmsted County, MN from 1935 to 1984. The relative risk of seizures was 1.5 (95% confidence interval 1.0–2.2) after mild injuries, but with no increase after 5 years; 2.9 (95% confidence interval 1.9–4.1) after moderate injuries; and 17.2 (95% confidence interval 12.3–23.6) after severe injuries. Significant risk factors for the development of posttraumatic seizures were brain contusion with subdural hematoma, skull fracture, loss of consciousness, or amnesia of greater than 24 h, and age over 65 years. Englander et al. (2003) found a 12% incidence of posttraumatic seizures in 647 TBI patients followed over 24 months (15). The highest cumulative probability for late seizures included biparietal contusions (66%), dural penetration (62.5%), multiple intracranial procedures (36.5%), multiple subcortical contusions (33.4%), evacuated subdural (27.8%), midline shift >5 mm (25.8%), and multiple cortical contusions (25%). In addition GCS was correlated with seizure incidence: GCS 3–8 had a cumulative seizure probability of 16.8%, whereas GCS 9–12 had 24.3% and GCS 13–15 had 8.0%. In a large prospective, randomized, double-blind seizure prophylaxis study from Seattle, Temkin et al. (2003) reported independent risk factors from Cox regression multivariate models. Five factors emerged as increasing seizure risk in this population: early seizures (within 7 days), coma for over 1 week, dural penetration, depressed skull fracture not surgically treated, and one or more nonreactive pupil (23). These findings are in agreement with Jennett (1975) who described that intracranial hemorrhage, linear and depressed skull fractures, focal/penetrating injuries, presence of focal neurological deficit, and prolonged amnesia (>24 h) are injury patterns associated with a higher incidence of seizures (10). Figure 4.1 shows examples of injuries associated with significant seizures.

Other factors that can predispose to the development of post-traumatic seizures include age (incidence is higher in the pediatric population (24)), history of alcohol abuse, previous seizures, and a family history of seizures (4). Genetic predisposition to post-TBI seizures is an interesting issue that has not been well-addressed to date. Similar injuries lead to a wide variety of seizure incidence and frequency. Not all studies agree on the genetic predisposition. Jennet found that family history of epilepsy was more common in patients aged less than 16 years with late post-TBI seizures (25). In the Vietnam Head Injury Study this factor was not predictive of either early or late seizures (7). In another study examining genetic susceptibility to epilepsy, seizure incidence among relatives of patients with post-TBI seizures was not higher than among the general population (26). In a prospective study of late post-traumatic seizures after moderate and severe TBI, 106 patients were examined for the ApoE locus by restriction fragment length polymorphism analysis

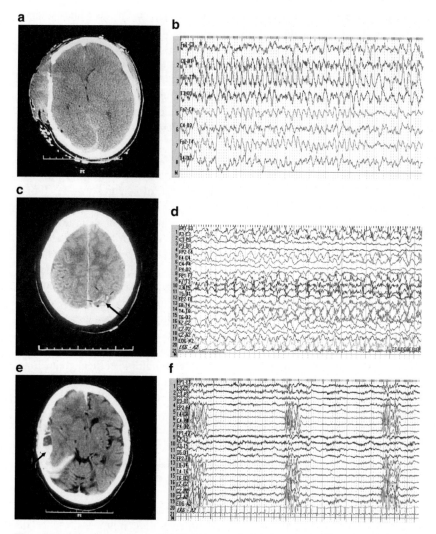

Fig. 4-1. Clinical examples of TBI patients admitted to the NICU, who developed seizures. Case 1: (**a**) A 26-year-old woman involved in a rollover MVC with prolonged extraction. The patient had a generalized tonic-clonic seizure on arrival in the trauma bay. She underwent an emergent craniotomy for large subdural hematoma, and postoperatively remained in coma. At some point the next day, she was noted to have some involuntary left and right leg movements. A single routine EEG at that time showed generalized slowing. The CT of the head after the surgery demonstrates diffuse cerebral edema and midline shift. (**b**) A continuous EEG was started to exclude nonconvulsive seizures. This shows sustained left sided epileptiform activity (runs of spike-slow waves), which, interestingly, did not correlate with any clinical movements. The patient was treated with benzodiazepines and phenytoin and slowly regained function, to the level of walking with assistance. Case 2: (**c**) A 20-year-old man brought to the trauma center with a gunshot wound to the head. He had GCS of 15 both at the scene and in the trauma bay. On CT of the head, the bullet had barely penetrated the calvarium, but he did have an area of contusion in the left parietal cortex (*arrow*). After admission for observation he was found at one point to be unresponsive. He quickly regained his level of consciousness, but was found to be having continued right sided facial twitching. (**d**) A representative strip of EEG from this patient showing left sided epileptiform activity (runs of polyspikes-slow waves), correlating with right face and arm twitches. He was successfully treated with a load of phenytoin. Case 3: (**e**) A 59-year-old woman with a history of atrial fibrillation, hypertension, and coumadin therapy was found on the

(27). Twenty-one patients had at least one late post-TBI seizure. The relative risk of late post-TBI seizures for patients with the e4 allele was 2.41 (95% CI 1.15–5.07, $p=0.03$). It is to be noted that the presence of this allele was not associated with an unfavorable outcome.

In studies examining posttraumatic seizures, an arbitrary definition of early and late is commonly used. Early seizures are defined as occurring in the first 7 days after injury and late seizures occur after this point. Early seizure incidence ranges from 2.1 to 16.9% (5, 25, 28). The incidence of late seizures ranges from 1.9 to 30% (16). However, this classification is potentially too restrictive. Many TBI patients remain critical in the ICU for longer than 7 days; it would be unreasonable to consider a seizure on the tenth hospital day a 'late' seizure. Some studies have extended the acute period to include the first month post-injury. This approach, however, is not ideal, as the underlying cause of seizures in the first week after injury is most likely different from the cause of seizures occurring in the first month or indeed in the first year after injury. Seizures in the first week are more likely related to neurochemical and metabolic derangements, whereas later seizures may be related to the formation of glial scar leading to cortical irritation. Also, there is a significant occurrence of seizures at the scene of both mild and severe TBIs (29, 30). These immediate seizures are more likely related to the direct disruption of cortical and subcortical connections as a result of percussive forces on the brain, and less likely the result of neurochemical or metabolic derangements. However, classifying the timing of onset of post-traumatic seizures is important for both trying to understand their pathophysiology and also in trying to define factors that can predict their occurrence.

A second important goal of dividing seizures by time of occurrence is to evaluate whether early seizures can predict the occurrence of late seizures, or the development of a long-term seizure problem. Early seizures are linked with late seizure development. The increased risk for late seizures after early seizures is independent of the actual number of seizures occurring during the first week after TBI (16). Not all studies however, report an increased incidence of late seizures after early pot-TBI seizures. In one large retrospective study from Olmsted County in Minnesota that examined 4,541 civilians with TBI during 1935–1984, Annegers et al. (1998), utilizing multivariate analysis, found that early seizures are not an independent risk factor for late post-traumatic epilepsy, and most likely early seizures are a marker of injury severity sufficient to cause late epilepsy (5). Another interesting observation is that the incidence of late seizures after early post-TBI seizures was dependent on the age of the patient. Children less than 16 years old may not be at increased risk for late seizures regardless of the early seizure type (4, 16). Studies have also indicated

---

Fig. 4-1. (continued) ground, unresponsive, after an unwitnessed fall. On arrival in the trauma bay, she was hypotensive, unresponsive, and flaccid to noxious stimuli but with preserved brainstem reflexes. CT of the head demonstrated a large right subdural hematoma (*arrow*). Following admission to the ICU, she was noted clinically to be having left sided intermittent twitching. (**f**) An EEG demonstrated runs of right hemispheric polyspikes or spikes and slow waves, separated by periods of relatively depressed background activity. The patient developed extensive cerebral edema and became brain dead despite medical treatment

Table 4-1. Risk Factors for Developing Early and Late Post-Traumatic Seizures. (Adapted from Frey (16)).

Risk factor	Increased risk for seizures	
	Early	Late
Acute intracerebral hematoma	+	+
Acute subdural hematoma	+	+
LOC or post-TBI amnesia >30 min	+	
LOC or post-TBI amnesia >24 h		+
Younger age (children)	+	
Older age (>65 years)		+
Diffuse cerebral edema (children)	+	
Depressed/Linear skull fracture	+	+
Metal fragment retention	+	+
Focal neurological deficits	+	+
Persistent EEG changes (>1 month)		+
Early post-TBI seizures		+
Chronic alcoholism		+

LOC loss of consciousness, + risk factor has been shown to increase the risk of seizures at the specified time-point.

that seizures at the scene of the trauma (i.e., immediate seizures) are not linked with any increased risk of developing late seizures (10, 29).

The incidence of posttraumatic seizures differs in the pediatric population. The overall incidence is higher than in adults (5, 24, 28). Early posttraumatic seizures occur slightly more commonly (13), with reported incidence rates of 9–15% (13, 24, 31–33). As with adults, there is a close correlation between injury severity and the incidence of any type of seizures. Hahn et al. (1988) demonstrated that the incidence of posttraumatic seizures was seven times greater in children with severe TBI and GCS <8, compared with milder injury and higher GCS (31). Young age is also an important risk factor for seizures, with younger age having higher risk (32–34). The occurrence of early seizures in severe TBI is also higher than that in the adult population, with reported incidences as high as 38.7% in one study (32). Furthermore, early seizures tend to occur even earlier in children; up to 50–80% of early seizures in the pediatric population occur in the first 24 h after injury (24, 35). Table 4-1 summarizes the risk factors for early and late seizures.

4.3. Experimental Approaches to Posttraumatic Seizures

Immediate posttraumatic seizures have been described in several experimental models of traumatic brain injury including the impact acceleration model of diffuse TBI and models of cortical contusion (36, 37). One study monitored EEG for 2 h post-injury in rodents exposed to a cortical contusion, and generalized seizure activity was recorded in 14 out of 17 cases, at a mean time of 67 s after trauma (37). Concurrent microdialysis measured a consistent increase in aspartate, taurine, glutamate, and glycine; however, it is not clear if this represented a cause or a consequence of the seizures. Longer term behavioral studies in experimental TBI have not demonstrated any significant evidence of clinical seizure activity (38, 39). This finding is at odds with the clinical behavior of TBI and it may relate to differences in seizure thresholds between rodents and humans.

The origin of posttraumatic seizures is not known and improved understanding requires a good experimental model. Studies have evaluated in vivo seizure activity, in vitro seizure activity in brain tissue from injured animals, and in vitro seizure activity in brain tissue injured in vitro. In vivo models have focused on either direct observation of seizures, or stimulation of seizures by cortical injection of ferrous chloride (40); the latter technique is thought to mimic cortical accumulation of blood breakdown products, and causes recurrent focal epileptiform discharges. One of the in vitro approaches used isolated hippocampal slices from the brains of injured animals, followed by in vitro electrophysiological recording (41). In vitro models of traumatic brain injury have difficulty in reproducing a meaningful level of trauma. Models have included scraping hippocampal slices or stretching neurons grown in culture (42, 43). Combining all these techniques, Golarai et al. (2001) examined changes in the rodent brain after weight drop injury to the somatosensory cortex (44). They found an early selective cell loss in the dentate gyrus and area CA3 of the hippocampus, a persistently enhanced susceptibility to pentylenetetrazole-induced seizures for up to 15 weeks after injury and an abnormal hyperexcitability in the granule cell and molecular layers of the dentate gyrus.

4.4. Pathophysiology of Posttraumatic Seizures

The pathophysiological mechanisms causing posttraumatic seizures are not well-understood, and there is likely some variation depending on the time of onset after injury. Posttraumatic seizures should be thought of as primary and secondary. Primary post-traumatic seizures are those caused by direct effects of the brain injury itself. Secondary seizures are caused by other epileptogenic factors not directly related to the injury, such as fever, metabolic and electrolyte abnormalities, or drug reactions. Primary and secondary seizures are related in that the injury itself may contribute to a reduction in the seizure threshold, thereby increasing the epileptogenicity of the factors that can cause secondary seizures.

Traumatic brain injury is characterized by a cascade of metabolic and neurochemical events which start at the time of injury and continue throughout the acute and subacute phases of injury of which many are potentially epileptogenic. Examples include hyperglycolysis (45), pH changes, extracellular elevation of glutamate (and other amino acids) (46, 47), transient flux of ions including sodium and potassium, (48), altered cerebral blood flow (49), and loss of the inhibitory neuronal pool.

Elevations in extracellular excitatory amino acids can cause widespread depolarization that may reach seizure threshold. Loss of inhibitory neurons may promote generation of a seizure focus. Ionic transients may shift the cell membrane equilibrium potential either causing action potential generation or a reduction in the stimulus threshold required to generate an action potential.

Changes in extracellular pH can also shift the membrane potential; alkalosis tends to cause depolarization. Seizures arising in the more chronic phases of injury are less likely caused by acute changes in cellular physiology. These late seizures are more likely related to the influence of glial scars, breakdown products of hemoglobin, death of inhibitory interneurons, or disruption of neuronal connections with formation of abnormal neosynapses with greater excitatory potential (50).

Epileptogenesis may not be entirely a neuronal phenomenon. It is known that glial membrane channels participate in ionic homeostasis (51) especially at times of neuronal activity. In particular, glial cells buffer levels of extracellular potassium, and failure of this mechanism can result in increased neuronal excitability and seizures (52). Electrophysiological recordings in hippocampal slices from experimentally injured brains have demonstrated reductions in inward and outward potassium currents, and abnormal accumulation of extracellular potassium. Abnormal glial buffering of potassium may represent one mechanism of posttraumatic seizure development (41).

Seizures themselves also place a stress on both the brain and organism, and these stresses may contribute to the injury forming a vicious cycle of repeated injury and further seizure generation. In particular, seizures have been shown to cause hyperglycolysis, elevated extracellular amino acids including glutamate (53), elevated extracellular glycerol levels (suggestive of cell membrane breakdown (54)), hyperperfusion (55), changes in extracellular levels of bioactive lipids (56), alterations in neurotransmitter receptor expression (57), alterations in neurotransmitter uptake mechanisms (58), and changes in synaptic morphology (59).

The impact of seizures on macroscopic physiological parameters in traumatic brain injury has not been well studied. In a study using continuous EEG monitoring in ICU patients with severe TBI (20), the incidence of raised ICP was similar in both seizure and non-seizure patients. The mean ICP was higher in the seizure group (15.6 vs. 11.8 mm Hg, $p < 0.001$); however, this finding may simply reflect seizures occurring in the most severely injured patients. A separate analysis comparing ICP values in individual patients on seizure days and non-seizure days demonstrated no significant difference. Furthermore serial trends of ICP in the hours before and after seizure events did not demonstrate a clear seizure-related effect. Seizures can cause profound hypotension and hypoxia (in the nonventilated patient) and prolonged myoclonic and tonic/clonic activity can lead to excess tissue and serum lactate levels and acidosis. These factors may constitute secondary insults, known to worsen outcome after TBI (60).

4.5. Diagnosis of Seizures

The occurrence of seizures can be suspected by clinical activity, but EEG confirmation is required. The clinical appearance of early seizures in the ICU includes generalized tonic-clonic, and focal seizures. Complex partial seizures may also occur, but documentation of these in an intubated, sedated patient is difficult. Focal seizures can appear as rhythmic myoclonic activity or as a more subtle finding, such as a facial twitch (20). Seizures may also manifest as a decrease in mental status, and any work up for this problem after TBI should include an evaluation for seizures. Seizures may be masked in the ICU population by the use of neuromuscular blocking agents and therefore, caution should be taken when using these agents in patients who are at higher risk of posttraumatic seizures. If prolonged paralysis is needed, one should consider continuous EEG monitoring in high risk patients.

The EEG can be utilized in different ways for diagnosing posttraumatic seizures. The simplest method is to obtain an EEG in a patient clinically suspected of having seizures. However, this EEG is a snapshot of the injured brain's electrical activity. If it does not capture a single seizure event or nonconvulsive status, then seizure diagnosis relies on being able to identify abnormal interictal activity. If there is a significant delay in obtaining the EEG then seizure activity may not be seen and the diagnostic yield of the study is compromised. Few studies have examined the benefit of frequent screening of EEGs or continuous EEG monitoring. Dawson et al. (1951) obtained serial short-duration EEGs in 45 brain injured patients every few days during the first 14 days and found a 25% incidence of seizures by EEG criteria (61). Vespa et al. (1999) examined the role of continuous EEG monitoring in moderate to severe TBI and found a 22% incidence of seizures among 94 patients admitted to the ICU (20). More importantly, 52% of the patients with seizures had no clinical evidence of seizure activity. Additionally in the subgroup with no clinical or electrographic seizures, 10% of patients had epileptiform and nonepileptiform activity. Epileptiform activity included isolated spikes or sharp waves and/or repetitive sharp waves. Pseudoperiodic lateralized epileptiform discharges (PLEDs) were also seen in patients without other evidence of seizures. Nonepileptiform EEG abnormalities observed in these patients included symmetric disorganized slowing, asymmetrical disorganized delta waves with a focus, intermittent rhythmic delta activity, absence of sleep potentials, and progressive loss of EEG amplitude with burst suppression. The latter was associated with impending brain death. Other EEG abnormalities were observed, including increased beta activity, amplitude suppression and burst suppression. These patterns were seen in both the seizure and non-seizure groups and are related to sedative hypnotics, such as midazolam or propofol. Other studies have described a loss of EEG reactivity to external stimuli and loss of spontaneous variability (62–65). Alpha coma is a term used to refer to coma in the presence of widespread alpha (8–12 Hz) activity in anterior-central cortical areas. This finding is associated with a poor prognosis in TBI patients (66–69).

The findings of the aforementioned study on continuous EEG monitoring in TBI support the use of longer monitoring in severely brain injured patients for early diagnosis and treatment of seizures (20). Analysis of the EEG is also important in making determinations regarding seizures. Many studies have focused on compressed spectral array and other quantitative methods, whereas the highest yield of information comes from both trend analysis and examination of the raw EEG data. Vespa et al. (1999) used frequency analysis by fast Fourier transformation in the ICU, followed by examination of 2 min epochs that were evaluated for any increases in total power (20). Any epochs in which increased spectral power was observed had the raw EEG data analyzed for evidence of seizures. The trend analysis was therefore used to flag periods where seizures might have occurred and this approach allowed a more focused examination of the raw EEG. Power spectral analysis has also been used to examine prognosis in TBI. Poor prognosis is frequently associated with unvarying activity, and a predominance of delta band activity (1–3 Hz) (62). Variable spectral patterns are associated with better prognosis (62, 70), as are persistence or return of a peak in the alpha or theta frequency (71, 72). Finally, the urgency of ordering the EEG when seizures are suspected after TBI has to be considered. In one recent study, 23 emergent EEGs (EmEEG), defined as studies performed in less than 1 h from request, were ordered mainly in post-TBI ICU patients (73). The reason for ordering the test was to rule out convulsive status epilepticus in 12 patients, non-convulsive status epilepticus in six, and seizures in another six patients. Clinical seizures before the test was performed were observed in three patients and suspicious clinical activity (unclear to the observers if it represented seizures) was observed in 12 additional patients. The EmEEG showed convulsive status epilepticus in three patients, non-convulsive status in two patients, and epileptiform activity or electrographic seizures in four patients. Half of the patients were already on antiepileptic therapy when the test was performed.

4.6. Treatment of Posttraumatic Seizures

There are two principal goals of treating posttraumatic seizures in the ICU. Firstly, in the acute posttraumatic period the goal should be rapid cessation of seizure activity in order to prevent secondary physiological and biochemical insults and worsening injury. Secondly, further episodes of seizure activity should be prevented. There has been some debate about whether prevention of early seizures can result in a lower incidence of late posttraumatic seizures. Studies have also addressed whether long-term prophylaxis with antiepileptic agents is indicated (11, 74).

The initial management of seizures in the critically ill brain injured patient should include close observation of vital signs to ensure adequate oxygenation and end-organ perfusion, and adherence to ACLS and ATLS guidelines for assessment of ABCs. In the nonintubated TBI patient, intubation and mechanical ventilation should be considered depending on the severity of the injury, the duration of mental status change, and the ability to protect the airway. An assessment of the seizure's origin should also be made. It should not always be assumed that seizures are primarily related to the brain injury. Critically ill patients are exposed to a wide variety of metabolic and pharmacological stressors that may trigger seizures independently of any brain injury. Such stressors include hypoglycemia, hyponatremia, hypocalcemia, hypophosphatemia, hypoxemia, hypocarbia, alcohol/recreational drug withdrawal, fever, meningoencephalitis, and hepatorenal failure. If seizures are newly diagnosed in a brain injured patient, any of these complicating factors should be evaluated for and corrected as needed. Furthermore, a combination of these factors may interact in an additive fashion with the injury to trigger seizures, where each factor by itself would be insufficient.

A patient not currently on antiepileptics should be started on either phenytoin (15–18 mg/kg IV loading dose and 300–400 mg/day IV or enteral, with frequent assessment of serum levels and a goal of 10–20 mg/dl), valproic acid (15–20 mg/kg IV loading dose and 600–3,000 mg/day IV or enteral) or carbamazepine (600–1,200 mg/day via enteral route). Phenytoin has benefits over other agents including the ability to load rapidly, the ability to titrate dose to effect, the widespread ability to follow serum levels, and a long standing clinical experience with the agent. Negative factors against dilantin is the risk of Stevens-Johnson syndrome, reliance on hepatic clearance and variability in serum levels due to complex pharmacokinetics, and therefore difficulty targeting the therapeutic range. Newer antiepileptic agents such as levetiracetam are becoming available in intravenous form and levels can be checked. These are promising agents for future use, but with limited data so far.

Prolonged seizures should be stopped rapidly using one of the sedative hypnotic agents at higher dose, such as lorazepam (1–2 mg IV), diazepam (10–20 mg IV), midazolam (2–5 mg IV), sodium thiopentone (100–300 mg IV), or propofol (50–200 mg IV). Seizures that are recurrent or ongoing despite the above measures should be treated as status epilepticus. Higher doses of benzodiazepines should be given (lorazepam 5–10 mg, diazepam 20–40 mg, or midazolam 5–20 mg, all as IV slow boluses), and if the seizures remain refractory to those measures, then a propofol (150 mcg/kg/min), thiopental (0.3–0.4 mg/kg/min), or pentobarbital (0.2–0.4 mg/kg/min) infusions should be started with continuous EEG monitoring and a goal of achieving EEG burst suppression (see Chapter on Treatment of Seizures in Critical Care).

Several studies have examined the efficacy of antiepileptics in preventing early seizures. The largest prospective, randomized, double-blind, placebo controlled trial to date examined 404 brain injured patients given phenytoin prophylaxis or placebo for 1 year after traumatic brain injury (11). The follow-up was continued for 2 years and phenytoin levels were maintained in the high therapeutic range. A significant reduction in early seizures (<7 days) was observed. Patients receiving phenytoin had a 3.6% incidence of seizures as compared with 14.2% in the placebo group ($p<0.001$, risk ratio 0.27, 95% CI 0.12–0.62). No significant reduction in the development of late seizures was reported. By the end of the first year 21.5% of phenytoin treated patients and 15.7% of the placebo patients had seizures. By the end of the second year, these numbers had increased to 27.5% and 21.1% respectively ($p>0.2$). In addition, the incidence of adverse drug effects in the first two weeks of treatment was low (75). Hypersensitivity reactions occurred in 2.5% of the phenytoin treated patients as compared to 0% of the placebo patients ($p=0.12$) during the first two weeks of treatment. On the basis of these findings, the Seattle group advocates the use of prophylactic phenytoin administration for the first 1–2 weeks after injury. Other studies have also confirmed the ability of phenytoin to reduce the incidence of early seizures (76).

Other antiepileptics have been evaluated; Glotzner et al. (1983) found in a group of 139 TBI patients that carbamazepine can significantly reduce seizure incidence (77). Temkin et al. (1999) conducted another randomized, double-blind study comparing phenytoin to valproic acid for the prevention of post-TBI seizures. In this study, 132 patients were randomized to receive either phenytoin or valproic acid (78). Incidence of early and late seizures did not differ between the phenytoin and valproic acid groups.

Several studies have examined the role of seizure prophylaxis in preventing late onset posttraumatic seizures and only one study has found a beneficial effect of long-term seizure prophylaxis (76). This study was not blinded or placebo controlled, however. Thirty four patients with severe TBI were randomized to receive phenytoin for 3 months and were compared with 52 untreated severe TBI patients. After 2 years, 6% of patients treated with phenytoin developed posttraumatic epilepsy as compared with 42% of the untreated group. McQueen et al. (1983) evaluated 164 patients in a prospective, randomized double blind study comparing phenytoin and placebo, and found no beneficial effect in the reduction of late seizure (74). Temkin et al. (1990) in their large well controlled study of 404 patients did not find any reduction in late posttraumatic seizures (11). Studies of other agents including carbamazepine (77) and phenobarbital (79) have also been unable to demonstrate any clear benefit on the incidence of late seizures. Glotzner et al. (1983) evaluated carbamazepine in a prospective, randomized, double-blind study of 139 patients and found no significant reduction in late posttraumatic seizures (77). Manaka et al. (1992) conducted a prospective, randomized, double-blind study of 126 patients receiving placebo or phenobarbital and found no reduction in late seizures in the treatment group (79).

There is very little information available regarding the use of levetiracetam in traumatic brain injury. Jones et al. (2008) reported on data collected from 32 cases of severe TBI treated with levetiracetam and compared with a historical cohort of 41 cases treated with phenytoin monotherapy (80). Their data suggest that levetiracetam has an equivalent protective benefit as compared with dilantin within the numbers of patients analyzed, but that it might be associated with a higher number of abnormalities on EEG and therefore may be associated with a higher tendency for seizures. A larger cohort would be required to evaluate whether this translates into reduced seizure protection.

Clearly the occurrence of seizures needs to be rapidly treated in brain-injured patients. The clinical evidence at present supports the use of seizure prophylaxis for the prevention of early seizures (<7 days from injury), but does not support long term administration of antiepileptics for the prevention of late onset seizures (81, 82) (Table 4-2). Specific risk factors for developing posttraumatic seizures have been identified including GCS <10, depressed skull fracture, cortical contusion, subdural/epidural hematomas, intracerebral hematoma, penetrating injury, focal deficit, or prolonged amnesia (>24 h) (10, 11, 23).

Table 4-2. Summary of Studies in the Literature that Examine Prophylaxis Against the Risk of Early and Late Seizures Following Traumatic Brain Injury, and the Antiepileptic Drug Used.

Study	Drug used	Early seizures	Late seizures
Young et al. 86)	DPH	0.99 (0.27–3.61)	
Young et al. (83)	DPH		1.29 (0.56–3.0)
McQueen et al. (74)	DPH		1.09 (0.41–2.86)
Glotzner et al. (77)	CBZ	0.37 (0.18–0.78)*	0.71 (0.39–1.3)
Temkin et al. (11)	DPH	0.25 (0.11–0.57)*	1.3 (0.82–2.08)
Pechadre et al. (76)	DPH		0.14 (0.03–0.55)
Manaka (79)	PB		1.38 (0.54–3.5)
Temkin (78)	VPA	2.9 (0.7–13.3)	1.4 (0.8–2.4)

Values represent relative risk with the 95% confidence interval in parentheses.
*Significant with $p < 0.05$.

It is recommended that particular attention is given to seizure prophylaxis in the subgroup of brain injured patients with these pathologies.

4.7. Outcome of Seizures Complicating TBI

It is pertinent to ask whether the benefits of seizure prophylaxis on early seizures reported in the literature translates into improved mortality or morbidity. Few studies have specifically addressed outcomes in relation to seizure prophylaxis (11, 74, 76, 77, 83). No study to date has demonstrated any improvement in mortality as a result of administering anticonvulsants. A meta-analysis of several studies described a pooled relative risk of 1.15 (95% CI 0.89–1.51) for mortality in treated vs. untreated patients implying treatment has no effect on mortality (84). Two studies have examined outcome in surviving patients in relation to seizure prophylaxis. Glotzner et al. (1983) found a worse outcome in the treated group (RR 1.49, 95% CI 1.06–2.08, $p = 0.183$) (77) and Temkin et al. (1990) found no overall effect of seizure prophylaxis on patient outcome (RR 0.96, 95% CI 0.72–1.39, $p = 0.75$) (11). One study comparing the efficacy of phenytoin and valproate actually found a trend to a higher mortality in the valproate treated group (RR 2.0, 95% CI 0.9–4.1, $p = 0.07$), but it is unclear whether this is clinically significant (78). A recent study using continuous EEG monitoring in critically ill ICU patients did not find any differences in either mortality or outcome at the time of discharge between the groups of patients with or without seizures (20). However, six patients with status epilepticus were identified, of whom three were found to be in nonconvulsive status. All six of the patients ultimately died, two due to sepsis after control of status epilepticus, three of them from progressive neurological deterioration and brain death, and one patient from late respiratory arrest. Clearly the occurrence of status epilepticus is a grave prognostic sign in the traumatically brain injured patient, and the high risk of non-convulsive status suggests that EEG recording should be more frequently utilized in this patient population. Finally the potential benefit for using antiepileptic drug prophylaxis after TBI has to be weighed against the potential risk for impeding recovery of brain function from these compounds in addition to safety and cost (85).

4.8. Conclusions

Seizures may occur in up to 22% of ICU patients with severe traumatic brain injury. There is a relatively high risk of nonconvulsive seizures in this population. Seizures may exacerbate the injury process and disrupt both patient care and family coping. Therefore, seizures should be recognized quickly and treated promptly. The clinician should have a high index of suspicion for seizures, especially in patients with clearly defined risk factors for seizure development. Continuous EEG monitoring should be considered in those patients who are considered to be at high risk of clinical or subclinical seizures. Seizure prophylaxis with antiepileptics is supported by the literature for the prevention of early seizures (defined as <7 days post-injury) but not for late seizures. Phenytoin and carbamazepine have been used in this setting and both found to be efficacious in preventing early seizures. More experience is being gained with newer agents, such as levetiracetam.

Anticonvulsants have not been found to reduce the incidence of developing late post-traumatic seizures, and therefore, prolonged prophylaxis with antiepileptics is not currently supported.

References

1. Sosin DM, Sniezek JE, Thurman DJ (1996) Incidence of mild and moderate brain injury in the United States, 1991. Brain Inj 10(1):47–54
2. Thurman D, Guerrero J (1999) Trends in hospitalization associated with traumatic brain injury. JAMA 282(10):954–957
3. Sosin DM, Sniezek JE, Waxweiler RJ (1995) Trends in death associated with traumatic brain injury, 1979 through 1992. Success and failure. JAMA 273(22):1778–1780
4. Annegers JF, Grabow JD, Kurland LT, Laws ER Jr (1980) The incidence, causes, and secular trends of head trauma in Olmsted County, Minnesota, 1935–1974. Neurology 30(9):912–919
5. Annegers JF, Hauser WA, Coan SP, Rocca WA (1998) A population-based study of seizures after traumatic brain injuries. N Engl J Med 338(1):20–24
6. Lee ST, Lui TN, Wong CW, Yeh YS, Tzaan WC (1995) Early seizures after moderate closed head injury. Acta Neurochir (Wien) 137(3–4):151–154
7. Salazar AM, Jabbari B, Vance SC, Grafman J, Amin D, Dillon JD (1985) Epilepsy after penetrating head injury. I. Clinical correlates: a report of the Vietnam Head Injury Study. Neurology 35(10):1406–1414
8. Hauser WA (1990) Prevention of post-traumatic epilepsy. N Engl J Med 323(8):540–542
9. Hauser WA, Tabaddor K, Factor PR, Finer C (1984) Seizures and head injury in an urban community. Neurology 34(6):746–751
10. Jennett WB (1975) Epilepsy after nonmissile head injuries, 2nd edn. Heinemann, London
11. Temkin NR, Dikmen SS, Wilensky AJ, Keihm J, Chabal S, Winn HR (1990) A randomized, double-blind study of phenytoin for the prevention of post-traumatic seizures. N Engl J Med 323(8):497–502
12. Kollevold T (1976) Immediate and early cerebral seizures after head injuries. Part I. J Oslo City Hosp 26(12):99–114
13. Black P, Shepard RH, Walker AE (1975) Outcome of head trauma: age and post-traumatic seizures. Ciba Found Symp (34):215–226
14. Scholtes FB, Renier WO, Meinardi H (1994) Generalized convulsive status epilepticus: causes, therapy, and outcome in 346 patients. Epilepsia 35(5):1104–1112
15. Englander J, Bushnik T, Duong TT, Cifu DX, Zafonte R, Wright J et al (2003) Analyzing risk factors for late posttraumatic seizures: a prospective, multicenter investigation. Arch Phys Med Rehabil 84(3):365–373
16. Frey LC (2003) Epidemiology of posttraumatic epilepsy: a critical review. Epilepsia 44(Suppl 10):11–17
17. Vespa PM, Miller C, McArthur D, Eliseo M, Etchepare M, Hirt D, Glenn TC, Martin N, Hovda D (2007) Nonconvulsive electrographic seizures after traumatic brain injury results in intracranial pressure and metabolic crisis. Crit Care Med 35(12):2830–2836
18. Wiedemayer H, Triesch K, Schafer H, Stolke D (2002) Early seizures following non-penetrating traumatic brain injury in adults: risk factors and clinical significance. Brain Inj 16(4):323–330
19. Annegers JF, Grabow JD, Groover RV, Laws ER Jr, Elveback LR, Kurland LT (1980) Seizures after head trauma: a population study. Neurology 30(7 Pt 1):683–689
20. Vespa PM, Nuwer MR, Nenov V, Ronne-Engstrom E, Hovda DA, Bergsneider M et al (1999) Increased incidence and impact of nonconvulsive and convulsive seizures after traumatic brain injury as detected by continuous electroencephalographic monitoring. J Neurosurg 91(5):750–760

21. Young GB, Jordan KG, Doig GS (1996) An assessment of nonconvulsive seizures in the intensive care unit using continuous EEG monitoring: an investigation of variables associated with mortality. Neurology 47(1):83–89

22. Ronne-Engrstrom E, Winkler T (2006) Continuous EEG monitoring in patients with traumatic brain injury reveals a high incidence of epileptiform activity. Acta Neurol Scand 114(1):47–53

23. Temkin NR (2003) Risk factors for posttraumatic seizures in adults. Epilepsia 44(Suppl 10):18–20

24. Mansfield RT (1997) Head injuries in children and adults. Crit Care Clin 13(3):611–628

25. Jennett WB, Lewin W (1960) Traumatic epilepsy after closed head injuries. J Neurol Neurosurg Psychiatry 23:295–301

26. Ottman R, Lee JH, Risch N, Hauser WA, Susser M (1996) Clinical indicators of genetic susceptibility to epilepsy. Epilepsia 37(4):353–361

27. Diaz-Arrastia R, Gong Y, Fair S, Scott KD, Garcia MC, Carlile MC et al (2003) Increased risk of late posttraumatic seizures associated with inheritance of APOE epsilon4 allele. Arch Neurol 60(6):818–822

28. Desai BT, Whitman S, Coonley-Hoganson R, Coleman TE, Gabriel G, Dell J (1983) Seizures and civilian head injuries. Epilepsia 24(3):289–296

29. McCrory PR, Bladin PF, Berkovic SF (1997) Retrospective study of concussive convulsions in elite Australian rules and rugby league footballers: phenomenology, aetiology, and outcome. BMJ 314(7075):171–174

30. McCrory PR, Berkovic SF (2000) Video analysis of acute motor and convulsive manifestations in sport- related concussion. Neurology 54(7):1488–1491

31. Hahn YS, Fuchs S, Flannery AM, Barthel MJ, McLone DG (1988) Factors influencing posttraumatic seizures in children. Neurosurgery 22(5):864–867

32. Lewis RJ, Yee L, Inkelis SH, Gilmore D (1993) Clinical predictors of post-traumatic seizures in children with head trauma. Ann Emerg Med 22(7):1114–1118

33. Ong LC, Dhillon MK, Selladurai BM, Maimunah A, Lye MS (1996) Early posttraumatic seizures in children: clinical and radiological aspects of injury. J Paediatr Child Health 32(2):173–176

34. Hahn YS, Chyung C, Barthel MJ, Bailes J, Flannery AM, McLone DG (1988) Head injuries in children under 36 months of age. Demography and outcome. Childs Nerv Syst 4(1):34–40

35. Hendrick EB, Harris L (1968) Post-traumatic epilepsy in children. J Trauma 8(4):547–556

36. Marmarou A, Foda MA, van den Brink W, Campbell J, Kita H, Demetriadou K (1994) A new model of diffuse brain injury in rats. Part I: Pathophysiology and biomechanics. J Neurosurg 80(2):291–300

37. Nilsson P, Ronne-Engstrom E, Flink R, Ungerstedt U, Carlson H, Hillered L (1994) Epileptic seizure activity in the acute phase following cortical impact trauma in rat. Brain Res 637(1–2):227–232

38. Beaumont A, Marmarou A, Czigner A, Yamamoto M, Demetriadou K, Shirotani T et al (1999) The impact-acceleration model of head injury: injury severity predicts motor and cognitive performance after trauma. Neurol Res 21(8):742–754

39. Hamm RJ, Pike BR, Temple MD, O'Dell DM, Lyeth BG (1995) The effect of postinjury kindled seizures on cognitive performance of traumatically brain-injured rats. Exp Neurol 136(2):143–148

40. Willmore LJ (1990) Post-traumatic epilepsy: cellular mechanisms and implications for treatment. Neurology 31(Suppl 3):S67–S73

41. D'Ambrosio R, Maris DO, Grady MS, Winn HR, Janigro D (1999) Impaired K(+) homeostasis and altered electrophysiological properties of post-traumatic hippocampal glia. J Neurosci 19(18):8152–8162

42. Rzigalinski BA, Weber JT, Williughby KA, Ellis EF (1998) Intracellular free calcium dynamics in stretch-injured astrocytes. J Neurochem 70(6):2377–2385

43. Yang L, Benardo LS (2000) Valproate prevents epileptiform activity after trauma in an in vitro model in neocortical slices. Epilepsia 41(12):1507–1513

44. Golarai G, Greenwood AC, Feeney DM, Connor JA (2001) Physiological and structural evidence for hippocampal involvement in persistent seizure susceptibility after traumatic brain injury. J Neurosci 21(21):8523–8537

45. Bergsneider M, Hovda DA, Shalmon E, Kelly DF, Vespa PM, Martin NA et al (1997) Cerebral hyperglycolysis following severe traumatic brain injury in humans: a positron emission tomography study. J Neurosurg 86(2):241–251

46. Bullock R, Zauner A, Myseros JS, Marmarou A, Woodward JJ, Young HF (1995) Evidence for prolonged release of excitatory amino acids in severe human head trauma. Relationship to clinical events. Ann N Y Acad Sci 765:290–297

47. Goodman JC, Valadka AB, Gopinath SP, Cormio M, Robertson CS (1996) Lactate and excitatory amino acids measured by microdialysis are decreased by pentobarbital coma in head-injured patients. J Neurotrauma 13(10):549–556

48. Nilsson P, Hillered L, Olsson Y, Sheardown MJ, Hansen AJ (1993) Regional changes in interstitial K+ and Ca2+ levels following cortical compression contusion trauma in rats. J Cereb Blood Flow Metab 13(2):183–192

49. DeWitt DS, Prough DS, Taylor CL, Whitley JM (1992) Reduced cerebral blood flow, oxygen delivery, and electroencephalographic activity after traumatic brain injury and mild hemorrhage in cats. J Neurosurg 76(5):812–821

50. McKinney RA, Debanne D, Gahwiler BH, Thompson SM (1997) Lesion-induced axonal sprouting and hyperexcitability in the hippocampus in vitro: implications for the genesis of posttraumatic epilepsy. Nat Med 3(9):990–996

51. Ballanyi K, Grafe P, ten Bruggencate G (1987) Ion activities and potassium uptake mechanisms of glial cells in guinea- pig olfactory cortex slices. J Physiol 382:159–174

52. Janigro D, Gasparini S, D'Ambrosio R, McKhann G, DiFrancesco D (1997) Reduction of K+ uptake in glia prevents long-term depression maintenance and causes epileptiform activity. J Neurosci 17(8):2813–2824

53. Carlson H, Ronne-Engstrom E, Ungerstedt U, Hillered L (1992) Seizure related elevations of extracellular amino acids in human focal epilepsy. Neurosci Lett 140(1):30–32

54. Vespa P, Martin NA, Nenov V, Glenn T, Bergsneider M, Kelly D et al (2002) Delayed increase in extracellular glycerol with post-traumatic electrographic epileptic activity: support for the theory that seizures induce secondary injury. Acta Neurochir Suppl 81:355–357

55. Duncan R (1992) Epilepsy, cerebral blood flow, and cerebral metabolic rate. Cerebrovasc Brain Metab Rev 4(2):105–121

56. Bazan NG, Tu B, Rodriguez de Turco EB (2002) What synaptic lipid signaling tells us about seizure-induced damage and epileptogenesis. Prog Brain Res 135:175–185

57. Doi T, Ueda Y, Tokumaru J, Mitsuyama Y, Willmore LJ (2001) Sequential changes in AMPA and NMDA protein levels during Fe(3+)- induced epileptogenesis. Brain Res Mol B

58. Samuelsson C, Kumlien E, Flink R, Lindholm D, Ronne-Engstrom E (2000) Decreased cortical levels of astrocytic glutamate transport protein GLT- 1 in a rat model of posttraumatic epilepsy. Neurosci Lett 289(3):185–188

59. Ben Ari Y (2001) Cell death and synaptic reorganizations produced by seizures. Epilepsia 42(Suppl 3):5–7

60. Chesnut RM, Marshall LF, Klauber MR, Blunt BA, Baldwin N, Eisenberg HM et al (1993) The role of secondary brain injury in determining outcome from severe head injury. J Trauma 34(2):216–222

61. Dawson RE, Webster JE, Gurdjian ES (1951) Serial electroencephalography in acute head injuries. J Neurosurg 8:613–630

62. Bricolo A, Turazzi S, Faccioli F, Odorizzi F, Sciaretta G, Erculiani P (1978) Clinical application of compressed spectral array in long-term EEG monitoring of comatose patients. Electroencephalogr Clin Neurophysiol 45(2):211–225

63. Hutchinson DO, Frith RW, Shaw NA, Judson JA, Cant BR (1991) A comparison between electroencephalography and somatosensory evoked potentials for outcome prediction following severe head injury. Electroencephalogr Clin Neurophysiol 78(3):228–233

64. Rumpl E, Lorenzi E, Hackl JM, Gerstenbrand F, Hengl W (1979) The EEG at different stages of acute secondary traumatic midbrain and bulbar brain syndromes. Electroencephalogr Clin Neurophysiol 46(5):487–497

65. Synek VM (1990) Revised EEG coma scale in diffuse acute head injuries in adults. Clin Exp Neurol 27:99–111

66. Hari R, Sulkava R, Haltia M (1982) Brainstem auditory evoked responses and alpha-pattern coma. Ann Neurol 11(2):187–189

67. Obeso JA, Iragui MI, Marti-Masso JF, Maravi E, Teijeira JM, Carrera N et al (1980) Neurophysiological assessment of alpha pattern coma. J Neurol Neurosurg Psychiatry 43(1):63–67

68. Stockard JJ, Bickford RG, Aung MH (1975) The electroencephalogram in traumatic brain injury. In: Vinken RJ, Bruyn GW (eds) Handbook of clinical neurology. Elsevier, Amsterdam, pp 317–367

69. Westmoreland BF, Klass DW, Sharbrough FW, Reagan TJ (1975) Alpha-coma. Electroencephalographic, clinical, pathologic, and etiologic correlations. Arch Neurol 32(11):713–718

70. Sironi VA, Ravagnati L, Signoroni G (1982) Diagnostic and prognostic value of EEG compressed spectral analysis in post-traumatic coma. In: Villani R, Papo I, Giovanelli M (eds) Advances in neurotraumatology. Excerpta Medica, Amsterdam, pp 328–330

71. Cant BR, Shaw NA (1984) Monitoring by compressed spectral array in prolonged coma. Neurology 34(1):35–39

72. Steudel WI, Kruger J (1979) Using the spectral analysis of the EEG for prognosis of severe brain injuries in the first post-traumatic week. Acta Neurochir Suppl (Wien) 28(1):40–42

73. Varelas PN, Spanaki MV, Hacein-Bey L, Hether T, Terranova B (2003) Emergent EEG: indications and diagnostic yield. Neurology 61(5):702–704

74. McQueen JK, Blackwood DH, Harris P, Kalbag RM, Johnson AL (1983) Low risk of late post-traumatic seizures following severe head injury: implications for clinical trials of prophylaxis. J Neurol Neurosurg Psychiatry 46(10):899–904

75. Haltiner AM, Newell DW, Temkin NR, Dikmen SS, Winn HR (1999) Side effects and mortality associated with use of phenytoin for early posttraumatic seizure prophylaxis. J Neurosurg 91(4):588–592

76. Pechadre JC, Lauxerois M, Colnet G, Commun C, Dimicoli C, Bonnard M et al (1991) [Prevention of late post-traumatic epilepsy by phenytoin in severe brain injuries. 2 years' follow-up]. Presse Med 20(18):841–845

77. Glotzner FL, Haubitz I, Miltner F, Kapp G, Pflughaupt KW (1983) Seizure prevention using carbamazepine following severe brain injuries. Neurochirurgia (Stuttg) 26(3):66–79

78. Temkin NR, Dikmen SS, Anderson GD, Wilensky AJ, Holmes MD, Cohen W et al (1999) Valproate therapy for prevention of posttraumatic seizures: a randomized trial. J Neurosurg 91(4):593–600

79. Manaka S (1992) Cooperative prospective study on posttraumatic epilepsy: risk factors and the effect of prophylactic anticonvulsant. Jpn J Psychiatry Neurol 46(2):311–315

80. Jones KE, Puccio AM, Harshman KJ, Falcione B, Benedict N, Jankowitz BT et al (2008) Levetiracetam versus phenytoin for seizure prophylaxis in severe traumatic brain injury. Neurosurg Focus 25(4):E3

81. Chang BS, Lowenstein DH (2003) Practice parameter: antiepileptic drug prophylaxis in severe traumatic brain injury: report of the Quality Standards Subcommittee of the American Academy of Neurology. Neurology 60(1):10–16
82. The Brain Trauma Foundation, The American Association of Neurological Surgeons, Congress of Neurological Surgeons, The Joint Section on Neurotrauma and Critical Care (2007) Guidelines for the management of severe traumatic brain injury. XIII Antiseizure prophylaxis. J Neurotrauma 24(Suppl 1):S83–S86
83. Young B, Rapp RP, Norton JA, Haack D, Tibbs PA, Bean JR (1983) Failure of prophylactically administered phenytoin to prevent late posttraumatic seizures. J Neurosurg 58(2):236–241
84. Schierhout G, Roberts I (1998) Prophylactic antiepileptic agents after head injury: a systematic review. J Neurol Neurosurg Psychiatry 64(1):108–112
85. Hernandez TD (1997) Preventing post-traumatic epilepsy after brain injury: weighing the costs and benefits of anticonvulsant prophylaxis. Trends Pharmacol Sci 18(2):59–62
86. Young B, Rapp RP, Norton JA, Haack D, Tibbs PA, Bean JR (1983) Failure of prophylactically administered phenytoin to prevent early posttraumatic seizures. J Neurosurg 58(2):231–235

Chapter 5

Brain Tumors and ICU Seizures

Efstathios Papavassiliou and Panayiotis Varelas

Abstract Seizures are a common presentation of brain neoplasms. Both primary brain tumors and metastases can present with seizures, which are more commonly focal depending on the location and the pathology of the lesion. In general, more benign tumors have higher incidence of seizures than more malignant ones. These patients are admitted to an intensive care unit (ICU) either for preoperative monitoring or in the postoperative period. They should be treated with antiepileptics, if seizures are witnessed. The question remains whether they should be prophylactically treated with antiepileptic medications, if seizures have not occurred yet in the preand postoperative period and for how long. More recent data do not seem to support such prophylactic administration.

Keywords Brain tumors, Seizures, Intensive care unit, Malignant, Benign

5.1. Introduction

Primary and metastatic brain tumors are frequently associated with epilepsy. In the intensive care unit (ICU), three categories of patients with brain tumors related to seizures may be brought to the intensivist's attention. In up to one-third of patients with brain tumors, seizures may be the initial presenting symptom, and some of these patients, especially if the seizures recur or they are associated with significant cerebral edema, hemorrhage or signs of increased intracranial pressure (ICP), or pending herniation, will end up being admitted to the ICU and spend anywhere from 1 day to few days of monitoring. In all these cases, the members of the ICU team will be the first ones to address at least the acute, short-term management of the seizures. The second large category includes postoperative patients of brain tumor resection, who spend at least 1 day in the ICU for observation. These patients may have one or more seizures in the ICU, and appropriate treatment should be prescribed. An important issue to be addressed in the postoperative period, if patients are seizure-free, is whether they need prophylactic antiepileptic drug treatment during their ICU or hospital stay. The third category includes patients with

From: *Seizures in Critical Care: A Guide to Diagnosis and Therapeutics*: Current Clinical Neurology, Second Edition, Edited by: P. Varelas, DOI 10.1007/978-1-60327-532-3_5,
© Humana Press, a part of Springer Science+Business Media, LLC 2005, 2010

known and already-treated brain tumors, who are admitted because of refractory seizures or status epilepticus (SE) or who have an unexplained change in mental status and have been found to be in a nonconvulsive state.

There are not many data regarding the ICU stay and management of these patients. A recent study by Ziai et al. addressed only postoperative issues. In this retrospective study, only 23/158 (15%) postoperative tumor patients had a >24 day stay in the NICU at the Johns Hopkins Hospital [1]. Predictors of >1-day stay in the Neurosciences ICU (NICU) in a logistic regression model were a tumor severity index, comprising preoperative radiologic characteristics of tumor location, mass effect, and midline shift, (odds ratio (OR), 12.5; 95%confidence interval (CI), 3.1–50.5); an intraoperative fluid score, comprising estimated blood loss, total volume of crystalloid, and other colloid/hypertonic solutions administered (1.8, 1.2–2.6); and postoperative intubation (67.5, 6.5–702.0). Seizures were preoperatively present in 15/158 (9.5%) patients. There was no difference in their incidence between group 1 (£24 h NICU stay) or group 2 (>24 h NICU stay) (11/135 vs. 4/23, $p=0.6$). Five patients (3.2%) had postoperative seizures. More patients who stayed longer had seizures postoperatively (2/135 patients in group 1 vs. 3/23 patients in group 2, OR, 95% CI: 10, 1.6–62.5, $p = 0.02$). NICU resource use was reviewed in detail for 134 of 135 patients who stayed in the unit for £1 day. A total of 226 NICU interventions were performed in 69 (51%) patients. Fifteen (6.6%) were related to IV antiepileptic administration, but this was never done after the first 16 postoperative hours. This study provides valuable information regarding incidence of ICU seizures in brain tumor patients and use of ICU resources to treat them, but the results cannot be necessarily generalized to other ICUs.

5.2. Incidence

Overall, the incidence of brain tumors is 4% in patients with epilepsy [2]. Conversely, seizure occurrence remains a major morbidity problem in patients with intracranial tumors. Approximately 30–70% of patients with primary brain tumors will have seizures at some point throughout their disease [3–6]. About 40% of all the patients with metastatic brain tumors will have a seizure during their disease [7, 8]. Half of these seizures will be simple or partial complex seizures, and the other half will be secondary generalized seizures [9, 10]. Brain tumors are rarely associated with primary generalized seizures. SE can also occur in patients with brain tumors, either convulsive or nonconvulsive. In a recent study from the University of Virginia, 555 patients were admitted with a diagnosis of SE over a 7-year period. Fifty patients had a concurrent diagnosis of cancer, 28 (5%) of whom had SE related to the tumor or treatment [11].

Among the primary brain tumors, the higher incidence of seizures is found in patients with oligodendroglioma (92%) and dysembryoplastic neuroectodermal tumors (DNET, 100%) [2]. Astrocytomas and meningiomas have an incidence of about 70%, and glioblastomas have an incidence of about 35% [3]. Other studies by Whittle and Beaumont [12], Rasmussen and Blundell [13], and Hoefer et al. [14] have reported oligodendrogliomas with seizure frequency of 89–90%, astrocytomas of 60–66%, glioblastomas of 31–40%, meningiomas of 29–41%, and metastatic tumors of 35%. Melanoma, choriocarcinoma, lung cancer, and breast cancer are tumors frequently metastasizing to the brain and associated with hemorrhage and seizures. Among metastatic tumors, melanoma seems to have the highest incidence of seizures. Conversely, based on a study from the Cleveland Clinic, among patients with intractable chronic epilepsy the most common types of tumors discovered are ganglioglioma in 49/127 (39%) of cases and low-grade astrocytoma in 48/127 (38%) of cases [15]. Pleomorphic xanthoastrocytoma, dysembryoplastic neuroectodermal tumors, and oligodendroglioma are also tumors frequently associated with chronic epilepsy. Overall, it seems likely that low-grade, well-differentiated gliomas have higher incidence of seizures than more aggressive glioblastomas or anaplastic astrocytomas [2, 16]. A similar distinction may be true for age: children have low-grade tumors and epilepsy as the primary if only sign compared to middle-aged or elderly adults who have higher grade tumors and more neurological focality [2].

Different brain areas are also characterized by varying susceptibility to seizures. For example, among patients with gliomas, seizures occur in 59% of frontal tumors, 42% of parietal tumors, 35% of temporal tumors, and 33% of occipital tumors [17]. Similar observations suggest that the limbic and temporal lobe, primary and supplementary motor (M-I, M-II) areas, and primary and secondary somatosensory (S-I, S-II opercula and insula) areas have the lowest thresholds for seizures [16]. In contrast, the occipital lobe has a much higher threshold [18]. Tumors in the subcortical areas, such as thalamus and posterior fossa, are much less epileptogenic as well. It is noteworthy that 4% of patients without primary or metastatic brain tumors have seizures, usually due to electrolyte abnormalities, organ dysfunction, or chemotherapeutic agent toxicity [2].

5.3. Clinical Presentation

Besides focal neurological deficits, altered mental status, headache, and signs of increased ICP (nausea, vomiting, papilledema), seizures are one of the most common presentations in patients with brain tumors. A first, unprovoked seizure in an adult is always suggestive of an intracranial tumor, until proven otherwise [19].

The timing of their presentation is important to know. Seizure onset is usually within the first 24 h postoperatively [20, 21] and, therefore, may be witnessed during the patient's stay in the ICU. However, in a double-blind trial by North et al. of phenytoin versus placebo following craniotomy, 45% of the seizures occurred within the first week and 64% within the first month [22]. Patients who had seizures preoperatively are at a higher risk of developing postoperative seizures [23]. The type of the seizures does not seem to be different pre and postoperatively [21, 23].

SE occurs either at the time of tumor diagnosis (29%) or during tumor progression (23%). However, an almost equal percentage of SE occurred while the tumor was stable (23%), as shown in a recent study [11].

Not all seizures have the same presentation: several seizure types have been reported and mainly reflect the location of the lesion. Most characteristic are the hypothalamic hamartomas, which are associated with gelastic seizures and precocious puberty. Parasagittal meningiomas may present with generalized seizures when located in the anterior one-third of the sagittal sinus, whereas meningiomas of the middle third usually present with focal seizures, at times following a Jacksonian marching pattern. Choroid plexus tumors in children may have seizures as the presenting symptom in 18% of the cases [24]. Simple or partial seizures characterized by olfactory, gustatory, and epigastric auras, depersonalization, and feelings of fear and pleasure are usually an indication of temporal lobe pathology. Complex partial seizures with repetitive psycho-motor movements (for example, masticatory), impairment of consciousness, or déjà-vu phenomena are also associated with the temporal lobe. Delusions and psychotic behavior have been reported with frontal lobe tumors [25]. Lesions involving the frontal eye fields are associated with turning of the eyes and head to one side (contraversive or ipsiversive, depending on the side of turning compared to the lesion). Parietal lobe tumors are associated with sensory seizures, and occipital lobe tumors can cause seizures with lights, colors, and geometric patterns [19].

Because some tumors present with nonconvulsive seizures or SE, a clinical presentation of decreased or altered mental status, including coma, should not be attributed to the tumor per se, but an evaluation with electroencephalography (EEG) should be undertaken to exclude this treatable cause. Drislane reported six patients with systemic cancer, whose EEGs showed nonconvulsive SE (NCSE). Three patients were confused, and the other three were stuporous or comatose. The possibility of paraneoplastic encephalopathy was raised in three of them. Antiepileptic treatment led to an improved mental status in four of these patients [26]. Five patients out of 84 (6%) with cancer and altered mental status (coma or delirium) were found to be with NCSE by EEG in an Italian study. None of these patients had brain metastases: one was aphasic, two patients treated with ifosfamide had absence, and two patients treated with cisplatin had complex partial SE. All had rapid recovery after antiepileptic treatment [27]. In a recent study, four patients never diagnosed before with metastatic central nervous system (CNS) disease presented with altered mental status. All patients had abnormal neuroimaging of the brain, were in NCSE by EEG, and were treated with fosphenytoin IV. In two patients, the NCSE resolved, but in the other two, despite an initial mental status improvement, status recurred, and both eventually died after 5 and 20 days, respectively [28].

5.4. Pathophysiology

The pathogenic mechanism of epileptogenesis in patients with brain tumors is not fully understood [16] and is beyond the scope of this Chapter. A recent excellent review by van Breemen et al. is available for the interested reader [2]. The location, as well as the histopathology, which correlates with the infiltrative potential, is an important factor determining the clinical presentation of the tumors [29]. Tumors that tend to cause hemorrhage, necrosis, inflammation, and ischemia have a higher incidence of seizures. Focal hypoxia, mass effect and edema, and altered levels of excitatory amino acids, all have been postulated to play a role in epileptogenesis. Different types of tumors may cause seizures through different mechanisms. Some tumors, like DNETs and gangliogliomas, with significantly higher seizure frequencies, have been associated with intrinsic epileptogenic properties.

Brain tumors are thought to alter the dendritic, axonal, and synaptic plasticity of the neurons and in this way contribute to epileptogenesis [30, 31]. Echlin proposed that brain tumors cause partial isolation and deafferentation of the cerebral cortex, resulting in denervation hypersensitivity [32], but there is no definite proof of that theory.

Sodium channels in tumor cells may play a role in epileptogenesis, since these channels are responsible for generating action potentials more frequently than others [33, 34]. Inhibitory (GABA, taurine) as well as excitatory amino acid (glutamate, aspartate) deregulation may also contribute to the process [35–37]. Changes in extracellular Mg^{2+} ions and their effect on the ionotropic NMDA receptors have also been implicated [38]. Increased levels of Fe^{2+} in peritumoral brain tissue also convey a potential for paroxysmal epileptogenic activity. Alterations in the glial gap junctions have been observed in the cortex surrounding glial tumors [16]. Alkaline pH with increased lactate levels has also been observed in brain tumors [39]. Enzymatic changes and immune differences among individuals have also been implicated. Positron emission tomography (PET) imaging has shown increased glucose metabolism and cerebral blood flow in epileptogenic cortex [40].

All these mechanisms may be present and may work in parallel in the process of epileptogenesis. However, the individual's susceptibility to different homeostatic changes (systemic or regional) and their contribution in reducing the seizure threshold, probably make up for the extensive variability noted in patients with similar findings, but different clinical presentations.

Iatrogenic contribution is another entity that ICU specialists should be aware of. The route of ICU drug administration is important, besides their epileptogenic potential (see Drug-Induced Seizures in Critically Ill Patients, Chapter 13). For example, patients with primary brain lymphoma receiving intrathecal chemotherapy have a 47% incidence of seizures [41]. Even IV contrast has been implicated in the generation of seizures in a patient with primary brain tumor [42].

Systemic cancer can metastasize to the brain and produce seizures as their first manifestation. The intracranial metastases usually originate from embolization of neoplastic cells to the brain, commonly in terminal arterial supply territories, such as the gray/white matter junction. However, systemic cancer may induce seizures through additional noninvasive mechanisms: coagulopathy and stroke (sinus thrombosis); nonbacterial thrombotic endocarditis with cerebral emboli; systemic metabolic derangements, such as hypomagnesemia [43] or hyponatremia [44]; opportunistic infections after chemotherapy; or direct toxicity of chemotherapeutic agents to the brain [45, 46]; these are few of the potential pathogenetic mechanisms for which treatment is available. Paraneoplastic syndromes, such as limbic encephalopathy with anti-Hu antibodies, can be associated with seizures preceding the diagnosis of cancer [47]. Some patients with cancer and altered mental status may be in NCSE (Fig. 5-1). EEG or continuous video-EEG may be necessary to evaluate these patients and reach the correct diagnosis.

If seizures become refractory to antiepileptic treatment, development of multidrug-resistance proteins in tumor beds may be the cause. The multidrug-resistance gene MDR1 (ABCB1, P-glycoprotein) and multidrug-resistance-related protein (MRP, ABCC1) are expressed in the cells forming many blood–brain and blood–cerebrospinal fluid (CSF) barriers and contribute to

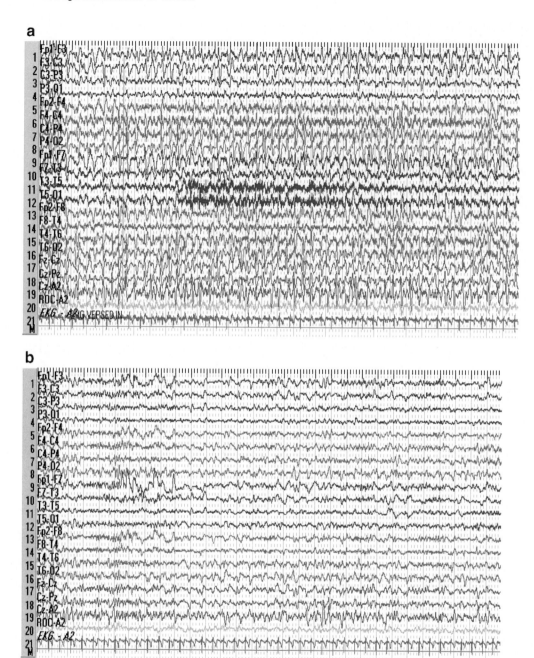

Fig. 5-1. Sixty-three-year-old man with metastatic squamous cell carcinoma of the tonsils to the brain. Patient had two large metastases, one in the right parieto-occipital area (resected, with recurrence) and one in the left frontal area, status post whole brain radiation and chemotherapy. He was admitted to the NICU for change in mental status: drowsy, able to say only "Eeeh" with minimal stimulation, moving all four extremities, but not following commands. No toxic or metabolic reason present in the work-up. Patient was on phenytoin with therapeutic levels. (**a**) EEG: nearly continuous triphasic waves over both frontal regions on a theta/delta background. (**b**) EEG after 2 mg of midazolam IV were administered: marked attenuation of the background, including the triphasic waves. The patient was placed on lorazepam 1 mg po tid. Two days later his mental status had improved and he was able to carry some conversation. Despite that, he was transferred to palliative care where he expired 9 days later

decreased transport into the brain parenchyma of drugs such as phenytoin, carbamazepine, phenobarbital, lamotrigine, and felbamate (levetiracetam is not a substrate for MDR1, and gabapentin may be moved out of the brain via a nonspecific transporter) [2]. These proteins are overexpressed in the cells of patients with glioma [48], focal cortical dysplasia, and ganglioglioma [49].

5.5. Evaluation of Patients with ICU Seizures

Most of the seizures associated with primary or metastatic CNS tumors are of focal onset (Figs. 5-2 and 5-3) with or without secondary generalization. These patients may progress to convulsive status and permanent neurologic damage. Brain tumors are not intrinsic and can lead to seizures associated with increased blood volume, ICP, and tissue displacement, resulting in cerebral herniation. Posturing in this case has to be differentiated from a seizure. Seizures due to brain tumors must also be differentiated form intermittent episodes of increased ICP with plateau waves, which cause headaches, diplopia and other visual disturbances, fluctuation of mental status, motor deficits, or dystonic or opisthotonic postures.

A patient who has a sudden change of mental status postoperatively after brain tumor resection will need to be evaluated for hemorrhage, edema, infarction, as well as seizures, clinical or subclinical. In parallel with a head computed tomography (CT), magnetic resonance imaging (MRI), or MR spectroscopy and the appropriate workup for other common critical care causes of encephalopathy (see above), an EEG will confirm whether the patient is having nonconvulsive seizure activity and may also help in assessing the appropriate response to treatment. In a study of 102 patients with meningioma resection, Rothoerl et al., reported normal preoperative 30-min EEGs in 49% and normal postoperative EEGs in 33.3%. Thirty-two percent of patients had preoperative and 15% postoperative seizures. Of those with preoperative seizures, 53% had complete seizure resolution postoperatively. Dominant hemispheric localization and pre or postoperative headache were associated with postoperative seizures. Interestingly, the pre- or postoperative EEG findings were not associated with postoperative seizures in this series [50]. This may be due to the short period of EEG recording, which may have missed significant abnormalities more easily picked on a longer or continuous EEG. The role of continuous EEG monitoring (CEEGM) in this ICU population has not been well established, but there is growing evidence of its utility in diagnosing NCSE in tumor patients. Jordan monitored 124 NICU patients with CEEGM and reported that 34% of them had nonconvulsive seizures and 27% were in NCSE. Among the 11 patients with brain tumors, 6 (54%) had nonconvulsive seizures. Overall, CEEGM played a decisive or contributing role in the ICU management in 13/16 (81%) of brain tumor patients in a later report with additional patients by the same author [51, 52]. NCSE was reported in two patients with non-Hodgkin's lymphoma presenting with mutism and confusional state after ifosfamide (an alkylating agent, structurally an isomer of cyclophosphamide) infusion [53]. Another patient with glioblastoma multiforme was treated with IV tirapazamine and brain irradiation. After CT scan was performed with intravenous contrast medium, the patient became aphasic and the EEG showed NCSE. IV lorazepam and a loading dose of phenytoin returned the patient to normal state the next morning [42].

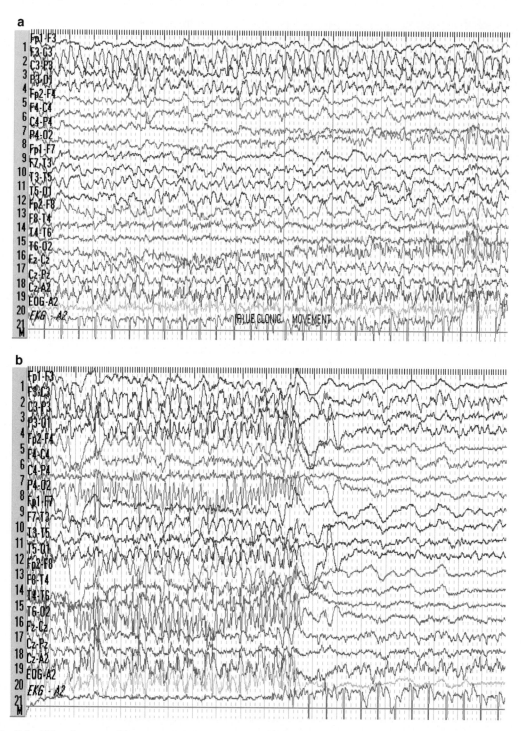

Fig. 5-2. Fifty-nine-year-old man post left frontal oligodendroglioma resection 7 days earlier, and readmitted to the NICU because of significant edema, presents with intermittent episodes of right upper extremity clonic activity lasting for 15–60 s. (**a**) EEG revealing left frontocentral epileptiform discharges at a frequency of 2–3 Hz progressing to involve the right occipital head region (right side of the epoque). (**b**) EEG 30 s later: abrupt cessation of spike and slow-wave activity with subsequent attenuation of the record. The patient responded to IV lorazepam 1 mg and extra phenytoin to correct the low levels

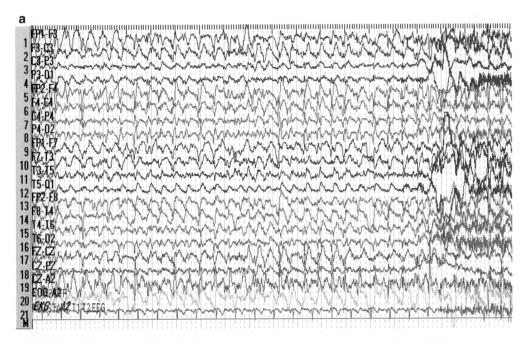

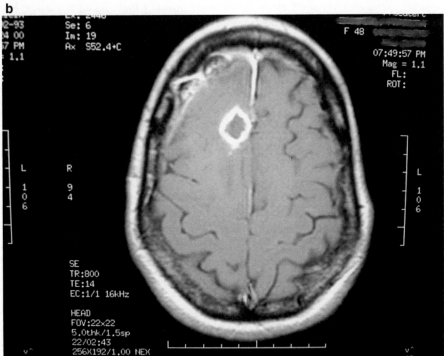

Fig. 5-3. Forty-eight-year-old woman admitted for frequent paroxysmal episodes of staring and found to host a lesion on the CT of the head. (**a**) EEG showing rhythmic sharp waves maximally over the right frontocentral region. The patient was unresponsive with head and eyes turned to the left during this event. (**b**). Gadolinium enhanced T-1 weighted MRI of the head showing a ring-enhancing lesion on the right frontal lobe. The lesion was resected and found to be a metastasis

If an EEG is not considered, and MRI is performed in a patient with cancer and mental status change, abnormalities that may be attributed to seizures can be found. These may alarm the intensivists and, after an EEG is performed, the intensivists may reach the correct diagnosis. This is the case of four patients with primary or metastatic brain tumors from Memorial Sloan-Kettering cancer Center, who had been intermittently confused or unresponsive 1–7 days before the MRI: the MRI showed cortical hyperintensity on FLAIR, T2-weighted, or diffusion-weighted images, with or without leptomeningial enhancement on T1 with gadolinium. In two of these patients who had 18 F PET, hypermetabolism was shown in the abnormal cortical MRI locations. All patients and another eight were in NCSE on the EEG, and all except for one improved clinically after receiving antiepileptic drugs. Repeat MRI 1–4 weeks later showed complete resolution of abnormalities in three patients and improvement in the fourth patient [54]. These results emphasize the need for electroencephalographic emergent evaluation of tumor patients with unexplained change in the neurological examination in the ICU.

5.6. Treatment

5.6.1. Prophylactic Administration of Antiepileptics

The issue of prophylactic treatment of patients with brain tumors is very complex. If a seizure has already occurred, there is little doubt for the value of antiepileptics [55], but when the patient has never exhibited epileptic phenomena, such a treatment becomes more controversial. Efficacy of the treatment has to be balanced with adverse events associated with the chosen drugs. Despite the best efforts, a significant percentage of patients still have breakthrough seizures and the response to the treatment is very unpredictable. Several reasons have to be considered: lack of antiepileptics to have an effect on a vast range of physiologic derangements induced by brain tumors, difficulty maintaining appropriate antiepileptic levels, and tumor progression or recurrence [16, 56]. On the other hand, antiepileptic treatment is not without adverse effects, some of them potentially serious. The case report by Cockey et al. is revealing of our inability to predict complications in those medically complex patients: severe Stevens–Johnson syndrome, documented by biopsy, occurred in a patient with metastatic squamous cell carcinoma receiving phenytoin, whole-brain radiation therapy, and a tapering steroid dose [57]. Moreover, there is growing evidence supporting increased frequency and severity of side effects from antiepileptics in this population: in a meta-analysis of studies examining prophylactic treatment in patients with newly diagnosed brain tumors, 23.8% (range 5–38%) of treated patients experienced side effects that were severe enough to lead to change or discontinuation of the medications. This incidence is higher than that in the general population and should make physicians skeptic about the real need for using them [55]. The bottom line is that the personal preference and previous training or experience of physicians may be more important in making the decision than clinical evidence for pros and cons. According to a study conducted in Rhode Island, 55% of participating physicians gave antiepileptic prophylaxis, but the percentage differed according to the subspecialty: 33% of radiation oncologists, 50% of oncologists, 53% of neurologists, and 81% of neurosurgeons [55, 58].

Additional morbidity by the treatment directed at the tumor may be of some help in making the appropriate decision. Tumor resection is still the cornerstone of brain tumor management. Seizures after tumor resection may pose a serious problem. Extensive intraoperative retraction and cortical injury associated with tumor invasion and aggressive resection are probably associated with increased seizure frequency postoperatively. Residual anesthetic agents may prevent early diagnosis of seizures, as well as neurologic complications. Seizures may compromise the airway and cause limb injuries or structural brain injury, possibly predisposing the patient to more seizures or even status [59]. Seizures can also cause cerebral acidosis, cerebral edema, and increased ICP (which may already be elevated), all of them challenging the compensatory mechanisms of the brain [60]. Metabolic disturbances, such as hyponatremia or hypernatremia, hypoxia, pain-induced hyperventilation, and hyperglycemia, which are frequently noted postoperatively, may also contribute to increased seizure frequency and should be treated aggressively. Lee et al. found that 80% of patients before having a seizure had metabolic acidosis and 20% had hyponatremia [21]. The altered rate of metabolism, especially by the liver, during surgery, also affects the levels of anticonvulsants. More than one study has shown that inadequate levels of phenytoin were the leading cause of postcraniotomy seizures [7, 22].

The effect of surgery on seizures has been studied in numerous trials. Overall, surgical excision of the tumor results in improved control of seizures, and the more extensive the resection of gliomas, the lower the postoperative seizure frequency, although this last notion is not supported by all studies [16]. The effect of craniotomy *per se*, with the meningeal or parenchymal injury that ensues, on seizure occurrence cannot be easily separated from the very effect the tumor induces. Most of the available studies were performed in mixed tumor and nontumor patients; therefore, the conclusions may not be applicable to the former. In the next sections, we will mention some of the most important studies regarding craniotomy, all including tumor patients, because these data are pertinent to the decisions that an intensivist has to make. Subsequently, we will present the data regarding prophylactic antiepileptic use specifically in patients with brain tumors.

Kvam et al. showed that out of 538 postcraniotomy patients, 23 had postoperative seizures. Out of these 23 patients, only 5 had seizures preoperatively. The authors suggested a preoperative loading dose of 10 mg/kg of phenytoin, followed by a postoperative dose of 5 mg/kg/day [20]. A study more pertinent to the ICU was conducted in Taiwan [60]. Three hundred and seventy-four patients postcraniotomy were randomized to receive phenytoin (15 mg/kg IV during surgery, followed by 3–6 mg/kg/day for 3 days) or placebo. The group receiving phenytoin had two early postoperative seizures and the placebo nine, but the difference was not statistically significant. Eighty percent of the seizures occurred within 20 min after surgery. Thus, the authors recommended that prophylactic anticonvulsant medication be given at least 20 min before completion of wound closure. This view was not shared by the authors of a subsequent large prospective study, who did not recommend prophylactic antiepileptics after supratentorial craniotomy. In this study, 276 postcraniotomy patients were randomized to receive carbamazepine or phenytoin for 6 or 24 months, or no treatment [61]. The three treatment groups did not overall differ in the risk of seizures, but there was a nonsignificant 10% reduction of seizures in the two groups that received antiepileptic medications. Meningiomas had the highest risk for seizures (75% by 4 years) and pituitary tumors the lowest (21% by 4 years). Longer operations, those associated with dissection of the lesion away from the surface of the brain, and left-sided or bilateral lesions also carried a higher risk. Early seizures (within 1 week) after craniotomy did not increase the likelihood of late epilepsy. Adding to the debate are the results of a prospective, stratified, randomized, double-blind Dutch study, which compared 300-mg phenytoin/day to 1,500-mg valproate/day given for 1 year in 100 postcraniotomy patients. Fourteen patients had postoperative seizures, but there was no difference in seizure incidence between the two groups [62]. Finally, a meta-analysis of six controlled studies addressing the issue showed a tendency of prophylactic antiepileptics to prevent postoperative convulsions in patients without pre-existing seizures, but this effect did not reach statistical significance ($p=0.1$ one-tailed) [63].

Several studies have examined the need for antiepileptic use, either prophylactically or after surgery, usually in mixed primary or metastatic brain tumor populations. In a double-blind, randomized study of phenytoin (100 mg tid) versus placebo in 281 postcraniotomy patients, the phenytoin group had significantly less seizures (12.9% vs. 18.4%) and highest protection was present between days 7 and 72. Routine prophylaxis with phenytoin (in a dosage of 5–6 mg/kg/day) was recommended by the authors in high-risk patients postcraniotomy. Preferably, treatment should be started 1 week preoperatively, and therapeutic levels of phenytoin should be maintained [22]. However, the subgroup analysis of 81 patients with brain tumors and craniotomy showed that 21% of patients treated with phenytoin had seizures versus only 13% of nontreated (OR 1.8, 95%CI 0.6–6.1). Only the meningioma subgroup in this study had slightly lower risk for seizures in the treated versus placebo patients. Therefore, based on these results, the recommendations for phenytoin prophylaxis should not apply to brain tumors.

In a subsequent Italian study, 65/128 (51%) patients with supratentorial brain tumors had preoperative seizures and were treated with antiepileptic drugs. Those without preoperative seizures were randomized to receive phenobarbital or phenytoin as prophylactic treatment or no treatment. No significant difference in seizure incidence was found between patients treated (7%) and those not treated (18%). The authors suggested short-term preventive antiepileptic treatment after surgery in patients without preoperative seizures and continuation of postoperative treatment in patients with preoperative epilepsy [64].

Other antiepeileptics have also been used. Glantz et al. conducted a well-designed randomized, double-blind, placebo-controlled study comparing the incidence of first seizures in 74 valproate and placebo-treated patients with newly diagnosed supratentorial brain tumors. The drug and placebo groups did not differ significantly in the incidence of seizures (35% in the valproate and, surprisingly, 24% in the placebo-treated group (OR 1.7, 95%CI 0.6–4.6, $p=0.3$)). Based on these results, no prophylactic treatment with valproate could be recommended [58].

Finally, a prospective, randomized, unblinded study from Canada examined the effect of prophylactic phenytoin administration in newly diagnosed patients with primary and metastatic brain tumors without prior seizures. Seizures occurred in 26 (26%) of all patients, eleven (24%) in the treated, and 15 (28%) in the nontreated group (OR 0.82, 95%CI 0.3–2) [65].

Similarly, reports on patients exclusively with metastatic brain tumors do not support the use of prophylactic anticonvulsants [7, 66]. In a large retrospective analysis of 195 patients with metastatic brain tumors, Cohen et al. reported that 18% of patients presented with seizures. Of the remaining seizure-free patients, 40% were treated prophylactically with antiepileptics (phenytoin in >90%). In a follow-up period of up to 59 weeks, 10% of patients developed late seizures. The incidence of seizures did not differ between treated (13.1%) and untreated (11.1%) groups. However, this study is flawed by the fact that two-third of patients with seizures had subtherapeutic antiepileptic levels. The authors did not advocate antiepileptic use, unless the patient had the first seizure [7].

More recently, a meta-analysis evaluated five trials with inclusion criteria (patients with a neoplasm, either primary glial tumors, cerebral metastases, or meningiomas, but no history of epilepsy, who were randomized to either an antiepileptic drug or placebo). The three antiepileptics studied were phenobarbital, phenytoin, and valproic acid. This meta-analysis confirmed the lack of antiepileptic benefit at 1 week and at 6 months of follow-up. In addition, the antiepileptics had no effect on seizure prevention for specific tumor pathology 67.

Summarizing the above information, the Quality Standards Subcommittee of the American Academy of Neurology published a meta-analysis of 12 studies, which had addressed the issue of prophylactic antiepileptic treatment for newly diagnosed brain tumor patients. Four were randomized and eight were cohorts. Only one study showed significant difference between treated and untreated groups and, actually, favored the untreated. The overall OR from the randomized trials was 1.09, 95% CI 0.63–1.89 ($p=0.8$) for seizure incidence and 1.03, 0.74–1.44 ($p=0.9$) for seizure-free survival. Therefore, the Subcommittee recommended no prophylactic use of antiepileptics on patients with newly diagnosed brain tumors. Tapering and discontinuing the antiepileptics was appropriate after the first postoperative week in those patients without a seizure (who were, nevertheless, treated). Although not excluding the possibility that some subgroups of brain tumor patients may be at a higher risk for seizures (melanoma, hemorrhagic or multiple metastatic lesions, tumors located near the Rolandic fissure, slow-growing primary CNS tumors), the Subcommittee did not find any reason for prophylaxis in those patients [55].

5.6.2. Treatment of Seizures in the ICU

Treatment of seizures or SE in patients with brain tumors follows the general guidelines that are presented in Chap. 15. There are, however, several important details regarding these complex patients, which the intensivist should master.

Firstly, one should not forget that surgery may be a potent treatment modality in patients with refractory epilepsy and brain tumors, because studies have shown that resection of the epileptogenic zone due to brain tumors may lead to seizure-freedom or significant control of seizures in 70–90% of patients [68, 69].

Secondly, interaction between the various medications is the most important problem and can lead to unforeseen complications. Antiepileptics, especially those affecting the cytochrome P450 system, may affect the metabolism of

Table 5-1. Hepatic Metabolism of Common Chemotherapeutic Agents and Older Antiepileptics (Modified from [72]).

	Hepatic cytochrome P system used
Chemotherapeutic drug	
Corticosteroids	CYP3A4
Vinca alkaloids	CYP3A4
Etoposide/teniposide	CYP3A4
Tamoxifen	CYP1A2, CYP2D6
Cyclophosphamide	CYP2B
Nitrosoureas	CYP3A4, CYOC19, CYP2D6
Taxanes	CYP3A4, CYP2C8
Irinotecan	CYP3A4
Busulfan	CYP3A4
Doxorubicin	CYP3A4
Cisplatin	CYP3A4, CYP2E1
Methotrexate	80–90% renally excreted unchanged
Antiepileptic drug	
Phenytoin	CYP3A4, inducer
Phenobarbital	CYP3A4, inducer
Carbamazepine	CYP3A4, inducer
Valproic acid	CYP3A4, inhibitor

chemotherapeutic agents used for the treatment of metastatic or primary CNS tumors (Table 5-1). These agents have a narrow therapeutic window and real potential for toxicity or lethal side effects, if their activity is increased by an additional agent, or to lose their anticancer efficacy, if their activity is decreased, and to reduce the chance for remission. Usually, the addition of phenytoin, carbamazepine, Phenobarbital, and other inducers reduces the levels or efficacy of cyclophosphamide, methotrexate, adriamycin, nitrosoureas, paclitaxel, etoposide, topotecan, irinotecan, thiotepa, and corticosteroids [55, 70]. Valproic acid, being an inhibitor, can have the opposite effect and increase the chemotherapeutic agents' levels. Despite these interactions, valproic acid may be safer to be used with chemotherapy. It not only has antitumor properties (see below), but can also suppress the multidrug-resistance gene MDR1, leading to less refractoriness [71].

In addition, competition for binding to plasma proteins may be important with several of those medications, especially in states of hypoalbuminemia, not uncommon in the ICU or during chemotherapy. Measuring the free levels of drugs and adjusting the dose can be useful in order to avoid toxicity or subtherapeutic levels.

Regarding the steroids, either their dose should be increased or the patient should be switched to one of the newer, noninducing antiepileptic agents (lamotrigine, tiagabine, levetiracetam, zonisamide, vigabatrin, and gabapentin). These newer drugs are either renally excreted (levetiracetam, zonisamide, gabapentin, vigabatrin) or, if hepatically metabolized, are either noninducers of the cytochrome P system (lamotrigine, tiagabine) or mild inducers (oxcarbazepine) [72]. Of note, all these new antiepileptic drugs, except lamotrigine and oxcarbazepine, have been approved only as adjuncts to other antiepileptics. Overall, the intensivist should be cautious because no data from large studies are available reporting the interaction of chemotherapeutic agents with the newer antiepileptics [70], nor is the efficacy of the latter in controlling seizures in patients with brain neoplasms known. Emerging data, however, have shown that the addition of levetiracetam (1–4 g/day) to older antiepileptics in patients with refractory seizures can lead to reduction of seizures by 65–90%. In fact, 44–46% of patients in these small case series (a total 86 patients included) were switched to levetiracetam monotherapy later on [73–75]. In another older small study of 14 patients with brain tumors, addition of gabapentin (0.3–2.4 g/day) to phenytoin, carbamazepine, or clobazam led to 100% seizure reduction and 57% seizure freedom [76].

Chemotherapeutic agents or corticosteroids can also affect the metabolism of several antiepileptics, increasing or decreasing their levels [77–79]. This may explain the subtherapeutic levels of these drugs in the studies that evaluated their prophylactic use [7, 58, 64, 65]. Phenytoin concentrations may become toxic after withdrawal of dexamethesone [80], probably due to slower hepatic metabolism of the former. Poor seizure control may result from the combinations of phenytoin with cisplatin or corticosteroids and valproic acid with methotrexate. Increased toxicity of antiepileptics can occur when phenytoin is combined with 5-fluorouracil [81]. In addition, several chemotherapeutic agents may have proconvulsant activity on their own [27, 53] (see Drug-Induced Seizures in Critically Ill Patients, Chapter 13) and the intensivist should be aware that the aforementioned studies of prophylactic antiepileptic treatment did not control for the presence of specific chemotherapeutic agents. Newer chemotherapeutic agents, however, such as temozolomide, may decrease seizure frequency in 50–60% or lead to seizure freedom in 20–40% of treated patients, but the mechanism is unclear [82, 83].

An interesting aspect of the antiepileptic drug use in patients with cancer is their potential for antineoplastic or immunosuppressive effect [84–87]. Valproate exhibits inherent antitumor activity through inhibition of histone deacetylase (which leads to cell differentiation, growth arrest, and apoptosis of cancer cells, including gliomas) [81, 88]. Phenytoin, on the other hand, may lead to immunosuppression, but clinical studies are not available. Neutropenia secondary to myelosuppressive chemotherapy may worsen with carbamazepine, an adverse effect that should be monitored very carefully [89]. Gabapentin may also ameliorate chemotherapeutic-induced nausea and this may be of additional benefit in patients with seizures and breast cancer [90].

Interaction between antiepileptics and irradiation treatment offered to the brain or spine may lead to dermatologic complications. Skin rash in patients treated with phenytoin and brain irradiation may herald Stevens–Johnson syndrome [57, 91], and valproic acid has been implicated in Rowell's syndrome (lupus erythematosus associated with erythema multiforme-like lesions) [92]. One retrospective study, however, of 289 patients with brain tumors treated with antiepileptics and radiation, found only one (0.3%) patient who developed erythema multiforme. Phenytoin was associated with milder rashes in 22% of patients, a higher incidence than the usual 5–10%. These rashes did not appear to be related to radiation, because they usually occurred before its initiation [93].Individualizing the treatment in the ICU and afterwards is probably best. Factors that should be considered before one decides if and when to treat the patient and which medications to use include the histopathology of the tumor, the location of the mass, the presence of pre-existing epilepsy, the extent of additional injury incurred by craniotomy, the involvement of other important organs metabolizing the drugs, the nutritional state of the patient, the pharmacological interactions between the agents, and the ability of the patient to tolerate side effects of the treatment.

5.7. Outcome

Although not pertinent to the ICU management, one should be aware that there are data supporting a better outcome in patients with brain tumors and seizures [16]. In a retrospective analysis of 560 patients with primary supratentorial tumors, the median survival of the 164 (29%) patients presenting with epilepsy was 37 months compared to 6 months of those presenting with other symptoms ($p < 0.0001$) [94]. In the study by Whittle and Beaumont of 34 supratentorial oligodendrogliomas, 17% of patients who presented with seizures and 67% of those who presented with other symptoms had died in the follow-up. However, in a multivariate model, young age and not epilepsy was a favorable independent predictor [12]. In a recent study of 35 patients with SE, 8 (23%) died within 30 days after the status. More patients with systemic cancer (50%) than with primary brain tumors (14%) died within 30 days, implying that the tumor histology is a more important factor for mortality than SE *per se* [11]. This information can be of some help in the discussions the intensivist may have with the patients or relatives in the ICU.

References

1. Ziai WC, Varelas PN, Zeger SL, Mirski MA, Ulatowski JA (2003) Neurologic intensive care resource use after brain tumor surgery: an analysis of indications and alternative strategies. Crit Care Med 31:2782–2787
2. van Breemen MS, Wilms EB, Vecht CJ (2007) Epilepsy in patients with brain tumours: epidemiology, mechanisms, and management. Lancet Neurol 6:421–430
3. LeBlanc F, Rasmussen T (1974) Cerebral seizures and brain tumors. In: Vinken PJ, Bruyn GW (eds) Handbook of clinical neurology. Elsevier, Amsterdam, pp 295–301
4. Cascino G (1990) Epilepsy and brain tumors: implications to treatment. Epilepsia 31(Suppl 3):S37–S44
5. Bartolomei J, Christopher S, Vives K, Spencer DD, Piepmeier JM (1997) Low grade gliomas of chronic epilepsy: a distinct clinical and pathological entity. J Neurooncol 34:79–84
6. McKeran R, Thomas DGT (1980) The clinical study of gliomas. In: Thomas D, Graham DL (eds) Brain tumors: scientific basis, clinical investigation and current therapy. Lippincott, Baltimore, pp 194–230
7. Cohen N, Strauss G, Lew R, Silver R, Recht L (1988) Should prophylactic anticolvusants be administered to patients with newly diagnosed cerebral metastases? A retrospective analysis. J Clin Oncol 6:1621–1624
8. Simonescu M (1960) Metastatic tumors of the brain. A follow-up study of 195 patients with neurosurgical considerations. J Neurosurg 17:361–373

9. Ketz E (1974) Brain tumors and epilepsy. In: Vinken P, Bruyn GW (eds) Handbook of clinical neurology. Elsevier, Amsterdam, pp 254–269

10. Moots P, Moots P, Maciunas RJ, Eisert DR, Parker RA, Laporte K, Abou-Khalil B (1995) The course of seizure disorders in patients with malignant gliomas. Arch Neurol 52:717–724

11. Cavaliere R, Farace E, Schiff D (2006) Clinical implications of status epilepticus in patients with neoplasms. Arch Neurol 63:1746–1749

12. Whittle I, Beaumont A (1995) Seizures in patients with supratentorial oligodendroglial tumours; clinicopahtological features and management considerations. Acta Neurochir 135:19–24

13. Rasmussen T, Blundell J (1959) Epilepsy and brain tumours. Clin Neurosurg 7:138–158

14. Hoefer P, Schlesinger EB, Peress HH (1947) Seizures in patients with brain tumours. Res Nerv Ment Dis Proceed 26:50–58

15. Morris H, Estes ML, Prayson RA et al (1996) Frequency of different tumor types encountered in the Cleveland Clinic epilepsy surgery program. Epilepsia 37:96

16. Beaumont A, Whittle IR (2000) The pathogenesis of tumour associated epilepsy. Acta Neurochir 142:1–15

17. Scott G, Gibberd FB (1980) Epilepsy and other factors in the prognosis of gliomas. Acta Neurol Scand 61:227–239

18. Mahaley MJ, Dudka L (1981) The role of anticonvulsant medications in the management of patients with anaplastic gliomas. Surg Neurol 16:399–401

19. Victor M, Ropper AH (2001) Principles of Neurology. McGraw-Hill, New York

20. Kvam D, Loftus CM, Copeland B, Quest DO (1983) Seizures during the immediate postoperative period. Neurosurgery 12:14–17

21. Lee S, Lui TN, Chang CN, Cheng WC (1990) Early postoperative seizures after posterior fossa surgery. J Neurosurg 73:541–544

22. North JB, Penhall RK, Hanieh A, Frewin DB, Taylor WB (1983) Phenytoin and postoperative epilepsy - a double blind study. J Neurosurg 58:672–677

23. Fukamachi A, Koizumi H, Nukui H (1985) Immediate postoperative seizures - incidence and computed tomographic findings. Surg Neurol 24:671–676

24. Ellenbogen R, Winston KR, Kupsky WJ (1989) Tumors of the choroid plexus in children. Neurosurgery 25:327–335

25. Sato T, Takeichi M, Abe M, Tabuchi K, Hara T (1993) Frontal lobe tumor associated with late-onset seizure and psychosis: a case report. Jpn J Psychiatry Neurol 47:541–544

26. Drislane FW (1994) Nonconvulsive status epilepticus in patients with cancer. Clin Neurol Neurosurg 96:314–318

27. Cocito L, Audenino D, Primavera A (2001) Altered mental state and nonconvulsive status epilepticus in patients with cancer. Arch Neurol 58:1310

28. Blitshteyn S, Jaeckle KA (2006) Nonconvulsive status epilepticus in metastatic CNS disease. Neurology 66:1261–1263

29. Ettinger A (1994) Structural causes of epilepsy. Tumors, cysts, stroke, and vascular malformations. Neurol Clin 12:41–56

30. McKinney R, Debanne D, Gahwiler BH et al (1997) Lesion induced axonal sprouting and hyperexcitability in the hippocampus in vitro. Implications for the genesis of posttraumatic epilepsy. Nat Med 3:990–996

31. Gray W, Sundstrom LE (1998) Kainic acid increases the proliferation of granule cell progenitors in the dentate gyrus of the rat. Brain Res 790:52–59

32. Echlin F (1959) The supersensitivity of chronically "isolated" cerebral cortex as a mechanism in focal epilepsy. Electroencephalog Clin Neurophysiol 11:697–732

33. Patt S, Labrakakis C, Bernstein M et al (1996) Neuron-like physiological properties of cells from human oligodendroglial tumors. Neuroscience 71:601–611

34. Labrakakis C, Patt S, Weydt P et al (1997) Action potential generating cells in human glioblastoma. J Neuropath Exp Neurol 56:243–254

35. Goldstein D, Nadi NS, Stull R, Wyler AR, Porter RJ (1988) Levels of catechols in epileptogenic and nonepileptogenic regions of the human brain. J Neurochem 50:225–229
36. Kish S, Dixon LM, Sherwin AL (1988) Aspartic acid aminotransferase activity is increased in actively spiking compared with non-spiking cortex. J Neurol Neurosurg Psychiatry 51:552–556
37. Sherwin A, Vernet O, Dubeau F, Olivier A (1991) Biochemical markers of excitability in human neocortex. Can J Neurol Sci 18:640–644
38. Avoli M, Drapeau C, Pumain R, Olivier A, Villemure J-G (1991) Epileptiform activity induced by low extracellular magnesium in the human cortex maintained in vitro. Ann Neurol 30:589–596
39. Okada Y, Kloiber O, Hossman KA (1992) Regional metabolism in experimental brain tumors in cats: relationship with acid/base, water and electrolyte homeostasis. J Neurosurg 77:917–926
40. Alger J, Frank JA, Bizzi A et al (1990) Metabolism of human gliomas: assessment with H-1 MR spectroscopy and F-18 fluorodeoxyglucose PET. Radiology 177:633–641
41. Neuwelt E, Goldman DL, Dahlborg SA et al (1991) Primary CNS lymphoma treated with osmotic blood-brain barrier disruption: prolonged survival and preservation of cognitive function. J Clin Oncol 9:1580–1590
42. Lukovits TG, Fadul CE, Pipas JM, Williamson PD (1996) Nonconvulsive status epilepticus after intravenous contrast medium administration. Epilepsia 37:1117–1120
43. van de Loosdrecht AA, Gietema JA, van der Graaf WT (2000) Seizures in a patient with disseminated testicular cancer due to cisplatin-induced hypomagnesaemia. Acta Oncol 39:239–240
44. McDonald GA, Dubose TD Jr (1993) Hyponatremia in the cancer patient. Oncology (Huntingt) 7:55–64; discussion 67–58; 70–51
45. Meropol NJ, Creaven PJ, Petrelli NJ, White RM, Arbuck SG (1995) Seizures associated with leucovorin administration in cancer patients. J Natl Cancer Inst 87:56–58
46. Delanty N, Vaughan CJ, French JA (1998) Medical causes of seizures. Lancet 352:383–390
47. Dalmau J, Graus F, Rosenblum MK, Posner JB (1992) Anti-Hu—associated paraneoplastic encephalomyelitis/sensory neuronopathy. A clinical study of 71 patients. Medicine (Baltimore) 71:59–72
48. Calatozzolo C, Gelati M, Ciusani E et al (2005) Expression of drug resistance proteins Pgp, MRP1, MRP3, MRP5 and GST-pi in human glioma. J Neurooncol 74:113–121
49. Aronica E, Gorter JA, Jansen GH et al (2003) Expression and cellular distribution of multidrug transporter proteins in two major causes of medically intractable epilepsy: focal cortical dysplasia and glioneuronal tumors. Neuroscience 118:417–429
50. Rothoerl RD, Bernreuther D, Woertgen C, Brawanski A (2003) The value of routine electroencephalographic recordings in predicting postoperative seizures associated with meningioma surgery. Neurosurg Rev 26:108–112
51. Jordan KG (1999) Nonconvulsive status epilepticus in acute brain injury. J Clin Neurophysiol 16:332–340; discussion 353
52. Jordan KG (1999) Continuous EEG monitoring in the neuroscience intensive care unit and emergency department. J Clin Neurophysiol 16:14–39
53. Primavera A, Audenino D, Cocito L (2002) Ifosfamide encephalopathy and nonconvulsive status epilepticus. Can J Neurol Sci 29:180–183
54. Hormigo A, Liberato B, Lis E, DeAngelis LM (2004) Nonconvulsive status epilepticus in patients with cancer: imaging abnormalities. Arch Neurol 61:362–365

55. Glantz MJ, Cole BF, Forsyth PA et al (2000) Practice parameter: anticonvulsant prophylaxis in patients with newly diagnosed brain tumors. Report of the Quality Standards Subcommittee of the American Academy of Neurology. Neurology 54:1886–1893

56. Schaller B, Ruegg SJ (2003) Brain tumor and seizures: pathophysiology and its implications for treatment revisited. Epilepsia 44:1223–1232

57. Cockey GH, Amann ST, Reents SB, Lynch JW Jr (1996) Stevens-Johnson syndrome resulting from whole-brain radiation and phenytoin. Am J Clin Oncol 19:32–34

58. Glantz MJ, Cole BF, Friedberg MH et al (1996) A randomized, blinded, placebo-controlled trial of divalproex sodium prophylaxis in adults with newly diagnosed brain tumors. Neurology 46:985–991

59. Deutschman C, Haines SJ (1985) Anticonvulsant prophylaxis in neurological surgery. Neurosurgery 17:510–516

60. Lee S, Lui TN, Chang CN, Cheng WC, Wang DJ, Heimbarger RF, Lin CG (1989) Prophylactic anticonvulsants for prevention of immediate and early postcraniotomy seizures. Surg Neurol 31:361–364

61. Foy PM, Chadwick DW, Rajgopalan N, Johnson AL, Shaw MD (1992) Do prophylactic anticonvulsant drugs alter the pattern of seizures after craniotomy? J Neurol Neurosurg Psychiatry 55:753–757

62. Beenen LF, Lindeboom J, Kasteleijn-Nolst Trenite DG et al (1999) Comparative double blind clinical trial of phenytoin and sodium valproate as anticonvulsant prophylaxis after craniotomy: efficacy, tolerability, and cognitive effects. J Neurol Neurosurg Psychiatry 67:474–480

63. Kuijlen JM, Teernstra OP, Kessels AG, Herpers MJ, Beuls EA (1996) Effectiveness of antiepileptic prophylaxis used with supratentorial craniotomies: a meta-analysis. Seizure 5:291–298

64. Franceschetti S, Binelli S, Casazza M et al (1990) Influence of surgery and antiepileptic drugs on seizures symptomatic of cerebral tumours. Acta Neurochir (Wien) 103:47–51

65. Forsyth PA, Weaver S, Fulton D et al (2003) Prophylactic anticonvulsants in patients with brain tumour. Can J Neurol Sci 30:106–112

66. Hung S, Hilsenbeck S, Feun L (1991) Seizure prophylaxis with phenytoin in patients with brain metastasis. Proc Am Soc Clin Oncol 10:327

67. Sirven JI, Wingerchuk DM, Drazkowski JF, Lyons MK, Zimmerman RS (2004) Seizure prophylaxis in patients with brain tumors: a meta-analysis. Mayo Clin Proc 79:1489–1494

68. Zentner J, Hufnagel A, Wolf HK et al. (1997) Surgical treatment of neoplasms associated with medically intractable epilepsy. Neurosurgery 41:378–386; discussion 386–377

69. Britton JW, Cascino GD, Sharbrough FW, Kelly PJ (1994) Low-grade glial neoplasms and intractable partial epilepsy: efficacy of surgical treatment. Epilepsia 35:1130–1135

70. Patsalos PN, Froscher W, Pisani F, van Rijn CM (2002) The importance of drug interactions in epilepsy therapy. Epilepsia 43:365–385

71. Vecht CJ, Wagner GL, Wilms EB (2003) Interactions between antiepileptic and chemotherapeutic drugs. Lancet Neurol 2:404–409

72. Rios O, French JA (2004) Interactions between antiepileptic drugs and chemotherapeutic agents. Profiles Seizure Manage 3:5–8

73. Newton HB, Dalton J, Goldlust S, Pearl D (2007) Retrospective analysis of the efficacy and tolerability of levetiracetam in patients with metastatic brain tumors. J Neurooncol 84:293–296

74. Wagner GL, Wilms EB, Van Donselaar CA, Vecht Ch J (2003) Levetiracetam: preliminary experience in patients with primary brain tumours. Seizure 12:585–586

75. Maschio M, Albani F, Baruzzi A et al (2006) Levetiracetam therapy in patients with brain tumour and epilepsy. J Neurooncol 80:97–100
76. Perry JR, Sawka C (1996) Add-on gabapentin for refractory seizures in patients with brain tumours. Can J Neurol Sci 23:128–131
77. Sylvester RK, Lewis FB, Caldwell KC, Lobell M, Perri R, Sawchuk RA (1984) Impaired phenytoin bioavailability secondary to cisplatinum, vinblastine, and bleomycin. Ther Drug Monit 6:302–305
78. Neef C, de Voogd-van der Straaten I (1988) An interaction between cytostatic and anticonvulsant drugs. Clin Pharmacol Ther 43:372–375
79. Gattis WA, May DB (1996) Possible interaction involving phenytoin, dexamethasone, and antineoplastic agents: a case report and review. Ann Pharmacother 30:520–526
80. Ruegg S (2002) Dexamethasone/phenytoin interactions: neurooncological concerns. Swiss Med Wkly 132:425–426
81. Vecht CJ, Wagner GL, Wilms EB (2003) Treating seizures in patients with brain tumors: drug interactions between antiepileptic and chemotherapeutic agents. Semin Oncol 30:49–52
82. Brada M, Viviers L, Abson C et al (2003) Phase II study of primary temozolomide chemotherapy in patients with WHO grade II gliomas. Ann Oncol 14:1715–1721
83. Pace A, Vidiri A, Galie E et al (2003) Temozolomide chemotherapy for progressive low-grade glioma: clinical benefits and radiological response. Ann Oncol 14:1722–1726
84. Bittigau P, Sifringer M, Genz K et al (2002) Antiepileptic drugs and apoptotic neurodegeneration in the developing brain. Proc Natl Acad Sci USA 99:15089–15094
85. Blaheta RA, Cinatl J Jr (2002) Anti-tumor mechanisms of valproate: a novel role for an old drug. Med Res Rev 22:492–511
86. Bardana EJ Jr, Gabourel JD, Davies GH, Craig S (1983) Effects of phenytoin on man's immunity. Evaluation of changes in serum immunoglobulins, complement, and antinuclear antibody. Am J Med 74:289–296
87. Kikuchi K, McCormick CI, Neuwelt EA (1984) Immunosuppression by phenytoin: implication for altered immune competence in brain-tumor patients. J Neurosurg 61:1085–1090
88. Li XN, Shu Q, Su JM, Perlaky L, Blaney SM, Lau CC (2005) Valproic acid induces growth arrest, apoptosis, and senescence in medulloblastomas by increasing histone hyperacetylation and regulating expression of p21Cip1, CDK4, and CMYC. Mol Cancer Ther 4:1912–1922
89. Weissman DE (1988) Glucocorticoid treatment for brain metastases and epidural spinal cord compression: a review. J Clin Oncol 6:543–551
90. Guttuso T Jr, Roscoe J, Griggs J (2003) Effect of gabapentin on nausea induced by chemotherapy in patients with breast cancer. Lancet 361:1703–1705
91. Eralp Y, Aydiner A, Tas F, Saip P, Topuz E (2001) Stevens-Johnson syndrome in a patient receiving anticonvulsant therapy during cranial irradiation. Am J Clin Oncol 24:347–350
92. Esteve E, Favre A, Martin L (2002) Post-radiotherapy eruption in a patient treated with valproic acid. Rowell's syndrome? Ann Dermatol Venereol 129:901–903
93. Mamon HJ, Wen PY, Burns AC, Loeffler JS (1999) Allergic skin reactions to anticonvulsant medications in patients receiving cranial radiation therapy. Epilepsia 40:341–344
94. Smith DF, Hutton JL, Sandemann D et al (1991) The prognosis of primary intracerebral tumours presenting with epilepsy: the outcome of medical and surgical management. J Neurol Neurosurg Psychiatry 54:915–920

Chapter 6

Global Hypoxia–Ischemia and Critical Care Seizures

Matthew A. Koenig and Romergryko Geocadin

Abstract Seizures after cardiopulmonary arrest are a common problem in the intensive care unit, occurring in as many as one-third of these patients during hospitalization. The etiology, treatment, and prognostic importance of seizures in this setting have not been well delineated in the literature. Whether seizures exacerbate global hypoxic–ischemic brain injury in humans remains unclear, which raises uncertainty about how aggressively they should be treated. Some pathological data suggest that anoxic brain injury is worsened by generalized tonic-clonic (GTC) status epilepticus. When the prognosis remains uncertain, GTC status epilepticus should be treated in the conventional manner described elsewhere in this book. Partial seizures and simple myoclonus are unlikely to exacerbate neuronal damage, and treatment should probably be reserved for those seizures that are traumatic to family members or interfere with mechanical ventilation. Status myoclonus in hypoxic–ischemic coma is particularly troublesome because it can be highly refractory to conventional anticonvulsants and appears to portend an extremely poor prognosis, regardless of its management. Care should be taken to distinguish true SM from postanoxic action myoclonus (Lance–Adams Syndrome), which does not carry the same prognostic significance. It is also important to distinguish SM occurring after pure respiratory arrest from cardiac arrest, as there are several case reports of patients making good neurological recoveries after respiratory arrest despite SM. The decision to use anesthetic agents and paralytics in the setting of SM must be individualized.

Keywords Hypoxic, Ischemic encephalopathy, Seizures, Status epilepticus, Postanoxic myoclonus

6.1. Introduction

The increasing success of cardiopulmonary resuscitation (CPR) in reviving individuals from cardiac and respiratory arrest has generated an upsurge in hospital admissions for patients in postresuscitative coma. As many

From: *Seizures in Critical Care: A Guide to Diagnosis and Therapeutics*: Current Clinical Neurology, Second Edition, Edited by: P. Varelas, DOI 10.1007/978-1-60327-532-3_6,
© Humana Press, a part of Springer Science+Business Media, LLC 2005, 2010

as one-third of comatose CPR survivors experience seizure activity at some time during the hospital course, most commonly within the first 24 h (1–3). The immediate postresuscitation period is also marked by the highest risk of hemodynamic instability, recurrent arrest, and prognostic uncertainty. Cardiac intensive care units in the United States have become accustomed to facing the challenge of managing seizures and myoclonus in the setting of hypoxic–ischemic coma. Despite the common occurrence of this problem, clinical and basic science research in this area has been sparse and several important questions remain unanswered. Do seizures exacerbate brain damage in hypoxic–ischemic coma? How aggressively should they be treated and with which agents? Can some seizure types offer prognostic information that impacts the decision to withdraw care? This review will provide a comprehensive presentation of existing literature related to this problem.

6.2. Epidemiology

Community-based population data are not currently available. The epidemiologic information related to this problem is primarily based on reports from highly selected patient populations. Several small studies describe the epidemiology of various seizure types in the setting of hypoxic–ischemic insults. In a referral population of 114 patients who survived CPR for over 24 h, Krumholz et al. (1) described seizures in 44%. Thirty-five percent of patients had myoclonus alone or in association with other seizure types. Status epilepticus was found in 32%, the majority of which was either status myoclonus (SM) alone or a combination of SM and GTC status epilepticus, which the authors termed myoclonic status epilepticus. In prospective (2) and retrospective (3) studies of all comatose patients admitted after CPR, Snyder et al. found that one-third of patients experienced seizures, the majority of whom had more than one seizure type. Myoclonic seizures were described in 19%, partial seizures in 19%, and GTC seizures in 6% of the total population. The incidence of myoclonic seizures was bimodal, with the majority beginning within 12 h after CPR and the remainder delayed by several days (2). In the classic outcome study by Levy et al. (4), 15% of patients in hypoxic–ischemic coma experienced generalized convulsions, while 10% had isolated myoclonus. The posthypoxic syndrome of action myoclonus described by Lance and Adams (5) can occur within a few days of cardiac arrest, but the incidence rate among survivors has never been studied.

6.3. Pathophysiology

6.3.1. Pathological and Chemical Changes in Hypoxic–Ischemic Injury and Seizures

Experimental animal studies have provided insights into the mechanism of epileptogenesis in hypoxic–ischemic coma. Adenosine triphosphate (ATP)-sensitive potassium channels (K_{ATP}) are activated by hypoxic stress, resulting in protective cellular hyperpolarization by inward rectifying potassium currents

(6). K_{ATP} knockout mice subjected to brief episodes of hypoxia are more susceptible to generalized seizures (6). The highest concentration of K_{ATP} channels is located within the substantia nigra-pars reticulata (SN_{PR}), which acts as a central gating system for the propagation of generalized seizures (6). In prolonged hypoxia–ischemia, SN_{PR} may be damaged and the gating function of the K_{ATP} receptors may be lost. Alternatively, hypoxic depletion of ATP could result in loss of the inward rectifying potassium current and failure to block seizure propagation at the SN_{PR} (6).

Prolonged generalized seizures induce permanent neuronal injury that shares some characteristics with global hypoxia. Excess glutamate release activates N-methyl-D-aspartate (NMDA) receptors resulting in intracellular accumulation of calcium and early apoptosis (7). When mitochondrial energy stores are depleted during hypoxic and ischemic states, the cytotoxicity of NMDA receptor activation is markedly potentiated (8). Experimental blockade of the NMDA receptor inhibits neuronal toxicity even though it does not shorten the duration of the seizure (9).

Pathological studies of uncomplicated seizures in humans report neither neuronal injury nor ischemic cell changes limited to the hippocampus, particularly the Sommer sector (H1) (10). After prolonged status epilepticus, the cortex may show laminar ischemic changes similar to hypoxic–ischemic encephalopathy with or without involvement of the cerebellar Purkinje cells (10). Experimental data from well-oxygenated baboons with chemically induced status epilepticus showed cortical damage but limited cerebellar pathology (11). In mechanically ventilated rats, prolonged seizures produced cellular changes limited to the substantia nigra pars reticulata (SN_{PR}), hypothalamus, and globus pallidus (12, 13). Damage to the white matter and deep gray matter structures other than the hippocampus is not typically demonstrated in adult humans in the absence of concomitant hypoxia or ischemia (10). Pathological changes demonstrated in global hypoxia–ischemia, on the other hand, involve all neuronal layers of the cortex, subcortical gray matter structures, cerebellum, and spinal cord in human autopsy series (14).

Animal data have been important in studying whether seizures exacerbate hypoxic–ischemic neuronal injury. Young et al. studied extracellular inhibitory and excitatory amino acid concentrations in juvenile rabbits with hypoxia alone, seizures alone, and seizures after hypoxia (15). They found no increase in glutamate or GABA with hypoxia or seizures. When seizures were preceded by a period of hypoxia, however, there was a dramatic increase in both glutamate and GABA (15). Concomitant hypoxia and seizures potentiate neuronal excitotoxicity and excess glutamate release may lower the seizure threshold. In neonatal rats subjected to 3 h of unilateral stagnant hypoxia, CSF concentrations of glutamate and GABA were elevated (16). When these rats were subjected to prolonged status epilepticus, the concentration of GABA increased further but glutamate did not (16). These findings suggest that glutamate neurotoxicity in the setting of hypoxia–ischemia was not enhanced by seizures. Several pathological studies of global hypoxic–ischemic insults in neonatal rats found no further increase in lesion size after status epilepticus (16–18). In newborn rats with limited hypoxic–ischemic lesions from unilateral carotid ligation, however, status epilepticus resulted in heightened neuronal injury (19). It is believed that prolonged global hypoxia–ischemia results in such devastating neurological injury that the additional damage caused by seizures, if present, may be pathologically undetectable (19).

6.3.2. Myoclonus in Hypoxic–Ischemic Coma

Many clinicians ascribe SM in the setting hypoxic–ischemic coma to agonal neuronal firing that is a fragment of GTC status epilepticus (20–22). Celesia et al. (22) speculated that hypoxic–ischemic destruction of the neocortex, cerebellum, and subcortical gray matter disrupt the normal propagation and regulation of tonic-clonic seizure activity, resulting in SM. They note that hypoxic damage to the neocortical laminar and intralaminar nuclei disrupts Jacksonian seizure progression while destruction of the thalamic relay system prevents generalization to GTC convulsions (22).

Pathological data were provided in several case series of patients with SM in postanoxic coma (20–22). In the Young et al. series (20), damage was seen in all layers of the cerebral cortex, hippocampus, basal ganglia, cerebellar Purkinje cells, and spinal cord gray matter. These findings are more reflective of severe hypoxic–ischemic injury than neuronal damage from status epilepticus (20). In the Celesia et al. series (22), the only two patients with Ammon's horn sclerosis – reflective of neuronal damage from status epilepticus – had GTC status epilepticus prior to the development of SM. In the study by Wijdicks et al. (21), postanoxic patients with SM showed significantly greater involvement of all cortical laminae than those who died without SM. The damage in the hippocampus and cerebellum was not significantly different between the two groups. These data were interpreted to reflect that patients with SM had suffered greater anoxic brain injury (21), but the study was not designed to discern whether or not myoclonic seizures contributed to this injury.

6.3.3. Lance–Adams Syndrome

Although, in their classic paper describing the posthypoxic syndrome of action myoclonus, Lance and Adams (5) implicated damage to the ventrolateral thalamic nuclei as the causative lesion, subsequent reports have focused on impaired serotonin neurotransmission and lesions in the caudal medulla and cortex. Many patients with Lance–Adams syndrome have low cerebrospinal fluid (CSF) concentrations of serotonin metabolites (23, 24). Rat models of posthypoxic myoclonus demonstrate impaired neurotransmission at 5-HT_{1B} and $5\text{-HT}_{2A/2B}$ receptors (25, 26). Myoclonus is often attenuated by treatment with 5-hydroxytryptophan (5-HTP), valproic acid, and clonazepam – substances which are known to enhance serotonergic neurotransmission – in both the rat (27) and human (28). Excess CSF serotonin metabolites, exacerbation of myoclonus with serotonin agonists, and amelioration with the serotonin antagonist methysergide were reported in a single patient with severe hypercarbic respiratory arrest (29). The exact role of serotonin in Lance–Adams syndrome remains unclear.

6.4. Clinical Presentation

6.4.1. Generalized Tonic-Clonic Seizures

GTC seizures following CPR were reported in 16 of 114 cardiac arrest survivors in the Krumholz prospective series (1). GTC status epilepticus occurred in conjunction with myoclonus in 17% of patients, a constellation Krumholz et al. termed myoclonic status epilepticus. The majority of these seizure episodes began within 5 h (range 1–12) of cardiac arrest and lasted an average of 17.5 h (range 2–48). All patients were profoundly comatose at seizure onset. In the same series, respiratory arrests were more frequently implicated in myoclonic status epilepticus than cardiac arrests (1). Snyder et al. (3) reported GTC seizures in 4 of their 63 patients in coma after CPR in another prospective series. The majority of these seizure episodes occurred in close proximity to the administration of lidocaine. One of these patients had GTC convulsions simultaneous with myoclonus.

6.4.2. Focal and Complex Partial Seizures

Focal and complex partial seizures following CPR have not been extensively reported in the literature. Krumholz et al. (1) mention that 3 of the 114 cardiac arrest survivors studied developed focal motor seizures. Snyder et al. (3) reported complex and simple partial seizures in 12 of their 63 patients in hypoxic–ischemic coma. Most patients were profoundly comatose at the onset of seizures. Partial seizures typically began within the first 12 h after arrest, but could be delayed 2–4 days (3). The majority of seizure episodes lasted less than 48 h, but a few patients had recurrence of partial seizures after 4–6 days. The majority of patients with partial seizures had other types of seizures as well, including GTC seizures and myoclonus.

6.4.3. Myoclonus

Cortical, reticular, segmental, generalized, reflex, and action myoclonus have all been described as sequelae to hypoxic–ischemic encephalopathy (1, 3, 5, 20–22, 30–37). Cortical myoclonus is felt to be a fragment of focal seizures, with myoclonic jerks involving only a small number of adjacent muscle groups (38). It preferentially involves distal appendicular structures, typically affecting agonist and antagonist muscle groups simultaneously, and may be multifocal (38). Cortical myoclonus occurs spontaneously, but may be accentuated by volitional movement (action myoclonus) or somatosensory stimulation (reflex myoclonus) (38). The movements are typically preceded by time-locked EEG discharges at the sensorimotor cortex. Reticular myoclonus is felt to be a fragment of generalized epilepsy, with myoclonic jerks involving the entire body (38). Axial structures and proximal muscle groups are preferentially involved and the jerks may also be triggered by movement or somatosensory stimuli (38). Reticular myoclonus is believed to result from lesions of the nucleus reticularis gigantocellularis in the caudal medulla (38). EEG spikes are generalized and follow the movement, suggestive of a subcortical discharge referred to the cortex (38). Primary generalized myoclonus involves synchronous jerks of the distal appendicular muscles time-locked to generalized cortical discharges on EEG (38). SM is any form of epileptic myoclonus that persists for greater than 30 min. Segmental myoclonus is felt to be a nonepileptic brainstem or spinal cord reflex resulting in isolated, nonrhythmic jerks of axial structures with no EEG correlate.

Snyder et al. (3) reported myoclonic seizures in 12 of their 63 CPR survivors. Most patients had synchronous, symmetric jerks involving the face, adductors of the thighs, and flexors of the arms. Others had asynchronous, asymmetric jerks involving the extremities alone. Myoclonus occurred in 30% of CPR survivors in the Krumholz et al. series (1), the majority of whom (78%) had generalized or multifocal cortical myoclonus with co-occurrence of other seizure types. Segmental myoclonus involving the eyes, palate, and pharynx was noted in several patients. In the Young et al. series (20), myoclonic jerks were always bilaterally synchronous and involved the face, particularly the eyelids. The extraocular muscles could be involved as well (20, 21). Limb jerks occurred variably and simultaneous to facial movements. Myoclonic jerks occasionally involve the diaphragm and interfere with mechanical ventilation (20). Myoclonus typically begins within 12 h of cardiopulmonary arrest with a mean duration around 24 h (1, 3, 21, 22). A subgroup of patients develops myoclonus only 3–5 days after arrest and it persists for days to weeks (3). Spontaneous myoclonus typically occurs at a frequency of a jerk every 1–5 s (22). Stimulus sensitivity has been reported in many patients (3, 20–22, 31, 32, 34), with increased jerks on tracheal suctioning, touch, painful stimuli, or loud noise. Stereotyped myoclonic jerks have also been reported with episodic hypotension (21). One group reported reticular myoclonus in synchrony to the carotid pulse that was ablated by carotid sinus massage (37).

6.4.4. Lance–Adams Syndrome

Some mention must be made of Lance–Adams syndrome because it may evolve while the patient remains in the intensive care unit (5, 39, 40). In the original Lance and Adams case series (5), three of the four patients began experiencing myoclonus during the first few days after resuscitation while they remained in postanoxic coma. "Generalized myoclonus was a feature of the early stages of the illness soon after the episode of hypoxia but after a few days, when consciousness was regained and the patients' condition stabilized, the movements became restricted in site and all tendency to rhythmicity was lost (5)." In one series, 9 of 14 patients first experienced myoclonus within days of the hypoxic event, and – in all but one – myoclonic jerks were first noted during coma (40). After arousal from coma, Lance and Adams' (5) patients had normal or near-normal intellect, subtle cerebellar signs, and lability of mood. The myoclonic jerks were brief, variable in amplitude, and typically comprised a series of contractions of agonist and antagonist groups. Myoclonus was usually limited to the activated limb, but occasionally spread contralaterally or ipsilaterally. It could be enhanced by emotional states or sensory stimuli such as pinprick, touch, tendon tap, or loud noise. Postanoxic myoclonus can share characteristics of both cortical and reticular myoclonus (40–45). The majority of patients in one series (40) had cortical discharges on EEG preceding and time-locked to myoclonic jerks. These jerks were predominantly distal and limited to the part of the body involved in the volitional movement. Myoclonic jerks involved the facial muscles in several patients, interfering with swallowing and speaking. Other patients had stimulus-sensitive myoclonic jerks that were bilateral, synchronous, and predominantly involving axial structures, suggestive of reticular reflex myoclonus (40). One case report (42) described a patient who developed both cortical action myoclonus and reticular reflex myoclonus after CPR.

6.5. Laboratory Investigation

6.5.1. Electroencephalography

EEG has been the mainstay of clinical investigation in postanoxic seizures. In a recent study (46) from a single university center, cardiorespiratory arrest was the indication for ordering an EEG in 11% (29 out of 261) of emergent studies. EEG was ordered to rule out status epilepticus in 23 patients and seizures in 3 patients. Suspicious clinical activity was reported in 65% and previously witnessed seizures in 10%. Twenty-one patients were already receiving antiepileptic medications when the study was ordered. Generalized slowing was the most common EEG finding (11 cases), followed by convulsive status epilepticus (8 cases), epileptiform discharges (4 cases), and nonconvulsive status epilepticus as seen in Fig. 6-1 (3 cases). In the multivariate analysis of all emergent EEGs in this study, history of cardiopulmonary arrest was the only independent predictor of convulsive or nonconvulsive status epilepticus (46).

Krumholz et al. (1) found epileptiform discharges in 58% of survivors with clinical seizures or myoclonus and 88% of those with myoclonic status epilepticus. Epileptiform discharges were rare in CPR survivors without clinical seizures or myoclonus (9%, $p < 0.001$). Burst suppression (Fig. 6-2) was also seen more frequently (76%, $p < 0.001$) in patients with myoclonic status epilepticus (1). EEG characteristics of the various types of seizures after HI injury have also been described. Snyder et al. (3) commented that the most common finding in patients with partial seizures was diffuse slowing, with spike activity and rhythmic slowing occurring in a minority of patients. The EEG findings in comatose patients with myoclonus are highly variable. The most frequently reported patterns include burst-suppression, diffuse slowing, isoelectric tracing, periodic spikes and polyspike/slow wave complexes, and alpha coma (1, 3, 20–22, 30–32). The most common tracing in most series is diffuse slowing with or without periodic spikes or polyspike complexes (30). The interval between complexes is stable for a given patient, but ranges from 0.5 to 5 s (30). The complexes may or may not be time-locked to the myoclonic jerks (20, 22). In stimulus-sensitive myoclonus, tactile, and auditory stimulation elicit bursts of generalized spike-polyspike complexes that precede and are time-locked to clinical myoclonus (22, 32). Burst-suppression is the second most-frequently reported pattern (30). The bursts typically last 1–10 s and are separated by prolonged periods of suppression ranging 5–25 s (30). One series reported periods of inter-burst suppression lasting as long as 2–4 min (32). Burst-suppression patterns in hypoxic–ischemic coma without myoclonus have typical intervals around 15 s (47) and prolonged suppression in this scenario may reflect more profound brain injury (32). As described above, patients with Lance–Adams syndrome follow 3 EEG patterns: focal time-locked spikes that precede the myoclonus (cortical myoclonus), generalized nontime-locked spike-and-slow-wave complexes that follow the myoclonus (reticular myoclonus), and no abnormal EEG activity (segmental myoclonus) (40–45). EEG has also been used for prognostic purposes after cardiopulmonary arrest (48–50). In a systematic review of EEG data (51), five out of six studies demonstrated 100% specificity for poor outcome in CPR survivors with burst-suppression or isoelectric patterns within the first week. The likelihood ratio for poor outcome with these EEG patterns was 9.0 (95% CI 2.5–33.3) (51).

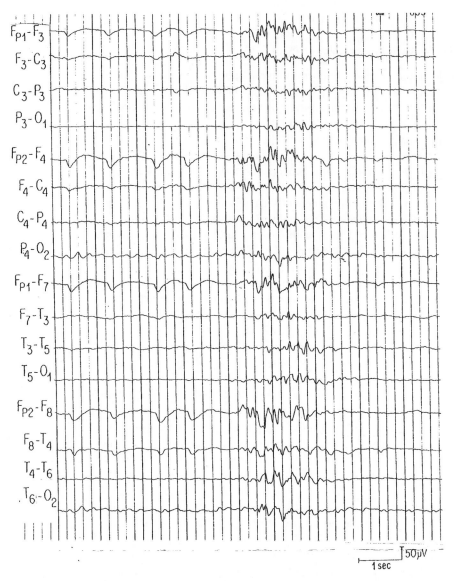

Fig. 6-1. Burst-suppression EEG pattern in a 62-year-old man with generalized myoclonus, arising from coma after resuscitation from cardiac arrest

6.5.2. Electromyography

Electromyography (EMG) may be useful in delineating reticular myoclonus from cortical myoclonus in patients with Lance–Adams syndrome, especially in conjunction with EEG. Patients with cortical myoclonus demonstrate EMG discharges that occur in a rostrocaudal distribution, are time-locked to cortical spikes on EEG, and have conduction delays similar to direct cortical stimulation of the motor tract (5, 38). Patients with reticular myoclonus involving the cranial nerves demonstrate a caudorostral distribution of EMG discharges originating in the caudal medulla that are not time-locked and normally precede cortical EEG spikes (38, 41, 43).

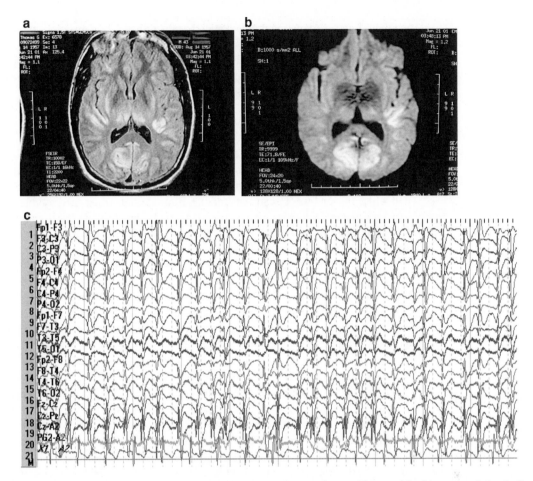

Fig. 6-2. Nonconvulsive status in a patient with postanoxic myoclonus: 43-year-old white man admitted after drowning. He was found in the bottom of a lake, where he stayed for approximately 15 min. He was initially pulseless and without breathing. In the ICU he developed continuous bilateral and synchronous myoclonic jerks in the upper and lower extremities. In addition, the patient had several generalized tonic-clonic convulsions, which were suppressed by phenytoin and valproic acid. The patient regained only brainstem reflex function and eventually expired in palliative care 12 days after extubation. (**a, b**) DWI MRI of the brain 29 h later demonstrating diffuse abnormalities, especially in the basal ganglia, thalamus, and insular and occipital cortex. (**c**) Continuous EEG monitoring demonstrating bihemispheric continuous runs of sharp and slow waves, which did not correlate with myoclonic jerking or clinical convulsions

6.5.3. Somatosensory-Evoked Potentials

Somatosensory-evoked potentials (SSEP) have prognostic utility in postanoxic coma and have contributed to clinical research in Lance–Adams syndrome. It has not been studied in acute postanoxic myoclonus per se. Bilateral absence of early cortical SSEP responses portends poor outcome in hypoxic–ischemic coma (47, 52–58). In a systematic review of SSEP data (51), bilateral absence of N20 cortical responses measured in the first week of hypoxic–ischemic coma was 100% specific for poor outcome with a pooled 95% confidence interval for a false positive test of 0–2.0%. It is the most precise means of predicting poor outcomes in these patients, likely related to the minimal influence of medications and metabolic derangement (51). SSEP has also been useful in studying Lance–Adams syndrome. Patients with cortical action myoclonus often demonstrate abnormally large evoked potentials in the sensorimotor cortex, whereas patients with reticular myoclonus do not (38, 40, 42, 43). These data have been used to support the hypothesis that cortical reflex myoclonus results from hyperexcitability of the sensory input to a cortical reflex arc (38).

6.5.4. Brain Imaging

Brain Imaging has been extensively studied in patients after cardiopulmonary arrest, but not in the subpopulation with hypoxic–ischemic seizures and myoclonus. Torbey et al. (59) demonstrated loss of distinction between the grey and white matter on CT scan immediately after cardiac arrest. A gray matter to white matter Hounsfield unit ratio <1.18 at the level of the basal ganglia predicted death in this small retrospective study (59). In one series, brain CT scans done at various times after cardiopulmonary arrest were grossly normal in 77% of all comatose patients with or without subsequent seizures (21). Cerebral edema and hypodensities in the deep cortical white matter, cerebellum, thalamus, and cortical watershed areas occurred more frequently in those patients with myoclonus than in those without myoclonus.

Brain MRI has been studied in survivors of cardiac arrest and in status epilepticus, but not in the subpopulation with both seizures and cardiorespiratory arrest. One small study of CPR survivors (60) showed restricted diffusion in the basal ganglia, cerebellum, and cortex on the day of arrest. Diffusion was restricted mostly in the cortical and subcortical gray matter between 24 h and 13 days and in the white matter between 14 and 20 days. After 21days, diffusion-weighted imaging was normal (60). In the absence of hypoxic or ischemic insults, status epilepticus is known to induce T2- and diffusion-weighted hyperintensities and T1-weighted hypointensities as well as contrast enhancement in the involved cortex, adjacent subcortical white matter, and hippocampus (61). These changes represent cortical cytotoxic edema and subcortical vasogenic edema that typically reverses when seizures are controlled (61) (Fig. 6-3).

Brain imaging is poorly studied in CPR survivors with seizures. In one series, brain MRI and CT in patients with Lance–Adams syndrome were normal in one-third of patients, showed cortical or cerebellar infarcts in one-third, and showed mild cortical and cerebellar atrophy in the remaining third (40).

6.5.5. Cerebrospinal Fluid Analysis

Cerebrospinal fluid has not been studied in the setting of acute hypoxic–ischemic seizures in humans. In Lance–Adams syndrome, conflicting data have been reported with regard to concentrations of serotonin metabolites, as described above. The majority of patients have depressed serotonin metabolites and often respond clinically and biochemically to serotonin precursors and agonists like 5-HTP, clonazepam, and valproic acid (24, 28). Those patients with elevated CSF serotonin metabolites tend to respond to serotonin antagonists like methysergide (29).

6.6. Differential Diagnosis

Many conditions that cause cardiopulmonary arrest may also lower the seizure threshold. This understanding is especially important if prolonged seizures are

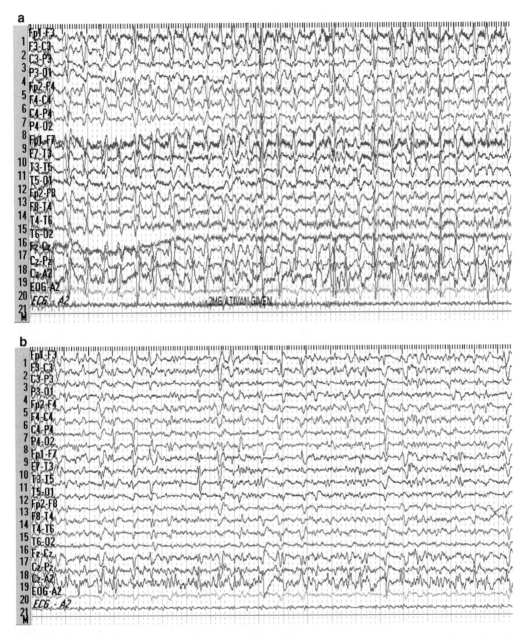

Fig. 6-3. Nonconvulsive status epilepticus. Seventy-five-year-old woman involved in a car accident, with admission GCS of 15, developed multiorgan failure after a protracted ICU stay. She had a cardiac arrest in the ICU, after which she never regained consciousness. An EEG was performed to rule out nonconvulsive status epilepticus. (**a**) Continuous bursts of triphasic wave activity at a rate of 1–2 Hz, occasionally intermixed with bursts of spike activity. (**b**) Significant decrease of the epileptiform activity after intravenous administration of 2-mg lorazepam. The patient did not have any clinical improvement and remained in coma

taken as an indication of severe irreversible brain injury that may influence the decision to limit medical care. Patients with a previous diagnosis of epilepsy may present in status epilepticus after a relatively brief episode of hypoxia. Pre-existing epilepsy may not be known at the initial point of care and baseline antiepileptic drug levels may be helpful in this regard. Drugs given to patients during the resuscitation may trigger or lower seizure threshold. Lidocaine, used as part of the standard Advanced Cardiac Life Support protocol, is well known to induce seizures at serum levels >9 μg/ml (62–64). Propafenone, although rarely used in cardiac arrest, has also been reported to lower the seizure threshold (65). Streptokinase, prourokinase, and tissue-type plasminogen activator given during acute myocardial infarction may also induce seizures (66). Although rarely used in the modern management of asthma, theophylline administered for respiratory arrest secondary to status asthmaticus is epileptogenic (67). Stimulants, tricyclic antidepressants, and cocaine can potentially cause arrhythmic cardiac arrest and seizures (59, 63, 68, 69). Alcohol-, barbiturate-, and benzodiazepine-withdrawal seizures must be considered in the first few days of admission in alcoholics and sedative users who present with respiratory or cardiac arrest. Penicillins, fluoroquinolones, and other antibiotics may trigger seizures. Rapid withdrawal of anesthetic agents, such as propofol and barbiturates, may also precipitate prolonged seizures. For more details on drug-induced seizures, please review chapter 12.

Metabolic derangements, such as hyponatremia and hypomagnesemia, are common in patients with congestive heart failure, intrinsic renal disease, the syndrome of inappropriate antidiuretic hormone release (SIADH), and diuretic users. If severe, hyponatremia may produce obtundation – with or without focal neurological deficits – and seizures. Profound hypoglycemia in insulin users may also precipitate coma and seizures in the setting of cardiopulmonary arrest. Seizures in encephalopathic patients may be difficult to clinically distinguish from shivering, rigors, hyperekplexia, and reflex startle responses (38, 42). EEG, with or without paralytic medications, may be helpful in this regard. Specific discussion on the role of metabolic and systemic derangement in seizure disorder is provided elsewhere in this book.

6.7. Treatment

6.7.1. General Considerations

Seizures are most likely to occur during the first day after cardiopulmonary arrest. This is a period of hemodynamic instability, prognostic uncertainty, and high risk of recurrent arrest. Cardiac arrest and profound hypotension often cause hepatic and renal damage, which may alter the metabolism and excretion of resuscitative and anticonvulsant medications. Drugs used to control these – often highly refractory – seizures may have untoward effects on cardiac rhythm, blood pressure, and level of consciousness. Intravenous phenytoin is well known to induce hypotension and may trigger arrhythmias such as ventricular fibrillation, complete heart block, bradycardia, and asystole. Divalproex sodium, phenytoin, and barbiturates can precipitate hepatic injury that may be especially problematic in the setting of shock liver. Divalproex sodium and phenytoin also have significant interactions with many antiarrhythmic agents, including lidocaine and amiodarone. Intravenous benzodiazepines and barbiturates may also induce hypotension and may interfere with neurological examination, such that a falsely poor prognosis is given.

6.7.2. Simple and Complex Partial Seizures

Simple and complex partial seizures have not been demonstrated to cause neuronal injury in most case series and may not require aggressive management in postanoxic coma. In the Snyder et al. case series (3), few patients had partial seizures in isolation and most patients had good seizure control with phenytoin alone, Phenobarbital alone, or both. The decision to treat partial seizures in comatose patients must be individualized, weighing the ease of treatment versus the low risk of exacerbated neuronal injury in this setting.

6.7.3. Generalized Tonic-Clonic Seizures

GTC seizures are well known to cause progressive neuronal injury after 30 min (6, 9, 10). They typically begin during the first day after cardiopulmonary arrest, a period in which the ultimate prognosis remains unclear. The pathological data in postanoxic patients with GTC status epilepticus is limited, but one series (22) did demonstrate Ammon's horn sclerosis – typical of epileptic neuronal injury – in two such patients. GTC status epilepticus should be managed aggressively in these patients – particularly when it occurs early in the hospital course – as detailed elsewhere in this book (Chapter 15)

6.7.4. Myoclonus

Isolated epileptic myoclonus and segmental myoclonus are not harmful and do not require treatment unless they interfere with mechanical ventilation or clinical care. Whether or not SM exacerbates the brain damage caused by hypoxic–ischemic encephalopathy remains unclear. Most clinicians argue that SM represents agonal neuronal activity that reflects neurological devastation. A review of the literature for this publication found five patients (5, 22, 36, 70) who developed SM in postanoxic coma and had good neurological outcomes. Importantly, all of these patients appear to have suffered respiratory arrest as opposed to cardiac arrest. Several case series focused purely on cardiac arrest (1, 3, 20, 21, 30, 35) report uniform mortality or vegetative state in postanoxic SM. It is unclear, however, whether these results reflect a "self-fulfilling prophesy" as SM itself may be used as an argument to withdraw supportive care (21, 35). Although pathological studies from patients with SM after cardiopulmonary arrest show greater cortical involvement than similar patients without SM (21), it is unclear whether SM is reflective or causative of this injury. SM is often refractory to treatment short of pharmacological coma. Medications employed with varying degrees of success include phenytoin, phenobarbital, levetiracetam, valproic acid, and benzodiazepines (1, 3, 20–22, 30, 32, 33, 35).

6.7.5. Prophylactic Anticonvulsant Use

Prophylactic use of anticonvulsants in postanoxic coma has not been rigorously studied outside of thiopental in the Brain Resuscitation Clinical Trial I (71). In this study, comatose survivors of cardiac arrest were randomized to standard care with or without a loading dose of thiopental. There was no statistically significant difference in outcome between the two groups (71). A subgroup analysis of seizure activity demonstrated a trend toward fewer seizures, lower mortality, and better neurological outcomes in the treatment arm, but the difference failed to reach statistical significance. No description of the seizure activity is given in this study (71).

6.7.6. Lance–Adams Syndrome

Lance–Adams syndrome may develop while the patient remains in the intensive care unit and may interfere with physical rehabilitation, swallowing, and weaning from the ventilator. Various treatment strategies have been employed for the amelioration of action myoclonus in Lance–Adams syndrome (5, 23, 24, 26, 28, 29, 40, 42–45, 72–77). Clinical improvement has been reported with 5-HTP (23, 24, 28, 76), valproic acid (73), carbamazepine (74), gabapentin (72), clonazepam (24), levodopa (75), monoamine oxidase inhibitors (24), piracetam (40), and methysergide (29). In a recent study of levetiracetam (77), two patients with Lance–Adams syndrome responded to doses of 750–1,500 mg per day. As discussed above, many patients with Lance–Adams syndrome have depleted serotonin metabolites in the CSF and respond to serotonin precursors and agonists (24, 28). Others have elevated CSF serotonin precursors and improve with methysergide, a serotonin antagonist (29). If clinical response to medications involving serotonergic neurotransmission is unclear, it may be reasonable to use CSF serotonin metabolite concentrations as a guide to therapy – although this approach has not been rigorously studied. Lance–Adams syndrome has been shown to improve several years after the anoxic event (40). In one series (40), 14 patients were followed for 3.7 years. Three patients were eventually able to discontinue antimyoclonic medications and five patients were able to ambulate independently. Subtle improvement was the rule in the remaining patients.

6.7.7. Supportive Management

A relatively benign intervention in any seizure type is the optimization of factors that affect systemic function such as electrolytes, medications, and infections. Correction of hypoglycemia, hyponatremia, hypocalcemia, and hypomagnesemia may reduce the risk of recurrent cardiac events and seizures. As with any severe neurological injury, serum glucose levels should be normalized using insulin as needed. Acid-base disturbances should be optimized with appropriate adjustments to the mechanical ventilator. Discontinuation of proconvulsant medications should be undertaken if possible.

6.8. Prognosis and Outcomes

The prognostic significance of seizures in hypoxic–ischemic coma has been a source of controversy in the literature. Levy's classic study of a general population of patients in hypoxic–ischemic coma failed to demonstrate poorer outcomes in the subpopulation with seizures of any type (4). Although Snyder et al. (2) showed 17% survival in hypoxic–ischemic coma patients with myoclonus and 32% survival with seizures versus 43% survival without any seizure activity, the difference failed to reach statistical significance. Likewise, there was only a trend toward higher incidence of excellent outcome in survivors without seizure than in patients who had any form of seizure activity (2). Another large study by Krumholz et al. (1) showed that seizures

Table 6-1. Survival and Consciousness at Discharge of Comatose Patients after Cardiopulmonary Resuscitation (Modified from (1)).

	N	Alive at discharge	Conscious at discharge
All patients	114	30 (26%)	21 (18%)
No seizure or myoclonus	64	21 (33%)	15 (23%)
Any seizure or myoclonus	50	9 (18%)	6 (12%)
All status epilepticus (SE)	36	4 (11%)*	1 (3%)*
SE without myoclonus	10	1 (10%)	1 (10%)
SE with myoclonus	19	3 (16%)	0[a]
Status myoclonus alone	7	0	0

[a]Significantly different from patients without this condition ($P < 0.01$).

or myoclonus per se are not significantly related to outcome, but convulsive status epilepticus and myoclonic status epilepticus confer poor outcome as judged by survival and recovery of consciousness (Table 6-1).

In 2006, the American Academy of Neurology (AAN) published a practice parameter for prediction of outcome in comatose survivors of cardiac arrest (78). This evidence-based review determined level A evidence that absence of pupillary light responses or corneal reflexes, and extensor or no motor response to pain after 72 h was a specific indicator of poor prognosis for meaningful recovery (78). They found that single seizures and sporadic focal myoclonus do not accurately predict poor prognosis, but there was level B evidence to suggest that the presence of SM within the first 24 h was invariably associated with in-hospital death or poor outcome even in patients with motor responses or intact brainstem reflexes (78). The authors also mentioned reports of patients with SM making good neurological outcomes in the setting of respiratory arrest as opposed to cardiac arrest (78). Bilateral absence of cortical N20 potentials was also found to have level B evidence for predicting poor outcomes, but only level C evidence was found for the predictive value of malignant EEG patterns (78). Prognostication after cardiac arrest should be rendered using evidence-based practices as provided by the AAN consensus statement algorithm. In the case of SM, if continued supportive management is desired because of family choice or prognostic uncertainty and standard anticonvulsant medications have failed to ameliorate SM, the decision to pursue pharmacological coma or neuromuscular blockade must be individualized. Because most SM abates within 48 h, it may be practical to use anesthetic agents and paralytics for this period of time without prolonged loss of the ability to examine the patient (1).

6.9. Hypothermia and Seizures after Resuscitation from Cardiac Arrest

All the current knowledge about the frequency and prognostic impact of seizures in comatose survivors of cardiac arrest was acquired prior to the hypothermia era. Two well-designed clinical trials have demonstrated that therapeutic hypothermia improves neurological recovery (79, 80). Current treatment protocols for hypothermia after cardiac arrest have been based on the study designs of the major clinical trials and typically involve initiation of hypothermia within 4 h of CPR, a target temperature of 32–34°C, maintenance of therapy for 12–24 h, and a period of gradual re-warming (80, 81). The majority of patients experience shivering during the hypothermia maintenance period that requires both sedation and/or paralysis (80). The use of long-acting paralytic agents has the obvious potential to mask convulsive seizures, leading some to recommend continuous EEG monitoring during the hypothermia period to aid seizure recognition (82, 83). Recommendations for continuous EEG monitoring, however, would require the expense of providing 24-h EEG services, which may be difficult to justify while it remains uncertain that there is a benefit to recognizing and treating nonconvulsive seizure activity in this population.

Because hypothermia, like anesthetic agents, has the ability to decrease cerebral metabolism and neuronal activity, hypothermia has been studied for treatment of refractory seizures (84–86). Animal models have shown that focal brain cooling increases the seizure threshold in rats treated with proconvulsant agents (87, 88). Based on these findings, it is reasonable to speculate that the frequency of seizures in cardiac arrest survivors treated with hypothermia is likely to be lower than normothermic controls. The major clinical trials of hypothermia for cardiac arrest survivors, however, were not designed to study seizure frequency. In the European multicenter trial (79), the incidence of seizures during the first 7 days after cardiac arrest was 8% in the normothermia group and 7% in the hypothermia group. The protocol included paralytic agents, however, so convulsive seizures may have been missed during the hypothermia maintenance period. Because EEG monitoring was not routinely undertaken, nonconvulsive seizures also may not have been recognized. Other clinical trials of hypothermia for cardiac arrest have not reported seizure frequency.

Aside from the frequency of seizures in patients treated with hypothermia, the prognostic impact of seizures remains unstudied in this population. If seizures worsen ischemic neuronal injury, there is animal data that suggests that treatment with hypothermia may lessen this injury (89). In a rat model of flurothyl-induced status epilepticus, animals cooled to 32.5°C had significantly less epileptic neuronal injury to the neocortex and striatum than normothermic controls (90). In a separate study using a rat model of global ischemia, postischemic hypothermia had no impact on seizure frequency but resulted in decreased epileptic neuronal injury (91). In a fetal sheep model of hypoxic arrest, epileptiform activity on EEG and neuronal injury were both reduced in animals treated with hypothermia after resuscitation (92). In humans, a recent case report described a patient treated with hypothermia after cardiac arrest who achieved a favorable outcome despite prolonged status epilepticus (93). The authors speculated that hypothermia may have altered the normal association between refractory status epilepticus after cardiac arrest and poor outcomes.

In the AAN practice parameter, the authors were careful to note that "current indicators of poor prognosis in comatose survivors are derived from patients not treated with induced moderate hypothermia. If this treatment becomes standard care, these indicators may need revision." (78). In fact, a few recent studies have addressed the impact of hypothermia on the prognostic accuracy of SSEP and EEG. In a recent study of 60 comatose survivors of cardiac arrest

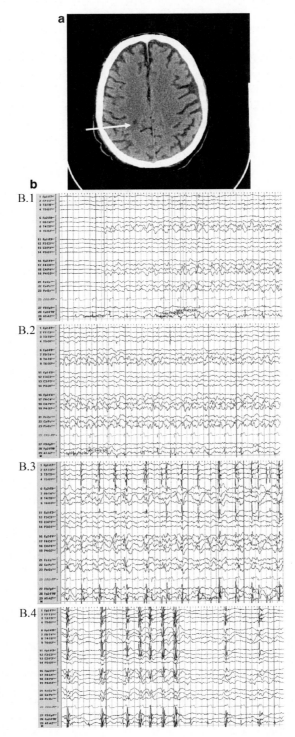

Fig. 6-4. Seventy-year-old man s/p coronary artery bypass (×3 vessels), with complicated course in the cardiac-ICU (hemodynamic instability with prolonged hypotension). Four days after his surgery, he developed generalized tonic-clonic status epilepticus and was placed on pentobarbital coma under continuous EEG monitoring. He never regained consciousness, but the status epilepticus resolved after more than a month in barbiturate coma. Because of skin ulceration under the electrode placement areas, the continuous EEG had to be stopped. (**a**) CT of the head showing a small centrum semiovale subacute lacune (*white arrow*), but paucity of other significant radiologic injuries. No MRI was ever performed due to the prolonged and severe critical condition of the patient. (**b**) Electrographic seizure, beginning from the parieto-temporo-occipital areas of the right hemisphere (**b**.1), evolving (**b**.2), spreading to the left (**b**.3) and ending (**b**.4)

randomized to hypothermia for 24 h or normothermia, bilateral absence of cortical N20 responses remained 100% specific to poor outcomes (94). Use of EEG for prognostication in patients undergoing therapeutic hypothermia, however, has been more problematic. In a recent study of continuous amplitude-integrated EEG, although EEG had predictive value after re-warming, the presence of electrocerebral silence during the hypothermia period had poor predictive specificity (82). The authors speculated that EEG interpretation was confounded by use of sedative agents. Further studies need to be done to confirm these findings and to determine whether the prognostic importance of seizures and myoclonic status epilepticus is altered by therapeutic hypothermia.

Acknowledgments The authors would like to acknowledge Dr. Ernst Niedermeyer and Dr. Peter Kaplan for their helpful suggestions and EEG tracings.

References

1. Krumholz A, Stern BJ, Weiss HD (1988) Outcome from coma after cardiopulmonary resuscitation: relation to seizures and myoclonus. Neurology 38:401–405
2. Snyder BD, Ramirez-Lassepas M, Lippert DM (1977) Neurologic status and prognosis after cardiopulmonary arrest: I. a retrospective study. Neurology 27:807–811
3. Snyder BD, Hauser WA, Loewenson RB, Leppik IE, Ramirez-Lassepas M, Gumnit RJ (1980) Neurologic prognosis after cardiopulmonary arrest: III. Seizure activity. Neurology 30:1292–1297
4. Levy DE, Caronna JJ, Singer BH, Lapinski RH, Frydman H, Plum F (1985) Predicting outcome from hypoxic-ischemic coma. JAMA 253:1420–1426
5. Lance JW, Adams RD (1963) The syndrome of intention or action myoclonus as a sequel to hypoxic encephalopathy. Brain 86:111–136
6. Yamada K, Ji JJ, Yuan H, Miki T, Sato S, Horimoto N, Shimizu T, Seino S, Inagaki N (2001) Protective role of ATP-sensitive potassium channels in hypoxia-induced generalized seizure. Science 292:1543–1546
7. Meldrum BS (1997) Epileptic brain damage: a consequence and cause of seizures. Neuropathol App Neurobiol 23:185–202
8. Novelli A, Reilly JA, Lysko PG, Henneberry RC (1988) Glutamate becomes neurotoxic via the N-methyl-D-aspartate receptor when intracellular energy levels are reduced. Brain Res 451:205–212
9. Fariello RG, Golden GT, Smith GG, Reyes PF (1989) Potentiation of kainic acid epileptogenicity and sparing from neuronal damage by an NMDA receptor antagonist. Epilepsy Res 3:206–213
10. Norman RM (1964) The neuropathology of status epilepticus. Med Sci Law 4:46–51
11. Meldrum BS, Brierley JB (1973) Prolonged epileptic seizures in primates: ischemic cell change and its relation to ictal physiological events. Arch Neurol 28:10–17
12. O'Connell BK, Towfighi J, Kofke WA, Hawkins RA (1988) Neuronal lesions in mercaptopropionic acid-induced status epilepticus. Acta Neuropathol 77:47–54
13. Nevander G, Ingvar M, Auer R, Siesjö BK (1985) Status epilepticus in well-oxygenated rats causes neuronal necrosis. Ann Neurol 18:281–290
14. Brierley JB (1976) Cerebral hypoxia. In: Blackwood W, Corsellis JAN (eds) Greenfield's neuropathology. Edward Arnold, Edinburgh, pp 43–85
15. Young RSK, During MJ, Aquila WJ, Tendler D, Ley E (1992) Hypoxia increases extracellular concentrations of excitatory and inhibitory neurotransmitters in subsequently induced seizure: in vivo microdialysis study in the rabbit. Exp Neurol 117:204–209
16. Cataltepe O, Vannucci RC, Heitjan DF, Towfighi J (1995) Effect of status epilepticus on hypoxic-ischemic brain damage in the immature rat. Ped Res 38:251–257

17. Hayakawa T, Higuchi Y, Nigami H, Hattori H (1994) Zonisamide reduces hypoxic-ischemic brain damage in neonatal rats irrespective of its anticonvulsant effect. Eur J Pharmacol 257:131–136

18. Towfighi J, Housman C, Mauger D, Vannucci RC (1999) Effect of seizures on cerebral hypoxic-ischemic lesions in immature rats. Dev Brain Res 113:83–95

19. Wirrell EC, Armstrong EA, Osman LD, Yager JY (2001) Prolonged seizures exacerbate perinatal hypoxic-ischemic brain damage. Ped Res 50:445–454

20. Young GB, Gilbert JJ, Zochodne DW (1990) The significance of myoclonic status epilepticus in postanoxic coma. Neurology 40:1843–1848

21. Wijdicks EFM, Parisi JE, Sharbrough FW (1994) Prognostic value of myoclonus status in comatose survivors of cardiac arrest. Ann Neurol 35:239–243

22. Celesia GG, Grigg MM, Ross E (1988) Generalized status myoclonicus in acute anoxic and toxic-metabolic encephalopathies. Arch Neurol 45:781–784

23. Guilleminault C, Tharp BR, Cousin D (1973) HVA and 5-HIAA CSF measurements and 5-HTP trials in some patients with involuntary movements. J Neurol Sci 18:435–441

24. Chadwick D, Hallet M, Harris R, Jenner P, Reynolds EH, Marsden CD (1977) Clinical, biochemical, and physiological features distinguishing myoclonus responsive to 5-HTP, tryptophan with monoamine oxidase inhibitor, and clonazepam. Brain 100:455–487

25. Jaw SP, Hussong MJ, Matsumoto RR, Truong DD (1994) Involvement of 5-HT2 receptors in posthypoxic stimulus-sensitive myoclonus in rats. Pharmacol Biochem Behav 49:129–131

26. Pappert EJ, Goetz CG, Vu TQ, Ling ZD, Leurgans S, Raman R, Carvey PM (1999) Animal model of posthypoxic myoclonus: effects of serotonergic antagonists. Neurology 52:16–21

27. Truong DD, Matsumoto RR, Schwartz PH, Hussong MJ, Wasterlain CG (1994) Novel rat cardiac arrest model of posthypoxic myoclonus. Movement Disorders 9:201–206

28. De Lean J, Richardson JC, Hornykiewicz O (1976) Beneficial effect of serotonin precursors in postanoxic action myoclonus. Neurology 26:863–868

29. Gimenez-Roldan S, Mateo D, Muradas V, De Yeben JG (1988) Clinical, biochemical, and pharmacologic observation in a patient with postasphyxial myoclonus: association with serotonin hyperactivity. Clin Neuropharmacol 11:151–160

30. Jumao-as A, Brenner RP (1990) Myoclonic status epilepticus: a clinical and electroencephalographic study. Neurology 40:1199–1202

31. Niedermeyer E, Bauer G, Burnite R, Reichenbach D (1977) Selective stimulus-sensitive myoclonus in acute cerebral anoxia. Arch Neurol 34:365–368

32. Van Cott AC, Blatt I, Brenner RP (1996) Stimulus-sensitive seizures in postanoxic coma. Epilepsia 37:868–874

33. Wolf P (1977) Periodic synchronous and stereotyped myoclonus with postanoxic coma. J Neurol 215:39–47

34. Kanemoto K, Ozawa K (2000) A case of post-anoxic encephalopathy with initial massive myoclonic status followed by alternating Jacksonian seizures. Seizure 9:352–355

35. Wijdicks EFM, Young GB (1994) Myoclonus status in comatose patients after cardiac arrest. The Lancet 343:1642–1643

36. Arnoldus EPJ, Lammers GJ (1995) Postanoxic coma: good recovery despite myoclonus status. Ann Neurol 38:697–698

37. Hanakawa T, Hashimoto S, Iga K, Segawa Y, Shibasaki H (2000) Carotid brainstem myoclonus after hypoxic brain damage. J Neurol Neurosurg Psychiatry 69:672–674

38. Hallett M (1987) The pathophysiology of myoclonus. TINS 10:69–73

39. Harper SJ, Wilkes RG (1991) Posthypoxic myoclonus (the Lance-Adams syndrome) in the intensive care unit. Anaesthesia 46:199–201

40. Werhahn KJ, Brown P, Thompson PD, Marsden CD (1997) The clinical features and prognosis of chronic posthypoxic myoclonus. Mov Disord 12:216–220

41. Hallett M, Chadwick D, Adam J, Marsden CD (1977) Reticular reflex myoclonus: a physiological type of human post-hypoxic myoclonus. J Neurol Neurosurg Psychiatry 40:253–264

42. Brown P, Thompson PD, Rothwell JC, Day BL, Marsden CD (1991) A case of postanoxic encephalopathy with cortical action and brainstem reticular reflex myoclonus. Mov Disord 6:139–144

43. Witte OW, Niedermeyer E, Arendt G, Freund HJ (1988) Post-hypoxic action (intention) myoclonus: a clinico-electroencephalographic study. J Neurol 235:214–218

44. Lance JW, Adams RD (2001) Negative myoclonus in posthypoxic patients: historical note. Mov Disord 16:162–163

45. Fahn S (1986) Posthypoxic action myoclonus: literature review update. Adv Neurol 43:157–169

46. Varelas PN, Spanaki MV, Hacein-Bey L, Hether T, Terranova B (2003) Emergent EEG: Indications and diagnostic yield. Neurology 61:702–704

47. Beydoun A, Yen CE, Drury I (1991) Variance of interburst intervals in burst suppression. Electroencephalogr Clin Neurophysiol 79:435–439

48. Chen R, Bolton CF, Young GB (1996) Prediction of outcome in patients with anoxic coma: a clinical and electro-physiologic study. Crit Care Med 24:672–678

49. Binnie CD, Prior PF, Lloyd DSL, Scott DF, Margison JH (1970) Electroencephalographic prediction of fatal anoxic brain damage after resuscitation for cardiac arrest. Br Med J 4:265–268

50. Møller M, Holm B, Sindrup E, Lyager Nielsen B (1978) Electroencephalographic prediction of anoxic brain damage after resuscitation from cardiac arrest in patients with acute myocardial infarction. Acta Med Scand 203:31–37

51. Zandbergen EGJ, de Haan RJ, Stoutenbeek CP, Koelman JHTM, Hijdra A (1998) Systematic review of early prediction of poor outcome in anoxic-ischaemic coma. The Lancet 352:1808–1812

52. Ahmed I (1988) Use of somatosensory evoked responses in the prediction of outcome from coma. Clin Electroencephalogr 19:78–86

53. Bassetti C, Bomio F, Mathis J, Hess CW (1996) Early prognosis in coma after cardiac arrest: a prospective clinical, electrophysiological, and biochemical study of 60 patients. J Neurol Neurosurg Psychiatry 61:610–615

54. Brunko E, Zegers de Beyl D (1987) Prognostic value of early cortical somatosensory evoked potentials after resuscitation from cardiac arrest. Electroencephalogr Clin Neurophysiol 66:14–24

55. Kano T, Shimoda O, Morioka T, Yagishita Y, Hashiguchi A (1992) Evaluation of the central nervous function in resuscitated comatose patients by multilevel evoked potentials. Resuscitation 23:235–248

56. Rothstein TL, Thomas EM, Sumi SM (1991) Predicting outcome in hypoxic-ischemic coma. A prospective clinical and electrophysiologic study. Electoencephalogr Clin Neurophysiol 79:101–107

57. Walser H, Mattle H, Keller HM, Janzer R (1985) Early cortical median nerve somatosensory evoked potentials. Prognostic value in anoxic coma. Arch Neurol 42:32–38

58. Madl C, Kramer L, Yeganehfar W (1996) Detection of nontraumatic comatose patients with no benefit of intensive care treatment by recording of sensory evoked potentials. Arch Neurol 53:512–516

59. Torbey MT, Selim M, Knorr J, Bigelow C, Recht L (2000) Quantitative analysis of the loss of distinction between gray and white matter in comatose patients after cardiac arrest. Stroke 31:2163–2167

60. Arbelaez A, Castillo M, Mukherji SK (1999) Diffusion-weighted MR imaging of global cerebral anoxia. Am J Neuroradiol 20:999–1007

61. Kim JA, Chung JI, Yoon PH, Kim DI, Chung TS, Kim EJ, Jeong EK (2001) Transient MR signal changes in patients with generalized tonic-clonic seizure or status epilepticus: periictal diffusion-weighted imaging. Am J Neuroradiol 22:1149–1160

62. Ye JH, Ren J, Krnjevic K, Liu PL, McArdle JJ (1999) Cocaine and lidocaine have additive inhibitory effects on GABA A current of acutely dissociated hippocampal pyramidal cells. Brain Res 821:26–32

63. Barat SA, Abdel-Rahman MS (1997) Decreased cocaine- and lidocaine-induced seizure response by dextromethorphan and DNQX in rat. Brain Res 756:179–183

64. DeToledo JC (2000) Lidocaine and seizures. Ther Drug Monit 22:320–322

65. Kerns W, English B, Ford M (1994) Propafenone overdose. Ann Emerg Med 81:35–39

66. Caramelli P, Mutarelli EG, Caramelli B, Tranchesi B, Pileggi F, Schaff M (1992) Neurological complications after thrombolytic treatment for acute myocardial infarction: emphasis on unprecedented manifestations. Acta Neurol Scand 85:331–333

67. Cooling DS (1993) Theophylline toxicity. J Emerg Med 11:415–425

68. Hollander JE (1995) The management of cocaine-associated myocardial ischemia. N Eng J Med 333:1267–1272

69. Koppel BS, Samkoff L, Daras M (1996) Relation of cocaine use to seizures and epilepsy. Epilepsia 37:875–878

70. Goh WC, Heath PD, Ellis SJ, Oakley PA (2002) Neurological outcome prediction in a cardiorespiratory arrest survivor. Br J Anaesth 88:719–722

71. Brain Resuscitation Clinical Trial I Study Group (1986) Randomized clinical study of thiopental loading in comatose survivors of cardiac arrest. N Eng J Med 314:397–403

72. Kanthasamy AG, Vu TQ, Yun RJ, Truong DD (1996) Antimyoclonic affect of gabapentin in a posthypoxic animal model of myoclonus. Eur J Pharmacol 297:219–224

73. Fahn S (1978) Post-anoxic action myoclonus: improvement with valproic acid. N Eng J Med 299:313–314

74. Hirose G, Singer P, Bass N (1971) Successful treatment of posthypoxic action myoclonus with carbamazepine. JAMA 218:1432–1433

75. Coletti A, Mandelli A, Minoli G, Tredici G (1980) Post-anoxic action myoclonus (Lance-Adams syndrome) treated with levodopa and gabaergic drugs. J Neurol 223:67–70

76. Beretta E, Regli F, de Crousaz G, Steck AJ (1981) Postanoxic myoclonus: treatment of a case with 5-hydroxytryptophane and a decarboxylase inhibitor. J Neurol 225:57–62

77. Krauss GL, Bergin A, Kramer RE, Cho YW, Reich SG (2001) Suppression of posthypoxic and post-encephalitic myoclonus with levetiracetam. Neurology 56:411–412

78. Wijdicks EFM, Hijdra A, Young GB, Bassetti CL, Wiebe S (2006) Practice parameter: prediction of outcome in comatose survivors after cardiopulmonary resuscitation (an evidence-based review). Neurology 67:203–210

79. The Hypothermia After Cardiac Arrest Study Group (2002) Mild therapeutic hypothermia to improve the neurologic outcome after cardiac arrest. N Eng J Med 346:549–556

80. Bernard SA, Gray TW, Buist MD et al (2002) Treatment of comatose survivors of out-of-hospital cardiac arrest with induced hypothermia. N Eng J Med 346:557–563

81. Nolan JP, Morley PT, Vanden Hoek TL, Hickey RW (2003) Therapeutic hypothermia after cardiac arrest: ILCOR advisory statement. Resuscitation 57:231–237

82. Rundgren M, Rosén I, Friberg H (2006) Amplitude-integrated EEG (aEEG) predicts outcome after cardiac arrest and induced hypothermia. Intensive Care Med 32:836–842

83. Hovland A, Nielsen EW, Kluver J, Salvesen R (2006) EEG should be performed during induced hypothermia. Resuscitation 68:143–146

84. Schmitt FC, Buchheim K, Meierkord H, Holtkamp M (2006) Anticonvulsant properties of hypothermia in experimental status epilepticus. Neurobiol Dis 23:689–696

85. Orlowski JP, Erenberg G, Lueders H, Cruse RP (1984) Hypothermia and barbiturate coma for refractory status epilepticus. Crit Care Med 12:367–372

86. Corry JJ, Dhar R, Murphy T, Diringer MN (2007) Hypothermia for refractory status epilepticus. Neurocrit Care 9:189–197

87. Karkar KM, Garcia PA, Bateman LM, Smyth MD, Barbaro NM, Berger M (2002) Focal cooling suppresses spontaneous epileptiform activity without changing the cortical motor threshold. Epilepsia 43:932–935

88. Imoto H, Fujii M, Uchiyama J et al (2006) Use of a Peltier chip with a newly devised local brain-cooling system for neocortical seizures in the rat. J Neurosurg 104:150–156

89. Takei Y, Nishikawa Y, Tachibana M et al (2004) Hypothermia during kainic acid-induced seizures reduces hippocampal lesions and cerebral nitric oxide production in immature rabbits. Brain Dev 26:176–183

90. Lundgren J, Smith ML, Blennow G, Siesjo BK (1994) Hyperthermia aggravates and hypothermia ameliorates epileptic brain damage. Exp Brain Res 99:43–55

91. Siemkowicz E, Haider A (1995) Post-ischemic hypothermia ameliorates ischemic brain damage but not post-ischemic audiogenic seizures in rats. Resuscitation 30:61–67

92. Bennet L, Dean JM, Wassink G, Gunn AJ (2007) Differential effects of hypothermia on early and late epileptiform events after severe hypoxia in preterm fetal sheep. J Neurophysiol 97:572–578

93. Sunde K, Dunlop O, Rostrup M, Sandberg M, Sjøholm H, Jacobsen D (2006) Determination of prognosis after cardiac arrest may be more difficult after introduction of therapeutic hypothermia. Resuscitation 69:29–32

94. Tiainen M, Kovala TT, Takkunen OS, Roine RO (2005) Somatosensory and brainstem auditory evoked potentials in cardiac arrest patients treated with hypothermia. Crit Care Med 33:1736–1740

Chapter 7

Seizures in Fulminant Hepatic Failure, Multiorgan Failure, and Endocrine Crisis

Andrew Beaumont and Paul M. Vespa

Abstract Fulminant hepatic failure and other causes of multiorgan dysfunction can be associated with seizures. These seizures can be convulsive or nonconvulsive, and may significantly affect the pathobiology of the patient's critical condition. The use of continuous electroencephalography has become very important in the identification and treatment of seizures in critically ill patients with hepatic or other metabolic disorders. Seizures arise either as a direct result of the organ failure, or as a result of a secondary metabolic disturbance. Correction of the underlying metabolic syndrome may result in the prevention and treatment of the seizures. Secondary organ failure and endocrine abnormalities are commonly seen in the neurocritically ill population, and these patients are more prone to seizures. Organ failure can influence the treatment of both new onset and preexisting seizure disorders by altering the pharmacokinetics of major anticonvulsants. Alternatively, anticonvulsants can precipitate organ failure. Therefore, pharmacotherapy of seizures in these settings should be undertaken cautiously.

Keywords Hepatic failure, Renal failure, Endocrinopathy, Diabetes, Dialysis, Encephalopathy, Seizures

7.1. Introduction

Seizures are a common complication of organ failure and endocrine disease, either as a result of general biochemical and metabolic abnormalities, or as a specific syndrome related to the primary disease process. Critically ill patients may be hospitalized as a result of the organ failure or endocrine disease, or these conditions may arise as complications of another disease process. The acuity of onset of these problems may determine the overall response of the organism to the factors that alter seizure threshold. Even acute organ failure typically occurs in progressive stages, each of which may be associated with differing susceptibility to seizures. Endocrine disease is typically more indolent in onset but the effects are dependent on the hormone cascade

From: *Seizures in Critical Care*: *A Guide to Diagnosis and Therapeutics*: Current Clinical Neurology, Second Edition, Edited by: P. Varelas, DOI 10.1007/978-1-60327-532-3_7,
© Humana Press, a part of Springer Science+Business Media, LLC 2005, 2010

involved and the organism's natural storage of the relevant hormone, i.e., hypothyroidism is rarely acute unless there is sudden loss of large amounts of thyroid tissue, whereas Addisonian crisis may develop quickly because of the daily requirements for steroid hormone production.

The principles of seizure management in this group of patients follow an algorithm common to seizures complicating other medical conditions. Acute seizures should be controlled, seizure prophylaxis with antiepileptics should be instituted, and any causative factors, including biochemical/metabolic abnormalities and the primary disease process, should be corrected.

This chapter will review the features of seizures in fulminant hepatic failure, hepatorenal failure, and endocrine crisis, including their incidence, treatment, and clinical implications for critical care. Seizure medications are metabolized and excreted by the hepatorenal system and therefore, management of seizures in the setting of renal or hepatic failure must be undertaken cautiously.

7.2. Organ Failure

7.2.1. Hepatic Failure

Hepatic failure is a common indication for ICU admission; in addition, hepatic failure frequently complicates other serious illnesses. More than 2,000 cases of acute hepatic failure occur in the US every year, with an estimated mortality of 80% (1). Acute fulminant hepatic failure is most commonly caused by toxins such as acetaminophen (39%), acute drug reaction (17%), viral hepatitis (12%), and less commonly, acute hypotension, sepsis, and fulminant primary liver disease. The biochemical effects of hepatic failure include significant alterations in glucose metabolism, and build up of tissue and serum ammonia, with the resulting formation of glutamine and subsequent severe, excitotoxic brain edema (2). This combined with the activation of excitatory amino acids and the impairment of astrocyte function leads to malignant brain edema, and elevated intracranial pressure. Systemic build up of toxins in the circulation occurs as a result. This combination of events can cause progressive encephalopathy, a spectrum of neurological dysfunction classically divided into four stages. Stage I is euphoria or depression, with mild confusion, slurred speech, and disordered sleep; stage II is lethargy and moderate confusion; stage III is marked confusion, incoherent speech, and somnolence; stage IV is coma with cerebral edema formation and elevated intracranial pressure (ICP).

Seizures can arise in any of the stages of hepatic failure, either as a result of the encephalopathic process or secondary to other changes in serum levels of electrolytes, glucose, or other metabolites. The incidence of seizures in hepatic encephalopathy has been reported as varying from 2 to 33% (3). Ellis et al. (2000) enrolled 42 patients with stage III and stage IV hepatic encephalopathy in a controlled trial to evaluate the benefit of prophylactic phenytoin administration (4). Subclinical seizure activity, as documented by continuous EEG, was seen in 3/20 patients in the treated group, compared with 10/22 in the untreated group. One study has reported the incidence of status epilepticus in hepatic encephalopathy that was refractory to anticonvulsants but responded to lactulose therapy with a reduction in the serum ammonia levels (5). The pathophysiology of hepatic encephalopathy is unclear, but it has been postulated to arise from a combination of hyperammonemia, abnormal glutamine metabolism, elevated glutamate levels, enhanced GABAergic effects, and the contribution of false neurotransmitters.

Bickford and Butt (6) have described three classical phases of EEG changes in hepatic encephalopathy, the incidence of which is directly related to arterial ammonia levels. The first stage involves a diffuse theta pattern, the second stage involves triphasic waveforms with often sharp or spike morphology, and the third stage consists of arrhythmic delta activity with poor bilateral synchrony. The majority of seizures are reported to occur with the second stage EEG pattern. Ficker et al. (1997) reviewed EEG data from 120 patients at the Mayo Clinic with hepatic encephalopathy (7). Epileptiform abnormalities were identified in 18 patients (15%). Interictal discharges were observed in 13 patients consisting of focal spike and sharp wave discharges. Ten patients had electrographic seizures, either focal (6 patients) or generalized (5 patients), and 12 patients had clinical seizures (focal in 4 and generalized in 8 patients). Most patients with epileptiform activity died or deteriorated; the authors suggested that the presence of seizures is associated with a poor prognosis. Special care must be taken in patients with asterixis, which can cause a rhythmic artifact on the EEG that could be mistaken for ictal activity.

The occurrence of nonconulsive seizures in patients with fulminant hepatic failure has been documented (5, 8–10). These seizures may be manifested only by continuous electroencephalopgraphy (cEEG) (11). cEEG is a useful modality as it provides temporal assessment of the EEG rather than a cross-sectional analysis of the EEG at a single point in time. Most studies of critically ill patients have demonstrated a much higher incidence of seizures using cEEG as compared with a one-time, 30 min EEG (12). The incidence of seizures is higher, around 25% when the serum ammonia level >124 mmol/L (13). Routine monitoring of cEEG in the acute phase of fulminant hepatic failure is highly recommended by these authors.

Seizures may occur after the initial crisis of fulminant hepatic failure is over. In several studies (13–15), seizures have occurred in the early posttransplant period of time. The reasons for these seizures are not clear, but may relate to exposure to immunosuppressants that are known to lower seizure thresholds, such as acyclovir. Hence, a change in mental status may require repeat testing for the presence of nonconvulsive seizures.

Special cases of liver failure with associated neurological dysfunction include Wilson's disease, Reye's syndrome, and the hepatic porphyrias. Wilson's disease (hepatolenticular degeneration) is a rare autosomal recessive disease, occurring between the first and third decades, characterized by failure of copper metabolism leading to copper deposits in the liver and brain. The disease has been localized to an abnormal gene (ATP7B) on chromosome 13q14.3 that codes for a copper transporting ATPase. The condition usually presents as either liver disease and/or neuropsychiatric disease. Seizures occur infrequently, and more commonly movement disorders predominate. Dening et al. (1988) reviewed the incidence of seizures in Wilson's disease in both a series of 200 of their own patients, and the literature (16). They found a seizure prevalence of 6.2%, ten times higher than in the general population. Seizures were recorded at any stage of the disease but most commonly after beginning treatment. They found that seizures responded well to therapy with 60% of cases remaining seizure free at 7 years. The authors also concluded that penicillamine-induced pyridoxine deficiency was only responsible for seizures in a few cases, and that the most likely etiology of the seizures was copper deposition in the brain.

Reye's syndrome is a disorder of children associated with aspirin use in the context of a viral illness (typically influenza A/B or varicella). The disorder is characterized by rapid hepatic failure, encephalopathy presenting as seizures or coma, and fatty infiltration of the viscera. The majority of reported cases occurred in the pediatric population, but adult cases have been also described (17, 18). The incidence of Reye's syndrome has declined dramatically since 1986, when the FDA required that all aspirin products have labels warning about the possible association. The pathophysiology of the condition is poorly understood but it is probably related to hepatic mitochondrial dysfunction. There is little data about the absolute prevalence of seizures in Reye's syndrome, however seizures may relate to progressive cerebral edema, raised ICP, and cerebral hypoperfusion. Some studies have recorded the EEG in Reye's syndrome and reported increased delta activity with overall EEG suppression and 14 Hz positive burst discharges (19, 20). The prognostic significance of seizures in Reye's syndrome is unclear, as some patients with seizures recover completely. Some patients, however, are left with epilepsy, including West and Lennox-Gastaut syndromes.

The hepatic porphyrias include acute intermittent porphyria, variegate porphyria, and hereditary coproporphyria resulting from different enzymatic deficiencies in heme synthesis with similar neurologic manifestations. Neurological manifestations include abnormal behavior, confusion, agitation, anxiety, hallucinations, and seizures. It has been estimated that 3.7% of patients with acute intermittent porphyria have seizures, including generalized and focal with secondary generalization (21). In some cases seizures can be related to hyponatremia (21). Porphyria may complicate the treatment of seizures. Acute exacerbations of porphyria can be triggered by a large number of anticonvulsant drugs including phenytoin, barbiturates, ethosuximide, diazepam, valproate, carbamazepine, and lamotrigine. Management of seizures in porphyric patients requires management of the porphyria with hematin infusions, removal of any precipitants including antiepileptics, and the use of antiepileptics that will not exacerbate the porphyric state. The effect of newer anti-epileptics on chicken embryo cultured cells treated with deferoxamine (blocking heme synthesis) was reported by Hahn et al. (1997) (22). Anti-epileptic drug concentrations representative of doses used in humans were achieved. Felbamate, lamotrigine, and tiagabine, but not gabapentin or vigabatrin, increased mRNA levels of aminolevulinic acid synthase, the rate controlling enzyme for porphyrin synthesis and levels of porphyrins. Therefore, anticonvulsants clinically recommended in this situation include gabapentin and vigabatrin (22, 23). Alternatively, isoflurane anesthesia can be used.

7.2.1.1. Treatment of Seizures in Hepatic Failure

Several other aspects of hepatic failure can influence seizure activity (14). In patients with a pre-existing seizure disorder, hepatic failure may alter serum levels of anticonvulsants normally cleared by the liver. Table 7-1 lists the common antiepileptics and outlines the role of hepatic and renal function in their metabolism and clearance, and also the known effects of the agents on hepatic and renal function. The degree of hepatic failure can also play a role in the

Table 7-1. Antiepileptic Medications: Characteristics Related to Hepatic or Renal Failure.

	Protein binding	Liver metabolism	Renal clearance	Dialyzable	Adverse hepatic effects	Adverse renal effects
Phenobarbital	20–60	metabolized – inactive	21% including metabolites	Y	Hepatotoxicity	Nephrotoxicity
Phenytoin	88–93	metabolized – inactive	2% and inactive metabolites	N	Hepatitis/ hepatic necrosis	Interstitial nephritis, nephrotoxicity, renal failure
Clonazepam	86	metabolized	0.5–1.0% including inactive metabolites	N/A	Transient elevation LFT's	None
Ethosuximide	minimal	80% metabolized – inactive	20% – unchanged	Y	None	None
Carbamazepine	75	98% metabolized, some active	72% including metabolites	Y	Hepatitis, cholangitis, abnormal LFT's, hepatic failure, bile duct injury	Renal failure, tubulointerstitial nephritis (rare)
Valproate	90	metabolized – some active	70–80% including metabolites	Y	Elevated LFTs (common), hepatic failure, hepatitis, hepatotoxicity (0.02%)	Renal failure (rare)
Lamotrigine	55	metabolized – inactive	94% including metabolites	Y	Elevated LFT's (rare), acute hepatitis (rare), hepatic failure (rare)	Renal failure (rare)
Gabapentin	<3	not metabolized	76–84% unchanged	Y		
Topiramate	9–17	minimal	55–97% unchanged	Y	1% incidence of elevated LFT's, hepatic failure (rare)	2% incidence of renal calculi
Vigabatrin	none	small amount	65% unchanged	Y	Hepatic failure (rare)	None
Levetiracetam	none	small amount	66% unchanged, 25% inactive metabolites	Y	None	None
Tiagabine	96	metabolized – inactive	2% unchanged, 25% inactive metabolites	N	None	None

(continued)

Table 7-1. (continued)

	Protein binding	Liver metabolism	Renal clearance	Dialyzable	Adverse hepatic effects	Adverse renal effects
Felbamate	22–25	unknown	90%, with 40% metabolites of unknown activity	N/A	5% incidence of elevated LFT's, 6/75,000 patient years incidence of hepatic failure	None
Zonisamide	40–60	metabolized – inactive	35% unchanged, some metabolites	N/A	None	1.9% incidence of renal calculi, transient increase BUN (common)

Y yes, *N* no, *LFT* liver function tests.

metabolism of drugs. In early hepatitis there may be increased blood flow to the liver with relatively normal hepatocytes, a situation that may increase hepatic clearance of drugs. In more advanced hepatic failure with liver necrosis, hepatocellular tissue decreases and therefore, serum levels of drugs cleared by the liver may rise (24). In addition, hepatic failure is associated with hypoalbuminemia; this state can lead to increased serum free levels of drugs of those antiepileptics that are highly bound to serum protein. Hypoalbuminemia, a common finding in the ICU even outside of the context of hepatic failure, can therefore increase the risk of antiepileptic toxicity (25). Certain anticonvulsants, such as phenytoin, barbiturates, topiramate, felbamate, valproate, and lamotrigine, can also have a direct toxic effect on the liver (26). The interested reader should refer to the Chapter 15 for more details.

7.2.2. Renal Failure

7.2.2.1. Introduction
Renal failure represents a decline in the glomerular filtration rate that can occur acutely or chronically. Acute and chronic renal failures influence outcome in critical illness. In the critically ill population, it usually arises acutely as a result of sepsis, drug toxicity, hypotension, or as part of multiple organ failure. Chronic renal failure is a gradual and progressive loss of renal function that can ultimately result in end stage renal disease. ICU admission as a result of chronic renal failure is usually related to secondary complications such as respiratory distress, hyperkalemia, uremic encephalopathy, and postcardiopulmonary resuscitation. Estimates of the incidence of acute renal failure in the ICU population are approximately 3–4% (27, 28). Schwilk et al. (1997) examined 3,591 ICU admissions and found a 4.3% incidence of acute renal failure (ARF), as compared with 0.6% of the remaining hospital population (28). The incidence of ARF is proportional to the American Society of Anesthesiologists (ASA) score; ASA 5 patients had an incidence of 20.7% compared with 0.2% in ASA 2 patients. Electrolyte abnormalities are common in acute and chronic renal failure and include hyperkalemia,

hyponatremia, acidosis secondary to loss of bicarbonate, and secondary hyperparathyroidism.

In one study, seizures were reported in 5 of 13 patients with acute renal failure, typically occurring in the second week of illness (29). Seizures in chronic renal failure are often a late manifestation and occur in approximately 10% of patients (30). Even in patients on chronic hemodialysis with no known evidence of seizures, bilateral spike-and-wave patterns have been reported on EEG in 8–9% of cases (31). Pediatric renal failure patients are also seizure prone; analysis of 108 children with renal failure revealed a 15% incidence of seizures; all of the patients with seizures had received dialysis at some point (32).

7.2.2.2. Uremic Encephalopathy

Uremic encephalopathy is characterized by a waxing and waning neurological decline that can occur in both acute and chronic renal failure. A more rapid deterioration in renal function leads to a more severe and rapidly progressive encephalopathy. Early symptoms include apathy, fatigue, and decreased attention span. Frontal lobe symptoms follow with impaired abstract thinking, behavioral changes, and frontal lobe release signs, such as paratonia and the palmomental reflex. Seizures occur late after delirium, hallucinations, agitation, and torpor. They are usually a preterminal finding, and are typically generalized tonic-clonic in nature (33). The degree of azotemia correlates poorly with neurological dysfunction (34). The pathophysiology of uremic encephalopathy is poorly understood but is thought to relate to disruption in synaptic function possibly related to a parathormone (PTH) dependent enhancement of calcium transport leading to increased levels of calcium in the cortex (35). In both clinical and experimental studies, EEG abnormalities have been improved by parathyroid resection (36, 37). Various organic byproducts of renal failure have been implicated as uremic neurotoxins. In experimental studies it has been shown that neurotoxic organic acids share a common transport mechanism between the proximal renal tubule and the cerebral vasculature in the form of the transmembrane proteins OAT 1 and 3 (organic anion transporters) (38). There is evidence of decreased synaptic function and neurotransmission, leading to an overall decrease in the cerebral oxygen consumption and metabolic rate of cerebral tissue. Accumulation of guanidino-compounds, like guanidine succinate, that inhibit release of GABA and glycine in animal models of uremia has been implicated (33). The EEG in uremic encephalopathy typically shows non-specific changes of encephalopathy, with large amounts of predominantly theta and delta activity. It is important to distinguish this activity from seizures, especially when these waveforms become rhythmic. Tanimu et al. (1998) reported a patient with end-stage renal disease undergoing hemodialysis that became confused and was thought to have uremic encephalopathy. The EEG revealed generalized spike and wave discharges at 2–3 Hz that responded to intravenous diazepam with immediate resolution of the confusion (39). Thus, nonconvulsive absence of status epilepticus must also be considered in acutely encephalopathic hemodialysis patients. EEG abnormalities are most often seen in the acute encephalopathic state within 48 h of the onset of renal failure. Later in the course, when the encephalopathy becomes more chronic, the EEG changes are less prominent. There is a correlation between slow frequencies (<7 Hz) and increases in serum creatinine. In addition, bilateral spike and wave complexes without clinical seizures have been reported in up to 14% of patients with chronic uremic encephalopathy (33).

7.2.2.3. Dialysis Dysequilibrium Syndrome

Seizures can also occur during hemodialysis as part of the dialysis dysequilibrium syndrome (DDS). DDS is a syndrome first described in the 1960s; in its mildest form, it presents as restlessness, nausea, muscle cramps, and headache. In more severe forms, it is characterized by delirium, myoclonus and subsequently, generalized seizures, papilledema, and raised ICP. Symptoms typically arise towards the end of hemodialysis and usually resolve within hours to days (40). DDS is seen less commonly at present because of slower dialysis rates and more frequent sessions. It has become a diagnosis of exclusion, and other disorders including intracranial bleeding or infection have to be excluded first. The origin of DDS is thought to be due to rapid shifts of water into the brain as a result of the presence of idiogenic osmoles in the tissue (41) and intracellular acidosis (42). Before dialysis the tissue is protected from osmotic stress by idiogenic osmoles. With dialysis serum osmoles are removed. Therefore, the tissue becomes hyperosmotic compared with serum, and water enters the tissue causing edema.

7.2.2.4. Subdural Hematoma

Subdural hematoma (SDH), another possible cause of seizures in uremic patients, should also be considered, especially in the ICU population (43, 44). It occurs in 1–3.3% of patients undergoing dialysis and rarely is associated with head trauma. In an autopsy series of chronic dialysis patients who had sudden death, acute subdural hematoma was the third most common cause of death, occurring in 8.6% of patients (45). It can be bilateral in 20% of cases and may clinically present as obtundation, ataxia, and hemiparesis. The absolute incidence of seizures with SDH in the chronic renal failure population is unknown.

7.2.2.5. Dialysis Dementia

Dialysis dementia was first described by Alfrey in 1972 (46). This disorder is characterized by a progressive decline in cerebral function that can ultimately result in death. Dialysis dementia occurs in 0.6–1.0% of all dialysis patients and occurs at a mean age of 50 years, with a mean time of onset at 35 months after the start of dialysis, and a mean survival of 6–9 months after symptom onset (47). Early symptoms are dysarthria, dysphasia, lethargy, and depression. Seizures occur in 60% of patients in the advanced stages, along with psychosis and hallucinations, and should be distinguished from myoclonus that can occur in up to 80% of cases (48). EEG abnormalities may precede symptoms by months, and they include intermittent high voltage slowing and spike/wave activity, particularly in frontal leads (49). Elevated aluminum levels are reported in the cerebral cortex in dialysis dementia, and therapy with chelating agents such as desferrioxamine can reverse the dementia in up to 70% of cases.

7.2.2.6. Drug Induced Seizures

In the last few years, there have been several reports of drug-induced seizures. These tend to occur more commonly in patients with renal dysfunction. Noteworthy among these drugs are cephalosporins (50–53). Cefepime appears to be the most toxic drug, and this toxicity is often manifested as nonconvulsive seizures. Caution should be exercised when using these agents in patients with renal failure.

7.2.2.7. Treatment of Seizures Related to Renal Failure

Treatment of seizures in renal failure focuses on three approaches. Firstly, seizure prophylaxis should be initiated with an anticonvulsant, ideally one that has no renal clearance. Secondly, reversible epileptogenic electrolyte abnormalities should be corrected including hyponatremia and hypercalcemia. Thirdly, the underlying renal condition should be aggressively corrected and renal replacement therapy initiated where appropriate. In the case of uremic encephalopathy, correction of the uremia usually resolves neurological dysfunction including seizures.

Renal failure has important implications for anticonvulsant pharmacokinetics. Changes in the clearance of renally excreted anticonvulsants can affect the dosing requirements for both seizure prophylaxis in patients with preexisting seizure disorders and seizure prophylaxis in new onset seizures associated with renal failure (see Table 7-1 for renal clearance of common antiepileptics). Anticonvulsants with significant renal clearance include gabapentin, topiramate, and oxcarbazepine. They have to be avoided in renal failure or used in markedly reduced doses. Jones et al. (2002) reported that gabapentin dosing in a patient who missed hemodialysis led to ICU admission for desaturation and respiratory failure. Gabapentin normally has a half-life of 5–7 h. In patients with renal failure not undergoing hemodialysis, the half-life can increase to 132 h, but with hemodialysis it may decrease to 3.8 h (54). Other factors connected to renal failure can influence the pharmacokinetics of anticonvulsants. Edema from renal failure increases the volume of distribution of the bound drug, thereby reducing the effective concentration; also drugs that are significantly bound to proteins in plasma have higher effective serum concentrations if plasma protein concentration is reduced because of protein losing nephropathy. As an example, the accepted therapeutic range of phenytoin in patients with normal renal function is 10–20 mg/L, and this is reduced to 5–10 mg/L in patients with end-stage renal disease (55). Falsely elevated phenytoin levels can be detected by certain immunoassays after fosphenytoin administration due to cross-reactivity with fosphenytoin metabolites in critically ill patients with renal insufficiency (56). In addition to these issues, dialysis itself can remove quantities of anticonvulsants from the blood and anticonvulsant dosing may need to be adjusted relatively to the dialysis session. The intensivist should remember that the amount of drug removed during dialysis is typically inversely related to its protein bound fraction, and that the renally excreted drugs are the ones that are more dialyzed. Up to 35% of phenobarbital is removed during a session of continuous ambulatory peritoneal dialysis (57). Although phenytoin is not dialyzable and no supplemental dose is required after dialysis, high flux dialysis can result in up to 48.5% reduction in total body phenytoin. The intensivist has to be aware of this possibility in patients receiving dialysis, especially if a seizure disorder is exacerbated (58). Gabapentin is cleared by renal excretion only and 35% of the drug is removed during a dialysis session (59). For patients undergoing dialysis on gabapentin, an initial loading dose of 300–400 mg has been recommended. After each dialysis session an additional dose of 200–300 mg of the drug may be enough to maintain steady-state plasma concentration (59). Table 7-1 outlines the extent to which common antiepileptics are dialyzable. The interested reader should refer to the Chapter 15 for more details.

7.3. Endocrine Disease

7.3.1. Thyroid Disease

Thyroid disease usually causes reversible neurological change. Marked derangement of thyroid dysfunction, both hyper- and hypo-thryroidism can cause seizures (60, 61); however, it is more usual for thyroid disease to worsen seizures in a patient with a preexisting seizure disorder. Several derangements in thyroid hormone can occur in the context of critical illness. Most commonly seen is the sick euthyroid syndrome, characterized by reduced T3 levels, normal or low T4 levels, and decreased TSH levels (62). Critical illness is associated with reduced TSH secretion and pulsatility. In addition low TSH may be found in patients who received glucocorticoids and dopamine (63).

Generalized and focal seizures can be rarely seen in thyrotoxicosis and thyroid storm (64–66), and approximately 66% of hyperthyroid patients exhibit an abnormal EEG. These abnormalities include generalized slow wave activity, focal spike or focal slow waves, and triphasic waves. These abnormal EEG patterns reverse after treatment of the hyperthyroidism (67, 68). Liu et al. (1992) reviewed the literature in 1992, and found only 13 cases of thyrotoxicosis associated with seizures since 1956 (69). Recurrent encephalopathy and generalized seizures associated with relapses of thyrotoxicosis have also been reported (70). The mechanism of hyperthyroidism causing these changes is unknown; however, possibilities include a direct effect of thyroxine on cerebral metabolism, changes in ion channels, and up-regulation of catecholamine receptors. In experimental hyperthyroidism, seizure thresholds to epileptogenic drugs have been shown to be reduced (71). Correction of the thyrotoxicosis prevents seizure onset, and returns observed EEG abnormalities to normal (68). Another possible etiology is cerebral sinus thrombosis, a state highly associated with seizures. Siegert et al. (1995) reported two patients with Grave's disease, who presented with seizures and hemiplegia, and were found to have sagittal sinus thrombosis (72). They were controlled with phenytoin, oral anticoagulants, and prednisone. The authors attributed the sinus thrombosis to either a thyrotoxicosis induced hypercoagulable state (with increased factor VIII activity) or venous stasis in the neck due to compression of a large goiter.

Seizures are unusual in myxedema (73), although in some cases they may be the presenting sign (74). Psychiatric symptoms, encephalopathy, and coma are more common manifestations. It has been reported, however, that up to 20–25% of patients with myxedema coma may experience generalized convulsions or complex partial seizures. The EEG in myxedema typically has nonspecific generalized slowing and impaired photic driving (75). Non-convulsive seizures or status occasionally has to be distinguished from the unusually prolonged post-ictal state and an EEG is mandatory in that case. Seizures due to severe myxedema respond to replacement therapy. The low voltage slow patterns on the EEG may normalize before the clinical state of the patient and can be used as a prognostic index during treatment. Chronic antiepileptic drug administration is not indicated. Recurrence of seizures is suggestive of inadequate treatment or cessation of treatment, but in such cases the intensivist has to rule out other intracranial pathology. Because carbamazepine increases the metabolism of thyroid hormones, its use in hypothyroid patients has to be

carefully followed by additional thyroid replacement therapy to avoid precipitation of a hypothyroid crisis (76). The same is true with other antiepileptic
drugs such as phenytoin and phenobarbital.

Hashimoto's encephalopathy is a complication of Hashimoto's thyroiditis,
a steroid-responsive, relapsing thyroid disorder characterized by high titers of
thyroid auto-antibodies (77). A common feature of Hashimoto's encephalopathy is seizures and diffuse EEG abnormalities. The seizures may be generalized (77, 78) or partial (78, 79), and the EEG abnormalities include generalized
slowing, rhythmic bifrontal or temporal triphasic waves, and periodic sharp
waves (80). Clinically, myoclonus may also be seen, and this usually responds
to thyroxine replacement therapy. The incidence of seizures is independent
of the degree of thyroid dysfunction, and may even occur in the presence of
elevated antibodies alone. When a lumbar puncture is done for diagnostic purposes, the intensivist can expect abnormal results in up to 60% of cases with
leukocytosis, elevated protein, and IgG index or oligoclonal bands (81). The
pathophysiology of the disease is autoimmune, but the mechanism underlying
the seizures is not clear; autoimmune cerebral vasculitis or direct anti-neural
antibodies have been implicated.. Immunosuppressive therapy with steroids
improves the clinical picture.

7.3.2. Diabetes Mellitus and Glycemic Homeostasis

Disturbances in glycemic control are commonly seen in critically ill patients,
irrespective of a prior history of diabetes. Van den Berghe et al. (2001) (82)
examined 1,548 ICU admissions and found that 1,155 patients had mildly elevated serum glucose, and 182 had moderate glucose elevation. Only 204 had
a prior history of diabetes. In this study aggressive control of serum glucose
was associated with improved outcome.

Seizures have been reported to occur in 7–20% of all diabetic patients.
There is a paucity of data to support whether it is absolute serum levels of
glucose or rather rapid changes that are more important for epileptogenesis.
Anticonvulsants used at doses that control seizures in other disorders often
seem ineffective in treating seizures resulting from hypo or hyperglycemia
(83). Glucose transport across the blood brain barrier (BBB) is reduced during seizures and therefore, it is assumed that tissue hypermetabolism during
the ictus is independent of the plasma glucose level (84). It is unclear if this
presumed energy substrate deficiency may prolong the seizures.

Six percent of nonketotic hyperosmolar hyperglycemia (NHH) cases
present with focal motor seizures, and 25% of NHH patients eventually
develop seizures (85). Seizures in NHH occur early in hyperglycemia and
when osmolality is only modestly increased, with minimal reduction in
sodium levels and usually when consciousness is preserved. Seizures related
to NHH may occasionally have strange features. Reflex seizures (after limb
movement) have been well described (86, 87). They may present as speech
arrest (88) or have a visual component (89, 90). Transient subcortical T2 and
fluid-attenuated inversion recovery (FLAIR) hypointensity has been described
in the setting of status epilepticus and non-ketotic hyperglycemia and this has
been attributed to the accumulation of free radicals and iron deposition (91).
There is a lower incidence of seizures in ketotic hyperglycemia compared
with nonketotic hyperglycemia (83, 86). This is thought to occur as a result

of ketosis exerting an anticonvulsant effect through the production of GABA (92). GABA is thought to increase as a result of intracellular acidosis, which enhances GABA synthesis by glutamic acid decarboxylase. Ketogenic diets in patients with intractable epilepsy are thought to be effective through a similar mechanism.

Symptomatic hypoglycemia can occur in several endocrine disorders including primary hypothalamic-pituitary insufficiency (growth hormone, ACTH, TSH), primary adrenal insufficiency, primary hypothyroidism, and over-treated diabetes mellitus with either insulin or oral hypoglycemic agents such as sulfonylureas. Salicylates can also induce hypoglycemia by increasing glucose uptake in muscle tissue. Hypoglycemia can also be the result of pancreatic islet cell dysfunction such as islet cell hyperplasia or insulinoma (93). In such cases the seizures present during the night or early morning and are resistant to conventional anti-epileptic treatment. Seizures are the most common presenting neurological symptoms of hypoglycemia at any age. Hypoglycemic seizures usually occur at a serum glucose level of less than 40 mg/dL (94). Clinically, patients exhibit signs of sympathetic excitation before the seizures occur but not all the time. Tachycardia, palpitations, sweating, nervousness, hunger, headache, or tremor may be followed by a change in mental status, focal neurological signs, seizures, and coma. These symptoms and signs can be absent in patients with autonomic neuropathy such as chronic diabetics (95) or patients taking b-blockers such as propranolol.

Hart et al. (1998) retrospectively analyzed the clinical features of patients admitted to the hospital with hypoglycemia in a large teaching institution, and found seizures in 20% of all cases (96). EEG changes in hypoglycemia are non-specific. Bjorges et al. (1998) recorded quantitative EEG in 19 diabetic and 17 non-diabetic children exposed to a gradual reduction in serum glucose (97). Early changes in the EEG were increased amounts of delta and theta activity followed by epileptiform activity. At a specific serum glucose level diabetic children displayed significantly more EEG abnormalities than non-diabetic children. This suggests that seizure thresholds may be lower in diabetic patients, and factors other than absolute serum glucose levels are responsible for the seizures.

7.3.3. Pituitary Hormones

Pituitary dysfunction can result in several secondary endocrinopathies including alterations in thyroid and corticosteroid function. Seizures can arise as a result of any of these secondary endocrinopathies as detailed elsewhere. Conditions specific to the pituitary gland include diabetes insipidus and the syndrome of inappropriate antidiuretic hormone release (SIADH). SIADH by definition is caused by excess secretion of antidiuretic hormone (ADH) from the posterior pituitary, resulting in excess water retention in the distal renal tubule and collecting duct. SIADH can be caused by neoplasm, trauma, pain, infections, cavernous sinus thrombosis, cerebrovascular accident (CVA), multiple sclerosis (MS), hydrocephalus, psychosis, congenital lesions, drugs [carbamazepine, neuroleptics, tricyclics antidepressants, selective serotonin reuptake inhibitors (98)], postoperatively after transphenoidal surgery or endoscopic third ventriculostomy (99), and metabolic abnormalities.

Several of these conditions are seen in the critically ill patient population. Water retention results in acute hyponatremia, and this hyponatremia can lead to seizures. In contrast, the lack of ADH is diabetes insipidus (DI), characterized by polyuria, low urine specific gravity, and hypernatremia. Seizures do not typically occur in DI, although seizures can occur in any severe hyperosmolar state. Few studies have examined the absolute incidence of seizures in DI. Transient DI has been extensively reported in pregnancy (100). Combs et al. (1990) have reported a primigravida with transient DI, hypertension, and multiple seizures resistant to both magnesium sulfate and diazepam (101). They were successfully treated with phenytoin.

7.3.4. Sex Hormones

The role of sex hormones in the critically ill population has yet to be defined. The hypothalamic-pituitary axis is clearly disturbed in prolonged illness (102). Although endocrinopathies of the sex hormones per se are not associated with seizures in the ICU, sex steroid hormones have been found to have influence on seizure frequency in both experimental and clinical studies. In women, menarche, pregnancy, and the menopause can all influence seizure frequency, although these features are not common (103). The relationship between seizure frequency and the menstrual cycle (catamenial epilepsy) was first suggested by Locock (1857) (104), and more recent studies have reported perimenstrual exacerbation of seizures in up to 78% of women (105); an increase in the frequency of paroxysmal EEG discharges has also been observed perimenstrually (106).

The origin of menstrual variations in seizures is not clear; however, in animal studies, estrogen has been found to be proconvulsant and progesterone, anti-convulsant (107, 108). Estrogen has also been shown to be pro-convulsant in male animals (109). Logothetis et al. (1959) observed exacerbation of paroxysmal EEG abnormalities and seizures following intravenous estrogen in women with catamenial epilepsy (110). Clomiphene, an antiestrogen at the hypothalamic and pituitary levels, can also reduce seizure frequency (111), although whether this is related to clomiphene induced cycle changes or a direct effect on the hypothalamus/pituitary is not clear. Anovulatory menstrual cycles are characterized by lack of ovulation, and a lack of an increase in progesterone in the second half of the cycle. In a prospective study of 132 menstrual cycles from 35 patients, it was shown that a peri-menstrual increase in seizure frequency was only seen in ovulatory cycles (112). It is postulated that the change in seizure frequency relates to progesterone withdrawal immediately prior to the menses. In the perimenopausal period, estrogen/progesterone ratios become higher; therefore, it is not surprising that one study demonstrated that 64% of 39 women experienced a worsening of seizures peri-menopausally (113). During the menopause, there is an absolute reduction of all sex steroids, and it has been reported that 68% women report a clear reduction in seizure frequency (113).

7.3.5. Parathyroid Hormones

The role of parathyroid hormone in the critically ill has yet to be clearly defined. Hypocalcemia and hypercalcemia have both been documented in the critically ill population, and hypocalcemia is associated with worse outcomes (114, 115).

Hypocalcemia has been associated with elevated PTH levels early in non-surviving surgical ICU patients (115). Lind et al. (1992) examined 83 critically ill patients and found a 32% incidence of hypercalcemia. PTH levels were measured in 6 of these patients without renal failure, and PTH levels were found to be elevated (114). This suggests that a primary PTH dysfunction may cause hypercalcemia in the critically ill.

Seizures secondary to hypocalcemia in hypoparathroidism are common neurological manifestations, especially in children (75). Such seizures occur in 30–70% of patients and may be difficult to control (116). The seizure pattern may be generalized tonic-clonic (117), focal and less frequently atypical absence, and akinetic attacks (75). Seizures may be seen in chronic hypoparathyroidism late after thyroidectomy (118, 119). Some patients with familial hypoparathyroidism do not experience seizures, even with severe hypocalcemia (120). Some seizures in hypoparathyroidism are refractory to therapy, and are thought, in these cases, to be secondary to calcinosis of the brain. Idiopathic hypoparathyroidism can present with bilateral basal ganglia calcification, a useful imaging clue in a patient with seizures (121).

Antiepileptic drugs that induce hepatic enzymes, such as phenytoin and phenobarbital, can accelerate conversion of vitamin D and 25-hydroxyvitamin D into their inactive metabolites. These drugs can also impair calcium absorption from the gut and resorption from bone, contributing to hypocalcemia. Therefore, their use in cases of hypoparathyroidism could be questioned. Hyperparathyroidism can also cause seizures (122), which is most likely connected to hypercalcemia (123), as hypercalcemia has been shown to cause seizures in other settings (124).

7.3.6. Adrenal Glands

Adrenal dysfunction is well recognized in the critically ill population. Cortisol and catecholamines have both been shown to be elevated in this group of patients (125, 126). The incidence of absolute adrenal insufficiency is low. However, the concept of relative adrenal insufficiency has been introduced recently. This theory postulates that patients may not mount a level of corticosteroid response appropriate for the severity of their disease (127).

The adrenal gland is responsible for production of corticosteroid hormones and catecholamines. Alterations in corticosteroid function do not typically cause seizures; however, the secondary metabolic effects of these disorders can be epileptogenic. Adrenal insufficiency, including Addison's disease, may present with hypoglycemic seizures (128). Hypoglycemic seizures and coma due to isolated ACTH deficiency have been reported in children but rarely in adults (129). Addison's disease can also cause hyponatremia, another potential cause of seizures. However, the relatively gradual onset of hyponatremia in this setting less aggressively promotes seizure occurrence. The relationship between Cushing's syndrome and seizures is unknown. Hypercortisolism may potentially exacerbate seizure disorders. Some adrenocorticosteroids, including cortisol, are glutamatergic and may antagonize GABA-A receptors in the brain, thereby causing a proconvulsant effect. Herzog et al. (1998) reported 3 patients with Cushing's syndrome, seizures, and electromyographically confirmed myopathy. Their elevated serum ACTH and 24-h urinary cortisol concentration normalized after ketoconazole (200 mg 3–4 times/day) treatment, their seizure frequency decreased dramatically, and their weakness was improved (130). Dysfunction of the catecholamine function of the adrenal gland is typified by pheochromocytoma. Seizures may occur in patients with pheochromocytoma, and they are most commonly generalized. Their incidence appears to correlate with the degree of blood pressure elevation (131). In some cases, they can be the presenting complaint (132). The occurrence of seizures can be related either to the high catecholamines or to hypertensive encephalopathy. Cerebral vasospasm due to markedly elevated catecholamine levels can induce focal ischemia and seizure foci. Intracerebral hemorrhage during blood pressure elevation as a cause of seizures should be excluded by neuroimaging studies (132–134) (Figs. 7.1 and 7.2).

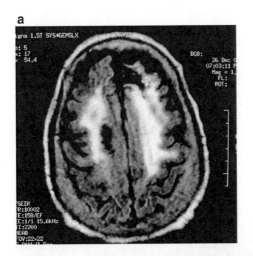

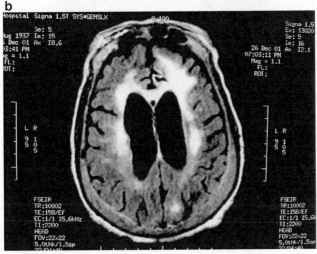

Fig. 7-1. (continued)

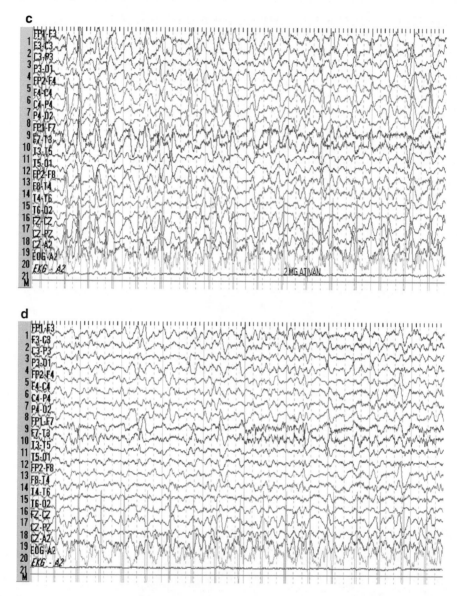

Fig. 7-1. *Case 1*: This 64 year-old woman with end-stage renal disease and history of previous strokes, on regular hemodialysis, was found down shaking and unresponsive by her daughter. The patient was admitted to the ICU and was intubated for aspiration pneumonia (**a**) and (**b**). MRI of the brain with FLAIR sequence showing diffuse periventricular white matter changes. (**c**) EEG, requested to rule out non-convulsive status epilepticus, showing runs of sharp triphasic waves. (**d**) EEG 2 min after the administration of 2 mg lorazepam IV demonstrating significant attenuation but no resolution of the triphasic waves. With additional 2 mg the triphasic waves were further suppressed. However, there was no clinical improvement on the patient's mental status, despite these measures and loading with phenytoin. She was extubated few days later and discharged to palliative care according to her wishes without regaining full consciousness

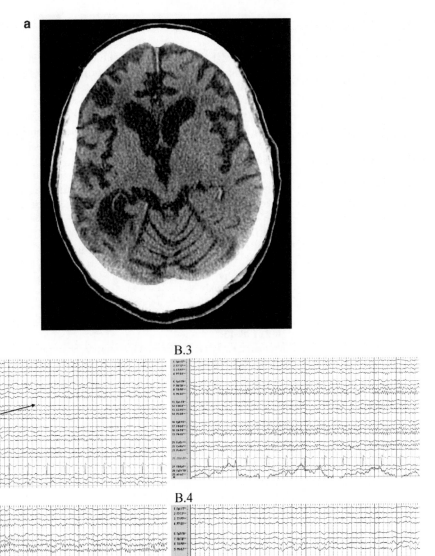

Fig. 7-2. *Case 2*: 65 year-old AA man admitted to the Neuro-ICU because of left facial twitching. He had end-stage liver disease from heavy alcohol abuse and hepatitis C, with an ammonia level of 74, ascites, and splenomegally. He was not a candidate for liver transplantation. He also had a history of seizures of unclear etiology. He was placed on continuous EEG monitoring and recorded 160 partial electrographic seizures during the first day of monitoring. He received levetiracetam (4 g/day), high dose topiramate (400 mg/day), and pregabalin (150 mg/day), and his seizures decreased to 60/day.A. CT of the head showing asymmetrical diffuse atrophy of the brain, right more than left.B. EEG showing the beginning from the right posterior parietal hemisphere (B.1, *black arrow*), the evolution (B.2 and B.3), and the end of a subclinical seizure

References

1. Lee WM (1993) Acute liver failure. N Engl J Med 329(25):1862–1872
2. Detry O, De Roover A, Honore P, Meurisse M (2006) Detry Brain edema and intracranial hypertension in fulminant hepatic failure: pathophysiology and management. World J Gastroenterol 12(46):7405–7412
3. Plum F, Posner JB (1984) Diagnosis of stupor and coma. TA Davis, Philadelphia
4. Ellis AJ, Wendon JA, Williams R (2000) Subclinical seizure activity and prophylactic phenytoin infusion in acute liver failure: a controlled clinical trial. Hepatology 32(3):536–541
5. Eleftheriadis N, Fourla E, Eleftheriadis D, Karlovasitou A (2003) Status epilepticus as a manifestation of hepatic encephalopathy. Acta Neurol Scand 107(2):142–144
6. Bickford RG, Butt HR (1955) Hepatic coma: the electroencephalographic pattern. J Clin Invest 34:790–799
7. Ficker DM, Westmoreland BF, Sharbrough FW (1997) Epileptiform abnormalities in hepatic encephalopathy. J Clin Neurophysiol 14(3):230–234
8. Tanaka H, Ueda H, Kida Y, Hamagami H, Tsuji T, Ichinose M (2006) Hepatic encephalopathy with status epileptics: a case report. World J Gastroenterol 12(11):1793–1794
9. Velioğlu SK, Gazioğlu S (2007) Non-convulsive status epilepticus secondary to valproic acid-induced hyperammonemic encephalopathy. Acta Neurol Scand 116(2):128–132
10. Engelhardt K, Trinka E, Franz G, Unterberger I, Spiegel M, Beer R, Pfausler B, Kampfl A, Schmutzhard E (2004) Refractory status epilepticus due to acute hepatic porphyria in a pregnant woman: induced abortion as the sole therapeutic option? Eur J Neurol 11(10):693–697
11. Jirsch J, Hirsch LJ (2007) Nonconvulsive seizures: developing a rational approach to the diagnosis and management in the critically ill population. Clin Neurophysiol 118(8):1660–1670
12. Vespa P (2005) Continuous EEG monitoring for the detection of seizures in traumatic brain injury, infarction, and intracerebral hemorrhage: "to detect and protect". J Clin Neurophysiol 22(2):99–106
13. Bhatia V, Singh R, Acharya SK (2006) Predictive value of arterial ammonia for complications and outcome in acute liver failure. Gut 55(1):98–104
14. Lacerda G, Krummel T, Sabourdy C, Ryvlin P, Hirsch E (2006) Optimizing therapy of seizures in patients with renal or hepatic dysfunction. Neurology 67(12 Suppl 4):S28–S33
15. Choi EJ, Kang JK, Lee SA, Kim KH, Lee SG, Andermann F (2004) New-onset seizures after liver transplantation: clinical implications and prognosis in survivors. Eur Neurol 52(4):230–236
16. Dening TR, Berrios GE, Walshe JM (1988) Wilson's disease and epilepsy. Brain 111(Pt 5):1139–1155
17. Atkins JN, Haponik EF (1979) Reye's syndrome in the adult patients. Am J Med 67(4):672–678
18. Chan ED (1993) Reye's syndrome in a young adult. Mil Med 158(1):65–68
19. Barr RE, Ackmann JJ, Harrington GJ, Varma RR, Lewis JD, Casper JT (1977) Computerized evaluation of electroencephalographic changes accompanying exchange transfusion in Reye's syndrome. Electroencephalogr Clin Neurophysiol 42(4):466–479
20. Yamada T, Tucker RP, Kooi KA (1976) Fourteen and six c/sec positive bursts in comatose patients. Electroencephalogr Clin Neurophysiol 40(6):645–653
21. Bylesjo I, Forsgren L, Lithner F, Boman K (1996) Epidemiology and clinical characteristics of seizures in patients with acute intermittent porphyria. Epilepsia 37(3):230–235

22. Hahn M, Gildemeister OS, Krauss GL, Pepe JA, Lambrecht RW, Donohue S et al (1997) Effects of new anticonvulsant medications on porphyrin synthesis in cultured liver cells: potential implications for patients with acute porphyria. Neurology 49(1):97–106

23. Zadra M, Grandi R, Erli LC, Mirabile D, Brambilla A (1998) Treatment of seizures in acute intermittent porphyria: safety and efficacy of gabapentin. Seizure 7(5):415–416

24. Rodighiero V (1999) Effects of liver disease on pharmacokinetics. An update. Clin Pharmacokinet 37(5):399–431

25. Boggs JG, Waterhouse EJ, DeLorenzo RJ (2000) The use of antiepileptic medications in renal and liver disease. In: Wyllie E (ed) The treatment of epilepsy: principles and practice. Williams & Wilkins, Baltimore

26. Asconape JJ (2002) Some common issues in the use of antiepileptic drugs. Semin Neurol 22(1):27–39

27. Schaefer JH, Jochimsen F, Keller F, Wegscheider K, Distler A (1991) Outcome prediction of acute renal failure in medical intensive care. Intensive Care Med 17(1):19–24

28. Schwilk B, Wiedeck H, Stein B, Reinelt H, Treiber H, Bothner U (1997) Epidemiology of acute renal failure and outcome of haemodiafiltration in intensive care. Intensive Care Med 23(12):1204–1211

29. Locke S, Merrill JP, Tyler HR (1961) Neurologic complication of uremia. Arch Intern Med 108:519–522

30. Tyler HR, Tyler KL (1994) Neurologic complications. In: Eknoyan G, Knochel JP (eds) The systemic consequences of renal failure. Grune & Stratton, New York

31. Hughes JR (1984) EEG in uremia. Am J EEG Technol 24:1–10

32. Rufo CM, Vazquez Florido AM, Madruga GM, Fijo J, Sanchez MA, Martin GJ (2002) Renal failure as a factor leading to epileptic seizures. An Esp Pediatr 56(3):212–218

33. Burn DJ, Bates D (1998) Neurology and the kidney. J Neurol Neurosurg Psychiatry 65(6):810–821

34. Fraser CL, Arieff AI (1988) Nervous system complications in uremia. Ann Intern Med 109(2):143–153

35. Smogorzewski MJ (2001) Central nervous dysfunction in uremia. Am J Kidney Dis 38(4 Suppl 1):S122–S128

36. Guisado R, Arieff AI, Massry SG, Lazarowitz V, Kerian A (1975) Changes in the electroencephalogram in acute uremia. Effects of parathyroid hormone and brain electrolytes. J Clin Invest 55(4):738–745

37. Cogan MG, Covey CM, Arieff AI, Wisniewski A, Clark OH, Lazarowitz V et al (1978) Central nervous system manifestations of hyperparathyroidism. Am J Med 65(6):963–970

38. Enomoto A, Takeda M, Taki K, Takayama F, Noshiro R, Niwa T et al (2003) Interactions of human organic anion as well as cation transporters with indoxyl sulfate. Eur J Pharmacol 466(1–2):13–20

39. Tanimu DZ, Obeid T, Awada A, Huraib S, Iqbal A (1998) Absence status: an overlooked cause of acute confusion in hemodialysis patients. J Nephrol 11(3):146–147

40. Raskin NH (1989) Neurological aspects of renal failure. In: Aminoff NJ (ed) Neurology and general medicine. Churchill Livingstone, New York, pp 231–246

41. Arieff AI, Massry SG, Barrientos A, Kleeman CR (1973) Brain water and electrolyte metabolism in uremia: effects of slow and rapid hemodialysis. Kidney Int 4(3):177–187

42. Arieff AI, Guisado R, Massry SG, Lazarowitz VC (1976) Central nervous system pH in uremia and the effects of hemodialysis. J Clin Invest 58(2):306–311

43. Maioriello AV, Chaljub G, Nauta HJ, Lacroix M (2002) Chemical shift imaging of mannitol in acute cerebral ischemia. Case report. J Neurosurg 97(3):687–691

44. Vujkovac B, Sabovic M (2000) Treatment of subdural and intracerebral haematomas in a haemodialysis patient with tranexamic acid. Nephrol Dial Transplant 15(1):107–109

45. Takeda K, Harada A, Okuda S, Fujimi S, Oh Y, Hattori F et al (1997) Sudden death in chronic dialysis patients. Nephrol Dial Transplant 12(5):952–955

46. Alfrey AC, Mishell JM, Burks J, Contiguglia SR, Rudolph H, Lewin E et al (1972) Syndrome of dyspraxia and multifocal seizures associated with chronic hemodialysis. Trans Am Soc Artif Intern Organs 18:257

47. Jack R, Rabin PL, McKinney TD (1983) Dialysis encephalopathy: a review. Int J Psychiatry Med 13(4):309–326

48. Chokroverty S, Bruetman ME, Berger V, Reyes MG (1976) Progressive dialytic encephalopathy. J Neurol Neurosurg Psychiatry 39(5):411–419

49. Hughes JR, Schreeder MT (1980) EEG in dialysis encephalopathy. Neurology 30(11):1148–1154

50. Primavera A, Cocito L, Audenino D (2004) Nonconvulsive status epilepticus during cephalosporin therapy. Neuropsychobiology 49(4):218–222

51. Alpay H, Altun O, Biyikli NK (2004) Cefepime-induced non-convulsive status epilepticus in a peritoneal dialysis patient. Pediatr Nephrol 19(4):445–447

52. Maganti R, Jolin D, Rishi D, Biswas A (2006) Nonconvulsive status epilepticus due to cefepime in a patient with normal renal function. Epilepsy Behav 8(1):312–314

53. Sonck J, Laureys G, Verbeelen D (2008) The neurotoxicity and safety of treatment with cefepime in patients with renal failure. Nephrol Dial Transplant 23(3):966–970

54. Jones H, Aguila E, Farber HW (2002) Gabapentin toxicity requiring intubation in a patient receiving long-term hemodialysis. Ann Intern Med 137(1):74

55. Brater DC (1996) Manual of drug use, 7th edn. Improved Therapeutics, Indianapolis

56. Roberts WL, De BK, Coleman JP, Annesley TM (1999) Falsely increased immunoassay measurements of total and unbound phenytoin in critically ill uremic patients receiving fosphenytoin. Clin Chem 45(6 Pt 1):829–837

57. Porto I, John EG, Heilliczer J (1997) Removal of phenobarbital during continuous cycling peritoneal dialysis in a child. Pharmacotherapy 17(4):832–835

58. Frenchie D, Bastani B (1998) Significant removal of phenytoin during high flux dialysis with cellulose triacetate dialyzer. Nephrol Dial Transplant 13(3):817–818

59. Wong MO, Eldon MA, Keane WF, Turck D, Bockbrader HN, Underwood BA et al (1995) Disposition of gabapentin in anuric subjects on hemodialysis. J Clin Pharmacol 35(6):622–626

60. Tonner DR, Schlechte JA (1993) Neurologic complications of thyroid and parathyroid disease. Med Clin North Am 77(1):251–263

61. Smith DL, Looney TJ (1983) Seizures secondary to thyrotoxicosis and high-dosage propranolol therapy. Arch Neurol 40(7):457–458

62. Docter R, Krenning EP, de Jong M, Hennemann G (1993) The sick euthyroid syndrome: changes in thyroid hormone serum parameters and hormone metabolism. Clin Endocrinol (Oxf) 39(5):499–518

63. Van den BG, de Zegher F, Lauwers P (1994) Dopamine and the sick euthyroid syndrome in critical illness. Clin Endocrinol (Oxf) 41(6):731–737

64. Aiello DP, DuPlessis AJ, Pattishall EG III, Kulin HE (1989) Thyroid storm. Presenting with coma and seizures. In a 3-year-old girl. Clin Pediatr (Phila) 28(12):571–574

65. Rangel-Guerra R, Martinez HR, Garcia HP, Alberto Sagastegui-Rodriguez J, Zacarias VJ, Antonio Infante CJ (1992) Epilepsy and thyrotoxicosis in a 4-year-old boy. Rev Invest Clin 44(1):109–113

66. Radetti G, Dordi B, Mengarda G, Biscaldi I, Larizza D, Severi F (1993) Thyrotoxicosis presenting with seizures and coma in two children. Am J Dis Child 147(9):925–927

67. Primavera A, Brusa G, Novello P (1990) Thyrotoxic encephalopathy and recurrent seizures. Eur Neurol 30(4):186–188

68. Jabbari B, Huott AD (1980) Seizures in thyrotoxicosis. Epilepsia 21(1):91–96
69. Lin CS, Yiin KT, Lin WH, Huang SY (1992) Thyrotoxicosis accompanied with periodic seizure attacks a case report and review of literature. Zhonghua Yi Xue Za Zhi (Taipei) 50(4):335–337
70. Li Voon Chong JS, Lecky BR, Macfarlane IA (2000) Recurrent encephalopathy and generalised seizures associated with relapses of thyrotoxicosis. Int J Clin Pract 54(9):621–622
71. Sandrini M, Marrama D, Vergoni AV, Bertolini A (1992) Repeated administration of triiodothyronine enhances the susceptibility of rats to isoniazid- and picrotoxin-induced seizures. Life Sci 51(10):765–770
72. Siegert CE, Smelt AH, de Bruin TW (1995) Superior sagittal sinus thrombosis and thyrotoxicosis. Possible association in two cases. Stroke 26(3):496–497
73. Gilmore RL (2003) Seizures associated with nonneurologic medical conditions. In: Wyllie E (ed) The treatment of epilepsy: principles and practice. Williams and Wilkins, Baltimore, pp 654–665
74. Bryce GM, Poyner F (1992) Myxoedema presenting with seizures. Postgrad Med J 68(795):35–36
75. Messing RO, Simon RP (1986) Seizures as a manifestation of systemic disease. Neurol Clin 4(3):563–584
76. De Luca F, Arrigo T, Pandullo E, Siracusano MF, Benvenga S, Trimarchi F (1986) Changes in thyroid function tests induced by 2 month carbamazepine treatment in L-thyroxine-substituted hypothyroid children. Eur J Pediatr 145(1–2):77–79
77. Bostantjopoulou S, Zafiriou D, Katsarou Z, Kazis A (1996) Hashimoto's encephalopathy: clinical and laboratory findings. Funct Neurol 11(5):247–251
78. Shaw PJ, Walls TJ, Newman PK, Cleland PG, Cartlidge NE (1991) Hashimoto's encephalopathy: a steroid-responsive disorder associated with high anti-thyroid antibody titers–report of 5 cases. Neurology 41(2 (Pt 1)):228–233
79. Ghika-Schmid F, Ghika J, Regli F, Dworak N, Bogousslavsky J, Stadler C et al (1996) Hashimoto's myoclonic encephalopathy: an underdiagnosed treatable condition? Mov Disord 11(5):555–562
80. Henchey R, Cibula J, Helveston W, Malone J, Gilmore RL (1995) Electroencephalographic findings in Hashimoto's encephalopathy. Neurology 45(5):977–981
81. Vasconcellos E, Pina-Garza JE, Fakhoury T, Fenichel GM (1999) Pediatric manifestations of Hashimoto's encephalopathy. Pediatr Neurol 20(5):394–398
82. Van den BG, Wouters P, Weekers F, Verwaest C, Bruyninckx F, Schetz M et al (2001) Intensive insulin therapy in the critically ill patients. N Engl J Med 345(19):1359–1367
83. Whiting S, Camfield P, Arab D, Salisbury S (1997) Insulin-dependent diabetes mellitus presenting in children as frequent, medically unresponsive, partial seizures. J Child Neurol 12(3):178–180
84. Cornford EM, Oldendorf WH (1986) Epilepsy and the blood-brain barrier. Adv Neurol 44:787–812
85. Grant C, Warlow C (1985) Focal epilepsy in diabetic non-ketotic hyperglycaemia. Br Med J (Clin Res Ed) 290(6476):1204–1205
86. Hennis A, Corbin D, Fraser H (1992) Focal seizures and non-ketotic hyperglycaemia. J Neurol Neurosurg Psychiatry 55(3):195–197
87. Siddiqi ZA, VanLandingham KE, Husain AM (2002) Reflex seizures and non-ketotic hyperglycemia: an unresolved issue. Seizure 11(1):63–66
88. Carril JM, Guijarro C, Portocarrero JS, Solache I, Jimenez A, Valera de Seijas E (1992) Speech arrest as manifestation of seizures in non-ketotic hyperglycaemia. Lancet 340(8829):1227
89. Harden CL, Rosenbaum DH, Daras M (1991) Hyperglycemia presenting with occipital seizures. Epilepsia 32(2):215–220
90. Tedrus GM, Fonseca LC (1995) Induced visual crisis and non-ketotic hyperglycemia: a case report. Arq Neuropsiquiatr 53(2):281–283

91. Seo DW, Na DG, Na DL, Moon SY, Hong SB (2003) Subcortical hypointensity in partial status epilepticus associated with nonketotic hyperglycemia. J Neuroimaging 13(3):259–263

92. Yudkoff M, Daikhin Y, Nissim I, Lazarow A, Nissim I (2001) Ketogenic diet, amino acid metabolism, and seizure control. J Neurosci Res 66(5):931–940

93. Service FJ, Dale AJ, Elveback LR, Jiang NS (1976) Insulinoma: clinical and diagnostic features of 60 consecutive cases. Mayo Clin Proc 51(7):417–429

94. Ehrlich RM (1971) Hypoglycaemia in infancy and childhood. Arch Dis Child 46(249):716–719

95. Lovvorn HN III, Nance ML, Ferry RJ Jr, Stolte L, Baker L, O'Neill JA Jr et al (1999) Congenital hyperinsulinism and the surgeon: lessons learned over 35 years. J Pediatr Surg 34(5):786–792

96. Hart SP, Frier BM (1998) Causes, management and morbidity of acute hypoglycaemia in adults requiring hospital admission. QJM 91(7):505–510

97. Bjorgaas M, Sand T, Vik T, Jorde R (1998) Quantitative EEG during controlled hypoglycaemia in diabetic and non-diabetic children. Diabet Med 15(1):30–37

98. Romerio SC, Radanowicz V, Schlienger RG (2000) SIADH with epileptic seizures and coma in fluoxetine therapy. Schweiz Rundsch Med Prax 89(10):404–410

99. Vaicys C, Fried A (2000) Transient hyponatriemia complicated by seizures after endoscopic third ventriculostomy. Minim Invasive Neurosurg 43(4):190–191

100. Yamamoto T, Ishii T, Yoshioka K, Yamagami K, Yamakita T, Miyamoto M et al (2003) Transient central diabetes insipidus in pregnancy with a peculiar change in signal intensity on T1-weighted magnetic resonance images. Intern Med 42(6):513–516

101. Combs CA, Walker C, Matlock BA, Crombleholme W (1990) Transient diabetes insipidus in pregnancy complicated by hypertension and seizures. Am J Perinatol 7(3):287–289

102. Van den BG, Weekers F, Baxter RC, Wouters P, Iranmanesh A, Bouillon R et al (2001) Five-day pulsatile gonadotropin-releasing hormone administration unveils combined hypothalamic-pituitary-gonadal defects underlying profound hypoandrogenism in men with prolonged critical illness. J Clin Endocrinol Metab 86(7):3217–3226

103. Herzog AG (1991) Reproductive endocrine considerations and hormonal therapy for women with epilepsy. Epilepsia 32(Suppl 6):S27–S33

104. Locock C (1857) Discussion of a paper by EH Sieveking: analysis of 52 cases of epilepsy observed by the author. Lancet 1:528

105. Rosciszewska D, Buntner B, Guz I, Zawisza L (1986) Ovarian hormones, anticonvulsant drugs, and seizures during the menstrual cycle in women with epilepsy. J Neurol Neurosurg Psychiatry 49(1):47–51

106. Newmark ME, Penry JK (1980) Catamenial epilepsy: a review. Epilepsia 21(3):281–300

107. Hom AC, Buterbaugh GG (1986) Estrogen alters the acquisition of seizures kindled by repeated amygdala stimulation or pentylenetetrazol administration in ovariectomized female rats. Epilepsia 27(2):103–108

108. Maggi A, Perez J (1985) Role of female gonadal hormones in the CNS: clinical and experimental aspects. Life Sci 37(10):893–906

109. Saberi M, Pourgholami MH, Jorjani M (2001) The acute effects of estradiol benzoate on amygdala-kindled seizures in male rats. Brain Res 891(1–2):1–6

110. Logothetis J, Harner R, Morrell F, Torres F (1959) The role of estrogens in catamenial exacerbation of epilepsy. Neurology 9(5):352–360

111. Herzog AG (1988) Clomiphene therapy in epileptic women with menstrual disorders. Neurology 38(3):432–434

112. Bauer J, Burr W, Elger CE (1998) Seizure occurrence during ovulatory and anovulatory cycles in patients with temporal lobe epilepsy: a prospective study. Eur J Neurol 5(1):83–88

113. Harden CL, Pulver MC, Ravdin L, Jacobs AR (1999) The effect of menopause and perimenopause on the course of epilepsy. Epilepsia 40(10):1402–1407

114. Lind L, Ljunghall S (1992) Critical care hypercalcemia – a hyperparathyroid state. Exp Clin Endocrinol 100(3):148–151

115. Burchard KW, Gann DS, Colliton J, Forster J (1990) Ionized calcium, parathormone, and mortality in critically ill surgical patients. Ann Surg 212(4):543–549

116. Panagariya A, Sharma A, Chhabria H (1990) Hypoparathyroidism-presenting as uncontrolled seizures. J Assoc Physicians India 38(6):442

117. Mithal A, Menon PS, Ammini AC, Karmarkar MG, Ahuja MM (1989) Spontaneous hypoparathyroidism: clinical, biochemical and radiological features. Indian J Pediatr 56(2):267–272

118. Reddy ST, Merrick RD (1999) Hypoparathyroidism, intracranial calcification, and seizures 61 years after thyroid surgery. Tenn Med 92(9):341–342

119. Cox RE (1983) Hypoparathyroidism: an unusual cause of seizures. Ann Emerg Med 12(5):314–315

120. Watanabe T, Bai M, Lane CR, Matsumoto S, Minamitani K, Minagawa M et al (1998) Familial hypoparathyroidism: identification of a novel gain of function mutation in transmembrane domain 5 of the calcium-sensing receptor. J Clin Endocrinol Metab 83(7):2497–2502

121. Unnikrishnan AG, Rajaratnam S (2001) A young man with seizures, abusive behaviour, and drowsiness. Postgrad Med J 77(903):54 58–59

122. Sallman A, Goldberg M, Wombolt D (1981) Secondary hyperparathyroidism manifesting as acute pancreatitis and status epilepticus. Arch Intern Med 141(11):1549–1550

123. Cherry TA, Kauffman RP, Myles TD (2002) Primary hyperparathyroidism, hypercalcemic crisis and subsequent seizures occurring during pregnancy: a case report. J Matern Fetal Neonatal Med 12(5):349–352

124. Kastrup O, Maschke M, Wanke I, Diener HC (2002) Posterior reversible encephalopathy syndrome due to severe hypercalcemia. J Neurol 249(11):1563–1566

125. Boldt J, Menges T, Kuhn D, Diridis C, Hempelmann G (1995) Alterations in circulating vasoactive substances in the critically ill–a comparison between survivors and non-survivors. Intensive Care Med 21(3):218–225

126. Vermes I, Beishuizen A, Hampsink RM, Haanen C (1995) Dissociation of plasma adrenocorticotropin and cortisol levels in critically ill patients: possible role of endothelin and atrial natriuretic hormone. J Clin Endocrinol Metab 80(4):1238–1242

127. Barquist E, Kirton O (1997) Adrenal insufficiency in the surgical intensive care unit patient. J Trauma 42(1):27–31

128. Ntyonga-Pono MP (1997) Addison's disease revealed by hypoglycemic convulsions. Med Trop (Mars) 57(3):311–312

129. Samaan NA (1989) Hypoglycemia secondary to endocrine deficiencies. Endocrinol Metab Clin North Am 18(1):145–154

130. Herzog AG, Sotrel A, Ronthal M (1998) Reversible proximal myopathy in epilepsy related Cushing's syndrome. J Neurol Neurosurg Psychiatry 65(1):134

131. Thomas JE, Rooke ED, Kvale WF (1966) The neurologist's experience with pheochromocytoma. A review of 100 cases. JAMA 197(10):754–758

132. Leiba A, Bar-Dayan Y, Leker RR, Apter S, Grossman E (2003) Seizures as a presenting symptom of phaeochromocytoma in a young soldier. J Hum Hypertens 17(1):73–75

133. Roberts AH (1967) Association of a phaeochromocytoma and cerebral gliosarcoma with neurofibromatosis. Br J Surg 54(1):78–79

134. Eclavea A, Gagliardi JA, Jezior J, Burton B, Donahue JP (1997) Phaeochromocytoma with central nervous system manifestations. Australas Radiol 41(4):373–376

Chapter 8

Seizures in Organ Transplant Recipients

Tarek Zakaria, Eelco F.M. Wijdicks, and Greg A. Worrell

Abstract Seizures are a nonspecific neurological manifestation of cerebral dysfunction and not indicative of any particular disease processes or pathology. As such, the evaluation and treatment of seizures in transplant patients generally follow the same clinical approach as for other patients. A seizure in a transplant patient is commonly unanticipated and entirely unexplained. The effects can be substantial with aspiration, loss of vascular catheters, and tissue trauma. Patients undergoing organ transplantation are at risk of seizures for multiple reasons, and while much of the neurological and transplantation literature reports on the incidence of seizures according to the particular organ transplanted, there are many similarities (e.g., Immunosuppression drugs) and we will try to concentrate on organ transplantation as a whole.

Keywords Organ transplant • Chemotherapy and seizures

8.1. Incidence of Seizures in Transplant Patients

The incidence of neurological complications and seizures in a given transplant population tends to decrease with time, presumably as familiarity and experience with immunosuppression regimens and their complications accumulate. This fact likely has been at least part of the wide range of seizure incidence reported in organ transplant (Table 8-1) (1). Reduction in the incidence of severe immunosuppression toxicity may have reduced the incidence of seizures.

8.1.1. Liver Transplant

The postoperative care of liver transplant patients is well established, and primarily focused on the management of hemodynamic function, pulmonary function, fluid balance, electrolyte status, and careful attention to transplant-related coagulopathy. Review of liver transplantation literature shows a wide range of incidence of seizures (1, 2) (3–7). Interestingly, while it was initially suggested that post-transplant seizures often heralded a poor outcome (4), a subsequent study of 630 OLT patients (5) found that only 28 (4%) patients

From: *Seizures in Critical Care: A Guide to Diagnosis and Therapeutics*: Current Clinical Neurology, Second Edition, Edited by: P. Varelas, DOI 10.1007/978-1-60327-532-3_8, © Humana Press, a part of Springer Science+Business Media, LLC 2005, 2010

Table 8-1. Incidence of Seizures in Organ Transplant Patients.

Transplant organ	Incidence of seizures (%)	Common etiologies (If available)
Liver	3–42%10%	Immunosuppression drug neurotoxicity
		Infection (5)
Bone marrow transplant	3–29%7%	Immunosuppression drug neurotoxicity
		Acute GVHD (11)
Heart	2–43%	New ischemic lesion(14)
Kidney	5–20%	Immunosuppression drug neurotoxicity (18)
Lung	22–27%	Immunosuppression drug neurotoxicity (20)
Pancreas	13%	See Ref. (22)

GVHD graft vs. host disease.

had generalized tonic-clonic seizures, and only in 7 (1%) patients did the seizure "herald a catastrophic neurological event" (5). In that study the cause of the seizures was varied, but immunosuppression toxicity defined as toxic blood levels or an increase of 100% or greater was the most common etiology (cyclosporine in 11 (40%) patients and FK506 in 6 (21%) patients). In addition to immunosuppressant drug toxicity, other causes of seizures included acute uremia (1 patient) and meningioma (1 patient), and the cause was unknown in 2 patients. In the 7 patients where seizures portended a poor prognosis, the etiology of seizures included: intracranial hemorrhage (1 patient), sepsis (1 patient), CNS infection (3 patients), anoxic encephalopathy (1 patient), and cerebral edema with fulminant hepatic failure (1 patient). The study did not attempt to distinguish between partial onset seizures that were secondarily generalized and generalized tonic clonic seizures. Partial seizures that did not generalize were not included. Seizures induced by immunosuppressive treatments might not be related to a toxic drug level. In a study of 132 patients with liver transplant treated with Tacrolimus, 12 (9%) developed generalized seizures despite therapeutic Tacrolimus range, and negative work-up for any predisposing factors. All patients were switched to cyclosporine or sirolimus with no recurrence of their seizure (8).

8.1.2. Bone Marrow Transplant

Bone marrow transplantation (BMT) is rapidly advancing as an effective treatment of lymphopoietic and hematopoietic disorders. The literature describing neurological complications of bone marrow transplant is limited, but seizures have been reported to occur in as many as 10% of patients (9). However, the incidence of seizures appears to depend on the patient population considered (1, 2), with 29% (6 of 21 patients) of sickle cell anemia patients having seizures compared to 3% (5 of 168 patients) for Hodgkin's disease (10). This difference may be due to pre-existing or peri-operative CNS lesions such as stroke in the patients with sickle cell anemia. In a prospective study from Italy, 115 patients were followed for a median period of 90 days after BMT for leukemia and 7% (8 of 115 patients) had seizures. Immunosuppression drug-related neurotoxicity and acute graft vs. host disease (GVHD) were found to be the most common etiology for seizures in this population (11). A case of non-convulsive status epilepticus has also been reported in a patient 2 years after autologous bone marrow stem cell transplantation for diffuse large cell non-Hodgkin's lymphoma. This patient with recurring episodes of altered mental status was found to have a left temporal lobe lymphoma (12). Other etiologies that may be more frequent in this patient population are strokes associated with thrombocytopenia, cerebral venous sinus thrombosis, and cardioembolic infarctions. The incidence of intractable chronic epilepsy related to cyclosporine toxicity after BMT has been reported recently. In a group of 185 children treated with cyclosporine after BMT, 15 (8%) presented with acute seizures, which were generalized in 7 and focal in 7 and with absent status in 1. After the first year, seizures persisted chronically in four cases and evolved to intractable epilepsy. Focal temporal epilepsy was diagnosed in three cases, whereas in the fourth case, multifocal epilepsy was observed. Magnetic resonance imaging (MRI) detected mesial temporal sclerosis in all of these cases. The risk factors associated with evolution to intractable epilepsy included lower age at transplantation (3–5 years), more than one relapsing seizure in the first year after transplantation, and longer treatment with cyclosporine (13).

8.1.3. Heart Transplantation

The primary medical concern following heart transplantation is focused on the hemodynamic status. The reported range of seizure incidence in heart transplantation patients is varied, ranging between 2 and 43% (1). In a report on consecutive orthotopic heart transplant patients, 15% (12 of 82 consecutive patients) had seizures (14), and the most frequent cause of seizures was a postoperative stroke. This is unique to heart transplantation, supporting a more extensive evaluation of seizures in these patients. In another recent report from Brazil, 69 patients underwent orthoptic heart transplantation. Neurologic complications occurred in 19 (31%) patients, including 11 (17.7%) with seizures. Seizures were seldom recurrent and no patient received long-term anti-epileptic drugs. All patients with seizures had normal brain CT or MRI, and the seizures were attributed to metabolic derangements (2 patients) and drug toxicity (cyclosporin in 8 patients and imipenem in 2 patients) (15).

Most reports identify a higher seizure incidence in pediatric heart transplant patients compared to adults. Whether this increase is secondary to an underlying increased seizure tendency in children, limited experience with immunosuppression, or another culprit is not known (1). A recent report contrasting the differences in seizure incidence in children (32%; 7 of 22 patients) and adults (13%; 7 of 77 patients) from a single institution supported the difference, although it did not reach statistical significance (16).

8.1.4. Kidney Transplantation

The kidney transplant patient is the least likely to have a prolonged intensive care stay. However, infrequently the transplanted kidney is slow to achieve adequate function and uremia can occur with progressive encephalopathy and seizures in the immediate post-transplant course. The range of seizure incidence in kidney transplantation is reported to be 5–20% (1). In a series of 109 pediatric renal transplant patients 20 patients (18%) had at least one seizure. The etiology in this series was multifactorial: hypertension (15 patients), fever/infection (4 patients) and acute allograft rejection (6 patients). Only 2 patients had significant intracerebral pathology (17). In a large series of 402 kidney transplants, significantly lower overall seizure incidence of 5% (20 of 402 patients) was reported (18).

A syndrome of rejection encephalopathy has also been described in renal transplant patients (19). Fifteen episodes of encephalopathy in 13 patients were described that occurred during an acute rejection crisis. The severity of the encephalopathy was found to be related to the severity of the rejection crisis, and not to other features such as blood pressure, fever, steroid therapy, or plasma electrolytes. The encephalopathy syndrome was associated with headache, papilledema, altered mental status, and generalized tonic clonic seizures in 6% of cases. The EEG showed generalized slowing with focal abnormalities in 25% of cases.

8.1.5. Lung Transplantation

Data are starting to accumulate on the incidence of seizures in lung transplantation. A study of 81 lung transplant patients reported an incidence of 22% (18 of 81 patients) of patients suffering seizures. In this study the occurrence of partial vs. GTC seizures was considered, and interestingly the majority of seizures had partial onset (89% 16 of the 18 patients). Reported etiologies included sustained hypertension (2 patients), stroke (4 patients), and imipenem toxicity (2 patients). Eleven patients had seizures within 10 days after initiation of methylprednisolone treatment for allograft rejection. Eight of the 9 patients who underwent MRI imaging had focal areas of T2 signal abnormality consistent with the localization of seizure semiology (20).

The reported incidence of seizures in pediatric lung transplantation can reach 27% (21).

8.1.6. Pancreas Transplantation

There are very few data on the neurological complications or seizures in pancreas transplantation. One report of 15 patients reported a 13% incidence of seizures (22).

8.2. Clinical Evaluation of Patients

The evaluation of the patient who is status post organ transplant begins with the clinical history. A prior seizure disorder is not a contraindication for organ transplantation, and patients with pre-existing seizure disorders are presumed to be at increased risk of post-operative seizures, because of metabolic/electrolyte abnormalities in the post-operative period. Knowledge of a pre-existing seizure disorder should allow measures to be taken to reduce the risk of perioperative seizures, for example, attention to maintenance of therapeutic Antiepileptic Drugs (AED) levels (Maintenance of AED levels can be challenging in the transplant patient as discussed in more detail below).

The first step is to establish the correct diagnosis. Simple partial motor seizures and GTC seizures are easily recognized. In an encephalopathic patient complex partial seizures are less readily identified by ICU personnel. Movement disorders, especially in the encephalopathic patient, can be confused with seizures. Nonepileptic myoclonus and tremor are commonly seen in patients with toxic and metabolic derangements. Nonepileptic myoclonus should not be confused with seizures, and is commonly due to drug toxicity or organ failure (e.g., Liver and Kidney failure). Persistent epileptic myoclonus is usually more focal (e.g., facial muscle twitching) and is frequently the manifestation of ischemic brain injury, often with associated laminar cortical necrosis. Non-convulsive status epilepticus can be especially difficult to diagnose, and usually requires a high index of suspicion before observing subtle clinical signs, such as eye movement irregularities. The incidence of non-convulsive status in critically ill patients is reported to be between 10 and 38% and the diagnosis should be suspected in any patient who is confused or comatose without clear etiology. Continuous EEG recording is required to confirm the presence of non convulsive status (23). Non-epileptic behavioral spells should also be considered. In these cases, the EEG is very helpful, and in most cases, recording during the movement or symptom in question yields a definitive answer. Similar to the evaluation of other patient populations with seizures, the classification of the seizure type is important, and in particular whether the seizure is of partial onset or generalized. Whether a generalized seizure is secondarily generalized or generalized from onset can have significant prognostic implications. While a new onset partial seizure can be an ominous sign of a focal CNS lesion, most GTC seizures in the post-transplant period do not portend a poor outcome (1, 5). The occurrence of new partial seizures, suggesting a possible structural etiology, may have greater prognostic significance compared to GTC, but this has never been investigated.

8.3. Etiology of Seizures in Transplant Patients

Some common etiologies for seizures in post-transplant patients are detailed in Table 8-2. The cause of seizures in post transplant population is often multifactorial, for example metabolic abnormalities coexisting with elevated levels of immunosuppression drugs, as well as antibiotics that can lower the seizure threshold. In transplantation patients, peri-operative seizures can result from immunosuppression drug neurotoxicity, metabolic and electrolyte abnormalities (commonly involving calcium, sodium, magnesium, and low serum glucose), CNS infections, sepsis, or can be related to CNS lesions, such as neoplasm or acute stroke. The development of a new CNS malignancy (usually a late complication of immunosuppression) or recurrence should be considered (*see* Case #1, below). The cause of seizures in some cases varies between transplant populations. For example, in a review of cardiac transplant patients Grigg et al. (14) found the most frequent cause of seizures was a peri-operative stroke. Patients undergoing BMT may have significant thrombocytopenia and associated cerebral hemorrhage, or leukocytosis and cortical venous thrombosis as an etiology for seizures. Liver transplant patients can have a significant coagulopathy with risk of cerebral hemorrhage. It has also been suggested that seizures may be related to steroid regimens that may disrupt the blood brain barrier making the patient more susceptible to the neurotoxic effects of immunosuppression drugs like cyclosporin and FK506 (20).

While the occurrence of seizures in the post-transplant patient may be the harbinger of an impending neurological catastrophe which usually initiates an emergency neurological consult and requires immediate evaluation and management, more often seizures are isolated events due to metabolic derangements and immunosuppression drug neurotoxicity. In fact, even the

Table 8-2. Possible Etiologies of Seizures in Post-transplant Patients.

Immunosuppression neurotoxicity-FK506 (Tacrolimus)	Cerebrovascular eventsIschemic and/or hemorrhagic infarcts
Cyclosporin A	Intracranial hematoma
OKT3 (muronmonab-CD3)	Cerebral sinus thrombosis
Metabolic Derangements	Hypoxic-ischemic event
Hyponatremia	Subarachnoid hemorrhage
Hypocalcemia	CNS Infection
Hypomagnesemia	Meningitis
Hyperglycemia (often hyperosmolar, nonketotic)	Encephalitis
	Abscess
	Consider fungal: Aspergillus, Nocardia, and Listeria
	Malignancy
	Lymphoma (complication of immuno-suppression or recurrence)
	Glioma
	Other metastatic cancer

ominous new partial seizure disorder may not have the same implication in transplant patients compared to the general population where new partial seizures often are the first manifestation of a new structural lesion, such as a neoplasm. Partial seizures were the most common seizure type in post lung transplant patients, and when not secondary to focal structural CNS lesions, they were believed to be due to focal immunosuppression drug neurotoxicity, and therefore possibly reversible (20).

8.3.1. Immunosuppression Drugs

From an immunological perspective, organ transplantation represents the introduction of a massive quantity of foreign antigenic substrate, which if recognized by the host system will initiate a robust immune response. Without immunosuppression drugs, organ transplantation would not be possible. However, immunosuppression drugs used in organ transplantation have a narrow therapeutic range (24, 25), and the myriad array of neurologic manifestations of neurotoxicity related to these drugs are established (24) (Table 8.3). Immunosuppression drug-related neurotoxicity should be high on the differential of possibilities for seizures in all post-transplant patients. The clinical profile of immunosuppression drug-related neurotoxicity is non-specific, but often fairly characteristic and readily diagnosed (Table 8-3). One of the most interesting neurological complications of immunosuppression agents is a posterior reversible leukoencephalopathy syndrome (PRES) reported with cyclosporin, and tacrolimus (24, 26–29). There is a propensity for immuno-suppression related neurotoxicity in the posterior circulation vascular territory, which may be related to blood brain barrier differences in the posterior circulation compared to anterior circulation.

Immunosuppression drugs used in organ transplantation clearly are an important etiology of seizures. In a series of patients undergoing liver

Table 8-3. Neurological and Psychiatric Complications from Immunosuppressive Drug Toxicity (In Order of Frequency).

Tremors
Psychiatric symptoms: anxiety, panic, maniac behavior, and delusions
Visual hallucinations
Vascular-type headaches
Generalized tonic-clonic seizures
Akinetic mutism
Speech apraxia
Cortical blindness
Cerebellar syndrome
Extrapyramidal syndrome
Coma

From (24). Used with permission.

transplantation at Mayo Clinic, 17 (61%) of 28 seizures were related to immunosuppression neurotoxicity (5).

8.3.2. Cyclosporin

The immunosuppression effect of cyclosporin is primarily achieved by inhibiting T-lymphocyte maturation and reducing interleukin-2 production. Cyclosporin-related neurotoxicity most commonly develops within weeks after transplantation and occurs frequently with intravenous loading (7) (24). The incidence of cyclosporine related neurotoxicity depends on the transplanted organ, occurring in approximately 10% of liver transplant patients who receive the drug intravenously in the postoperative period (7), but only ~5% of bone marrow transplants (30). This difference may be indicative of greater experience in use of the drug in long-established organ transplants, or possibly because of additional metabolic abnormalities seen in liver transplant patients. The risk of cyclosporin neurotoxicity has been reported to be increased by the presence of hypomagnesemia (31), hypocholesterolemia (32), corticosteroids (20), hypertension (33), and high drug concentrations (26) (27). Cyclosporin is well known to cause magnesium wasting, and levels must be followed closely.

The range of neurotoxicity-related complications is wide, and commonly can include psychiatric manifestations with agitation, manic behavior, bizarre delusions, panic, paranoia, and severe mood changes. The presentation of psychiatric symptoms usually resolves with reduction or discontinuation of cyclosporin. However, if these initial symptoms are not recognized, cyclosporin neurotoxicity can lead to actual structural abnormalities on MRI imaging primarily involving the cerebral white matter. Cyclosporin appears to have a propensity to involve the posterior circulation vascular territory, and neurological symptoms of visual hallucinations, cortical blindness, cerebellar syndrome, extrapyramidal syndrome, and coma have been described (24). Thus, cyclosporin is one of the agents causing a posterior reversible leukoencephalopathy syndrome (24, 26–29).

Seizures are commonly attributed to cyclosporin neurotoxicity (5). In fact, cyclosporin should be considered first in the differential when evaluating new seizures in the post-transplant patient.

8.3.3. Tacrolimus (FK-506)

The clinical experience with this drug is now comparable to cyclosporin, and the overall neurotoxicity profile is possibly better than cyclosporin, but the incidence of seizures is similar (34) (24). Most commonly, Tacrolimus neurotoxicity manifests with postural hand tremor (6), but similar to cyclosporin, cortical blindness and GTC seizures also occur. A posterior leukoencephalopathy syndrome with similar MRI abnormalities as seen with cyclosporin has also been reported (35).

8.3.4. Muromonab-CD3 (OKT3)

Muronmonab-CD3 (OKT3) achieves immunosuppression by inactivating CD3 lymphocytes, and is most often combined with corticosteroids, azathioprine, and cyclosporin. The most common neurologic symptom of OKT3 is headache, but neurotoxicity has been rarely reported to produce aseptic meningitis, seizures, cerebral edema, and vision loss (36–38).

8.3.5. Carmustine and Busulfan

These drugs are used in conditioning regimes in anticipation of BMT, and in high doses can cause seizures in 3–10% of patients (39, 40).

8.4. Diagnostic Evaluation

The clinical evaluation of a new seizure in the post-transplant patient should proceed within the overall clinical context. Generalized seizures are often the manifestation of gross electrolyte abnormalities or immunosuppression drug toxicity, and if such an abnormality is identified, additional studies requiring transport of a critically ill patient to the radiology suite, performing lumbar punctures and other invasive procedures may impose unnecessary risks with little potential diagnostic yield.

History and exam: Detailed list of medications should be obtained. Evidence of a focal abnormality on neurological exam necessitates neuroimaging with MRI.

Labs: Blood count and coagulation studies. Electrolytes, most importantly sodium, calcium, and magnesium. Glucose. Arterial blood gas, if clinically indicated. AED levels, Immunosuppression drug (e.g., cyclosporin, tacrolimus) and antibiotic levels (e.g., Imipenem). Blood cultures for bacteria, viruses, and fungi, if clinically indicated.

Imaging: CT and MRI: While the acutely ill patient may be evaluated with CT, the standard of care in the evaluation of new onset seizures is MRI (*see* Case #1, below). In patients with focal seizures or focal EEG abnormality, an MRI scan is indicated. The MRI characteristics of severe immunosuppression-related neurotoxicity are well described (24, 29).

CSF: If clinically indicated (consider risk of complications associated with coagulopathy or thrombocytopenia). The presence of increased intracranial pressure must be ruled out prior to lumbar puncture. Gram stain, differential cell count, protein, and glucose should be obtained on the CSF. When indicated, bacterial, viral, and fungal cultures should also be obtained.

EEG: Routine or prolonged video-EEG recording. EEG may be useful to rule out non-convulsive status in the encephalopathic patient. Video-EEG is very useful if there is uncertainty about whether an intermittent paroxysmal movement or spell is a seizure. Continuous video-EEG recording can also be used to assess efficacy of AED therapy. The presence of a focal abnormality on EEG raises the concern of a structural focal lesion.

8.5. Management of Seizures

Most seizures are self-limiting and cease spontaneously within 3–5 min. The majority of seizures do not require acute management and end spontaneously before acute therapy can be given. Seizures lasting longer than 4–5 min, recurring in a clustering pattern, or associated with prolonged periods of altered behavior or unresponsiveness may respond to the administration of a benzodiazepine and other AEDs.

The next step in the management of seizures is to correct any precipitating causes, with close attention to electrolyte and metabolic abnormalities and immunosuppression drug levels. In the case of immunosuppression drug neurotoxicity or electrolyte abnormality and a single brief GTC seizure, discontinuation of the drug for several days and correction of the electrolyte abnormality sometimes is all that is required.

The treatment with AED in the organ transplant patient population is often complicated by a number of factors (24, 25, 41), that can include a critically ill patient, viability of a transplanted organ, potential for drug-drug interactions (e.g., cyclosporin and phenytoin) and impairment of the organ system (e.g., liver and kidney) responsible for AED metabolism and clearance. While the concern for AED toxicity to the transplanted organ is often raised, there is little if any clinical evidence to support this. It is well known that idiosyncratic AED reactions can produce catastrophic organ failure, such as acute liver failure, and bone marrow suppression. However, we are not aware of data to support the fact that the transplant patient is at greater risk of these rare idiosyncratic reactions. Nonetheless, caution is indicated.

An important question to answer is whether long-term treatment with an AED is necessary. In our experience, if a clear provoking etiology can be identified and corrected (e.g., cyclosporin toxicity or electrolyte abnormality), then long-term treatment of a single convulsion with an AED is not indicated. In the setting of a metabolic derangement that cannot be corrected, a structural CNS lesion, CNS infection (where the probability of a recurrent seizure is high), or if the patient is critically ill and felt to be unable to tolerate further seizures, treatment with an AED should be initiated. A protocol has been developed (Fig. 8.1) (1) for treatment of seizures in the post-transplant patient. If GTC seizures are refractory, lasting beyond 5–8 min in this patient population, we proceed to a more aggressive protocol for status epilepticus. For GTC seizures that are refractory to lorazepam and phenytoin, we usually proceed to midazolam (Bolus 0.1 mg/kg: followed with 0.05–0.4 mg/kg/h) or propofol (5–10 mg/kg/h). Continuous EEG monitoring is indicated in this situation.

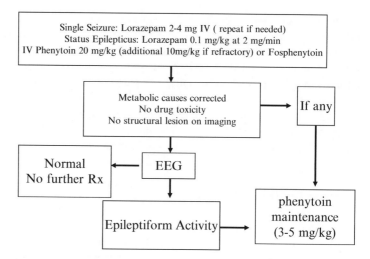

Fig. 8-1. Approach to a single seizure in a transplant patient

8.5.1. Antiepileptic Drugs

Phenytoin is the drug of choice for treatment of GTC seizures in the post-transplant patient. The standard loading dose is 18–20 mg/kg. For patients requiring rapid IV loading, we use Fosphenytoin because it is better tolerated with less risk of hypotension and can be safely infused at a faster rate (150 mg/min) compared to phenytoin (50 mg/min). Because many transplant patients have derangements in fluid status and may have hypoalbuminemia with associated decreased protein binding of phenytoin (and other protein bound AEDs, for example valproic acid and carbamazepine), both free and total phenytoin levels are used (Therapeutic range: Total phenytoin = 10–20 mg/mL and Free phenytoin = 1–2 mg/mL). The active drug is the unbound free phenytoin fraction, and it is not uncommon for patients to have toxic side effects with high free phenytoin level, but a subtherapeutic total phenytoin level.

Benzodiazepines are a class of drugs acting on GABA-ergic receptors with proven antiepileptic effect. Lorazepam has become a first-line drug for the emergent treatment of seizures because of longer duration of antiepileptic action compared to other benzodiazepines (42). The recommended lorazepam dose in status epilepticus is 0.07–0.1 mg/kg (infused at a rate of 2 mg/min). However, for the acute single seizure that is not prolonged in duration (not status epilepticus), we generally use approx 0.05 mg/kg IV to avoid respiratory depression. Midazolam is a short-acting benzodiazepine commonly used within the protocol for status epilepticus (42).

Phenobarbital is an effective older AED that is available in IV form and can be used if the patient is allergic to phenytoin. Phenobarbital has been suggested as the best choice (1) during the 2–6 weeks of bone marrow engraftment because, unlike phenytoin, valproic acid, and carbamazepine, phenobarbital has not been reported to cause bone marrow suppression. The IV loading dose of Phenobarbital is 10–20 mg/kg, which can be complicated by hypotension and respiratory depression. Thus, usually a smaller dose of 3 mg/kg can be tried first in patients who are not intubated and not in status epilepticus.

Valproic Acid is available as an IV preparation and has been demonstrated to be efficacious in the treatment of status epilepticus (43, 44). While limited data is available, valproic acid does not interfere with cyclosporin and tacrolimus metabolism. Our neurosurgical colleagues have commented on their impression of a coagulopathy associated with valproic acid, and some studies show a reduction in fibrinogen concentration, platelet count, and factor VIII-complex with this drug. In one oft-cited study, 63% of children treated with valproic acid had a history of bleeding, and 23% had prolonged bleeding (45). When compared to a control group, significant differences in coagulation parameters, similar to that seen in patients with congenital von Willebrand disease (vWD), were demonstrated. The decreases in coagulation parameters were not dependent on either valproic acid dose or time period of administration. For this reason, and not because of potential idiosyncratic reactions, caution is recommended in the acute transplant patient who may already have a coagulopathy.

Newer AEDS

Levetiracetam

Levetiracetam is the only new AED with IV formulation that can be used in the treatment of patients with status epilepticus. Levetiracetam is chemically unrelated to all the other AEDs. The exact mechanism of its antiseizure effect is unknown but its efficacy as adjunctive therapy for partial seizure disorders, with or without secondary generalization, myoclonic seizures, and primary generalized tonic clonic seizures has been demonstrated. The efficacy of levetiracetam begins after the first administration, with no appreciable therapeutic lag. There is, however, no literature comparing the efficacy of this treatment to standard therapies, nor has there been formal testing of its efficacy as monotherapy in a transplant patient population.

The pharmacokinetic properties of levetiracetam confer significant advantages compared with the older AEDs in the complicated setting of severely ill transplant patients. Unlike PHT and PB, levetiracetam is not protein-bound or liver cytochrome P450-dependent. Levetiracetam is only 10% protein bound and achieves maximal serum concentrations within 1–2 h and a steady-state concentration within 2 days. Sixty-six percent of the dose is excreted unchanged in the urine and 24% undergoes enzymatic hydrolysis. There are no known active metabolites or drug–drug interactions. The side-effect profile for levetiracetam is favorable, with only mild somnolence, coordination difficulties, or asthenia, and these typically occur at treatment onset and resolve with a reduction in dose. Neuropsychiatric adverse effects, consisting of mood or behavioral changes, or psychotic symptoms occur in about 13% of patients (compared with 6.2% after placebo in the seizure population). These are the most common reasons for withdrawal of levetiracetam therapy.

There are some data on the efficacy of levetiracetam in the transplant population. In a retrospective analysis of 17 patients with seizures after liver transplant treated with phenytoin or levetiracetam, only 6 of 11 (55%) of the phenytoin group had no more seizures at 30 days, whereas 6 of 6 (100%) in the levetiracetam-treated group were seizure-free at 30 days post-transplant (46).

8.5.2. AED Interaction with Immunosuppression

It is important to recognize that phenytoin, carbamazepine, and phenobarbital decrease serum cyclosporin and tacrolimus levels (47) (41) and discontinuation of these AEDs can lead to toxic immunosuppression drug concentrations, if appropriate dosing changes are not made. There is no known interaction with valproic acid or gabapentin. Interaction between immunosuppression drugs and the newer AEDs such as levetiracetam, lamotrigine, and topiramate have not been studied and they likely will provide useful alternatives. At this time they cannot be recommended as first line drugs, except for patients with known multi-drug allergies.

8.5.2.1. Management Considerations in Kidney Failure Patients

Renal failure may significantly perturb the clearance of AEDs, particularly gabapentin and levetiracetam, which are predominantly renally excreted. Hemodialysis will also clear up to about 50% of the body pool of these drugs during the standard 4-h procedure. Doses should therefore be reduced in patients with impaired renal function and supplemental doses should be given to patients after dialysis.

The more protein-bound a drug, the less dialyzable it is. PHT and VPA levels are not dramatically affected by dialysis, but PB and other AEDs with less protein binding will be affected. PHT dosing should be increased to every 6–8 h because of a shorter half-life in uremia, and lower loading doses should be used if protein binding is anticipated to be reduced.

8.5.2.2. Management Considerations in Liver Failure Patients

The most significant alterations in AED disposition occur in patients with chronic liver disease, acute hepatitis, drug-induced hepatotoxicity, cholestasis, and hepatic neoplastic disease.

Free fractions of diazepam, PHT, and VPA increase as a result of reduced circulating albumin concentrations. Frequent serum determinations of free fractions and gradual dose regulations are required. Close monitoring of serum CBZ and the 10,11-epoxide metabolite levels should be performed. Extreme caution should be taken if VPA is used in patients with liver disease. Hepatic dysfunction is less of a concern with PB, gabapentin, levetiracetam, topiramate, and zonisamide.

8.6. Case Studies

8.6.1. Case Study: #1

A fiftynine-year-old right-handed man with a history of non-Hodgkin's lymphoma. He was treated with BMT that was complicated by an acute reactivation of hepatitis B requiring antiviral treatment. Six months after transplantation, he complained of malaise, fatigue, and had low-grade fever. The following day he had a generalized tonic-clonic seizure. Within 15 min he had a second, and then a third generalized tonic-clonic seizure before recovering awareness. On arrival at Saint Marys Emergency Department, he had a GCS of 9, was not verbalizing, unable to follow commands, but had withdrawal to pain symmetrically. He was loaded with IV phenytoin and admitted to the Medical ICU. Detailed laboratory studies were unremarkable. His CT head was unremarkable. His EEG (Fig. 8.2) showed left frontal quasiperiodic lateralized epileptiform discharges (PLEDs) raising the possibility of herpes encephalitis, although the distribution of the interictal discharges would have been unusual for this diagnosis. The patient was covered with acyclovir as well as antibiotics. The spinal fluid examination was normal with only 1 nucleated cell, a protein of 44, glucose of 84, and negative herpes PCR.

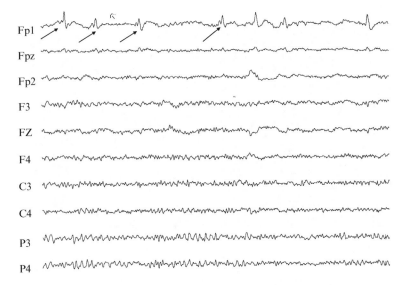

Fig. 8-2. EEG (Lapalcian Montage) showing quasi-periodic lateralized epileptiform discharges over the left frontal head region (Case #1)

The presence of a focal onset seizure, or focal EEG (left frontal PLEDs) is a cause for concern for a structural lesion involving the left frontal head region. The patient had a MRI the following morning that was felt to be normal. However, the MRI (Fig. 8.3a) quality was marginal because of movement artifact. By the following day the patient had a GCS 15, and was showing rapid improvement. A follow-up EEG one month later (not shown) continued to show the left frontal PLEDs, albeit in a more quasiperiodic pattern. Because of the persistence of the focal EEG abnormality the MRI was repeated, with attention to the left frontal region. The MRI, one month after presentation with new seizures, demonstrated a clear region of focal enhancement (Fig. 8.3b). The patient underwent brain radiation, but unfortunately the lymphoma did not respond and he died 2 months later. The important point demonstrated by this case is that a focal onset seizure or focal EEG abnormality can be an ominous sign, the etiology of which must be pursued vigorously.

8.6.2. Case Study: #2

A 36-year-old African-American female with a history of end-stage renal disease from focal segmental glomerulosclerosis and sickle cell disease, status post living-related renal transplant. Patient's immunosuppression regimen includes Tacrolimus and prednisone. One year post transplantation, the patient became fatigued and noticed dyspnea on exertion, sore throat, and had a productive cough with yellow sputum. The work-up demonstrated hemoglobin of 3.8, white cell count of 10,800 and stippling, teardrop, and fragmented red blood cells and serum creatinine of 4.4. The patient was admitted to the hospital and received a blood transfusion. Later that evening, she complained of confusion, blurred vision and subsequently had two GTC seizures, which lead to an ICU admission. Her Tacrolimus level was 10.2 (3.0–20.). The EEG showed generalized slowing, that was maximal over the posterior head region,

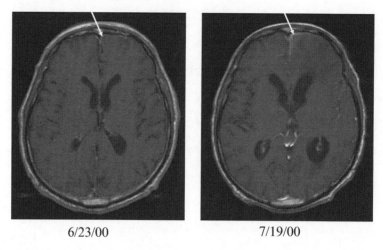

6/23/00   7/19/00

Fig. 8-3. MRI with contrast showing possible subtle area of left frontal meningeal enhancement on 6/23/00 and follow up scan one month later (Case #1)

but no epileptiform activity was appreciated. MR imaging demonstrated bilateral

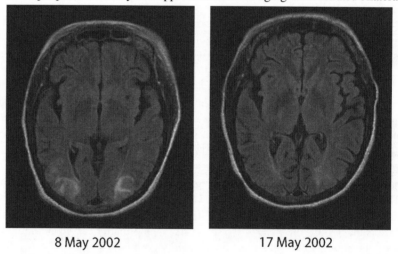

8 May 2002   17 May 2002

Fig. 8-4. Reversible Posterior Leukoencephalopathy Syndrome in renal transplant patient treated with Tacrolimus (Case #2)

subcortical T2 signal abnormalities in the occipital regions, suggestive of the posterior reversible leukoencephalopathy syndrome (Fig. 8.4a). Contrast and diffusion weighted images are not shown, but were unremarkable. She was loaded with IV fosphenytoin.

Later she had a renal biopsy thought to be suggestive of Tacrolimus toxicity and her immunosuppression regimen was changed to Sirolimus and her prednisone dose increased. Shortly after discontinuation of Tacrolimus a repeat MRI showed significant improvement (Fig. 8.4b). This case is an example of posterior reversible leukoencephalopathy syndrome due to Tacrolimus neurotoxicity (5).

References

1. Wszolek Z, Steg RE, Wijdicks EF (1999) Seizures. In: Wijdicks EF (ed) Neurologic complications in organ transplant recipients. Butterworth and Heinemann, Boston, pp 107–125
2. Wszolek ZK, Steg RE (1997) Seizures after orthotopic liver transplantation. Seizure 6:31–39
3. Martinez AJ, Estol C, AA F (1988) Neurologic complications of liver transplantation. Neurol Clin 6:327
4. Adams DH, Ponsford S, Gunson B et al (1987) Neurological complications after liver transplantation. Lancet 1:949–951
5. Wijdicks EF, Plevak DJ, Wiesner RH, Steers JL (1996) Causes and outcome of seizures in liver transplant recipients. Neurology 47:1523–1525
6. Wijdicks EF, Wiesner RH, Dahlke L, Krom R (1994) FK506-induced neurotoxicity in liver transplantation. Ann Neurol 35:498
7. Wijdicks EF, Wiesner RH, Krom R (1995) Neurotoxicity in liver transplant recipients with cyclosporine immunosuppresion. Neurology 45:1962
8. Sevmis S, Karakayali H, Emiroglu R, Akkoc H, Haberal M (2007) Tacrolimus-related seizure in the early postoperative period after liver transplantation. Transplant Proc 39(4):1211–1213
9. Patchell RA, White CL III, Clark AW, Beschorner WE, Santos GW (1985) Neurologic complications of bone marrow transplantation. Neurology 35:300–306
10. Snider S, Bashir R, Bierman P (1994) Neurologic complications after high-dose chemotherapy and autologous bone marrow transplantation for Hodgkin's disease. Neurology 44:681
11. Antonini G, Ceschin V, Morino S et al (1998) Early neurologic complications following allogeneic bone marrow transplant for leukemia: A prospective study. Neurology 50:1441–1445
12. Wszolek Z, Steg R, Armitage J Complex partial status epilepticus after bone marrow transplantation for non-Hodgkin's lymphoma. Bone Marrow Transplant 19:637–638
13. Gaggero R, Haupt R, Paola Fondelli M, De Vescovi R, Marino A, Lanino E, Dallorso S, Faraci M (2006) Intractable epilepsy secondary to cyclosporine toxicity in children undergoing allogeneic hematopoietic bone marrow transplantation. J Child Neurol 21(10):861–866
14. Grigg MM, Costanzo-Nordin MR, Celesia GG et al (1988) The etiology of seizures after cardiac transplantation. Transplant Proc 20(Suppl 3):937
15. Malheiros S, Almeida D, Massaro A et al (2002) Neurologic complications after heart transplantation. Arq Neuropsiquiatr 60:192–197
16. Mayer TO, Biller J, O'Donnell J, Meschia JF, Sokol DK (2002) Contrasting the neurologic complications of cardiac transplantation in adults and children. J Child Neurol 17:195–199
17. LM AAQ, Postlethwaite RJ, Webb NJ (1999) Seizures following renal transplantation in childhood. Pediatr Nephrol 13:275–277
18. Kahan BD, Flechner SM, Lorber MI, Golden D, Conley S, Van Buren CT (1987) Complications of cyclosporine-prednisone immunosuppression in 402 renal allograft recipients exclusively followed at a single center for from one to five years. Transplantation 43:197–204
19. Gross M, Sweny P, Pearson R, Kennedy J, Fernando O, Moorhead J (1982) Rejection encephalopathy. An acute neurological syndrome complicating renal transplantation. J Neurol Sci 56:23–34
20. Vaughn BV, Ali, II, Olivier KN et al (1996) Seizures in lung transplant recipients. Epilepsia 37:1175–1179
21. Wong M, Mallory GB Jr, Goldstein J, Goyal M, Yamada KA (1999) Neurologic complications of pediatric lung transplantation. Neurology 53:1542–1549

22. Kiok MC (1988) Neurologic complications of pancreas transplants. Neurol Clin 6:367–376

23. Alroughani R, Javidan M, Qasem A, Alotaibi N (2009) Non-convulsive status epilepticus; the rate of occurrence in a general hospital. Seizure 18(1):38–42

24. Wijdicks EF (1999) Neuologic Manesfestations of Immunosuppressive Agents. In: Wijdicks EF (ed) Neurologic complications in organ transplant recipients. Butterworth and Heinemann, Boston, pp 127–140

25. Gilmore RL (1988) Seizures and antiepileptic drug use in transplant patients. Neurol Clin 6:279–296

26. Kahan BD (1989) Cyclosporin. N Eng J Med 312:1725

27. Rubin AM, Kang H (1987) Cerebral blindness and encephalopathy with cyclosporin A toxicity. Neurology 37:1072

28. Wilson SE, de Groen PC, Aksamit AJ, Wiesner RH, Garrity JA, RA K (1988) Cyclosporin A-induced reversible cortical blindness. J Clin Neuroophthalmol 8:215–220

29. Truwit CL, Denaro CP, Lake JR, Demarco T (1991) MR imaging of reversible cyclosporin A-induced neurotoxicity. AJNR 12:651

30. Reece DE, Frei-Lahr DA, Shepard JD et al (1991) Neurologic complications in allogenic bone marrow transplant patients receiving cyclosporin. Bone Marrow Transplant 8:393

31. Thompson CB, June CH, Sullivan KM, Thomas ED (1984) Association between cyclosporin neurotoxicity and hypomagnesaemia. Lancet 2:1116

32. de Groen PC, Aksamit AJ, Rakela J et al (1987) Central nervous system toxicity after liver transplantation. The role of cyclosporin and cholesterol. N Eng J Med 317:861

33. Hauben M (1996) Cyclosporine neurotoxicity. Pharmacotherapy 16:576

34. Kelly PA, Burckart GJ, Venkataramanan R (1995) Tacrolimus: A new immunosuppressive agent. Am J Health Syst Pharm 53:1521

35. Shutter LA, Green JP, NJ Newman et al (1993) Cortical blindness and white matter lesions in a patient FK506 after liver transplantation. Neurology 43:2417

36. Parlevliet KJ, Bemelman FJ, Yong SL et al (1995) Toxicity of OKT3 increases with dosage: A controlled study in renal transplant recipients. Transplant Int 8:141

37. Seifeldin RA, Lawrence KR, Rahamtulla AF, AP M (1997) Generalized seizures associated with the use of muromonab-CD3 in two patients after kidney transplantation. Ann Pharmacother 31:586

38. Dukar O, Barr CC (1993) Visual loss complicating OKT3 monoclonal antibody therapy. Am J Opthalmol 115:781

39. De La Camara R, Tomas JF, Figuera A et al (1998) High dose busulfan and seizures. Bone Marrow Transplant 7:363

40. Jagannath S, Armitage JO, Dicke KA et al (1989) Prognostic factors for response and survival after high-dose cyclophosphamide, carmustine, and etoposide with autologous bone marrow transplantation for relapsed Hodgkins's disease. J Clin Oncol 7:179

41. Seifeldin RA (1995) Drug interactions in transplantation. Clin Ther 17:1043

42. Lowenstein DH, Alldredge BK (1998) Current concepts: status epilepticus. N Eng J Med 338:970–976

43. Sinha S, Naritoku DK (2000) Intravenous valproate is well tolerated in unstable patients with status epilepticus. Neurology 55:722–724

44. Manno EM (2003) New management strategies in the treatment of status epilepticus. Mayo Clin Proc 78:508–518

45. Kreuz W, Linde R, Funk M et al (1992) Valproate therapy induces von Willebrand disease type I. Epilepsia 33:178–184

46. Glass GA, Stankiewicz J, Mithoefer A, Freeman R, Bergethon PR (2005) Levetiracetam for seizures after liver transplantation. Neurology 64(6):1084–1085

47. Speeg KV, Halff GA, Schenker S (1995) Metabolsim of drugs before and after liver transplantation. In: Maddrey WC, MF S (eds) Transplantation of the liver, Appleton & Lange, Norwalk, CT, pp 427

Chapter 9

Extreme Hypertension, Eclampsia and Critical Care Seizures

Errol Gordon and Michel T. Torbey

Abstract The association between seizures and blood pressure elevation remains a common medical emergency encountered in an ICU setting. Syndromes such as pre-eclampsia or eclampsia, hypertensive encephalopathy, and posterior leukoencephalopathy commonly present with seizures. The primary treatment goal is to reduce the arterial blood pressure. In most cases seizure control is thus achieved, but unique medications, such as magnesium sulfate, may be needed. Fortunately, if treated immediately and aggressively, the pathophysiologic mechanism leading to seizures is reversible in most cases. Delayed treatment may result in irreversible brain injury or increased mother or fetus mortality.

Keywords Seizures, Eclampsia, Hypertensive encephalopathy, Leukoencephalo pathy, Magnesium

9.1. Introduction

> Most physicians are familiar with the syndrome of a sudden elevation of blood pressure, preceded by severe headache, and followed by convulsions, coma, or a variety of transitory cerebral phenomena. The pediatrician faces the problem with acute nephritis, the obstetrician with toxemia of pregnancy, and the internist with hypertensive vascular disease. (1)

Seizures have been reported in both chronic and acute hypertension (2). The association between hypertension and seizure occurrence is unclear. In chronic hypertension, seizures may be secondary to the effect of blood pressure elevation on the cerebral blood vessels and its association with higher risk of stroke. In acute hypertension, seizures may be secondary to disruption of blood brain barrier and secondary cerebral edema. In a population-based study from Rochester Minnesota 195 patients ³55 years with first unprovoked seizures were matched on age, gender, and duration of follow-up with patients without seizures (3). Blood pressure was obtained in the seizure patients before the first seizure occurrence. Overall, hypertension did not increase the risk of seizures, but the study found that a subgroup with left ventricular hypertrophy

From: *Seizures in Critical Care: A Guide to Diagnosis and Therapeutics*: Current Clinical Neurology, Second Edition, Edited by: P. Varelas, DOI 10.1007/978-1-60327-532-3_9, © Humana Press, a part of Springer Science+Business Media, LLC 2005, 2010

(LVH), a marker of severe, long-standing hypertension, without diuretic treatment had an 11-fold increased risk of unprovoked seizures. Interestingly, those patients with LVH treated with diuretics did not have an increased risk. This chapter will review the different acute hypertensive syndromes encountered in the ICU and emphasize the specific management of seizures associated with these disorders.

9.2. Hypertension and Pregnancy

Hypertensive disorders of pregnancy are common, affecting 7–15% of pregnant women (4). In the UK, 18.6% of maternal deaths are caused by hypertensive diseases (5). Five hypertensive disorders are commonly reported in pregnant women: (1) gestational hypertension; (2) pre-eclampsia (PREC); (3) eclampsia (EC); (4) PREC with superimposed chronic hypertension; and (5) chronic hypertension (6). Only PREC and EC are associated with seizures.

9.2.1. Pre-eclampsia and Eclampsia

Hippocrates was among the first to recognize fits occurring in pregnant women as early as the fourth century BC (7). This condition was termed eclampsia – a Greek word meaning "shine forth" – implying a sudden development (8). Pre-eclampsia and eclampsia are among the most common causes of maternal and fetal morbidity and mortality. In a retrospective review of 4,024 pregnancy-related deaths, 19.6% were related to PREC-EC (9).

Pre-eclampsia is hypertension in pregnancy diagnosed after 20 week with associated proteinurea (9). Eclampsia is defined as seizures occurring before, during, or after delivery. Although EC is usually preceded by PREC, in up to 38% of cases it can occur without symptoms or signs of PREC (8). Table 9-1 summarizes the definitions of both PREC and EC.

Table 9-1. Definition of PREC and EC.

PREC defined as:

- Newly diagnosed hypertension after 20 week gestation
- Relative increase of 15 mmHg diastolic or 30 mmHg systolic or absolute above >140/90 mmHg)
- Either or
- proteinuria (>300 mg/24 h or 1+ in dipstick testing)
- generalized edema (particularly in nondependent areas like hands and face)

Severe PREC is defined as:

- Blood pressure >160/110 mmHg
- Proteinuria 2 or 3+
- Serum creatinine >1.2 mg/dL
- Oliguria <500 mL/24 h
- Headache with or without visual symptoms, epigastric pain, pulmonary edema, thrombocytopenia <100,000/μL or increased aspartate or alanine transaminase

Eclampsia is defined as:

- Presence of seizures

9.2.1.1. Epidemiology

Preeclampsia affects up to 7% of pregnancies and <1% of these women develop EC (10). Approximately 1 in 50 women experiencing eclamptic seizures will die annually from complications (11). In a prospective survey of EC in the United Kingdom (UK), the incidence of EC was 4.9/1000 (12). The leading cause of death with PREC-EC patients is cerebrovascular accidents, particularly intracerebral hemorrhages. The mortality rate ranges from 2 to 24%. Table 9-2 summarizes the specific causes of death associated with EC and PREC. The case fatality in women with eclampsia is 71 per 10,000 (9). Although the incidence of PREC has not changed significantly over the past 6 decades, the rate of major complications from the disease has been on a marked decline (13).

Several risk factors for EC have been identified. Those include prima gravidity, lack of prenatal care, urinary tract infections, family history, diabetes mellitus, multiple gestation, extremes of age, obesity, black ethnicity, preexisting hypertension, vascular renal disease, prolonged labor, and hydatidiform moles (10, 14).

9.2.1.2. Pathophysiology

To date, the underlying pathophysiology of EC is not fully elucidated but vascular endothelial damage or dysfunction appears to be the common pathological feature in the placenta, kidneys, and brain (15). A recent hypothesis by Odent (16) proposed that PREC could be the result of maternal–fetal conflict. The developing fetal brain requires EPA, a long chain n-3 polyunsaturated fatty acid. The theory suggests that the fetus need for EPA override the maternal need. A decrease in maternal EPA in PREC and EC women as compared to their normotensive counterparts appears to play a role in the development of this condition (16). Other mechanisms suggested for eclamptic convulsions include cerebral vasospasm, hemorrhage or edema, metabolic or hypertensive encephalopathy (17).

9.2.1.3. Clinical Presentation

By definition, EC is characterized by the presence of seizures. They can occur before, during, or after labor (18). Antepartum EC refers to the onset of seizures before the start of labor. Intrapartum EC refers to seizures that occur during labor, and postpartum EC is the occurrence of seizures within 7 days of delivery of the fetus and placenta. Two percent of EC occur more than 7 days past delivery (19). In some women seizures can occur as late as 11 days (20). In the US, 53% of women had antepartum seizures, 36% intrapartum seizures

Table 9-2. Specific Causes of Death Among Pre-eclampsia or Eclampsia.

Cause of death	Pre-eclamsia (%)	Eclampsia (%)
Intracerebral hemorrhage	15.8	18.8
Cerebral edema	1.1	1.8
Cerebral embolism	0.4	0.8
Renal or hepatic failure	7.2	5.4
HELLP syndrome	4.8	2.3
Other	13.9	11.8

Adapted from (9).

and 11% postpartum seizures (19). In the UK 38% had antepartum seizures, 18% intrapartum seizures, 44% postpartum eclampsia (12).

The syndrome may also be associated with headaches, visual complaints, epigastric pain, oliguria, and depression of consciousness, thrombocytopenia, fetal growth retardation, and elevated liver enzymes.

9.2.1.4. Electrographic and Radiographic Features

Abnormal EEGs are reported with PREC (21). Diffuse slow activity (theta or delta waves) sometimes with focal slow activity are usually found on EEG (21). Paroxismal spike activity has been reported but this is not pathognomonic of PREC as similar patterns are found in other conditions (21). No correlation was found between EEG abnormalities and the degree of maternal arterial pressure (21).

The radiological features found in EC patients are certainly not unique. Diffuse cerebral edema (22), hemorrhages (23), and infarcts (24) have been demonstrated in patients with EC using computed tomography (CT) scan. Magnetic resonance image (MRI) studies of the brain of EC patients revealed focal changes characteristic of ischemia (25). MRI features consistent with reversible posterior leukoencephalopathy have also been reported (26).

9.2.1.5. Management

Early detection remains the mainstay of treatment in EC patients. The best treatment for PREC and EC is delivery. If delivery is not possible, then management of the patient should include hospitalization, close observation, and seizure prophylaxis until delivery can be performed. In a review of obstetric patients admitted to a medical-surgical ICU in a large tertiary referral center over a 5-year period, PREC was the single most common diagnosis, representing 22% of all patients (27).

Over the last two decades magnesium has emerged as the drug of choice for preventing eclampsia. Large randomized trials and systematic reviews have shown the usefulness of magnesium sulfate in treating recurrent eclamptic seizures and in the prophylaxis of EC (28–30).

In 1995 the Eclampsia Trial Collaborative Group showed unequivocally that magnesium given intramuscularly or intravenously is superior to phenytoin or diazepam in reducing recurrent eclamptic seizures (26). This international multi-center randomized study included 1,687 women with EC. The women allocated to magnesium sulfate therapy had a 52% (95% C.l. 37–64%) reduction in incidence of recurrent seizures than those given diazepam (13.2% vs. 27.9%). Maternal and perinatal morbidity were comparable between the two groups. In a second comparison between magnesium sulfate and phenytoin, the women randomized to receive magnesium sulfate had a 67% (95% C.I. 47–79%) reduced incidence of recurrent seizures (5.7% vs. 17.1%). Maternal mortality was non-significantly lower in the magnesium group compared with the phenytoin group (26). Women who received magnesium were also less likely to be ventilated when compared to phenytoin (14.9% vs. 22.5%). Women in the magnesium group were also less likely to develop pneumonia (3.9% vs. 8.8%) and less likely to be admitted to the ICU (16.7% vs. 25.1%) when compared to phenytoin.

The Magpie study, another randomized placebo-controlled trial, was designed to assess the value of magnesium for prophylaxis in EC (30). The study included approximately 10,000 women with PREC who were randomized to receive magnesium sulfate before or during labor, or after giving birth (30). Magnesium was effective in reducing seizures in 58% (95% C.I. 40–71%). Treatment was also safe for the neonate in this selling, and without any excess of serious maternal morbidity or mortality. Of the 5055 women who were randomized in each group, 46 (0.9%) had respiratory depression and 5 (0.1%) had respiratory arrest with magnesium compared to 27 (0.5%) and 2 (0.04%) in the placebo group. Respiratory arrest was responsible for one death in each group. (30).

Another multi-center randomized un-blinded study, compared magnesium to the calcium channel blocker nimodipine, a cerebral vasodilator, to prevent EC (31). PREC women who received nimodipine were more likely to have a seizure than those who received magnesium sulfate (2.6% vs. 0.8%, $p=0.01$). The antepartum risk for EC did not differ between the two treatment arms, but the nimodipine arm had a higher risk of post-partum seizures (1.1% vs.0%, $p=0.01$). Neonatal outcomes did not differ between the two groups (31).

Similar results were reported in a Cochrane review analysis that included published randomized studies between magnesium and placebo or anti-epileptics (29). After reviewing six studies, the authors concluded that Magnesium sulfate more than halves the risk of eclampsia, and probably reduces the risk of maternal death. A quarter of women had side effects, particularly flushing. The risk of placental abruption was reduced for women allocated to magnesium sulfate (RR 0.64, 95% C.l. 0.5–0.8). Women allocated to magnesium sulfate had a small, non-significant, increase (5%) in the risk of cesarean section. Magnesium sulfate was better than phenytoin and nimodipine in reducing the risk of eclampsia, but with an increased risk of cesarean section (RR I.2, 95% C.I. 1.05–1.4). The summary of the Cochrane review is detailed in Table 9-3.

The most commonly used magnesium protocol in EC is 4–6 g IV bolus over 5 min, followed by 1–2 g/h IV infusion for at least 48 h postpartum. If the treatment is used prophylactically in PREC, it can be stopped after 24 h (10). Half this dose should be used in patients with serum creatinine more than 1.3 mg/dL (10).

Patients should be admitted to the neurointensive care unit and monitored closely, particularly the respirations, patellar reflexes, and urine output. Magnesium is known to affect the neuromuscular junction, but it should not have any deleterious effect on a patient's mental status. If patellar reflexes are lost the next magnesium should be held and its level should be checked. It may be restarted at a lower dose when the reflexes return if still desired. If the urine output falls below 25 cc/h, then the rate of infusion of magnesium or the IM dose should be cut in half. In case of respiratory depression or arrest the patient airway must be first secured, (by endotracheal intubation if needed) and 1 g of calcium gluconate (10% solution) should be administered IV.

Table 9-3. Effect of Magnesium on Risk of Eclampsia.

Treatment compared with Magnesium Sulfate	Relative Risk (95% CI)
Placebo (30)	0.41(0.29–0.59)
Phenytoin (26)	0.05(0–0.84)
Nimodipine (31)	0.33(0.14–0.77)

In patients with refractory seizures several anticonvulsant regimens can be used. An additional dose 1–2 g IV of Mg can be given or a loading dose of phenytoin (18 mg/kg IV at a maximum rate of 50 mg/min) can be tried. A dark room with low noise, padded bed nails, and continuous fetal monitoring are additional measures.

9.2.2. HELLP Syndrome

Pritchard et al. first described the association between coagulation and liver enzymes abnormalities with PREC (32). In 1982, Weinstein coined this syndrome of hemolysis (anemia, increased bilirubin schistocytes in blood smear), elevated liver enzymes, and a low platelet count (<100,000/mm^3), as the HELLP syndrome (33). It can usually complicate up to 10% of eclamptic cases (17, 34). Mortality resulting from HELLP syndrome ranges from 2 to 24% of cases (9). Management of seizures in patients with HELLP syndrome is similar to EC patients. Magnesium should be initiated at seizures onset. Although no specific data exist regarding seizures, antepartum administration of corticosteroids (dexamethasone 10 mg every 13 h until delivery) has been shown to stabilize and improve laboratory values and clinical status of the mother and potentially the fetus (35, 36. The increase in liver enzymes may limit the use of some anticonvulsants such as phenytoin, carbamazepine, and or valproic acid. Levetiracetam may be used as a second line agent or as a second agent if magnesium failed to stop the seizures. The drug can be started as 500 mg P0 ql2h and increased to a maximum dose of 3,000 mg/day. If patients develop status epilepticus, phenobarbital or pentobarbital can be used as a therapeutic option. More details regarding treatment of seizures in patients with liver dysfunction can be found in the chapter on management of status epilepticus and critical care seizures.

9.3. Hypertensive Encephalopathy

Hypertensive encephalopathy (HE) is a complex cerebral disorder associated with a variety of conditions in which systemic BP rises acutely. The term was first coined by Oppenheimer and Fishberg in 1928 (37) and is defined as generalized or focal cerebral dysfunction which either partially or completely reverses with antihypertensive treatment (38).

9.3.1. Epidemiology

Hypertension is a prevalent disorder involving 20 to 30% of adults in developed countries (39). The definition of hypertension remains controversial. In the UK, hypertension is defined as blood pressure higher than 160/100 mmHg on two or more clinic readings whereas in the United States the cutoff is 140/90 mmHg. Although, improved treatment of chronic hypertension has lead to reduction in the incidence of hypertensive emergencies (40), the recognition and treatment of hypertension in the general population are still not adequate (41).

9.3.2. Clinical Features

Hypertensive encephalopathy is characterized by acute or subacute onset of lethargy, confusion, visual disturbances, and seizures (2). Other symptoms may include headache, stroke, and or papilledema (38). Symptoms may or may not be associated with proteinurea or hypertensive retinopathy (2). Seizures are often the initial presentation and they may be focal, generalized, or focal with secondary generalization (2). Initially, it was thought that the cerebral dysfunction associated with elevated blood pressure was related to the uremia from kidney disease (42). Table 9-4 summarizes the frequency of each of the presenting symptoms.

9.3.3. Pathophysiology

The endothelium plays an active role in controlling blood pressure by regulating the release of nitric oxide (NO) and other vasodilator molecules (2, 43). Although the pathophysiology of HE is not fully understood, an initial abrupt rise in vascular resistance seems to be a necessary initiating step (2). The sheer stress on the endothelial wall results in an initial burst of nitric oxide (NO) followed by steady stats release of NO promoting vasodilatation (2, 44). If the blood pressure remains elevated the compensatory mechanism may fail causing greater elevation in blood pressure and endothelial damage. A cascade follows which increases endothelial cell expression of adhesion molecules and makes the endothelium more permeable (2). Ultimately, the endothelial fibrinolytic activity may be inhibited and the coagulation cascade activated.

Cerebral blood flow (CBF) is regulated through a homeostatic mechanism referred to as autoregulation. Normotensive individuals maintain persistent CBF when their mean arterial pressure (MAP) stays in the range of 60–120 (2). Hyperperfusion of the cerebral vasculature is blunted by a compensatory vasoconstriction of the blood vessels. This compensatory mechanism is overwhelmed at MAP of 180 mmHg and cerebral autoregulation breaks down and vasodilatation occurs. This results in breakdown of the blood brain barrier (BBB), which causes edema and possible microinfarcts. Previously normotensive patients can develop signs of HE at blood pressures as low as 160/100 mmHg, whereas individuals with chronic hypertension will tolerate pressure as high as 220/110 mmHg before signs of HE ensues.

Table 9-4. Presenting Symptoms of Patients Admitted with Malignant Hypertension.

Symptoms	*N* (%)
Headache	10 (30%)
Stroke	9 (27%)
Cardiorespiratory	7 (21%)
Altered mental status	4 (13%)
Blurred vision	3 (9%)
Seizures	3 (9%)
Loss of consciousness	3 (9%)
Dizziness	1 (3%)
Asymptomatic	1 (3%)

Adapted from Ref. (38).

9.3.4. Electrographic and Radiographic Features

Currently, there is no known characteristic electroencephalographic feature of HE. Loss of posterior dominant alpha rhythm, generalized slowing, and posterior epileptiform discharges are seen on EEG. These findings usually resolve following clinical improvement (45, 46).

Imaging of the brain in a hypertensive, confused, lethargic patient who develops seizures in the ICU is crucial. Although the clinical presentation of HE is characteristic, the intensivist has to exclude the presence of intracranial hemorrhage or other mass (especially if there are focal neurological signs present), which induces the elevation of systemic blood pressure as a compensatory mechanism for cerebral perfusion. This is indeed a very common situation with ischemic or hemorrhage strokes and many times it is unclear if it is the cause or the effect. As a general statement, if the volume of the intraparenchymal blood is small or there is enough room inside the cranial cavity, due to coexisting brain atrophy, the hemorrhage is probably the result of hypertension, with additional effect from a probably abnormal underlying vasculature.

In uncomplicated cases cerebral imaging of individuals with HE shows edema in the cortex and sub-cortical white matter in the posterior areas of the brain, i.e., the occipital, the posterior parietal, and temporal lobes (47). The predilection for involvement of the posterior circulation may be due to paucity of sympathetic neural control in the posterior cerebral artery territory compared to the carotid artery territory (48). Schwartz et al.'s findings of increased apparent diffusion coefficient (ADC) values and lack of high signal on the diffusion-weighted images support the theory that the edema associated with HE is vasogenic (47).

9.3.5. Management of Hypertensive Encephalopathy

Patients should be admitted to the neuro-intensive care unit (NICU) for treatment and monitoring. An arterial line for continuous pressure monitoring should be placed immediately. If cerebral edema was present on the initial head CT and the patient has a Glasgow Coma Scale score £8, an intracranial pressure monitoring device should be placed. It is important to obtain a thorough past medical history for previous CVA's and renal disease. One should also inquire about anti-hypertensive medications and compliance. It is also paramount to ask for over-the-counter medication use (i.e., sympathomimetics) and illicit drug use, such as cocaine.

The goal of therapy in HE is to gradually decrease the MAP by approximately 25% or to reduce the diastolic BP to about 100 mmHg over a period of several minutes to hours. Precipitous reduction in BP to normotensive or hypotensive level should be avoided, as it may provoke cerebral hypoperfusion and ischemia. Sodium nitroprusside is the drug of choice for the initial treatment of HE. Due to the effect of nitroprusside on ICP, other agents such as B-blockers, Ca channel blockers, or ACE-inhibitors should be used after the initial control of BP. Hydralazine appears to be less effective in treating HE. Clonidine should be avoided because of its potential for CNS depression (47). Bed rest, sedation, and analgesia may further help BP control. Table 9-5 summarizes the most common antihypertensives used in the ICU and their side effects. Treatment of HE-induced seizures is not different from the general treatment of ICU seizures, outlined in the chapter of Management of Status Epilepticus and Critical Care Seizures.

Table 9-5. Commonly Used Parenteral Anti-hypertensive Drugs.

Medication	Mechanism of action	Bolus dose	Infusion rate	Pros	Cons
Sodium Nitroprusside	Vasodilator	No bolus dose	0.25–10.0 mg/kg/min	Short duration of actionImmediate onset of action	CBF, ↑↑ ICPCyanide toxicity
Nitroglycerin	Vasodilator	50 mcg IV	5–100 µg/kg/min	Short duration of actionRapid onset of action	CBF, ↑↑ ICPMethemoglobin production
Nicardipine	Vasodilator Ca++ Channel blocker	5 mg/h	5–15 mg/h	Short duration of action	Tachycardia
Clevidipine	Vasodilator, Ca++ Channel blocker	No bolus dose	2–32 mg/h	Ultra-short half-life: 1 min, easily titratable	Vial and tubing has to be changed q 4 h, 20% lipids emulsion
Hydralazine	Vasodilator	2.5–10 mg IV Q20-30 min for a max of 40 mg	No drip	Good anti-hypertensive effect	Longer duration of action CBF, ICP Glomerulonephritis, Lupus like syndrome, hemolytic anemia
Clonidine	α₂-agonist	0.1–0.2 mg PO	No drip	Might be helpful in alcohol withdrawal	CBF
Labetalol	α₁,β₁, β₂ receptor antagonist	5–20 mg IV q 15 min for a total of 340 mg	0.5–2 mg/min	Rapid onset of actionNo effect on ICP	CHFBronchospasm Bradycardia
Esmolol	β₁-selective	500 µg/Kg over 1 min	50–200 µg/Kg/min	Rapid onset of actionNo effect on ICP	Bradycardia
Enalaprilat	ACE inhibitor	0.625–5 mg IV q6 h	No drip	No effect on ICP or CBF	Could cause abrupt decrease in BPPotential ICP in patients with poor compliance Renal dysfunction

CBF Cerebral blood flow, *ICP* Intracranial pressure, *CHF* Congestive heart failure, *ACE* Angiotension converting enzyme.

9.4. Posterior Leukoencephalopathy Syndrome

Posterior leukoencephalopathy (PLE) is a recently recognized neurological disorder. It is characterized by white matter edema in the posterior parietal and occipital lobes of the brain (49). The term was first used by Hinchey et al., when they described 15 patients admitted with a wide variety of medical illnesses (49). Of these, seven were receiving immunosuppressive therapy, four had HE, and three were not hypertensive at all. In all patients, the neurological abnormalities resolved within 2 weeks. This syndrome has also been reported with uremia, hemolytic uremic syndrome, thrombotic thrombocytopenia purpura, cyclosporine A, cisplatin, interferon alpha, intrathecal methotrexate, severe hypercalcemia, and indinavir (50–52). For those patients who do not exhibit hypertension (children or adults), the syndrome of posterior reversible leukoencephalopathy has been coined, although some believe that a term such as reversible occipital-parietal encephalopathy is more appropriate, since both gray and white matter are involved (53 17).

9.4.1. Clinical Features

The most common presenting signs and symptoms include lethargy, confusion, and somnolence, paucity of speech, headaches and visual complaints. Lethargy and somnolence are often the first signs noted. Memory difficulties are not uncommon. Visual disturbances range from blurred vision to hemianopsia (49).

Seizures are common at onset: eleven out of 15 (73%) of the originally reported patients had one or more seizures. They are usually generalized tonic-clonic, but can also have a focal onset. Multiple seizures are more common than single seizures. Status epilepticus has also been reported (49). Seizures generally precede the other manifestations of the syndrome. Visual auras or visual hallucinations also precede the tonic-clonic or occipital seizures. Following a seizure, patients usually have prolonged mental status change and few end up in stupor or coma. (54)

9.4.2. Pathophysiology

This syndrome shares similar pathophysiological mechanisms with HE and eclampsia. Two pathophysiological mechanisms for PLS have been proposed (55). The first evokes cerebral vasospasm and cerebral ischemia as a cause for the changes seen on neuroimaging (56). The second suggests a breakdown in cerebrovascular autoregulation with secondary vasogenic edema. Recent MRI finding are in support of the autoregulation hypothesis (57). The pathological process is characterized by cerebral edema and petechial hemorrhages especially in the parieto-occipital and occipital lobes. Microscopically, these petechiae are ring hemorrhages around capillaries and precapillaries that are occluded by fibrinoid material (58).

9.4.3. Radiological Features

The most common neuroimaging abnormality on both MRI and CT is white matter edema in the posterior areas of the cerebral hemispheres. These changes are predominately symmetrical and specifically involve the occipital, parietal, and posterior temporal lobes (49). Other lesions are reported in the pons, thalamus, and the cerebellum. The gray matter is involved in some patients and hence the term Ieukoencephalopathy may not be the most appropriate (53, 57). Individuals with predominantly gray matter disease have a better course than those with predominantly white matter lesions. Brainstem lesions are found in 56% of patients (57). On MR images, the high signal on diffusion weighted imaging without the typical ADC dropout suggests vasogenic edema (47). This is referred to as pseudonormalization. Some patients with pseudonormalization can progress to having an infarct.

9.4.4. Management

Patients may need to be monitored in the NICU. Indications for transfer to the NICU include cerebral edema with midline shift and seizures. If the cause of PLE is found to be acute hypertension, then aggressive blood pressure management should be initiated. Treatment paradigms are similar to those for HE. If a particular drug was thought to be the inciting agent, then discontinuing the drug should be seriously considered. For seizures, benzodiazepines are indicated as first choice agents. If seizures are refractory or recurrent, then an additional anticonvulsant is indicated. The choice of anticonvulsant will depend on the patient's general clinical condition and associated renal or liver abnormalities. For more details regarding treatment of ICU seizures the reader should refer to the chapter Management of Status Epilepticus and Critical Care Seizures.

References

1. Finnerty FA Jr (1968) Hypertensive encephalopathy. Am Heart J 75(4):559–563
2. Delanty N (2002) Seizures: medical causes and management. Cur Clin Neurol. Humana Press, Totowa, N.J., pp xii, 368
3. Hesdorffer DC et al (1996) Severe, uncontrolled hypertension and adult-onset seizures: a case-control study in Rochester, Minnesota. Epilepsia 37(8):736–741
4. National High Blood Pressure Education Program Working Group Report on High Blood Pressure in Pregnancy (1990) Am J Obstet Gynecol 163(5 Pt 1):1691–1712
5. Deparment of Health (1994) Report on Confidential Enquiries into Maternal Deaths in the UK 1988–90, in DoH. London
6. Cunningham FG, Lindheimer MD (1992) Hypertension in pregnancy. N Engl J Med 326(14):927–932
7. O'Dowd MJ, Phillip EE (1994) The history of obstetrics and gynecology. Parthenon Publishing Group, New York
8. Mushambi MC, Halligan AW, Williamson K (1996) Recent developments in the pathophysiology and management of pre-eclampsia. Br J Anaesth 76(1):133–148
9. MacKay AP, Berg CJ, Atrash HK (2001) Pregnancy-related mortality from preeclampsia and eclampsia. Obstet Gynecol 97(4):533–538
10. Witlin AG et al (1997) Cerebrovascular disorders complicating pregnancy – beyond eclampsia. Am J Obstet Gynecol 176(6):1139–1145; discussion 1145–1148
11. Munro PT (2000) Management of eclampsia in the accident and emergency department. J Accid Emerg Med 17(1):7–11
12. Douglas KA, Redman CW (1994) Eclampsia in the United Kingdom. BMJ 309(6966):1395–1400
13. Leitch CR, Cameron AD, Walker JJ (1997) The changing pattern of eclampsia over a 60-year period. Br J Obstet Gynaecol 104(8):917–922

14. Ramin KD (1999) The prevention and management of eclampsia. Obstet Gynecol Clin North Am 26(3):489–503, ix

15. Lyall F, Greer IA (1994) Pre-eclampsia: a multifaceted vascular disorder of pregnancy. J Hypertens 12(12):1339–1345

16. Odent M (2001) Hypothesis: preeclampsia as a maternal-fetal conflict. MedGenMed 3(5):2

17. Usta IM, Sibai BM (1995) Emergent management of puerperal eclampsia. Obstet Gynecol Clin North Am 22(2):315–335

18. Lopez-Llera M (1992) Main clinical types and subtypes of eclampsia. Am J Obstet Gynecol 166(1 Pt 1):4–9

19. Katz VL, Farmer R, Kuller JA (2000) Preeclampsia into eclampsia: toward a new paradigm. Am J Obstet Gynecol 182(6):1389–1396

20. Dziewas R et al (2002) Late onset postpartum eclampsia: a rare and difficult diagnosis. J Neurol 249(9):1287–1291

21. Sibai BM et al (1984) Effect of magnesium sulfate on electroencephalographic findings in preeclampsia-eclampsia. Obstet Gynecol 64(2):261–266

22. Kirby JC, Jaindl JJ (1984) Cerebral CT findings in toxemia of pregnancy. Radiology 151(1):114

23. Milliez J, Dahoun A, Boudraa M (1990) Computed tomography of the brain in eclampsia. Obstet Gynecol 75(6):975–980

24. Gaitz JP, Bamford CR (1982) Unusual computed tomographic scan in eclampsia. Arch Neurol 39(1):66

25. Schwaighofer BW, Hesselink JR, Healy ME (1989) MR demonstration of reversible brain abnormalities in eclampsia. J Comput Assist Tomogr 13(2):310–312

26. Celik O, Hascalik S (2003) Reversible posterior leukoencephalopathy in eclampsia. Int J Gynaecol Obstet 82(1):67–69

27. Kilpatrick SJ, Matthay MA (1992) Obstetric patients requiring critical care. A five-year review. Chest 101(5):1407–1412

28. Which anticonvulsant for women with eclampsia? Evidence from the Collaborative Eclampsia Trial (1995) Lancet 345(8963):1455–1463

29. Duley L, Gulmezoglu AM, Henderson-Smart DJ (2003) Magnesium sulphate and other anticonvulsants for women with pre-eclampsia. Cochrane Database Syst Rev 2:CD000025

30. Altman D, Carroli G, Duley L, Farrell B, Moodley J, Neilson J, Smith D, Magpie Trial Collaboration Group (2002) Do women with pre-eclampsia, and their babies, benefit from magnesium sulphate? The Magpie Trial: a randomised placebo-controlled trial. Lancet 359(9321):1877–1890

31. Belfort MA et al (2003) A comparison of magnesium sulfate and nimodipine for the prevention of eclampsia. N Engl J Med 348(4):304–311

32. Pritchard JA et al (1954) Intravascular hemolysis, thrombocytopenia and other hematologic abnormalities associated with severe toxemia of pregnancy. N Engl J Med 250(3):89–98

33. Weinstein L (1982) Syndrome of hemolysis, elevated liver enzymes, and low platelet count: a severe consequence of hypertension in pregnancy. Am J Obstet Gynecol 142(2):159–167

34. Haddad B et al (2000) Risk factors for adverse maternal outcomes among women with HELLP (hemolysis, elevated liver enzymes, and low platelet count) syndrome. Am J Obstet Gynecol 183(2):444–448

35. Magann EF et al (1994) Postpartum corticosteroids: accelerated recovery from the syndrome of hemolysis, elevated liver enzymes, and low platelets (HELLP). Am J Obstet Gynecol 171(4):1154–1158

36. Magann EF et al (1994) Antepartum corticosteroids: disease stabilization in patients with the syndrome of hemolysis, elevated liver enzymes, and low platelets (HELLP). Am J Obstet Gynecol 171(4):1148–1153

37. Oppenheimer BS, Fishburg A (1928) Hypertensive encephalopathy. Arch Intern Med 41:264–278
38. Healton EB et al (1982) Hypertensive encephalopathy and the neurologic manifestations of malignant hypertension. Neurology 32(2):127–132
39. He J, Whelton PK (1997) Epidemiology and prevention of hypertension. Med Clin North Am 81(5):1077–1097
40. Bennett NM, Shea S (1988) Hypertensive emergency: case criteria, sociodemographic profile, and previous care of 100 cases. Am J Public Health 78(6):636–640
41. Berlowitz DR et al (1998) Inadequate management of blood pressure in a hypertensive population. N Engl J Med 339(27):1957–1963
42. Auer LM (1978) The pathogenesis of hypertensive encephalopathy. Experimental data and their clinical relevance with special reference to neurosurgical patients. Acta Neurochir Suppl (Wien) 27:1–111
43. Furchgott RF, Zawadzki JV (1980) The obligatory role of endothelial cells in the relaxation of arterial smooth muscle by acetylcholine. Nature 288(5789):373–376
44. Kuchan MJ, Frangos JA (1993) Shear stress regulates endothelin-1 release via protein kinase C and cGMP in cultured endothelial cells. Am J Physiol 264(1 Pt 2): H150–H156
45. Torocsik HV et al (1999) FK506-induced leukoencephalopathy in children with organ transplants. Neurology 52(7):1497–1500
46. Delanty N et al (1997) Erythropoietin-associated hypertensive posterior leukoencephalopathy. Neurology 49(3):686–689
47. Schwartz RB et al (1998) Diffusion-weighted MR imaging in hypertensive encephalopathy: clues to pathogenesis. AJNR Am J Neuroradiol 19(5):859–862
48. Vaughan CJ, Delanty N (2000) Hypertensive emergencies. Lancet 356(9227):411–417
49. Hinchey J et al (1996) A reversible posterior leukoencephalopathy syndrome. N Engl J Med 334(8):494–500
50. Covarrubias DJ, Luetmer PH, Campeau NG (2002) Posterior reversible encephalopathy syndrome: prognostic utility of quantitative diffusion-weighted MR images. AJNR Am J Neuroradiol 23(6):1038–1048
51. Kastrup O et al (2002) Posterior reversible encephalopathy syndrome due to severe hypercalcemia. J Neurol 249(11):1563–1566
52. Giner V et al (2002) Reversible posterior leukoencephalopathy secondary to indinavir-induced hypertensive crisis: a case report. Am J Hypertens 15(5):465–467
53. Pavlakis SG, Frank Y, Chusid R (1999) Hypertensive encephalopathy, reversible occipitoparietal encephalopathy, or reversible posterior leukoencephalopathy: three names for an old syndrome. J Child Neurol 14(5):277–281
54. Garg RK (2001) Posterior leukoencephalopathy syndrome. Postgrad Med J 77(903):24–28
55. Port JD, Beauchamp NJ Jr (1998) Reversible intracerebral pathologic entities mediated by vascular autoregulatory dysfunction. Radiographics 18(2):353–367
56. Trommer BL, Homer D, Mikhael MA (1988) Cerebral vasospasm and eclampsia. Stroke 19(3):326–329
57. Casey SO et al (2000) Posterior reversible encephalopathy syndrome: utility of fluid-attenuated inversion recovery MR imaging in the detection of cortical and subcortical lesions. AJNR Am J Neuroradiol 21(7):1199–1206
58. Donaldson JO (1994) Eclampsia. Adv Neurol 64:25–33

Chapter 10

Infection or Inflammation and ICU Seizures

Wendy C. Ziai and Mohammed Rehman

Abstract Effective treatment of seizures associated with CNS infection and inflammation depends on rapid diagnosis and early attainment of bactericidal activity within the CSF with appropriate antimicrobial agents, or appropriate management of vasculitis-induced cerebral complications. There is nothing specific regarding the management of ICU seizures in these situations, except for a high suspicion by the medical staff, as seizures are not uncommon in this setting. Improvement in long-term neurologic outcome depends on both the therapy of the infectious/inflammatory process and the intensive care multisystem monitoring commonly warranted in this patient population. The primary goal of preserving CNS function is shared by both the neurologist and the intensivist, making a multidisciplinary approach essential.

Keywords Central nervous system, Seizures, Infection, Inflammation, Intensive care unit, Lupus, Meningitis, Encephalitis

10.1. Introduction

Seizures in critically ill patients are potential markers or contributors of significant morbidity and mortality. Seizures are a relatively common neurologic manifestation in patients admitted to an intensive care unit and are not uncommonly associated with infection. Clinical seizures are a known complication of central nervous system (CNS) infection, particularly after viral infection (1) and less frequently after bacterial infections (2, 3). In patients with CNS infection, clinical seizures are associated with poor outcomes (4, 5). Of 217 patients admitted to a general medical/coronary intensive care unit with neurologic complications of a non-neurologic primary diagnosis, 28% of neurologic complications were seizures, second only to metabolic encephalopathy (6). Sepsis was the second most common cause of seizures after vascular lesions. In any patient presenting with fever and seizures, central nervous system (CNS) infection and inflammation need to be considered in the differential diagnosis. CNS infections are markedly different from systemic infections because of the

From: *Seizures in Critical Care: A Guide to Diagnosis and Therapeutics*: Current Clinical Neurology, Second Edition, Edited by: P. Varelas, DOI 10.1007/978-1-60327-532-3_10, © Humana Press, a part of Springer Science+Business Media, LLC 2005, 2010

closed anatomic space of the CNS, its immunological isolation from the rest of the body, and the often nonspecific nature of the key manifestations. Early recognition of seizure activity and aggressive management are essential to patient recovery and prevention of long-term neurologic sequelae. This review focuses on the significance of seizures in both systemic and CNS infection and inflammatory conditions.

The spectrum of clinical manifestations of central nervous system (CNS) infection and inflammation is vast. Seizures complicate many nervous system infections, some commonly, such as meningitis, herpes simplex encephalitis and cerebral malaria. The patient may present in a life-threatening state, as seen in full-blown meningoencephalitis, or in an asymptomatic state, as seen in the dormant stages of spirochete infections. Common CNS infections that may require critical care are meningitis, ventriculitis, encephalitis and brain abscess.

Recent studies emphasize the role of continuous electroencephalographic (EEG) monitoring (cEEG) because it can detect purely electrographic seizures (ESz) activity, including nonconvulsive status epilepticus, in approximately 18 to 40% of patients presenting with an unexplained decreased level of consciousness or clinical seizures (7). Moreover, ESz and other EEG findings, such as periodic epileptiform discharges (PEDs) are associated with worse outcome in patients with acute neurological injuries, such as in the aftermath of convulsive status epilepticus and in those with intracerebral (8) or sub-arachnoid (9) hemorrhages. In patients with CNS infections, recent guidelines recommend cEEG for patients with bacterial meningitis with seizures or fluctuations in the level of consciousness (10). In a retrospective cohort study by Carrera et al., it was noted that central nervous system infections undergoing cEEG monitoring, Esz and/or PEDs were frequent, occurring in 48% of the cohort, with more than half showing no clinical correlate (11).

10.2. CNS Infectious Disorders

10.2.1. Meningitis

Meningitis is the inflammation of the pia and arachnoid membranes (leptomeninges) that surround the brain and spinal cord (12). The classification of meningitis includes acute, aseptic and septic, syndromes (<4 weeks' duration), recurrent meningitis (multiple acute episodes of <4 weeks each), and chronic meningitis (>4 weeks' duration).

Acute aseptic meningitis, defined by negative routine screening cultures and stains of cerebrospinal fluid (CSF), is the most common form of meningitis (13). This usually starts with high-grade fever and severe headache. Associated problems such as nausea, vomiting, pharyngitis, diarrhea, neck stiffness and photophobia may occur. Seizures are not a common manifestation. Rapid and complete recovery is the usual course. Viral infection is commonly the cause of aseptic meningitis. Fifty-five percent to 70% of cases are caused by enteroviruses (echovirus, coxsackie A and B, poliovirus, and the numbered entero-viruses) (13, 14).

Other causes of aseptic meningitis include: human immunodeficiency virus (HIV), parasites, rickettsiae and mycoplasma, and autoimmune diseases such as Behçet's disease, Kawasaki disease and Vogt-Koyanagi-Harada disease (12). Malignancies and drug reactions have also been implicated. In a population-based study, the 20-year risk for unprovoked seizures was 2.1% after aseptic meningitis, not increased over the general population risk for unprovoked seizures (15).

Acute septic meningitis is the bacterial infection of the meninges. It is a neurologic emergency with mortality and morbidity rates as high as 25 and 60%, respectively (16). The classical presentation of septic meningitis includes fever, headache, reduced alertness and meningeal irritation. Seizures have been reported to occur in 5–28% of cases (17, 18, 20, 21). One retrospective review of 103 episodes of acute bacterial meningitis in adults found documentation of seizures in 29 cases (28%) (21). The relatively high incidence may reflect a large number of *L monocytogenes* cases which are more commonly associated with seizures. Seizures were usually observed within 24 h of presentation (76%). Seizure activity was an independent predictor of mortality in this series (34% mortality in patients with seizures compared to 7% without seizures; odds ratio 17.6, $p < 0.001$). Decreased level of consciousness on presentation was also predictive of death (26% vs. 2%). Coma can be a consequence of fulminant bacterial meningitis with diffuse cerebral edema leading to cerebral herniation. Multiple cerebral infarcts secondary to vasculitis have also been described (22). Systemic complications can occur in 22% patients (18), with septic shock in 12%, pneumonia in 8% and disseminated intravascular coagulation in 8%. In a univariate analysis, patients with bacterial meningitis had a poorer prognosis if the following were present: age greater than 60 years, coma at the onset or focal seizures within the first 24 h of admission (72% vs. 18% mortality among those without early onset seizures; $p < 0.001$) (17). This large retrospective study from the Massachusetts General Hospital evaluated 445 patients with acute bacterial meningitis between 1962 and 1988 (17). Seizures occurred in 23% of 493 episodes of meningitis. They were focal in 7%, generalized in 13% and not characterized in 3%. In two-thirds of cases, seizures occurred within 24 h of admission and more than one-third of early seizure patients had a history of alcoholism. *Streptococcus pneumoniae* was more frequently found in patients who developed seizures (58% vs. 30% in patients without seizures; $p < 0.001$), but alcoholism was a confounding factor. In a study by Zoon et al. Seizures occurred in 121 of 696 episodes (17%) with death occurring in 41% of patients with seizures, compared to 16% of patients without seizures ($p < 0.001$) (19).

Seizures in a patient with meningitis warrant a neuroimaging study (ideally, a contrast enhanced CT scan or MRI). Seizure is a manifestation of cortical irritation and its occurrence may indicate a cortically based complication (empyema, stroke, venous thrombosis). Cortical venous thrombosis usually presents with seizures and focal neurological signs. However, it is an uncommon event during bacterial meningitis: only 5.1% of autopsies of patients who died from meningitis had septic cortical vein thrombosis in a large series (23). Occurrence of seizures requires rapid treatment with anticonvulsants. Prophylactic anticonvulsants have no established benefit. Patients with persistent alteration in mental status or coma should undergo an EEG to rule out subclinical seizures. Continuous EEG monitoring (CEEGM) may be a better option in these cases. Using CEEGM, Jordan evaluated 200 patients admitted to a neurological intensive care unit. The study had decisive or contributing impact on clinical decision-making in 12/13 patients with intracranial infection (24).

Recurrent meningitis can be due to infectious and noninfectious causes. Viruses are the most likely infectious agents. The clinical presentation may resemble aseptic meningitis. Mollaret's meningitis is a type of recurrent aseptic meningitis associated with Epstein–Barr virus and herpes simplex type I virus (25, 26). Epileptic seizures are part of the clinical presentation of Mollaret's meningitis (27).

Chronic meningitis has a nonspecific presentation, with variable fever, headache, neck rigidity, and signs of parenchymal involvement, such as altered mental status, seizures or focal neurologic deficits (12). Infectious causes are commonly CNS tuberculosis and cryptococcus. Noninfectious causes include neoplasms, neurosarcoidosis and CNS vasculitis (12). Since the widespread use of the vaccine for Haemophilus influenzae type B, Streptococcus pneumoniae has replaced it as the most common cause of acute community-acquired bacterial meningitis in industrialized countries. The rising incidence of beta-lactam-resistant pneumococci has to be considered when choosing a regimen for empiric antibiotic therapy (28, 29). Empiric antibiotic therapy for a suspected bacterial CNS infection should be given in consideration with the patient's age, competence of the immune system and associated morbidities. An immune-competent adult should be started on a third-generation cephalosporin (ceftriaxone – 4g/d or cefotaxime – 8 to12g/d) with the addition of ampicillin(12g/d) for patients over age 50 who are more susceptible to *S. agalactiae* and *Listeria monocytogenes*. An immune compromised adult, such as patients with lymphoreticular tumors, receiving cytotoxic chemotherapy, or high-dose corticosteroid treatment, should be treated with ampicillin, vancomycin (2 to 3g/d) and a broad-spectrum cephalosporin such as ceftazidime (6g/d), which has more activity against gram-negative organisms (15). Neurosurgical patients, including those with CSF shunts, and head trauma patients require both gram-positive and gram-negative coverage with a recommended combination of vancomycin and ceftazidime (6g/d). (15) In areas with known high penicillin resistant *S. Pneumoniae* isolates, empiric therapy should also begin with vancomycin. Clinically significant S. *Pneumoniae* resistance to vancomycin has not been documented (28). Seizure treatment in the context of acute or chronic meningitis is not different from the treatment offered because of other causes and details can be found in the chapter "Management of status epilepticus and critical care seizures."

10.2.2. Encephalitis

Encephalitis is an acute infection of brain parenchyma and should be suspected in a febrile patient who presents with altered mental status and signs of diffuse cerebral dysfunction. Encephalitis is usually caused by viral infection, most commonly *Herpes simplex* virus (HSE) (15% of cases), varicella zoster virus (VZV), Epstein Barr virus (EBV), mumps, enteroviruses, lymphocytic choriomeningitis virus (LCM), and togaviruses (30). The route of invasion is varied and can be via the bloodstream, the skin through an insect bite, or via the respiratory or digestive route. Specific viruses can have characteristic presentations, such as parotitis associated with mumps and herpetic rash with HSE. Diplopia, dysarthria, and ataxia can be seen in immunocompromised patients with brainstem HSE (31, 32). Clinical presentation often includes a prodrome with fever, headache, and myalgia and mild respiratory infection. Changes in the level of consciousness, with focal neurological deficits may follow.

The majority of patients with encephalitis have abnormal EEG findings, the most frequent being diffuse, generalized high-amplitude delta or theta waves with occasional asymmetry (33–36). HSV encephalitis is typically associated with periodic lateralized epileptic discharges (PLEDs), although these have also been reported in St. Louis encephalitis (37) and in several conditions not associated with infection (35, 36). The periodic discharge pattern may be caused by the involvement of both cortical and subcortical areas (38). West Nile virus (WNV) CNS infection has been previously associated with frontally prominent slowing which is non-specific, but different from the pattern seen in HSV (34, 39, 40). This may reflect the fact that WNV affects both sub-cortical gray structures along with cortex distinguishing it from purely cortical viral syndromes (41).

Seizures, both focal and generalized, are a common manifestation of the encephalitides. They can occur in the acute infection stage, when the patient is admitted to an ICU, or later in life. They can be easily controlled with antiepileptic medications, but many times they become intractable. Epilepsy surgery may be a better option in cases where there is a clearly localized focus. In a series of 38 patients who developed medically intractable partial seizures, Marks et al. found that 16 of them had a history of meningitis and 22 had encephalitis. Meningitis was pathologically associated with mesial temporal sclerosis and encephalitis with neocortical foci. However, in patients with encephalitis at less than 4 years of age, seizures were also associated with mesial temporal sclerosis (42). In another population-based study, Annegers et al. found that the risk of developing unprovoked seizures within 20 years was 22% in patients with viral encephalitis and early seizures, 10% for those with viral encephalitis without early seizures, 13% in patients with bacterial meningitis and early seizures, and only 2.4% in patients with bacterial meningitis without early seizures (15).

10.2.2.1. Japanese Encephalitis

Japanese encephalitis (JE) is the most important epidemic viral encephalitis in the world, causing an estimated 50,000 cases annually and resulting in more than 10,000 deaths per year (43). Mortality is 30% and half of the survivors are left with severe neurologic sequelae (44, 45). Although JE virus is confined mainly to Asia, related neurotropic flaviviruses include West Nile virus, Murray Valley encephalitis virus and tick-borne encephalitis virus, which cause similar diseases in other geographical locations (46–48). JE virus is neurotropic and replicates rapidly in neurons, causing a perivascular inflammatory reaction, resulting in infection, neuronal dysfunction and death (49). Solomon prospectively studied 144 patients infected with JE virus (134 children and 10 adults) (50). JE virus was diagnosed using antibody detection, culture of serum and CSF, and immunohistochemistry of autopsy material. Forty patients (28%) had a witnessed seizure during the admission; of these, the majority (24/40; 62%) died or had a poor outcome compared to 26/104 (14%) in the group with no witnessed seizure (odds ratio [OR] 4.5; 95% confidence interval [CI]: 1.94–10.52). Patients with more than one witnessed seizure (29/40) were more likely to have a poor outcome (21/29; 72% died or had severe sequelae) compared to patients with a single seizure (4/11; 33% poor outcome; OR 5.25; 95% CI: 1.02–29.4). Ten of 18 patients who had generalized tonic–clonic seizures and all 15 patients with subtle clinical manifestations of seizures (twitching of a digit, eyebrow, nostrils, excess salivation, irregular breathing, eye deviation with or without nystagmus) were in status epilepticus. These patients had a higher mortality than those without the development of status (44% [11/25] vs. 0% of 15). The acute background EEG patterns were also associated with outcome in this study. Of 234 EEGs performed on 55 patients, poor outcome was associated with acute EEG findings of slow nonreactive, low-amplitude, burst suppression, or isoelectric patterns in 16/19 patients (84%) compared with poor outcome in 14/36 patients (39%) with findings of slow reactive, or normal EEG patterns (OR, 8.4; 95%CI: 1.8–44.5). Independent predictors of poor outcome by logistic regression in this patient cohort were comatose state, more than one witnessed seizure, herniation syndrome, and illness for 7 days or more. Patients with seizures were more likely to have elevated opening pressure on lumbar puncture ($p=0.03$) and to develop brainstem signs consistent with a herniation syndrome ($p<0.0001$). It is possible that these events are related. Seizures increase cerebral blood flow, and therefore intracranial volume, resulting in increased ICP (51). If seizures are prolonged, cerebral edema may occur secondary to a number of metabolic consequences including hypoxemia, hypoglycemia, increased lactate production, low CSF glucose, high CSF lactate, metabolic acidosis, and carbon dioxide retention if airway management is suboptimal (52, 53). Cerebral edema causes further increase in ICP, and may predispose an already inflamed brain to life-threatening compartmental shifts through the tentorium and foramen magnum, resulting in herniation syndromes. Although it is not possible from this study to determine whether seizures are a cause or a marker of severe disease, anti-convulsant prophylaxis in this patient population, and aggressive surveillance and management of seizures may improve the outcome. Over 30% of patients with seizures had subtle manifestations which could have been missed without EEG recording.

10.2.2.2. Herpes Simplex Encephalitis

Herpes simplex encephalitis (HSE), usually caused by HSV-1 is the most important form of treatable encephalitis. HSE is a medical emergency; prognosis depends on the patient's condition once treatment is started (54). HSE has a mortality rate of 50 to 70% with significant long-term morbidity in survivors including seizures, and cognitive and behavioral disorders (55). In a retrospective study from New Zealand, patients with HSE presented with acute stage seizures in 50% of cases and seizures constituted the fourth most common presenting symptom after headache, confusion and nausea/vomiting. Thirty-four of 49 initial patients were followed for an average of 2 to 6 years: 24% of them had developed epilepsy. In this series, the frequency of seizures was not different between patients with good and poor outcomes. The presence although of bilateral epileptiform abnormalities was more common among those with poor outcome (0/18 with good outcome vs. 5/10 with poor outcome; $p<0.01$) (57). HSE has a predilection for the temporal and orbitofrontal lobes, resulting in a clinical picture of altered consciousness, memory loss, personality change, and confusion or olfactory hallucinations, following a prodrome of headache and fever (54). MRI shows typical asymmetrical changes in the anterior and medial temporal lobe, inferior frontal lobe, insular cortex and splenium of the corpus callosum on fluid-attenuated inversion recovery (FLAIR) sequences as early as day 2 (55). Pathologically, HSE is an acute necrotising encephalitis with preferential involvement of the frontotemporal, cingulate, and insular cortex (56). Diagnosis of HSE is highly sensitive and specific using CSF polymerase chain reaction (PCR) to amplify viral DNA and MRI findings. EEG should be performed when suspecting encephalitis to distinguish focal encephalitis from generalized encephalopathy and to look for abnormal findings of HSE. Diffuse, bihemispheric slow waves and triphasic waves as in hepatic failure may suggest encephalopathy. Although no specific EEG patterns are pathognomonic of HSE, focal or lateralized EEG abnormalities in the presence of encephalitis are highly suspicious (58). Early changes in HSE may be nonspecific spike and slow-wave activity, delta waves, or triphasic waves which then evolve into the typical 2–3 Hz unilateral periodic lateralized epileptiform discharges (PLEDs), originating from the temporal lobes, seen in 84% of typical HSE. (60). Periodic discharges tend to occur only during the acute stage, and may disappear on the side of initial involvement before appearing on the newly involved side. When present bilaterally, they often occur in a time-locked relationship with each other (60). Their appearance later in the disease course may indicate a recurrence (59). EEG findings in either the acute or on long-term follow-up have not been shown to predict survival or severity of neurologic disability (58). In addition, the relationship between epileptiform abnormalities and occurrence of seizures has been reported as inconsistent (58). Lai and Gragasin found that among nine patients who had seizures in the acute stage of HSE, only four had epileptiform abnormalities on EEG; another four patients with no evidence of clinical seizure activity had nonperiodic epileptiform discharges on EEG (58).

Specific treatment with acyclovir is indicated in HSE, at a dosage of 10 mg/kg q8h for 10–14 days. Important factors influencing mortality and morbidity of HSE in a study by Jha et al. were; early acyclovir therapy, age, immune status of patient, duration of illness, and consciousness level before initiation of therapy (59). Supportive therapy also includes aggressive management of elevated intracranial pressure and treatment of seizures, usually with intravenous phenytoin. In patients with proven HSE, treatment with acyclovir significantly increases the likelihood of survival to 65 to 100% if disease is present for 4 days or less (61). Other studies still predict 25% mortality, even if acyclovir is started within 5 days of symptom onset (62). Cerebral edema, persistent vegetative state and systemic infection are the usual predictors of a fatal outcome. Other risk factors for poor prognosis include MRI abnormalities, bilateral EEG abnormalities and focal hyperperfusion on SPECT (63, 64). Only half of the patients return to their previous or similar level of productivity (65). Seizure prophylaxis should be instituted, in our opinion, in every patient with proven HSE although there are no randomized studies in humans. In a rabbit model, prophylactic administration of phenobarbital daily reduced mortality significantly (66). If treatment is started, it should be continued for at least 1 year (if acute stage seizures are present). Discontinuing the treatment may be decided on the basis of late seizures or EEG findings. Pathologically proven chronic HSV-1 encephalitis has been reported in patients with medically intractable seizures many years after the clinical acute encephalitis syndrome (67).

10.2.2.3. West Nile Virus Encephalitis

The incidence of seizures, status epilepticus and epilepsy in West Nile virus encephalitis (WNVE) is not yet well defined (72). Although early reports suggested seizures occurred in approximately 30% of patients with WNVE (68), reports from more recent epidemics suggest a much lower incidence of seizures ranging from 9% in a report from Israel (39) to 3% in a report from New York

(69), to absent in 2 cohorts of 326 patients and 32 elderly patients, respectively with WNV fever (70, 71). Klein (2002) reported that in 26 patients with neurologic involvement from WNV two had seizures, both of whom had encephalitis and normal CSF findings (39). The EEG was abnormal in 88% of patients with meningitis or meningo-encephalitis and in 74% with any neurological involvement. EEG abnormalities were most frequently diffuse symmetric slowing with frontal predominance although temporal predominant slowing and asymmetric frontal slowing were seen in some cases. These findings were confirmed by Gandelman-Marton et al. (2003) who reported EEG findings in 13 patients with WNV: in 8, generalized slowing was more prominent anteriorly; and in 3, more prominent temporally and was not associated with epileptiform discharges (40).

DellaBadia et al. reported a case of WNV encephalitis presenting with a simple partial seizure, focal motor, resulting from an occipital epileptogenic focus. The atypical epileptogenic location of the case and the observed frequency of seizures in WN encephalitis suggest that this virus is particularly irritative to cortical neuronal networks. Thus, when seizures, especially with atypical EEG patterns, present during an acute febrile illness in the warmer months, WN encephalitis should be considered (74).

10.2.3. Brain Abscess

A brain abscess is a purulent infection of brain parenchyma. It occurs most commonly in children aged 4–7 and in the third decade in adults (30). It commonly presents with site-specific focal neurological deficits such as aphasia and weakness. A focal exam may, however, be absent, and many patients present with signs of increased intracranial pressure (ICP). General manifestations of increased ICP include headache, change in mental status, and nausea and vomiting (73). Fever is less common. Neck rigidity may be present in 25% of cases and may indicate associated meningitis (75). Seizures, often generalized tonic–clonic, can occur in up to 40% of cases (74). The route of transmission is usually contiguous spread from a local primary focus such as paranasal sinusitis, otitis media, mastoiditis or penetrating head trauma. Ten percent of the cases spread hematogenously, usually from a pulmonary source such as bronchiectasis or lung abscess, but also from heart valves (infective endocarditis) or conditions causing a right to left shunt such as cyanotic heart disease in children, and Weber-Osler Rendu syndrome and patent foramen ovale in adults (75). While a single abscess is usual with contiguous spread, multiple abscesses are seen in 20% of cases of hematogenous seeding (76). Blood cultures in the presence of an intracranial abscess are usually negative. The cause of cerebral abscesses is polymicrobial in 30–60%, and anaerobic organisms are identified in about 30% of all isolates (76). The most common infectious agents are streptococcal species, especially *Streptococcus milleri*. Other organisms include *Bacteroides* species, the Enterobacteriaceae family and *Staphylococcus aureus* (30). *Listeria monocytogenes*, mycobacterial, fungal and parasitic agents may be causative in immunosuppressed patients. Brain abscesses with *Mycobacteria* and *Nocardia* often have associated pulmonary involvement (30).

The incidence of postoperative epilepsy in 56 patients with a supratentorial abscess was 38% in one study, of which 6 (11%) had seizures before operation (77). Although the first seizure occurred in 70% during the first year, the occurrence of late seizures was not uncommon. Preoperative epilepsy was not a risk for postoperative seizures (77). Parietal lobe location of abscess had the highest incidence of epilepsy (100%). In a population-based study from Olmstead County, Minnesota, epilepsy was found in 5/18 (28%) of surviving patients with brain abscess (78).

Treatment of brain abscess requires antibiotic therapy, prophylactic anticonvulsants and often surgical intervention. Empiric antibiotic coverage with a third-generation cephalosporin and metronidazole is acceptable, but with replacement of the metronidazole with oxacillin or vancomycin for staphylococcal species or with a history of trauma or a recent neurosurgical procedure (76). *Pseudomonas aeruginosa* should be treated with ceftazidime. Oral antibiotics for up to 3 months usually follow a 4 to 8 week course of intravenous antibiotics (30). Glucocorticoid therapy is recommended if cerebral edema is significant, especially with early signs of cerebral herniation (30). Definitive therapy with surgical excision and debridement of the abscess is recommended for posterior fossa lesions. The presence of a thick fibrotic capsule and impending rupture into the ventricles (79) implies a higher risk of residual neurologic deficits with this surgical approach, making aspiration a safer procedure although repeat operations may be required, including excision. Medical therapy alone may also be a reasonable option for poor surgical risk patients, multiple small abscesses, or high suspicion for Toxoplasma infection. Treatment of seizures due to a brain abscess is not different from the treatment of seizures due to other causes. More information is available in the chapter: "Treatment of ICU Seizures and Status Epilepticus." Prophylactic treatment is controversial and no randomized studies exist. Location of the abscess (parietal lobe), extension to the cortex, concurrent meningitis or surgical treatment (craniotomy) would make us strongly consider starting the ICU patient on prophylactic antiepileptic treatment. The duration of the treatment, either after a seizure or prophylactically, is also unknown, but we would recommend treating for at least the duration of the antimicrobial treatment (usually 3–6 months).

10.2.4. Intracranial Extra-Axial Pyogenic Infections

Epidural abscesses and subdural empyemas are bacterial infections within the extra cerebral spaces. Epidural abscesses, which usually occur in the frontal region can present with headache, fever and nausea, although neurological symptoms and complications are quite rare because of the protective effect of the tight adherence of dura to overlying skull. A subdural empyema, which is most commonly situated over the cerebral convexity, can cause altered level of consciousness, focal neurologic deficits and seizures. The spread of infection through the subdural space can cause inflammation of the brain parenchyma and result in edema, elevated intracranial pressure, septic thrombophlebitis, venous infarction or mass effect (30, 80). These extra-axial infections may result as a complication of trauma, neurosurgical procedures, meningitis, sinusitis, and other extracranial sources of infection. Otorhinogenic spread occurs mostly via the valveless emissary veins, allowing superficial infections to drain into the dural sinuses causing thrombophlebitis with infection of the subdural or epidural space (30). Subdural empyemas and epidural abscesses are commonly caused by staphylococcal species. Forty percent of the cases can be polymicrobial (30). *Streptococci*, followed by staphylococcal organisms and anaerobes such as *Propionebacterium* and *Peptostreptococcus* are the most common causes (30). Seizures are uncommon with epidural abscess and relatively common with subdural empyema. In a period of 14 years, 25 patients were retrospectively identified in a Taiwanese hospital (15 with subdural empyema and 9 with epidural abscess). Seizures were found in 54% of patients; only in one patient with epidural abscess and in 12/15 (80%) patients with subdural empyema (81). The same pattern of rarity of seizures with epidural abscess and relative frequency with subdural empyema is also encountered in children (82).

A study of 89 patients with subdural empyema was conducted to assess the incidence of late seizures (83). Mortality was 24/89 (27%). The incidence of early seizures was similar in those who died (62.5%) as in those who survived (63%). All patients received anticonvulsant prophylaxis which was continued for 12 to 18 months. Early seizures were more common in cases with parana-sal sinusitis, but did not correlate with occurrence of late epilepsy. Of those patients with follow-up, 29% who had early seizures had further attacks; of patients with no early seizures, 42% developed epilepsy during the follow-up period, most within the first 2 years (83). No factors were identified which predicted the occurrence of late seizures.

Subdural empyema can be treated with intravenous antibiotic therapy, with either a third- generation cephalosporin and metronidazole, or piperacillin with tazobactam, followed by early surgical evacuation (86). A prophylactic anticonvulsant is recommended. Craniotomy is generally preferred to multiple burr holes (83). Antibiotics should be continued for 2 to 6 weeks and may be considered as the only therapy for fluid collections <1 cm in diameter with rapid clinical improvement (84).

10.2.5. Ventriculitis

Ventriculitis is a pyogenic infection of the ventricular cavity. Arbitrary criteria for diagnosis include a CSF WBC >200/mm^3, or positive culture of the ventricular fluid (85). The ventricles may act as a reservoir for persistent inflammation, which may block the CSF outflow tracts and act as a brain abscess (85). The most common infecting organisms are Staphylococcal species. Thirty percent of all meningitis may be associated with ventriculitis while over 90% of neonatal meningitis is complicated by ventriculitis. (80, 86). It should be considered in patients with meningitis who do not quickly respond to antibiot-ics. Ventriculitis is frequently associated with CSF shunts. Intracranial devices, intrathecal chemotherapy, and rupture of a periventricular abscess through the ependyma can also increase the risk for ventriculitis. The incidence of seizures in ventriculitis is not known although it is probably similar to meningitis due to the frequent co-occurrence of both conditions.

A common cause of ventriculitis is shunt placement. Seizures are more frequent after shunt placement. In an older study, 18.2% of 99 patients with ventriculitis who were not shunted developed seizures vs. 65.4% of those receiving a shunt for hydrocephalus. EEG abnormalities were also more common in the shunted group (95%) vs. the nonshunted group (47%) (87). In another study, 15.2% of children <1 year with ventricular shunts devel-oped post-shunt epilepsy, in contrast with only 6.9% of patients >50 years old (88). Most studies evaluating seizures and hydrocephalus are in children. Patients with CNS malformations and mental retardation have the highest risk of post-shunt seizures (89). A large retrospective study of both children and adults from Oregon reported an increase in incidence of epilepsy (based on long-term administration of antiepileptic drugs) from 12% before shunt insertion to 33% 10 years later. The hazard rate was 2% per year. The cause of hydrocephalus was a strong determinant of epilepsy (patients with post-hemorrhagic hydrocephalus had the highest risk and those with myelomeningocele the lowest). Interestingly, CSF shunt infection was not associated in this series with increased risk for epilepsy (90). This finding was not confirmed in a later study in children shunted for hydrocephalus: children with shunt malformation, infection or a combination of these had higher incidence of epilepsy (91). Thus, shunt-related ventriculitis may or may not increase the incidence of seizures, but the independent effect of infection compared to purely ventricular catheter or shunt placement (which is generally agreed to increase the incidence of seizures) has not been studied.

Treatment of ventriculitis requires externalization or removal and replacement of the infected intraventricular device. Vancomycin is preferred in acute gram-positive ventriculitis because of the increasing resistance patterns to beta-lactam antibiotics (92). Although Vancomycin adequately penetrates the blood–brain barrier when the meninges are inflamed, CSF drug concentrations may be compromised in the case of ventriculitis or of an improving bacterial meningitis, where the meningeal inflammatory response may be less extensive (93). CSF penetration of vancomycin may be negligible under these conditions and intraventricular instillation of antibiotic may achieve adequate concentrations and be necessary for successful eradication (94). Treatment of gram-negative ventriculitis is more controversial as most studies show no significant clinical benefit with intrathecal administration of gentamycin or amikacin (95, 96). The intrathecal or intraventricular instillation of antimicrobials may be a risk factor for seizures. One should consider prophylactic antiepileptic drug use in such cases, especially if there is cortical irritation by periventricular drain catheter hematoma.

10.2.6. HIV Infection and Seizures

New onset seizures (NOS) are not uncommon in HIV patients, occurring in 3% of patients in a prospective study and between 11 and 17% of HIV patients in retrospective studies (99, 102–106). Seizures are usually seen in the advanced stages of the disease although they may occur early or as the presenting symptom of HIV infection (107). Von Paesschen found that out of 68 selected patients with seizures 62 had acquired immunodeficiency syndrome (AIDS) and only 6 patients had AIDS-related complex or just HIV seropositivity (107). Most patients have generalized seizures, although partial seizures, both simple and complex partial, may be seen in patients with diffuse brain disease such as HIV encephalopathy or meningitis (107). The reported incidence of convulsive status epilepticus is 8 to 18% and is often associated with poor prognosis (99, 101, 102). In a study by Lee et al., 42 patients with HIV infection and status epilepticus (SE), the median duration of SE was 2.0 ± 10 h. Most patients (37 [88%]) responded to IV benzodiazepine or phenytoin treatment. Nevertheless, 12 (29%) patients died and 15 (36%) developed new neurologic deficits (97). The most common EEG finding is nonspecific diffuse slowing; focal slowing and epileptiform activity is infrequent (97, 101). The pathophysiology of generalized seizures and status in HIV-infected patients may be related to lowered threshold for cortical excitability

Table 10-1. Common Causes of Seizures in HIV-Infected Patients.

Intracranial space-occupying lesions

    CNS lymphoma

    Brain abscess [tuberculoma, cryptococcus, nocardia]

Opportunistic infection

    Cerebral toxoplasmosis

    Cryptococcal meningitis, tuberculous meningitis

    CMV encephalitis

    Cysticercosis

    Progressive multifocal leukoencephalopathy

Metabolic derangements

    End-stage renal disease

Drugs

    Foscarnet

    Perinatal exposure to nucleoside analogues (febrile seizures)

Others

    Vascular infarction

    HIV-associated dementia

and impaired inhibitory mechanisms for terminating seizures once started (106). In the majority of patients, seizures are associated with an underlying intracranial mass lesion, infection, or metabolic disturbance (Table 10-1). Intracranial mass lesions, including opportunistic infections, neoplasms, and cerebrovascular disease make up almost half of neurological disorders in AIDS patients (101). These are all commonly associated with seizures. Wong et al. (101) reported on 70/630 (11%) HIV-positive patients, who presented with NOS. Generalized seizures occurred in 94% of patients, partial in 26 % and SE in 14%. An associated space-occupying lesion (SOL) or CNS infection was found in 38 patients (54%) with the following diagnoses: cerebral toxoplasmosis (11 patients), CNS lymphoma (8 patients), metabolic derangements (8 patients), cryptococcal meningitis (7 patients), and vascular infarction (4 patients). In this series, phenytoin was associated with adverse drug reactions in 16/62 (26%) of patients who received it. In a study by Kellinghaus et al. of 831 HIV-infected patients treated, 51 (6.1%) had seizures or epilepsy. Three of the 51 patients (6%) were diagnosed with epilepsy before the onset of the HIV infection. Fourteen patients (27%) only had single or few provoked seizures in the setting of acute cerebral disorders (eight patients), drug withdrawal or sleep withdrawal (two patients), or of unknown cause (four patients). Thirty-four patients (67%) developed epilepsy in the course of their HIV infection. Toxoplasmosis (seven patients), progressive multifocal leukencephalopathy (seven patients) and other acute or subacute cerebral infections (five patients) were the most frequent causes of seizures. EEG data of 38 patients were available. EEG showed generalized and diffuse slowing only in 9 patients, regional slowing in 14 patients and regional slowing and epileptiform discharges in 1 patient. Only 14 of the patients had normal EEG. At the last contact, the majority of the patients (46 patients, 90%) were on highly active antiretroviral therapy (HAART). Twenty-seven patients (53%) were on anticonvulsant therapy (gabapentin: 14 patients, carbamazepine: 9 patients, valproate: 2 patients, phenytoin: 1 patient, lamotrigine: 1 patient) (99).

Toxoplasmosis, the most common cause of intracranial mass lesion in AIDS presents with seizures as an early manifestation in 15 to 40% (98). The incidence of diagnosing toxoplasmosis in HIV-infected patients with new-onset seizures ranges from 12 to 28% (87, 93, 95). Timely identification and treatment of toxoplasmosis with sulfadiazine and pyrimethamine is important for clinical improvement.

The second most common intracranial mass lesion producing seizures in AIDS patients is CNS lymphoma. Other focal CNS lesions include brain abscess (tuberculous, cryptococcal, nocardial), tuberculomas, syphilitic gummas, and cerebrovascular diseases. Progressive multifocal leukoencephalopathy (PML), although a white matter disease without significant mass effect, can produce seizures, either partial or generalized (108). The mechanism may involve lesions adjacent to cerebral cortex, axonal conduction abnormalities, or disturbance of neuron–glia balance (108). Meningitis and encephalitis as a cause of NOS in HIV-infected patients ranges from 12 to 16%, with cryptococcal meningitis being the most frequent meningo-encephalitis producing seizures (97, 101, 102, 106, 107). Subacute sclerosing panencephalitis has emerged in HIV-infected children in developed countries and often presents with seizures and encephalopathy (106). Other less common infectious causes of seizures in AIDS patients include aseptic meningitis, neurosyphilis, herpes zoster leukoencephalitis, and cytomegalovirus encephalitis (107).

In 6 to 46% of reported HIV patients with NOS, no identifiable cause is found, and the etiology of seizures is attributed to the HIV infection itself (100–104). In one study HIV encephalopathy was responsible for seizures in 24% of patients (97). In another series, 41% of patients had cerebral atrophy identified as the only lesion on CT scan (102). Dore found that 18% of patients with NOS and no identifiable etiology were taking foscarnet, which was postulated to be epileptogenic (107). Modi et al. (104) studied 15 HIV-infected heterosexual patients from South Africa who presented with NOS as the sole neurologic manifestation and who were taking no medications. These patients were predominantly female with a mean age of 31 years and a mean latency of 1.6 months between discovery of HIV positivity and seizure onset. They had AIDS-defining CD4+ counts in 60%, and a high prevalence of pulmonary tuberculosis, and multiple non-neurologic illnesses. Thirteen patients had generalized seizures and two presented with status epilepticus. Their EEG findings were either normal (in one third), or showed a generalized epileptic disturbance (GED) in 40% of them. Despite normal neurologic exam excluding dementia, normal CSF analysis (apart from presence of HIV), and normal CT/MRI scans of the brain, single-photon emission computed tomography (SPECT) scans of the brain showed abnormal left or right temporal lobe perfusion deficits. The restricted temporal lobe hypoperfusion may represent a focal metabolic abnormality or encephalopathy induced by the HIV virus which is postulated to manifest as seizures. SPECT scan showing multiple or focal uptake defects is also reported as very sensitive in detecting the early stages of AIDS dementia (109). Postmortem neuropathological examination of the brain in 17 patients with NOS without identifiable cause showed microglial nodules or multinucleated cells or both in 6 patients, suggesting that the HIV infection was the likely cause of the seizures (101).

The likely pathophysiology of seizures in HIV-infected patients without identifiable etiology relates to the role of HIV infection in the brain. Specifically, HIV- or immune-related toxins produced by interactions between macrophages, microglia, monocytes, and astrocytes, may injure or kill neurons (106). Neurotoxic substances, including eicosanoids, platelet-activating factor, quinolate, cysteine, cytokines, and free radicals, increase glutamate release, activate voltage-dependent calcium channels and NMDA receptor-operated channels, leading to calcium influx and neuronal death. Neurotransmitter imbalances may also predispose to seizures.

Seizures are generally a poor prognostic indicator in HIV-infected patients and will likely recur. It is therefore recommended that patients experiencing a first seizure without a reversible cause be treated. In view of potential drug–drug interactions as a result of hepatic enzyme induction, and drug–disease interactions due to reduced concentrations of protease inhibitors and therefore antiviral efficacy (110), the choice of anticonvulsant is ideally one which has no effect on viral replication, has limited protein binding, and does not have effects on the cytochrome P450 system (111). These include gabapentin, topiramate and tiagabine. Most nucleoside reverse transcriptase inhibitors are renally metabolized through glucuronidation by enzyme systems different than the cytochrome P450, thus not affecting the hepatically metabolized antiepileptic drugs. On the other hand, the non-nucleoside reverse transcriptase inhibitors (like nerivapine, delaviradine and efivanenz) use the cytochrome P450 system and may lead either to induction (efivarenz) or inhibition (nevirapine and delaviradine), affecting the antiepileptics that use these systems (Table 10-2) (112). The intensivist should also remember that the HIV-protease inhibitors are substrates for and inhibitors of the hepatic CYP3A enzyme system and can affect antiepileptic drug concentrations.

Table 10-2. Antiepileptic and HIV-Protease Inhibitor Interactions – Adapted from (82).

Antiepileptic	Protease inhibitor	Interaction
Phenytoin	RI, SA, IN, NE	Increased Phenytoin levels; decreased PI efficacy
Phenobarbital	RI, SA, IN, NE	
Valproic Acid	RI	Decreased PI efficacy
Diazepam	RI, SA, IN, NE	Decreased valproate efficacy
Clonazepam	RI, SA, IN, NE	Increased diazepam toxicity, contraindicated
Lamotrigine	RI	Increased clonazepam toxicity, substitute clonazepam
Topiramate	RI	Decreased lamotrigine efficacy
Tiagabine	RI, SA, IN, NE	? Increased topiramate toxicity
Felbamate	RI, SA, IN, NE	Increased tiagabine toxicity
Ethosuximide	RI	Decreased PI efficacy
Gabapentin	–	Increased ethosuximide toxicity, substitute or decreased dose
Vigabatrin	–	–
		–

RI, ritonavir; *SA*, saquinavir; *IN*, indinavir; *NE*, nelfinavir.

Carbamazepine, at a dose of 200 mg/day for post-zoster meralgia, reached antiepileptic therapeutic levels in an HIV patient receiving triple anti-retroviral therapy (indinavir, zidovudine and lamivudine). On the other hand, indinavir plasma concentrations decreased significantly and HIV-RNA became detectable during the period of carbamazepine treatment (113). In addition to drug–drug metabolic interactions, the intensivist should also consider hypoalbuminemia, a common situation in the ICU and in the HIV-seropositive patients. Highly protein-bound antiepileptic (phenytoin, valproic acid, carbamazepine, clonazepam, and diazepam) may displace highly protein-bound anti-retroviral drugs (delaviradine, efivanez, saquinavir vitonavir, nelfinavir,lopinavir, and ampenavir) or vice versa, leading to toxic-free concentrations of either drug (114). The HIV-induced hypergammaglobulinemia may also predispose patients to hypersensitivity reactions from antiepileptics, especially phenytoin (115).

Phenytoin remains the most widely prescribed anticonvulsant for these patients although side effects are common, including skin rashes, leucopenia, thrombocytopenia and hepatic dysfunction (101, 106). Valproic acid should be avoided if possible since it has been shown to stimulate HIV replication in vitro (111, 116, 117). However, in a retrospective study of manic HIV(+) patients who were taking divalproex sodium and anti-retrovirals, the HIV-1 viral load did not increase. One patient who was not taking anti-retrovirals had a 0.17 log viral load increase (118).

10.3. Vasculitides

Vasculitides comprise a heterogeneous group of multisystem disorders characterized by inflammation and necrosis of blood vessel walls, resulting in a variety of sequelae including aneurysms, vessel wall rupture and hemorrhage, and occlusion and infarction (119, 120). Vasculitis affecting the central nervous system is both extremely variable and challenging because of lack of specific signs and symptoms, and lack of noninvasive diagnostic tests. Vasculitis isolated to the CNS is referred to as Primary CNS angiitis; secondary vasculitis is associated with numerous conditions, including infections, lymphoproliferative disease (lymphoma), drug abuse (amphetamines), connective tissue disease and other forms of systemic vasculitis (119). In most cases, the diagnosis is made based on clinical presentation, presence of specific serum markers and biopsy of lesions. A new era in neuroimaging diagnosis is also foreseen. Goerres et al. report a patient with refractory epilepsy evaluated with [^{11} C] CR-PK11195 PET (a specific ligand for the peripheral benzodiazepine binding site, abundant on cells of mononuclear phagocytic lineage). No gadolinium enhancement was found. PET showed several areas in the occipital and temporal lobes of abnormal PK11195 binding and a biopsy confirmed chronic vasculitis (121).

10.3.1. Necrotizing Vasculitides

This group of vasculitides includes classic polyarteritis nodosa (PAN), Wegner's granulomatosis (WG), allergic angiitis and granulomatosis (Churg–Strauss – CS), necrotizing systemic vasculitis-overlap syndrome, and lymphomatoid granulomatosis (119).

10.3.1.1. Wegner's Granulomatosis

WG is a necrotizing granulomatous vasculitis involving upper and lower respiratory tracts; three quarters of patients develop glomerulonephritis. Neurologic abnormalities are common and include cranial neuropathies due to contiguous extension of granulomas from the nasopharynx, encephalopathy, seizures, pituitary abnormalities and focal motor and sensory deficits due to small vessel vasculitis (109). Peripheral neuropathies are also common. Seizures are usually a late complication.

10.3.1.2. Polyarteritis Nodosa

CNS involvement in PAN ranges from 4 to 41% and is usually a late manifestation (120). Peripheral nervous system damage is much more common (50 to 75% of cases). CNS lesions include focal lesions causing TIA, stroke (ischemic or hemorrhagic), seizures and more commonly diffuse lesions causing, multifocal neurologic findings and encephalopathy (120, 122). Generalized or partial seizures have been described in 25 to 50% of patients with CNS complications and often occur together with acute diseases such as headache, acute confusional state and focal neurologic deficits (123). Seizures in PAN do not usually require long-term management. CNS disease is usually associated with systemic features such as fevers, cutaneous involvement and renal complications (124). Elevated ESR, leukocytosis, anemia, thrombocytosis, hematuria, proteinuria and circulating immune complexes may be found. Hepatitis B antigenemia is present in up to 30% of patients, and their treatment and outcome may be different from those with idiopathic PAN (119, 124). Angiography may demonstrate vasculitis as medium-sized vessels are involved. The presence of neurologic complications does not influence survival, which is significantly increased with treatment with corticosteroids and cytotoxic agents. Recommended treatment of seizures includes anticonvulsants as adjuncts to immunosuppressive therapy.

10.3.1.3. Churg–Strauss Syndrome

CS syndrome can involve multiple organs, particularly pulmonary vessels causing asthma and pulmonary infiltrates along with eosinophilia (109). Neurologic abnormalities are similar to PAN with early encephalopathy being frequent because of small vessel involvement. The CNS was involved in 62% of 47 cases from the Mayo Clinic. In this series, no patients had seizures (125).

10.3.2. Vasculitides Associated with Connective Tissue Disease

This group of vasculitides includes systemic lupus erythematosus (SLE), rheumatoid arthritis, scleroderma, Sjogren's syndrome and mixed connective tissue disease (MCTD). Whereas CNS involvement is common in SLE and MCTD, occurring in 20 to 50% of patients, it is rare in scleroderma and rheumatoid arthritis (120).

10.3.2.1. SLE

SLE is characterized by immunologically mediated damage to multiple organs, particularly skin, kidneys and joints, secondary to generation of autoantibodies and immune complexes (119). NMDA NR2A or NR2B autoantibodies, some of which cross-react with double-stranded DNA, have been detected in 30% of SLE patients, with or without neuropsychiatric impairments. Seizures unrelated to renal failure, hypertension or medications occur in approximately 14 to 17% of patients with SLE, usually in the early phases of illness and most are nonrecurrent (124). One large series reported 6/17 patients with a single seizure, and only 3 patients who continued to have seizures after 3 months (126). Seizures are the first and only manifestation of SLE in approximately 3% of patients (124). These patients have frequent laboratory abnormalities including antinuclear antibodies (92%), LE cells (76%), and hypocomplementemia (57%) (126). The presence of seizures does not alter mortality risk. However, during the terminal phases of disease, seizures may occur with increased frequency.

Seizures commonly occur together with neuropsychiatric (NP) findings, thrombocytopenia and cutaneous signs of vasculitis (124). NP disturbances are common in SLE. They often occur in the first year of disease, but are rarely the presenting symptom (127). One study of NP findings in a large cohort of southern Chinese patients with SLE followed for 16 years reported that seizure disorder was the most common event (occurring in 28% of patients), followed by cerebrovascular disease (19%), acute confusional state (14%) and psychosis (11%) (128). Seizures were mostly generalized tonic–clonic. Serological and other clinical associations with NP syndromes in SLE patients include vasculitis, antiphospholipid antibodies and hematological complications (thrombocytopenia, leukopenia) (128, 129), higher risk of renal failure (130), and history of cyclophosphamide treatment (128).

The pathogenesis of seizures and other NP syndromes in SLE is not well understood. Antiphospholipid antibodies are more frequently found in patients with SLE and seizures than in patients with SLE without seizures. In a study of 221 unselected patients with SLE, 43.8% of patients with epilepsy had detectable lupus anticoagulant versus 20.8% of patients without ($p=0.057$). A significant association was found between moderate to high titers of IgG anti-cardiolipin antibodies and the presence of seizures ($p=0.02$) (131). One important mechanism is likely an occlusive vasculopathy, suggested by the strong association between antiphospholipid antibodies and NP symptoms (128, 129). In a prospective study of 76 Indian women with SLE, a strong association was found between seizures and anti-cardiolipin and anti-beta 2 glycoprotein I antibodies (132). Circulating anti-cardiolipin antibodies from SLE patients with seizures decreased GABA-mediated responses in snail neurons in vitro (133). Pathologic studies of SLE patients with seizures have shown cerebral microinfarcts and subarachnoid hemorrhage (134). True vasculitis is actually rare in SLE and frequent findings include hyalinization, perivascular inflammation, and endothelial proliferation (119, 134). The most common pathological finding at autopsy is a noninflammatory small vessel vasculopathy (135). In vitro and in vivo studies suggest that antiphospholipid antibodies may activate vascular endothelial cells, leading to expression of leukocyte adhesion molecules and generating a prothrombotic state on the endothelial cell surface (136, 137). Evidence of disordered immune regulation is also present in the CNS in the form of immune complexes in the cerebrospinal fluid (CSF) (138) and choroid plexus (139), elevated IgG CSF/serum index, oligoclonal CSF IgG (140) and lymphocytotoxic antibodies that cross react with brain (141). More recently, autoantibodies to glutamate receptors, specifically NMDA NR2A or NR2B autoantibodies, some of which cross-react with double-stranded DNA, have been detected in 30% of SLE patients, with or without neuropsychiatric impairments (142). Glutamate receptor autoantibodies are also found in many patients with epilepsy, and encephalitis, and may contribute to seizures and brain damage.

In patients with SLE who present with seizures, it is important to consider several neurologic conditions, including infarction (cardioembolism from Libman-Sacks endocarditis, a mural thrombus, antibody-raised homocysteine levels, carotid dissection and hypertensive small vessel disease), cerebral venous sinus thrombosis, encephalitis, and cerebral vasculitis. In patients on immunosuppressants, it is crucial to rule out infections, including intracranial abscess, and cryptococcal meningitis. Widespread vascular abnormalities on angiography should suggest a cause other than SLE for seizures due to lack of large vessel involvement by this disease (124). EEG abnormalities are frequent, but with nonspecific findings (143). One small study of brain pathology in SLE patients reported the strongest association between the presence of cerebral microinfarcts and seizures (4/5 patients) (144). Patients with SLE (as well as WG and PAN), who are being treated with cytotoxic therapy, have also been reported to develop reversible posterior leukoencephalopathy syndrome (RPLS) with resulting seizures and other typical clinical and radiological manifestations (145). The etiology of RPLS in this context is believed to be dysfunction of the vascular endothelium secondary to several factors including hypertension, renal failure with fluid retention, and cytotoxic drugs. The condition is reversible with prompt antihypertensive, anticonvulsant, and correction of fluid overload management (145).

Treatment of seizures during a disease flare depends on the frequency of attacks and etiology. Most CNS complications occur in untreated patients or those on low-dose corticosteroids (124). Single seizures occurring during disease flares may respond to corticosteroids alone, but recurrent attacks should be treated with anticonvulsants (124). The risk of worsening disease with the use of hydantoins, ethosuximide, and trimethadione, causing drug-induced SLE is rare, and should not prevent the use of appropriate anticonvulsants (124). The intensivist is frequently perplexed when a patient on antiepileptics develops a rash. Possibilities include allergic reaction, unmasking of SLE by the drug or anti-convulsant hypersensitivity syndrome. The latter is characterized by the triad of fever, rash and internal organ involvement with incidence of 1:1,000 to 1:10,000 exposures. Aromatic antiepileptics (phenytoin, phenobarbital, carbamazepine) as well as lamotrigine, valproic acid, felbamate, primidone and trimethadione have been implicated (146–148). The reaction usually develops 1 to 12 weeks after initiation of therapy and is thought to be caused by insufficient detoxification of arene oxides (metabolites of aromatic antiepileptics). Lymphadenopathy, hypothyroidism (even 2 months later) and multiorgan involvement (skin, liver, kidney, lungs, CNS) can lead to fatal complications. Cross-reactivity among aromatic antiepileptics occurs in 75% of cases. Immediate discontinuation of the drug, hydration, anti-histamines, topical and systemic corticosteroids can be used. Because of their genetic predisposition, siblings of patients may be at increased risk. Drug-induced SLE is much more frequent with distinct clinical and laboratory abnormalities. Drugs such as phenytoin, carbamazepine, ethosuximide, trimethadione, primidone and valproate have been implicated, but rarely phenobarbital and benzodiazepines (148). The clinical presentation of drug-induced SLE is frequently abrupt onset of malaise and fever but overall the disease is milder than idiopathic SLE, and renal or neurological involvement is rare with pleuropulmonary and pericardial manifestations more common. The main difference between drug-induced SLE and hypersensitivity syndrome is the presence of autoanti-bodies in the former, including anti-histone, antinuclear antibodies, that may persist for months or years after discontinuation of the drug, as opposed to the symptoms that promptly remit.

10.3.2.2. Rheumatoid Arthritis

CNS involvement causing seizures in RA is uncommon (20% of patients with CNS involvement have seizures (149)), but can include isolated CNS vasculitis, involving small and intermediate sized vessels, blood hyperviscosity, meningeal infiltration with inflammatory cells, rheumatoid nodules and plaques, and choroid plexus infiltration (150–153). One report of RA of the CNS presenting with focal seizures was caused by a focal meningeal vasculitis (153). The patient responded to etanercept, cochicine, and anticonvulsant therapy.

10.3.2.3. Scleroderma

Neuropsychiatric symptoms have been reported in 5/32 (16%) of patients with systemic sclerosis and secondary generalized or focal motor seizures were noticed among them. EEG was normal in this series and primary CNS involvement could not be confirmed (154). Simple partial motor seizures associated with fibrosis of cerebral arterioles and arteritis involving middle cerebral artery branches and vasa vasorum of the carotid artery have been reported in scleroderma patients (155). These are thought to be the result of hypertension (119).

10.3.2.4. Sjogren's Syndrome (SS)

SS characterized by xerophthalmia and xerostomia may also present with CNS involvement, either focal or diffuse in 25% of cases (120). CNS manifesta-tions include seizures as well as focal motor, sensory and language deficits, movement disorders, brain stem syndromes, encephalopathy, dementia and recurrent aseptic meningitis (120, 156). Complex partial and simple partial motor seizures have been described. Cerebral findings are associated with antineuronal antibodies, or an autoimmune inflammatory cerebral vascu-lopathy affecting predominantly small vessels, and multiple areas of increased signal intensity on T2 and proton-density-weighted MRI (120, 157). Other common findings are peripheral neuropathy, elevated ESR, cutaneous vasculitis and renal tubular acidosis (156).

10.3.2.5. Mixed Connective Tissue Disease (MCTD)

Generalized motor seizures have been reported in association with ataxia, hemiparesis, meningeal signs, and psychiatric disturbances (158). The neu-ropathology of these findings is not well understood. Intractable temporal lobe seizures have been reported in patients with ulcerative colitis. Steroid tapering and abdominal surgery led to SE (159).

10.3.3. Vasculitis Associated with Other Systemic Diseases

This group of vasculitides includes Behçet's disease, ulcerative colitis, sarcoidosis, relapsing polychondritis and Kolmeier-Degos disease.

10.3.3.1. Behçet Disease

Behçet syndrome is a multisystem inflammatory disease of unknown cause which involves the central nervous system in approximately 5% of patients (160). Criteria for diagnosis (International Study Group for Behçet's syndrome) are recurrent oral ulceration plus two from recurrent genital ulceration, eye lesions, skin lesions, or positive pathergy test (hypersensitivity of the skin to nonspecific physiological insult (161)). Neurological involvement in Behçet syndrome usually manifests as a subacute brainstem meningoencephalitis, occasionally with hemispheric or spinal cord involvement, and MRI lesions in about 75% of cases (162). Seizures are observed independently, but are an important indication of CNS involvement, or can accompany cerebral venous sinus thrombosis or may be related to interferon-A treatment (163–166). In one review of 223 patients with neurologic Behçet disease, seizures were observed in 10 (4.5%) cases (163). Seizures occurred during neurologic exacerbation in only five patients, giving a prevalence of seizures due to BD of 2.2%. In the other five patients, seizures were not related to neurologic Behçet disease attacks. The most common seizure type was generalized tonic–clonic seizures with focal motor seizures, which were controllable in most cases. Seizures were associated with abnormal CSF findings (high protein, pleocytosis) in most cases, a poor prognostic factor in neuro-BD, indicating parenchymal involvement (160). It was postulated that seizure occurrence may indicate dissemination of the inflammatory process to involve cortex. They may also be associated with cerebral hypoperfusion; in a study of seven patients with Behçet's disease evaluated by SPECT, three of them had seizures and hypoperfusion in the temporal lobe, including the mesial portion (167). The occurrence of seizures also seemed to be associated with a high mortality rate, although it remains an unusual neurologic complication for this disease. Seizures are usually controlled with monotherapy with carbamazepine or phenytoin, but phenobarbital and oxcarbazepine have also been used successfully (163). Immunosuppressive therapy with intravenous steroids, and cyclophosphamide or chlorambucil may also help to control seizures (168).

10.3.3.2. Sarcoidosis

Sarcoidosis is localized in the central nervous system in 5 to 16% of the cases. Various neurological manifestations are observed, including: seizures, cognitive or psychic manifestations, hypothalamic and pituitary involvement, local pseudotumors, and hydrocephalus very frequently associated with asymptomatic lymphocytic meningitis and with cranial nerve palsy, particularly palsy of the seventh nerve, occurring less regularly. CNS localization is most often an early manifestation of the disease, unmasking sarcoidosis. It is often part of primary or secondary systemic polyvisceral sarcoidosis (169). The diagnostic process should first confirm nervous system involvement and then provide supportive evidence for the underlying disease; in the absence of any positive tissue biopsy, the most useful diagnostic tests are gadolinium-enhanced MRI of the brain and CSF analysis, although both are nonspecific. The mainstay of treatment is corticosteroids, but these often have to be combined with other immunosuppressants such as methotrexate, hydroxychloroquine or cyclophosphamide. There is increasing evidence that infliximab is a safe treatment with good steroid-sparing capacity (170).

Case

A 54-year-old African-American man was transferred to our Neuro-ICU for status epilepticus. He had a history of neurosarcoidosis, and epilepsy. This time he was found to be in complex partial status epilepticus, with recurrent seizures every 5–10 min emanating from the right centrotemporal regions (Fig. 10-1). Brain MRI showed several scattered enhancing lesions in both hemispheres (Fig. 10-2). He received several antiepileptic medications and steroids, and was placed on barbiturate coma without success for control-

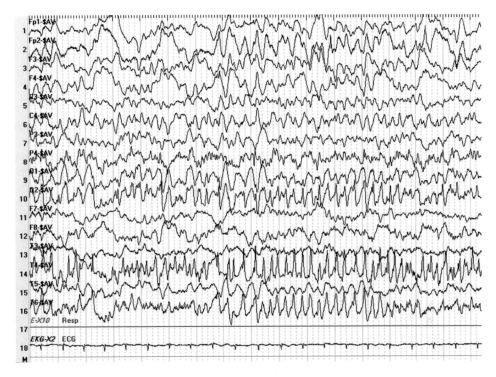

Fig. 10-1.

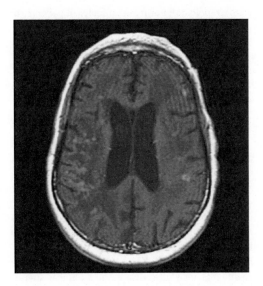

Fig. 10-2.

ling the seizures. Subsequently, intracranial electrodes were placed and 71 subclinical seizures were recorded from a right parietal epileptic focus, which was resected. His mental status improved significantly to the point that he was discharged to rehabilitation (171).

References

1. Tyler KL (2004) Herpes Simplex infections of the central nervous system: encephalitis and meningitis, including Mollaret's. Herpes 11(Suppl 2):57A–67A
2. Van De Beek D, De Gans J, Spanjaard L, Weisfelt M, Reistma JB, Vermeurlen M (2004) Clinical features and prognostic factors in bacterial meningitis. N Engl J Med 351(18):1849–1859
3. Whitley RJ, Soong SJ, Linneman C Jr, Liu C, Pazin G, Alford CA (1982) Herpes Simplex encephalitis: clinical assessment. JAMA 247(3):317–320
4. Wang KW, Chang WN, Chang HW et al (2005) The significance of seizures and other predictive factors during the acute illness for the long-term outcome after bacterial meningitis. Seizure 14(8):586–592
5. Aronin SI, Peduzzi P, Quagliarello VJ (1998) Community-acquired bacterial meningitis: risk stratification for adverse clinical outcomes and effect of antibiotic timing. Ann Intern Med 129(11):862–869
6. Bleck TP, Smith MC, Pierre-Louis SJC, Jares JJ, Murray J, Hansen C (1993) Neurologic compications of critical medical illnesses. Crit Care Med 21:98–103
7. Classen J, Mayer SA, Kowalski RG, Emerson RG, Hirsch LJ (2004) Detection of electrographic seizures with continious EEG monitoring in critically ill patients. Neurology 62(10):1743–1748
8. Claassen J, Jette N, Chum F et al (2007) Predictors and significance of electrographic seizures and periodic discharges after intracerebral hemorrhage. Neurology 69(13):1356–1365
9. Claasen J, Hirsch LJ, Frontera JA et al (2006) Prognostic significance of continious EEG monitoring in patients with poor-grade subarachnoid hemorrhage. Neuro Crit Care 4(2):103–112
10. Van De Beek D, De Gans J, Tunkel AR, Wijdicks EF (2006) Community-acquired bacterial meningitis in adults. N Engl J Med 354(1)L:44–53
11. Carrera E, Claassen J, Oddo M, Emerson RG, Mayer S, Hirsch LJ (2008) Continuous electrographic monitoring in critically ill patients with central nervous system infections. Arch Neurology 65(12):1612–1618
12. Coyle P (1999) Overview of acute and chronic meningitis. In: Marra CA (ed) Neurologic clinics: central nervous system infections, vol 17. W.B. Saunders Company, Philadelphia, pp 691–710
13. Townsend G, Shield W (1998) Infections of the central nervous system. Adv Intern Med 43:403–447
14. Rotbart H (1995) Enterviral infection of the central nervous system. Clin Infect Dis 20:971–981
15. Annegers JF, Hauser WA, Beghi E, Nicolosi A, Kurkland LT (1988) The risk of unprovoked seizures after encephalitis and meningitis. Neurology 38(9):1407–1410
16. Quagliarello VJ, Scheid WM (1997) Treatment of bacterial meningitis. N Engl J Med 336:708–716
17. Durand ML, Calderwood SB, Weber DJ, Miller SI, Southwick FS, Caviness VS, Swartz MN (1993) Acute bacterial meningitis in adults: a review of 493 episodes. N Engl J Med 328:21–28
18. Pfister HW, Feiden W, Einhaupl KM (1993) Spectrum of complications during bacterial meningitis in adults: Results of a clinical study. Arch Neurol 50:575–581
19. Zoons E, Weisfelt M, de Gans J, Spanjaard L, Koelman JH, Reitsma JB, van de Beek D (2008) Seizures in adults with bacterial meningitis. Neurology 70(22 Pt 2):2109–2115. Epub 2008 Feb 27
20. Sigurdardottir B, Bjornsson OM, Jonsdottir KE, Erlendsdottir H, Gudmundsson S (1997) Acute bacterial meningitis in adults: a 20-year overview. Arch Intern Med 157:425–430

21. Hussein AS, Shafran SD (2000) Acute bacterial meningitis in adults: a 12-year review. Medicine (Baltimore) 79(6):360–368

22. Igarashi M, Gilmartin RC, Gerald B et al (1984) Cerebral arteritis and bacterial meningitis. Arch Neurol 41:531

23. Dinubile MJ, Boom WH, Southwick FS (1990) Septic cortical thrombophlebitis. J Infect Dis 161(6):1216–1220

24. Jordan KG (1999) Continuous EEG monitoring in the neuroscience intensive care unit and emergency department. J Clin Neurophysiol 16(1):14–39

25. Graman P (1987) Mollaret's meningitis associated with acute Epstein-Barr virus mononucleosis. Arch Neurol 44:1204–1205

26. DR SJG, Barringer JR (1982) Isolation of herpes simplex virus type I in recurrent (Mollaret) meningitis. Ann Neurol 11:17–21

27. Barontini F, Ghezzi M, Marconi GP (1981) A case of benign recurrent meningitis of Mollaret. J Neurol 225(3):197–206

28. Doern GV, Brueggemann AB, Pierce G et al (1996) Antimicrobial resistance among clinical isolates of Stretococcus pneumoniae recovered from outpatients in the United States during the winter months of 1994 to 1995: results of a 30-center national surveillance study. Antimicrob Agents Chemother 40:1208

29. Ehrenstein BP, Salzberger B, Glück T (2005) New developments in the diagnosis and therapy of acute bacterial meningitis. Med Klin (Munich) 100(6):325–333

30. Armstrong WS, McGillicuddy JE (2000) Infections of the central nervous system. In: Crockard A, Hoff JT (eds) Neurosurgery: the scientific basis of clinical practice, vol. 2, 3rd edn. Blackwell Science, Oxford, pp 757–783

31. Chretien F, Belec L, Hilton DA et al (1996) Herpes simplex virus type I encephalitis in acquired immunodeficiency syndrome. Neuropathol Appl Neurobiol 22:394

32. Hamilton RL, Achim C, Grafe MR et al (1995) Herpes simpex virus brainstem encephalitis in an AIDS patient. Clin Neuropathol 14:45

33. Feki I, Marrakchi C, Ben Hmida M et al (2005) Epidemic West Nile virus encephalitis in Tunisia. Neuroepidemiology 24:1–7

34. Schmolck H, Maritz E, Kletzin I et al (2005) Neurologic, neuropsychologic, and electroencephalographic findings after European tickborne encephalitis in children. J Child Neurol 20:500–508

35. Vas GA, Cracco JB (1997) Diffuse encephalopathies. In: Daly DD, Pedley TA (eds) Current practice of clinical electroencephalography. Lippincott-Raven, Philadelphia, USA, pp 371–399

36. Westmoreland BF (1987) The EEG in cerebral inflammatory processes. In: Electroencephalography-basic principles, clinical applications and related fields. In: Niedermeyer E, Lopes da Silva E (eds) Electroencephalography: basic principles, clinical applications, and related fields. Urban & Schworzenberg, Baltimore-Munich, pp 259–273

37. Wasay M, Diaz-Arrastia R, Suss RA et al (2000) St Louis encephalitis: a review of 11 cases in a 1995 Dallas, Texas epidemic. Arch Neurol 57:114–118

38. Brenner RP, Schaul N (1990) Periodic EEG patterns: classification, clinical correlation, and pathophysiology. J Clin Neurophysiol 7:249–267

39. Klein C, Kimiagar I, Pollak L et al (2002) Neurological features of West Nile Virus infection during the 2000 outbreak in a regional hospital in Israel. J Neurol Sci 200:63–66

40. Gandelman-Marton R, Kimiagar I, Itzhaki A et al (2003) Electroencephalography findings in adult patients with West Nile virus associated meningitis and meningoencephalitis. Clin Infect Dis 37:1573–1578

41. Bagic A, Boudreau EA, Greenfield J, Sato S (2007) Electro-clinical evolution of refractory non-convulsive status epilepticus caused by West Nile virus encephalitis. Epileptic Disord 9(1):98–103

42. Marks DA, Kim J, Spencer DD, Spencer SS (1992) Characteristics of intractable seizures following meningitis and encephalitis. Neurology 42(8):1513–1518

43. Advisory Committee on Immunization Practices (1993) Inactivated Japanese encephalitis virus vaccine. Recommendations of the Advisory Committee on Immunization Practises (ACIP). MMWR Morb Mortal Wkly Rep 42(RR-1):1–15

44. Hoke CH, Nisalak A, Sangawhipa N, Jatanasen S, Laorakapongse T, Innis BL et al (1988) Protection against Japanese encephalitis by inactivated vaccines. New Engl J Med 319:608–614

45. Solomon T, Dung NM, Kneen R, Gainsborough M, Vaughn DW, Khanh VT (2000) Neurological aspects of tropical disease: Japanese encephalitis. J Neurol Neurosurg Psychiatry 68:405–415

46. Tsai TF (1997) Factors in the changing epidemiology of Japanese encephalitis and West Nile fever. In: Saluzzo JF, Dodet B (eds) Factors in the emergence of arbovirus diseases. Elseveir, Paris, pp 179–189

47. Kaiser R (1999) The clinical and epidemiological profile of tick-borne encephalitis in southern Germany 1994–98: a prospective study of 656 patients. Brain 122:2067–2078

48. Solomon T, Cardosa MJ (2000) Emerging arboviral encephalitis. Br Med J 321: 1484–1485

49. Johnson RT, Burke DS, Elwell M, Leake CJ, Nisalak A, Hoke CH et al (1985) Japanese encephalitis: immunocytochemical studies of viral antigen and inflammatory cells in fatal cases. Ann Neurol 18:567–573

50. Solomon T, Dung NM, Kneen R, Thao LTT, Gainsborough M, Nisalak A, Day NPJ, Kirkham FJ, Vaughn DW, Smith S, White NJ (2002) Seizures and raised intracranial pressure in Vietnamese patients with Japanese encephalitis. Brain 125:1084–1093

51. Minns RA, Brown JK (1978) Intracranial pressure changes associated with childhood seizures. Dev Med Child Neurol 20:561–569

52. Shorvon SD (1994) Status epilepticus: its clinical features and treatment in children and adults. Cambridge University Press, Cambridge

53. Simpson H, Habel AH, George EL (1977) Cerebrospinal fluid acid-base status and lactate and pyruvate concentrations after convulsions of varied duration and aetiology in children. Arch Dis Child 52:844–849

54. Bertram M, Schwarz S, Hacke W (1997) Acute and critical care in neurology. Eur Neurol 38:155–166

55. Osborn A (1994) Infections of the brain and its linings. Edition 1 In: Diagnostic neuroradiology. Mosby, St Louis, 673–715

56. Kennedy PGE (1988) A retrospective analysis of forty-six cases of herpes simplex encephalitis seen in Glasgow between 1962 and 1985. Q J Med 68:533–540

57. McGrath N, Anderson NE, Croxson MC, Powell KF (1997) Herpes simplex encephalitis treated with acyclovir: diagnosis and long term outcome. J Neurol Neurosurg Psych 63(3):321–326

58. Lai CW, Gragasin ME (1988) Electroencephalography in herpes simplex encephalitis. J Clin Neurophysiol 5(1):87–103

59. Jha S, Patel R, Yadav RK, Kumar V (2004) Clinical spectrum, pitfalls in diagnosis and therapeutic implications in herpes simplex encephalitis. J Assoc Physicians India 52:24–26

60. Smith JB, Westmoreland BF, Reagan TJ et al (1975) A distinctive clinical EEG profile in herpes simplex encephalitis. Mayo Clin Proc 50:469

61. Whitley RJ, Gnann JW (2002) Viral encephalitis: familiar infections and emerging pathogens. Lancet 359:507–514

62. Wijdicks E (2000) Acute encephalitis. Neurologic Catastrophes in the Emergency Department. Butterworth Heinemann, Boston, pp 195–214

63. Hokkanen L, Salonen O, Launes J (1996) Amnesia in acute herpetic and nonherpetic encephalitis. Arch Neurol 53:972

64. Launes J, Sirén J, Valanne L et al (1997) Unilateral hyperfusion in brain-perfusion SPECT predicts poor prognosis in acute encephalitis. Neurology 48:1347

65. Preiser W, Weber B, Klos G et al (1996) Unusual course of herpes simplex virus encephalitis after acyclovir therapy. Infection 24:384

66. Schlitt M, Bucher AP, Stroop WG, Pindak F, Bastian FO, Jennings RA, Lakeman AD, Whitley RJ (1988) Neurovirulence in an experimental focal herpes encephalitis: relationship to observed seizures. Brain Res 440(2):293–298

67. Jay V, Hwang P, Hoffman HJ, Becker LE, Zielenska M (1998) Intractable seizure disorder associated with chronic herpes infection. HSV1 detection in tissue by the polymerase chain reaction. Child's Nervous Syst 14(1–2):15–20

68. Pruzanski W, Altman R (1962) Encephalitis due to West Nile fever virus. World Neurol 3:524–527

69. Nash D, Mostashari F, Fine A et al (2001) West Nile Outbreak Response Working Group. The outbreak of West Nile virus infection in the New York City area in 1999. N Engl J Med 344:1807–1814

70. Chowers MY, Lang R, Nassar F et al (2001) Clinical characteristics of the West Nile fever outbreak, Israel, 2000. Emerg Infect Dis 7:675–678

71. Berner YN, Lang R, Chowers MY (2002) Outcome of West Nile fever in older adults. J Am Geriatr Soc 50:1844–1846

72. Petersen LR, Marfin AA (2002) West Nile virus: a primer for the clinician. Ann Intern Med 137:173–179

73. Sagher O, Hoff J (1997) Surgical management of CNS infections. In: Scheld WM, Whitley R, Durack DT (eds) Infections of the central nervous system, 2nd ed. Lippincott-Raven, Philadelphia, pp 945–972

74. DellaBadia J Jr, Jaffe SL, Singh J, Minagar A (2004) An occipital lobe epileptogenic focus in a patient with West Nile encephalitis. Eur J Neurol 11(2):111–113

75. Roos KL, Tunkel AR, Scheld WM (1997) Acute bacterial meningitis in children and adults. In: Scheld WM, Whitley R, Durack DT (eds) Infections of the central nervous system, 2nd ed. Lippincott-Raven Publishers, Philadelphia, pp 335–402

76. Wijdicks E (2000) Acute bacterial infections of the central nervous system. Neurologic Catastrophes in the Emergency Department. Butterworth Heinemann, Boston, pp 183–194

77. Calliauw L, de Praetere P, Verbeke L (1984) Postoperative epilepsy in subdural suppurations. Acta Neurochirurgica 71:217–223

78. Nicolosi A, Hauser WA, Musicco M, Kurland LT (1991) Incidence and prognosis of brain abscess in a defined population: Olmstead County, Minnesota, 1935–1981. Neuroepidemiology 10(3):122–131

79. Zeidman SM, Geisler FH, Olivi A (1995) Intraventricular rupture of a purulent brain abscess: case report. Neurosurgery 36:189

80. Zimmerman RA, Girard NJ (1997) Imaging of Intracranial Infections. In: Scheld WM, Whitley RJ, Durack DT (eds) Infections of the central nervous system, 2nd ed. Lippincott-Raven, Philadelphia, pp 923–944

81. Tsai YD, Chang WN, Shen CC, Lin YC, Lu CH, Liliang PC, Su TM, Ra CS, Lu K, Liang CL (2003) Intracranial suppuration: a clinical comparison of subdural empyemas and epidural abscesses. Surg Neurol 59(3):191–196

82. Smith HP, Hendrick EB (1983) Subdural empyema and epidural abscess in children. J Neurosurg 58(3):392–397

83. Bok AP, Peter JC (1993) Subdural empyema: burr holes or craniotomy? A retrospective computerized tomography-era analysis of treatment in 90 cases. J Neurosurg 78:574

84. Mauser HW, Ravijst R, Elderson A et al (1985) Nonsurgical treatment of subdural empyema. Case report. J Neurosurg 63:128

85. Salmon J (1972) Ventriculitis complicating meningitis. Amer J Dis Child 124:35–40

86. Barkovich A (1990) Infections of the nervous system. In: Barkovich AJ (ed) Pediatric neuroimaging. Raven Press, New York, pp 293–325

87. Ines DF, Marlkand ON (1977) Epileptic seizures and abnormal electroencephalographic findings in hydrocephalus and their relation to the shunting procedures. Electroencephalog Clin Neurophysiol 42(6):761–768

88. Dan NG, Wade MJ (1986) The incidence of epilepsy after ventricular shunting procedures. J Neurosurg 65(1):19–21
89. Sato O, Yamaguchi T, Kittaka M, Toyama H (2001) Hydrocephalus and epilepsy. Childs Nervous Syst 17(1–2):76–86
90. Piatt JH, Carlson CV (1995) Hydrocephalus and epilepsy: an actuarial analysis. Neurosurgery 39(4):722–728
91. Bourgeois M, Sainte-Rose C, Cinalli G, Maixner W, Malucci C, Zerah M, Pierre-Kahn A, Renier D, Hoppe-Hirsch E, Aicardi J (1999) Epilepsy in children with shunted hydrocephalus. J Neurosurg 90(2):274–281
92. Wilhelm M (1991) Vancomycin. Mayo Clin Proc 66:1165–1170
93. Redfield DC, Underman A, Norman D, Overturf GD (1980) Cerebrospinal fluid penetration of vancomycin in bacterial meningitis. In: Nelson JD, Geraci C (eds) Current chemotherapy and infectious disease. Proceedings of the International Congress of Chemotherapy and the 19th Interscience Conference on Antimicrobial Agents and Chemotherapy, vol 1. American Society for Microbiology, Washington, DC, pp 638–640
94. Luer MS, Hatton J (1993) Vancomycin administration into the cerebrospinal fluid: A review. Ann Pharmacther 27:912–921
95. BA GDJ, Kelly DL, Pegram S (1986) Gram-negative bacillary meningitis in the adult: review of 39 cases. Southern Med J 79:1499–1502
96. McCracken GH, Mize SG, Threlkeld N (1980) Intraventricular gentamycin therapy in gram-negative bacillary meningitis of infancy. Lancet 1:787–791
97. Holtzman DM, Kaku DA, So YT (1989) NOS associated with HIV infection: causation and clinical features in 100 cases. Am J Med 87:173–177
98. Lee KC, Garcia PA, Alldredge BK (2005) Clinical features of status epilepticus in patients with HIV infection. Neurology 65(2):314–316
99. Kellinghaus C, Engbring C, Kovac S, Möddel G, Boesebeck F, Fischera M, Anneken K, Klönne K, Reichelt D, Evers S, Husstedt IW (2008) Frequency of seizures and epilepsy in neurological HIV-infected patients. Seizure 17(1):27–33. Epub 2007 Jul 6
100. Aronow HA, Feraru ER, Lipton RB (1989) New-onset seizures in AIDS patients: etiology, prognosis, and treatment. Neurology 39:428(Suppl)
101. Wong MC, Suite NDA, Douglas RL (1990) Seizures in human immunodeficiency virus infection. Arch Neurol 47:640–642
102. Van Paesschen, Pesola GR, Westfal RE (1998) New-onset generalized seizures in patients with AIDS presenting to an emergency department. Acad Emerg Med 5(9):905–911
103. Pascual-Sedano B, Iranzo A, Marti-Fabregas J et al (1999) Prospective study of new-onset seizures in patients with immunodeficiency virus infection. Arch Neurol 56:609–612
104. Modi G, Modi M, Martinus J, Saffer D (2000) New onset seizures associated with human immunodeficiency virus infection. Neurology 55(10): 1558–1561
105. Van Paesschen W, Bodian C, Maker H (1995) Metabolic abnormalities and new onset seizures in human immunodeficiency virus – seropositive patients. Epilepsia 36:146–150
106. Garg RK (1999) HIV infection and seizures. Postgrad Med J 75:387–390
107. Dore GJ, Law MG, Brew BJ (1996) Prospective analysis of seizures occurring in human immunodeficiency virus type-1 infection. J Neuro AIDS 1:59–69
108. Moulignier A, Mikol J, Pialoux G, Fenelon G, Gray F, Thiebaut JB (1995) AIDS-associated progressive multifocal leukoencephalopathy revealed by new-onset seizures. Am J Med 99:64–68
109. Ajmani A, Habte-Gabr E, Zarr M, Jayabalan V, Dandala S (1991) Cerebral blood flow SPECT with Tc-99m exametamine correlates in AIDS dementia complex stages. A preliminary report. Clin Nucl Med 16(19):656–659

110. Barry M, Gibbons S, Back D, Mulcahy F (1997) Protease inhibitors in patients with HIV disease. Clinically important pharmacokinetic considerations. Clin Pharmacokinet 32:194–209

111. Romanelli F, Ryan M (2002) Seizures in HIV-seropositive individuals: epidemiology and treatment. CNS Drugs 16(2):91–98

112. Romanelli F, Pomeroy C (2003) Concurrent use of antiretrovirals and anticonvulsants in human immunodeficiency virus (HIV) seropositive patients. Curr Pharm Des 9(18):1433–1439

113. Hugen PW, Burger DM, Brinkman K, ter Hofstede HJ, Schuurman R, Koopmans PP, Hekster YA (2000) Carbamazepine-indinavir interaction causes antiretroviral therapy failure. Ann Pharmacotherapy 34(4):465–470

114. Toler SM, Wilkerson MA, Porter WH, Smith AJ, Chandler MH (1990) Severe phenytoin intoxication as a result of altered protein binding in AIDS. DICP 24(7–8):698–700

115. Romanelli F, Jennings HR, Nath A, Ryan M, Berger J (2000) Therapeutic dilemma: the use of anticonvulsants in HIV-positive individuals. Neurology 54(7): 1404–1407

116. Moog C, Kuntz-Simon G, Caussin-Schwemling C, Obert G (1996) Sodium valproate, an anticonvulsant drug, stimulates human immunodeficiency virus type 1 replication independently of glutathione levels. J Gen Virol 77(Pt 9): 1993–1999

117. Jennings HR, Romanelli F (2000) Comment: risk of drug-disease and disease-drug interactions with anticonvulsants in HIV-positive patients. Ann Pharmacotherapy 33(12):1373–13749

118. Maggi JD, Halman MH (2001) The effect of divalproex sodium on viral load: a retrospective review of HIV-positive patients with manic syndromes. Can J Psychiatry 46(4):359–362

119. Fieschi C, Rasura M, Anzini A, Beccia M (1998) Central nervous system vasculitis. J Neurol Sci 153:159–171

120. Ferro JM (1998) Vasculitis of the central nervous system. J Neurol 245:766–776

121. Goerres GW, Revesz T, Duncan J, Banati RB (2001) Imaging cerebral vasculitis in refractory epilepsy using [^{11} C](R)-PK11195 Positron emission tomography. AJR 176:1016–1018

122. Coblyn JS, McCluskey RT (2003) Case records of the Massachusetts General Hospital. Weekly clinicopathological exercises. Case 3-2003. A 36-year-old man with renal failure, hypertension, and neurologic abnormalities. New England J Med 348(4):333–342

123. Moore PM, Fauci AS (1981) Neurologic manifestations of systemic vasculitis. Am J Med 71:517–524

124. Messing RO, Simon RP (1986) Seizures as a manifestation of systemic disease. Neurol Clin 4(3):563–584

125. Sehgal M, Swanson JW, Deremee RA, Colby TV (1995) Neurologic manifestations of Churg-Strauss syndrome. Mayo Clinic Proc 70(4):337–341

126. Feinglass EJ, Arnett FC, Dorsch CA, Zizic TM, Stevens MB (1976) Neuropsychiatric manifestations of systemic lupus erythematosus: diagnosis, clinical spectrum, and relationship to other features of the disease. Medicine (Baltimore) 55:323–339

127. Van Dam AP (1991) Diagnosis and pathogenesis of CNS lupus. Rheumatol Int 11(1):1–11

128. Mok CC, Lau CS, Wong RW (2001) Neuropsychiatric manifestations and their clinical associations in southern Chinese patients with systemic lupus erythematosus. J Rheumatol 28(4):766–771

129. Karassa FB, Ioannidis JPA, Touloumi G, Boki KA, Moutsopoulos HM (2000) Risk factors for central nervous system involvement in systemic lupus erythematosus. Q J Med 93:169–174

130. Gibson T, Myers AR (1975) Nervous system involvement in systemic lupus erythematosus. Ann Rheum Dis 35:398–406

131. Herranz MT, Rivier G, Khamashta MA, Blaser KU, Hughes GR (1994) Association between antiphospholipid antibodies and epilepsy in patients with systemic lupus erythematosus. Arthritis Rheum 37(4):568–571

132. Shrivastava A, Dwivedi S, Aggarwal A, Misra R (2001) Anti-cardiolipin and anti-beta2 glycoprotein I antibodies in Indian patients with systemic lupus erythematosus: association with the presence of seizures. Lupus 10(1):45–50

133. Liou HH, Wang CR, Chou HC, Arvanov VL, Chen RC, Chang YC, Chuang CY, Chen CY, Tsai MC (1994) Anticardiolipin antisera from lupus patients with seizures reduce a GABA receptor-mediated chloride current in snail neurons. Life Sci 54(15):1119–1125

134. Ellis SG, Verity MA (1979) Central nervous system involvement in systemic lupus erythematosis: a review of neuropathologic findings in 57 cases, 1955–1977. Semin Arthritis Rheum 8:212–221

135. West SG (1994) Neuropsychiatric lupus. Rheum Dis Clin North Am 20:129–158

136. Simantov R, Lo SK, Gharavi A, Sammaritano LR, Salmon JE, Silverstein RL (1996) Antiphospholipid antibodies activate vascular endothelial cells. Lupus 5:440–441

137. Pierangeli SS, Colden-Stanfield M, Liu X, Barker JH, Anderson Gl, Harris EN (1999) Antiphospholipid antibodies from antiphospholipid syndrome patients activate endothelial cells in vitro and in vivo. Circulation 99:1997–2002

138. Seibold JR, Buckingham RB, Medsger TA et al (1982) Cerebrospinal fluid immune complexes in systemic lupus erythematosis involving the central nervous system. Semin Arthritis Rheum 12:68–76

139. Atkins CJ, Kondon JJ, Quismorio FP et al (1972) The choroid plexus in systemic lupus erythematosis. Ann Intern Med 76:65–72

140. Winfield JB, Shaw M, Silverman LM et al (1983) Intrathecal IgG synthesis and blood brain barrier impairment in patients with systemic lupus erythematosus and central nervous system dysfunction. Am J Med 74:837–844

141. Bluestein HG, Zvaifler NJ (1976) Brain-reactive lymphocytotoxic antibodies in the serum of patients with systemic lupus erythematosus. J Clin Invest 57:509–516

142. Levite M, Ganor Y (2008) Autoantibodies to glutamate receptors can damage the brain in epilepsy, systemic lupus erythematosus and encephalitis. Expert Rev Neurother 8(7):1141–1160

143. Cohen SB, Hurd ER (1981) Neurological complications of connective tissue and other "collagen-vascular" diseases. Semin Arthritis Rheum 11:190–212

144. Hanly JG, Walsh NM, Sangalang V (1992) Brain pathology in systemic lupus erythematosus. J Rheumatol 19(5):732–741

145. Primavera A, Audenino D, Mavilio N, Cocito L (2001) Reversible posterior leucoencephalopathy syndrome in systemic lupus and vasculitis. Ann Rheum Dis 60:534–537

146. Bessmertny O, Pham T (2002) Antiepileptic hypersensitivity syndrome: clinicians beware and be aware. Curr Allergy Asthma Rep 2(1):34–39

147. Vittorio CC, Muglia JJ (1995) Anticonvulsant hypersensitivity syndrome. Arch Int Med 155(21):2285–2290

148. Drory VE, Korczyn AD (1993) Hypersensitivity vasculitis and systemic lupus erythematosus induced by anticonvulsants. Clin Neuropharmacol 16(1):19–29

149. Beck DO, Corbett JJ (1983) Seizures due to central nervous system rheumatoid meningo-vasculitis. Neurology 33:1058–1061

150. Jan JE, Hill RH, Low MD (1972) Cerebral complications in juvenile rheumatoid arthritis. Can Med Assoc J 107:623–625

151. Makela A, Heikki L, Sillanpaa M (1979) Neurological manifestations of rheumatoid arthritis. In: Vinken PJ, Bruyen GW (eds) Handbook of clinical neurology, vol 38. Elsevier North Holland, Amsterdam, pp 479–503

152. Mandybur TI (1979) Cerebral amyloid angiopathy: possible relationship to rheumatoid vasculitis. Neurology 29:1336–1340

153. Neamtu L, Belmont M, Miller DC, Leroux P, Weinberg H, Zagzag D (2001) Rheumatoid disease of the CNS with meningeal vasculitis presenting with a seizure. Neurology 56:814–815

154. Hietaharju A, Jaaskelainen S, Hietarinta M, Frey H (1993) Central nervous system involvement and psychiatric manifestations in systemic sclerosis (scleroderma): clinical and neurophysiological evaluation. Acta Neurol Scand 87:382–387

155. Estey E, Lieberman A, Pinto R et al (1979) Cerebral arteritis in scleroderma. Stroke 10:595–597

156. Alexander E (1992) Central nervous system disease in Sjogren's syndrome. Rheum Dis Clin North Am 18:637–672

157. Spezialetti R, Bluestein HG, Peter JB, Alexander EL (1993) Neuropsychiatric disease in Sjogren's syndrome: anti-ribosomal P and anti-neuronal antibodies. Am J Med 95:153–160

158. Bennett RM, Bong DM, Spargo BH (1978) Neuropsychiatric problems in mixed connective tissue disease. Am J Med 65:955–962

159. Akhan G, Andermann F, Gotman MJ (2002) Ulcerative colitis, status epilepticus and intractable temporal seizures. Epileptic Disord 4(2):135–137

160. Akman-Demir G, Serdaroglu P, Tasci B et al (1999) Clinical patterns of neurological involvement in Behçet disease: evaluation of 200 patients. Brain 122:2171–2182

161. International Study Group for Behçet's Disease (1990) Criteria for diagnosis of Behçet's disease. Lancet 335:1078–1080

162. Kidd D, Steuer A, Denman AM et al (1999) Neurological complications in Behçet's syndrome. Brain 122:2183–2194

163. Aykutlu E, Baykan B, Serdaroglu P, Gokyigit A, Akman-Demir G (2002) Epileptic seizures in Behçet Disease. Epilepsia 43(8):832–835

164. Duran E, Chacon JR (2001) Behçet's disease with atypical double neurological involvement. Rev Neurol 33(4):333–334

165. El Bahri Ben Mvad et al (2002) Central venous thrombosis and Bechet's disease. Tunis Med 80(2):87–89

166. O'Duffy JD, Calamia K, Cohen S, Goronzy JJ, Herman D, Jorizzo J, Weyand C, Matteson E (1998) Interferon-alpha treatment of Behçet's disease. J Rheumatol 25(10):1938–1944

167. Vignola S, Nobili F, Picco P, Gattorno M, Buoncompagni A, Vitali P, Mariani G, Rodriguez G (2001) Brain perfusion spect in juvenile neuro-Behçet's disease. J Nucl Med 42(8):1151–1157

168. Mead S, Kidd D, Good C, Plant G (2000) Behçet's syndrome may present with seizures. J Neurol Neurosurg Psych 68(3):392–393

169. Valeyre D, Chapelon-Abric C, Belin C, Dumas JL (1998) Sarcoidosis of the central nervous system. Rev Med Interne 19(6):409–414

170. Joseph FG, Scolding NJ (2007) Sarcoidosis of the nervous system. Pract Neurol 7(4):234–244

171. Varelas PN (2008) How I treat status epilepticus in the Neuro-ICU. Neurocrit Care 9(1):153–157

Chapter 11

Electrolyte Disturbances and Critical Care Seizures

Jenice Robinson and Jose I. Suarez

Abstract Electrolyte disturbances in the ICU are extremely common. The electrolyte disorder most commonly associated with seizure is hyponatremia, although extremely low Mg^{2+}, phosphate, and both very low and high Ca^{2+} values can cause seizures. Critical care physicians must be vigilant to suspect and identify electrolyte disturbances in their patients, because a growing amount of information suggests that they are a marker and potentially a cause of poor prognosis. Electrolyte disturbances should never be uncritically accepted as the etiology of a seizure until a thorough investigation has been undertaken.

Keywords Electrolyte imbalance, Seizure, Hyponatremia, Hypernatremia, Hypocalcemia, Hypercalcemia, Hypophosphatemia, Hypoglycemia

11.1. Introduction

Electrolyte imbalances are very common in the intensive care unit (ICU). As will be reviewed, in some cases electrolyte disturbances may be associated with increased mortality in ICU patients. In patients with neurologic and neurosurgical disease, the added potential for disruption of the blood–brain barrier (BBB) exists and mechanisms for electrolyte homeostasis may break down.

As common as electrolyte disturbances are, they are still a relatively uncommon cause of seizure. A thorough search should be undertaken to identify other seizure etiologies prior to ascribing a seizure entirely to an electrolyte disturbance. As will be discussed further, both the seizure and the electrolyte disturbance may result from the same underlying cause; for example, encephalitis may cause both hyponatremia and seizure. A complete discussion of ion regulation in the brain and the pathogenesis of electrolyte-induced seizures is beyond the scope of this chapter, and has been covered well in recent reviews (1). We will review some major concepts in seizure pathogenesis and electrolytes.

From: *Seizures in Critical Care: A Guide to Diagnosis and Therapeutics*: Current Clinical Neurology, Second Edition, Edited by: P. Varelas, DOI 10.1007/978-1-60327-532-3_11,
© Humana Press, a part of Springer Science+Business Media, LLC 2005, 2010

11.2. Mechanisms for Ion Regulation and Effects of Concentration Changes

Ion concentrations in the cerebrospinal fluid (CSF) and the interstitial fluid of the brain differ from their concentrations in plasma: potassium (K^+), calcium (Ca^{2+}) and bicarbonate (HCO_3^-) concentrations are lower than in plasma, whereas magnesium (Mg^{2+}), sodium (Na^+), chloride (Cl^-) and hydrogen (H^+) concentrations are higher (1). The gradient between the brain and the plasma is maintained by active transport processes. The endothelial cells that form the BBB have a $3Na^+$ (sodium)/$2K^+$ ATP-ase pump that transports K^+ out of the brain against its gradient. Disease states that disrupt the BBB can cause failure of active transport mechanisms if the disruption is severe. We will briefly review the effects of changes on K^+ concentration, acid–base status, and osmolality on neuronal excitability.

11.2.1. Potassium

Raising the concentration of extracellular K^+ depolarizes the neuronal membrane. If the increase is mild, the membrane potential moves closer to firing threshold and the effect on transmission is excitatory. As the concentration of extracellular K^+ continues to rise, however, there is partial inactivation of Na^+ and Ca^{2+} currents in the presynaptic axon, leading to reduced action potential amplitude and decreased excitability, so that firing threshold forms a U-shaped curve with increasing K^+ concentrations. At the normal physiologic level of 2.7–3.5 mM, the low K^+ level provides a brake on neuronal excitation. Many in vitro experiments using slices of rat hippocampal cortex and baths containing various concentrations of K^+ have demonstrated this effect. When K^+ concentration is raised to 5.0–6.25 mM, synaptic transmission is increased; at higher levels synaptic transmission eventually becomes depressed. On the other hand, CA3 neurons in the hippocampus become spontaneously active once K^+ concentrations reach a level of 6.5–7 mM. If the concentration continues to increase, spreading depression occurs. The ongoing discussion of mechanisms involved in spreading depression has recently been reviewed (2).

11.2.2. Acid–Base Status

Alkalosis increases the excitability of the cortex, while acidosis decreases excitability (1). Clinically, severe alkalosis can induce tetany that resembles tetany seen with hypocalcemia. While this was once thought to occur because of an increase in the bound fraction of Ca^{2+}, the actual decrease in H^+ ion seems to be the major mechanism. H^+ inhibits voltage-gated channels, but in most brain tissue increased H^+ concentration inhibits Ca^{2+} channels and Na^+ channels greater than K^+ channels. Alkalosis (decreased H^+ concentration) therefore increases the inward Ca^{2+} and Na^+ currents more than it increases the outward K^+ current. The increased Ca^{2+} current results in increased neurotransmitter release and increased synaptic transmission.

An important factor to consider in management of acid–base disturbances is that carbon dioxide (CO_2) passes freely across the BBB, while H^+ does not; therefore, if an acute metabolic acidosis with increased H^+ results in respiratory compensation with a lowered partial arterial pressure of CO_2 (Pa CO_2), the brain may "see" just the lowered Pa CO_2 and a central alkalosis results. Patients with acute metabolic acidosis may have an increase in their central acidosis when treated with bicarbonate solutions by similar mechanisms.

11.2.3. Osmotic Effects

Even though little is known about the regulation of water transport across the BBB, it appears that water moves easily across this barrier. Ions do not move freely and need to be passed through channels in the capillary endothelium membrane, as discussed above. (1) When osmolality of plasma acutely drops compared with the osmolality of cerebral interstitial fluid (as in water intoxication), then water will move into the brain and cell and brain volumes increase. Compensatory mechanisms are significantly effective at restoring cell and brain volumes within 48 h.

An acute increase in plasma osmolality draws water from the brain, principally from the CSF and the interstitial fluid compartments. The most usual reason for large changes in plasma osmolality are changes in Na^+ concentration or addition of other osmolar substances such as keto acids in diabetic ketoacidosis. The issues involved in the treatment of hypo- and hypernatremia will be discussed in the next section.

Osmotic stresses have direct effects on synaptic transmission. In rat cortical slices, synaptic transmission is enhanced by lowering osmolality of the surrounding bath (3). Increasing osmolality decreases synaptic transmission. A decrease in the osmolality of the bathing fluid results in increased inward Ca^{2+} currents in the presynaptic neuron (4). This mechanism may explain the observed changes in synaptic transmission. For reasons that are not understood, if the osmolality of the fluid bath is kept equivalent with mannitol while the Na^+ is decreased, an increase in Ca^{2+} currents still occurs (4).

The physiology of Mg^{2+}, Ca^{2+} and phosphorus, and their effects on neuronal excitability, will be reviewed later.

11.3. Sodium Imbalance

11.3.1. Hyponatremia

Hyponatremia is a frequent and under-recognized cause of encephalopathy and seizures in the ICU. In one series of 55 patients from the Mayo Clinic with new-onset seizures in the medical and surgical ICUs, hyponatremia of <125 mEq/L was present in 18.2% of the patients (5). Seizures associated with hyponatremia are treated in a similar way to other seizures, but with the added need to determine and correct the source of the hyponatremia. The differential diagnosis of hyponatremia is broad, and a complete discussion is beyond the scope of this chapter (see Tables 11-1 and 11-2). The essential distinction that must be made is whether the hyponatremia is acute or chronic. This will determine the risk of cerebral edema, as well as how fast sodium may safely be corrected. Either acute or chronic hyponatremia can cause seizures, although seizures occur most often in the acute setting. Hyponatremia is considered acute if it develops over less than 48 h, since brain adaptation to reduced osmolarity occurs rapidly (6). Seizures, encephalopathy and other major neurologic manifestations can occur with even mild hyponatremia if

Table 11-1. Etiology of Hyponatremia in Patients with Low Plasma Osmolality.

Altered renal excretion of water

1. Decreased extracellular volume

Renal sodium loss: diuretics, adrenal insufficiency, SAH

Extra-renal sodium loss: diarrhea, vomiting, fluid sequestration ("third spacing")

2. Normal extracellular volume

SIADH, hypothyroidism, adrenal insufficiency, neoplasms, drugs, postoperative
  state, pain, acute respiratory failure, SAH, ischemic stroke, TBI

3. Increased extracellular volume

CHF, cirrhosis, renal failure

Excessive water intake

Psychogenic polydipsia

Hypo-osmolar irrigant solutions (such as those used during transurethral resection of
  the prostate)

SIADH syndrome of inappropriate secretion of ADH; *ADH* antidiuretic hormone; *SAH* subarachnoid
hemorrhage; *TBI* traumatic brain injury; *CHF* congestive heart failure.

Table 11-2. Drugs and Other Substances Reported to Cause Hyponatremia
(Drugs in Italics Reported to Cause Seizures) (Ref. 34–37, 86–101).

SIADH induction

Thiazides

Furosemide

Cyclophosphamide

Vincristine

Cisplatin

Barbiturates

Morphine

Clofibrate

Lisinopril

"Ecstasy" (3,4-methylenedioxymethamphetamine)

Carbamazepine

Oxcarbazepine

Lamotrigine

Tricyclic antidepressants

Serotonin-reuptake inhibitors (fluoxetine, sertraline)

Trazodone

Direct ADH-like effect

Desmopressin

Oxytocin

Increased Sensitivity to ADH

Chloropropamide

Tolbutamide

Indomethacin

Mechanism uncertain

(continued)

Table 11-2. (continued)

Neuroleptic drugs

Monoamine oxidase inhibitors

Hyperglycinemia following transurethral prostate resection

Laxatives containing polyethylene glycol

Visicol use during colonoscopy

ADH antidiuretic hormone; *SIADH* syndrome of inappropriate secretion of ADH.

the onset is rapid. Seizures may have focal or generalized onset. Reported electroencephalography (EEG) findings in hyponatremia are nonspecific, and frequently no changes are seen (7).

Acute, severe hyponatremia is associated with significant rate of death or morbidity because of cerebral edema if left untreated and should be rapidly corrected. Animal experiments have shown that following induced hyponatremia there is an initial phase of rapid ion transfers out of the cell (K^+, Na^+, Cl^- [chloride]), followed by a slow phase during which the intracellular concentrations of organic osmolytes decrease. Until the slow phase is complete, cellular edema exists. The mechanism by which hyponatremia produces seizures appears to have several components: low osmolarity and decreased Na^+ concentration have both been shown in vitro to increase neuronal excitability (4, 8). Additionally, if the onset of hyponatremia is acute, then cell and brain swelling can cause decreased cerebral perfusion pressure.

Clinically, acute hyponatremia poses the greatest danger when the rate of serum Na^+ decrease is greater than 0.5 mEq/L/h with a serum Na^+ concentration of less than 120 mEq/L (9). Some recommend that in the setting of acute, symptomatic hyponatremia serum Na^+ can be corrected using 3% saline solution as rapidly as 2.4 mEq/L/h until the range of mild hyponatremia is reached, when correction should be stopped for 24 h (10, 11). Other authors feel that this rapid correction represents an unnecessary risk, and recommend initial correction at a rate of 1–2 mEq/L/h to be stopped as soon as neurologic symptoms improve (12). Particularly if the exact duration of the hyponatremia is in doubt, caution should be used.

Patients with chronic hyponatremia frequently have mild symptoms and the urgency of correction is less. One series of hyponatremic patients from New York City (USA) and Oxford (UK) with serum Na^+ levels <120 mEq/L found that 76% had associated confusion, 6% had long tract signs, while only 3.3% developed seizures (13). Correction of chronic hyponatremia is generally recommended to be at the rate of less than 10 mEq/L/24 h to avoid central pontine myelinolysis (CPM), a deservedly famous complication of rapid Na^+ correction. Post-correction seizures can also occur, as in the aforementioned study, where the incidence was 1% (13). Even with slow correction, however, CPM has been reported to occur and patients with coexisting thiamine deficiency and multiple electrolyte abnormalities may be at increased risk (14). Liver failure and hypokalemia also are associated risk factors for CPM. A recent report suggests that uremia may protect against CPM, perhaps by resisting the movement of water out of the brain (15). The pathogenesis of CPM is still under investigation. An animal model of CPM has shown magnetic resonance imaging evidence of BBB disruption and complement deposition following rapid Na^+ sodium correction (16).

The exact rate of correction that can be tolerated by a patient with chronic hyponatremia is the subject of debate. Sterns et al. and other investigators reported patients who developed CPM following corrections of serum sodium of >0.5 mEq/L/h (17, 18). This number has become the accepted rate limit for safe correction, although critics have pointed out that many of the patients reported had multiple risk factors for CPM. Animal data show that in rats with chronic hyponatremia of <120 mEq/L lesions appear when the change in serum Na^+ is greater than 25mEq/L/24 h. The first lesions are noted at the level of 14–16 mEq/L/24 h (19). While this is animal data, it is supportive of the clinical observations in humans. From the same data, a high initial rate of correction was tolerated without resulting CPM as long as the total daily limit of Na^+ correction was respected.

Recently, a patient was reported who tolerated rapid reinduction of hyponatremia with hypotonic saline following a rise in serum Na^+ by 21 mEq/L over 24 h. The patient had neurologic deterioration subsequent to the overly rapid correction which improved when she was given hypotonic saline (20). The authors of this report previously published animal data suggesting that a window of 2–4 h exists following the onset of neurologic symptoms before irreversible CPM occurs, and a rescue therapy of hypotonic saline can be given during this window (21).

Other treatment modalities for hyponatremia have been explored. For instance, vasopressin (ADH) antagonists are currently in stages of clinical testing for hyponatremia involving the syndrome of inappropriate secretion of ADH (SIADH) (10). A suggested treatment algorithm for hyponatremia is shown in Fig. 11-1.

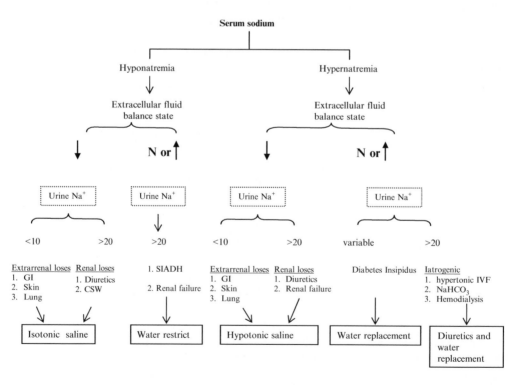

Fig. 11-1. Algorithm for the treatment of sodium imbalance. *CSW* cerebral salt wasting syndrome. Reprinted from: Diaz JL, Granados M, Suarez JI (2004) Management of medical complications in the Neurosciences Critical Care Unit. In: Suarez JI (ed) Critical care neurology and neurosurgery. Humana Press, Totowa, NJ

11.3.1.1. Acute Hyponatremia in the ICU

Common ICU settings for acute hyponatremia to occur include: the postoperative state, SIADH secondary to medications or other substances (see Table 11-2); SIADH or cerebral salt wasting from intracerebral processes such as meningitis, encephalitis, and subarachnoid hemorrhage (SAH); adrenal insufficiency; and potomania or psychogenic polydipsia. Some of these will be discussed in detail below.

Postoperative patients have a risk of developing hyponatremia that is frequently overlooked. One prospective study found that 4.4% of all postoperative patients develop hyponatremia of <130 mEq/L. The authors ascribed this mainly to hypotonic fluid administration and elevated serum ADH levels in their patients (22). In the ICU setting, however, the incidence may be higher. Of the 55 ICU patients with new-onset seizure reported by Widjicks, 8 of the 10 hyponatremic patients had undergone postoperative fluid loading (5). Hyponatremic encephalopathy resulting in death or persistent vegetative state following surgery in otherwise healthy patients has been reported (23). Probably, multiple mechanisms for postoperative hyponatremia occur, including iatrogenic free water loading and increased ADH levels secondary to volume loss, hypotension, and possibly other factors. A study of ADH levels in 16 patients undergoing uncomplicated cholecystectomy found that ADH levels increased on average 8.8 times their baseline levels during surgery and remained high for 2 additional days despite estimated blood losses of only 80–300 mL (24).

Patients with intracranial disease have a well-recognized risk of developing hyponatremia. Originally this was described as a salt-wasting syndrome caused by the inability of the renal tubule to reabsorb sodium secondary to the cerebral lesion (25). The syndrome is characterized by hyponatremia, natriuresis, and a decrease in the extracellular fluid volume. A natriuretic factor was hypothesized, but not found. Subsequently, SIADH was described, and most patients with hyponatremia following SAH were diagnosed clinically as having SIADH.(26) These patients had clinical diagnoses made on the basis of hyponatremia without dehydration (euvolemic or hypervolemic state), inappropriately elevated urine Na+, and urine osmolality higher than the serum osmolality. Fluid restriction was frequently used as a treatment for hyponatremia. A retrospective report of 134 patients with SAH found that one-third of patients had hyponatremia ([Na+] <135) during their hospital course, with 18% fulfilling criteria for SIADH. Of the patients with hyponatremia that were treated by fluid restriction, 21/26 developed cerebral infarctions (27). Subsequently, the same author reported that plasma volume decreased by >10% during the first week after SAH in 11/21 patients studied. Additionally, serum vasopressin levels were elevated at admission in 14/21 patients and fell during the first week in all patients (28). Other investigators have since reported that atrial natriuretic peptide (ANP) levels are elevated in patients with aneurysmal SAH and could account for natriuresis (29, 30). Most recently, a prospective observational study of 10 ICU patients with aneurysmal SAH who underwent clipping compared to a control group of patients who underwent craniotomy for resection of cerebral tumors had serum and urine electrolytes and plasma concentrations of brain natriuretic peptide (BNP), aldosterone, cortisol, ADH, and renin measured daily for 7 days postoperatively. None of the patients in either group developed hyponatremia, but all of the patients with SAH developed increased urine output, increased urinary excretion of Na^+, and increased fractional sodium filtration with elevated BNP and low aldosterone levels. None of the patients in the craniotomy group developed these findings. The authors suggested that their patients had salt-wasting syndrome associated with increased secretion of BNP and subsequent suppression of aldosterone synthesis (31). BNP in humans is mainly of cardiac origin, but is secreted by the hypothalamus as well. Further work remains to be done to define this syndrome.

Currently, most hyponatremia episodes in SAH are considered to be associated with hypovolemia, and are treated with volume expansion and mineralcorticoid supplementation when needed. If a patient is in symptomatic vasospasm, 3% NaCl may be given (32). A recent prospective study of patients with SAH did not find that hyponatremia was independently associated with poor outcome (33). Acute hyponatremia is also commonly observed following transurethral resection of the prostate (TURP) or endometrial resection when the operative field is irrigated with hypotonic glycine solutions (34–37). Neurological abnormalities include visual disturbances, seizures, confusion, and cerebral edema (on CT or MRI of the brain). In this instance, the administration of different irrigating solutions (i.e., sorbitol–mannitol), diuretics, and sodium reloading are measurements that should be undertaken to prevent or treat seizures. However, no randomized studies have been carried out and the role of anticonvulsant medications is uncertain.

Psychogenic polydipsia is a not-uncommon cause of severe, acute hyponatremia that deserves mention. Patients with polydipsia usually are considered able to tolerate large, rapid increases in Na^+ concentration and at are at high risk of dying if left untreated.(38) In a retrospective review of 10 years of institutional experience, one author reported 5 episodes of rapid Na^+ correction in this setting that resulted in neurologic complications out of 24 episodes of psychogenic polydipsia leading to hyponatremia. The complications included mild symptoms that resolved in two patients and clinical CPM in three patients. In two of these patients, hyponatremia was likely of subacute onset, and a third patient was chronically malnourished and abused alcohol (39). If the exact onset of the hyponatremia is in doubt, caution should be used.

In summary, hyponatremic patients with seizures should be treated with standard antiepileptic drugs, and the duration and underlying cause of their hyponatremia should be assessed to determine the appropriate rate of correction. Frequently, patients will have a single seizure without reccurrence, and the full differential diagnosis should be considered prior to ascribing the seizure to hyponatremia.

11.3.2. Hypernatremia

While hypernatremia is an extremely common problem in the ICU, especially in the elderly, associated seizures are rare. Other causes for the seizure such as meningitis, mass lesion, cortical vein or sinus thrombosis, subdural hemorrhage or nonketotic hyperglycinemia should be considered prior to ascribing a seizure to hypernatremia. In a neurologic patient, the possibility of neurogenic diabetes insipidus should be considered. This syndrome can occur after SAH, head trauma, intracranial tumors (i.e., transphenoidal pituitary tumor resection), or inflammation. Another common cause of hypernatremia in ICU patients is osmotic diuretics administration (such as mannitol) for the treatment of increased intracranial pressure. Finally, decreased response to thirst, in the presence of obtundation or lethargy, without adequate water access can be another cause of hypernatremia in hospitalized patients.

The acuity of the hypernatremia is important in deciding how fast to treat. Excessively fast rehydration can lead to cerebral edema, increased encephalopathy and seizures (40, 41). While seizures are rare, hypernatremia portends a poor prognosis: mortality ranges between 40 and 60% in hospitalized patients with hypernatremia (42). In a recent prospective, observational study of 298 patients with SAH, the incidence of hypernatremia was 19% and it was an independent predictor of poor prognosis (Odds Ration 2.7, 95% Confidence Intervals 1.2–6.1) (33). A different, retrospective study of 389 ICU patients showed the incidence of hypernatremia >150 mmol/L at admission to be 8.9%, with 5.7% of patients subsequently developing hypernatremia during the admission. The mortality rate for the patients with hypernatremia at admission was 20.3%, compared with 32% in patients who developed hospital-aquired hypernatremia ($p < 0.001$) (43).

11.4. Hypomagnesemia

Mg^{2+} deficiency is the most common electrolyte disturbance in hospitalized patients, and in the ICU its incidence has been found to be 20–65% (44, 45). As an isolated cause of seizure, it occurs rarely, but clinically has a large importance in the critically ill patient. Multiple studies have shown that low Mg^{2+} is a risk factor for poor prognosis. A prospective, observational study of 381 patients admitted to the regular floor and to the ICU showed that the mortality rates of patients with admission Mg^{2+} levels of <1.5 were twice the rates of non-hypomagnesemic patients with similar other variables (46). Other studies have failed to find an association between admission Mg^{2+} and mortality (47). A recently published prospective, observational study from Brussels (Belgium) of 446 consecutive ICU patients, which measured ionized and unionized Mg^{2+} levels, demonstrated an ionized hypomagnesemia (normal values 0.42–0.59 mmol/L) at admission in 18% of patients, and that there was no correlation with outcome. Ionized hypomagnesemia that developed during ICU admission was correlated with increased length of ICU stay, higher admission severity of illness (as determined by the APACHE II score), higher prevalence of sepsis and higher mortality rate (48). While the relative merits of measuring ionized or total serum Mg^{2+} levels remains under discussion, Mg^{2+} levels clearly are of significance.

Mg^{2+} is required for normal endocrine function, protein synthesis and enzymatic reactions. An average person has approximately 24 g of Mg^{2+} in their body, of which roughly two-thirds is stored in the bone, and one third in the cardiac muscle, skeletal muscle and liver. Normal Mg^{2+} homeostasis is entirely dependent on dietary intake. In normal circumstances, an adult person ingests 200–300 mg of Mg^{2+} daily and absorbs about one-half of this amount. Mg^{2+} is filtered by the kidney; in a day, around 2.5 g of Mg^{2+} enters the tubules and roughly 95% is reabsorbed in the proximal convoluted tubule and the loop of Henle. Mg^{2+} is almost entirely intracellular, but acidosis and ischemia promote release of magnesium from the cell. Among the activities Mg^{2+} is believed to support are the cell membrane Na^+/K^+ ATPase pump, proper selectivity of ion channels, and Ca^{2+} channel blockade. In a low Mg^{2+} state, intracellular Ca^{2+} concentrations rise and this may be the reason for the increased vasoconstrition seen with low Mg^{2+} (49).

Table 11-3. Causes of Clinical Hypomagnesemia.

Malnutrition and gastrointestinal factors

Alcoholism

Protein-calorie malnutrition

Total parenteral nutrition without magnesium replacement

Nasogastric suction

Intestinal bypass surgery

Short bowel syndrome

Diarrhea

Laxative abuse

Colonic neoplasm

Bulimia

Pancreatitis

Renal wasting

Diuretics

Antibiotics (aminoglycosides, foscarnet)

Cisplatin

Cyclosporine

Hypercalcemic states

Postobstructive diuresis

Acute tubular necrosis (diuretic phase)

Hereditary renal magnesium wasting (Bartter's and Gitelman's syndromes

Aldosteronism

Alcohol

Endocrine

Diabetic ketoacidosis

Hyperparathyroidism

Hyperthyroidism

Hyperaldosteronism

Acute intracellular shifts

Refeeding syndrome

Glucose infusions

Amino acid infusions

Insulin

Catecholamines

β_2 agonists

Metabolic acidosis

Other

Exchange transfusion

Acute intermittent porphyria

Citrated blood products

Phosphorus depletion

The situations in which Mg^{2+} deficiency arises are decreased nutritional intake, stress-induced catecholamine release, gastrointestinal malabsorption, failure of the kidney to reabsorb the filtered ion, as part of an endocrine disorder, and with acute shifts into the cell from the serum (Table 11-3) (50). All of these situations arise most frequently in the ICU (44). The clinical effects of Mg^{2+} depletion include the generation of cardiac arrhythmias (supraventricular tachycardias, atrial fibrillation, ventricular tachycardias), electrocardiographic changes (long QT interval, long PR interval, wide QRS, peaked T waves, ST segment depression), vasospasm and bronchospasm due to smooth muscle constriction, hypertension, endocrine and electrolyte effects (parathormone [PTH] stimulation or suppression, insulin resistance, refractory hypokalemia, hypocalcemia, and hypophosphatemia), and neurologic manifestations. Patients usually do not have neurologic manifestations until total serum levels drop below 1.0 mg/dL. The primary patient complaints may be tremor, fasciculations, spontaneous carpopedal spasm, or generalized muscle weakness. On exam, Chvostek's and Trousseau's signs may be elicited. Seizures when they occur are usually generalized. Because seizures also release catecholamines, which lowers the Mg^{2+} levels, low concentrations post-seizures may not be the cause, but rather the effect (51). Some controversy exists as to whether tetany ever occurs without coexisting severe hypocalcemia; reports exist, but in a prospective study of hypomagnesemic patients no tetany was observed, and tremor and fasciculations were only seen in patients who were also hypocalcemic (52, 53).

Mg^{2+} deficiency is a rare cause of intractable seizures in humans (54). In infants, these seizures occur with the rare condition of primary familial hypomagnesemia (55). These infants are supplemented for life with oral Mg^{2+} and this improves the outcome (56). In adult patients, the exact threshold level of Mg^{2+} necessary to cause intractable seizures is not well understood. The mechanism by which low Mg^{2+} causes seizures is under investigation. Mg^{2+} acts as a membrane stabilizer by screening the surface charge of the cell membrane, a property shared by it with Ca^{2+}. In contrast, at all synapses Mg^{2+} and Ca^{2+} antagonize each other; Mg^{2+} inhibits neurotransmitter release, while Ca^{2+} promotes it (1). Mg^{2+} present at normal levels antagonizes N-methyl-D-aspartate (NMDA)-receptor activation by undetermined mechanisms, helping to modulate the influx of Ca^{2+} into the cell. In rats, a neuroprotective effect of Mg^{2+} has been seen to NMDA-induced seizures (57). This may be one mechanism by which low Mg^{2+} facilitates seizures, but it does not appear to be the primary mechanism. In vitro, rat hippocampal slices suspended in an Mg^{2+}-free bath develop seizure-like discharges that evolve to late recurrent discharges approximately 2 h later that are not blocked by anticonvulsants (58). NMDA receptor blockade with antagonists aborts epileptiform discharges because of low Mg^{2+}, suggesting a role of the NMDA receptor activation for the generation of hypomagnesemix seizures (59). One investigator has found that seizure-like discharges induced in this manner are associated with an increase in the NADH/NAD ratio, unlike discharges elicited with 4-aminopurine, suggesting that failure of energy metabolism could be involved in the evolution of recurrent discharges in this model (60). An interesting feature in experimentally induced hypomagnesemia seizures is that they can be provoked by noise in several rat strains. By changing the intensity of the noise stimulus, one can change the susceptibility of these audiogenic seizures. This characteristic has been used to test the antiepileptic effect of drugs such as phenytoin, carbamazepine, phenobarbital, ethosuximide, and diazepam (61, 62).

Any seizing patient with the right clinical risks for hypomagnesemia must have the Mg^{2+} level done, as well as the levels of the other electrolytes that are commonly low in the presence of hypomagnesemia (K^+, Ca^{2+}, phosphorus). In the absence of renal failure and when clinical suspicion is strong, therapy may be started while Mg^{2+} levels are still pending. No clinical trial has demonstrated that Mg^{2+} infusion is the adequate therapy for seizures arising in the context of low Mg^{2+} levels, and standard anticonvulsants are used. Phenytoin may be preferred to valproate as there is animal data to suggest that it may have more sustained efficacy (62, 63). Mg^{2+} can be dosed at 4–6 g of magnesium sulfate intravenously and given rapidly at a rate not faster than 1 g/min. This dose can be repeated every 6 h until loss of patellar reflexes is seen (an early sign of Mg^{2+} intoxication).

11.5. Disorders of Calcium Homeostasis

11.5.1. Hypocalcemia

The classic setting for hypocalcemic seizures is in the newborn period. In the past, many newborns had hypocalcemic, hypomagnesemic seizures with onset at 4–14 days of life caused by the high phosphate content in cow's milk-based formulas (64). With improvement in formula composition, the most common time for neonatal hypocalcemic, hypomagnesemic seizures is now from birth to 3 days of age. By one recent retrospective series, these seizures occurred most frequently in infants with congenital heart disease (7 out of 15 patients) and only one had a mother with hyperparathyroidism. The author suggested that the heart defects could be associated with an incomplete form of DiGeorge's syndrome but no further information was available to support this. Prognosis depended on the severity of the associated medical conditions (65).

In adult patients, hypocalcemia usually presents with manifestations of neuromuscular irritability such as tetany, carpopedal spasms and perioral and limb paraesthesias (66). With very low Ca^{2+} levels such as those which occur following complete parathyroidectomy, papilledema, confusion and seizures can occur. Generalized convulsions and status epilepticus usually follow a generalized tetanic episode. Seizures secondary to alendronate-induced hypocalcemia have recently been reported (67). Although seizures purely due to hypocalcemia are rare, neurologists should be familiar with the many causes of hypocalcemia that occur in the ICU (see Table 11-4).

The mechanism of hypocalcemic seizures in rat hippocampal models appears to involve epileptiform discharges predominantly from area CA1 of the hippocampus. There appears to be ephaptic transmission that occurs in very low Ca^{2+} states (<0.3 mEq/L) as the epileptiform discharges could not be abolished by blockade of NMDA and non-NMDA receptors (68).

Treatment of hypocalcemic seizures includes intravenous Ca^{2+} and an antiepileptic medication. The usual dose is 2 ampules of Ca^{2+} gluconate (10 cc ampule contains 4.6 mEq of elemental Ca^{2+}) or 1 ampule of Ca^{2+} chloride (10 cc ampule contains 13.6 mEq of elemental Ca^{2+}) intravenou sly slowly (over 10–20 min). Additional continuous infusion can be started at a rate of 1–1.5 ampules of Ca^{2+} gluconate over 6–8 h with serum Ca^{2+} levels measurement every 4–6 h to maintain serum Ca^{2+} levels near 8 mg/dL. The patient should have Mg^{2+} replaced as well. Hyperphosphatemia should be treated,

Table 11-4. Causes of Hypocalcemia.

Post-thyroidectomy

Post-parathyroidectomy or autoimmune hypoparathyroidism

Pseudohypoparathyroidism

Repeated transfusions

Critical illness

Plasmapheresis

Sepsis

Acute Pancreatitis

Fat embolism

Crush injury

Rhabdomyolysis

Hypomagnesemia

Primary hypomagnesemia with secondary hypocalcemia

Vitamin D deficiency

Heparin

Other drugs (foscarnet, pentamidine)

Chronic renal failure

Acute renal failure

if present. Cardiac monitoring is usual because Ca^{2+} can occasionally cause bradyarrhythmias and first-degree heart block, particularly if the patient is already taking digoxin.

11.5.2. Hypercalcemia

Severe hypercalcemia (>13.5 mEq/L), such as that which occurs in primary hyperparathyroidism, has been reported to cause seizures in the setting of confusion and encephalopathy, although this is uncommon (69, 70). This presentation with generalized or focal seizures and coma is sometimes referred to as parathyroid storm. Hypercalcemia as the result of a neoplasm, either by direct invasion of bone, or as a result of PTH-related protein (PTHrP) release also can cause this presentation and is an oncologic emergency (71). Among drugs, lithium can cause hypercalcemia through PTH secretion (72).

Multiple cases of patients with severe hypercalcemia and a posterior leukoencephalopathy with visual loss, confusion, drowsiness, and seizures have been reported (73, 74). These patients had multiple areas of subcortical ischemia by neuroimaging, predominantly in the parieto-occipital regions. Cytotoxic edema is suggested by the presence of diffusin-weighted imaging abnormalities on MRI (73). EEG has revealed either occipital intermittent rhythmic delta activity (73) or periodic lateralizing epileptiform discharges (74). Symptoms resolved with treatment of the serum Ca^{2+}. One author suggests the partly reversible vasospasm of the cerebral vessels as an explanation (74).

The pathophysiology of hypercalcemia-induced seizures is still unclear, as in rat hippocampus the tendency for neurons to produce multiple spikes is reduced (75).

EEG findings in hypocalcemia include bursts of high-voltage slow waves, with sharp and spike waves and without triphasic waves (76). In hypercalcemia, bursts of high-voltage slow waves and triphasic waves have been reported, but periodic lateralized discharges (PLEDS) may be seen (74, 76).

The treatment of hypercalcemia requires vigorous intravenous hydration (6–10 L/day) to replete volume and avoid renal failure, and limitation of oral Ca^{2+} intake to 0.5–1.0 mg/day. Following this, intravenous furosemide can be given to encourage calciuresis. In the case of chronic hypercalcemia or when hydration and furosemide fails to normalize serum Ca^{2+}, agents such as intravenous mithramycin, pamidronate and etidronate are used. Calcitonin can also be used but tachyphylaxis reduces its utility for long-term treatment.

11.6. Hypophosphatemia

Low phosphate levels frequently accompany deficiencies in other electrolytes. The majority of serious complications occur with severe hypophosphatemia, defined as serum concentrations <1 mg/dL (<0.32 mmol/L). Moderate hypophosphatemia is considered to be 1.0–2.0 mg/dL (0.3–0.7 mmol/L). The reported incidence of hypophosphatemia in a general population of hospitalized patients is 2.5–3.1% (77). In the ICU setting, an incidence at admission of 17–45% has been reported (77, 78). A higher incidence among some neurologic patients may be present. In a recent report of 18 ICU patients with severe head injury, 61% had hypophosphatemia at admission along with other electrolyte abnormalities. There may be a yet undefined mechanism in cerebral injury causing phosphate wasting. A caveat, however, is that some of the patients had received a dose of mannitol prior to electrolyte measurements (79). Hypophosphatemia can arise because of insufficient intake or absorption, intracellular redistribution, or renal losses (see Table 11-5). The refeeding syndrome is a famous cause of hypophosphatemia in the ICU and can occur after starvation for as short as 48 h (80).

Phosphorus is a vital component of normal metabolism. Phosphorus is required for adenosine triphosphate (ATP) synthesis, and the neurologic symptoms are believed to arise from ATP deficiency. Phosphorus is also required for 2,3-DPG production, and hypophosphatemia therefore increases the affinity of the red blood cell for oxygen, decreasing peripheral oxygenation. Hemolytic anemia may occur in severe hypophosphatemia secondary to increased rigidity of the red blood cells, which require ATP to remain deformable. Leukocyte and platelet function is decreased. Cardiac and respiratory failure may occur.

Normal dietary intake of phosphorus is approximately 1.0–1.5 g. Phosphorus is absorbed in the jejunum of the small intestine and is in the serum as a free ion. Phosphorus is freely filtered by the kidney and 80–90% is reabsorbed in the proximal tubules. Of the daily phosphorus intake, approximately two-thirds is excreted in the urine with normal renal function. PTH and 1,25-dihydroxyvitamin D3 decrease phosphate reabsorption. Roughly, 80% of total body phosphorus is in the bone. Of the remaining 20%, almost all is in the intracellular space (81).

Classic neurologic findings of hypophosphatemia are muscle weakness, either symptomatic or asymptomatic. A painful myopathy may develop, which can progress to rhabdomyolysis (82). Paresthesias, tremors, and neuropathy have been reported. Acute hypophosphatemia has been reported to cause coma or seizures (83).

Table 11-5. Causes of Hypophosphatemia.

Decreased intake/absorption

Starvation

TPN formula without phosphorus

Alcoholism

Intracellular redistribution

Refeeding syndrome

Acute asthma

COPD

Respiratory alkalosis

Sepsis

Increased renal loss

Fanconi's syndrome

Cystinosis

Amyloidosis

Myeloma

Wilson's disease nephrosis

Cadmium toxicity

Acute lead toxicity

Acetaminophen toxicity

Hyperparathyroidism

Vitamin D-resistant rickets

Medications (acetazolamide, theophylline, steroids, dopamine, estrogen, cisplatin

TPN total parenteral nutrition; *COPD* chronic obstructive pulmonary disease.

Replacement of phosphorus has been associated with diarrhea, hypotension, cardiac arrhythmia, confusion, paresthesia, metastatic calcification, hyperkalemia, or hypernatremia from the salt used to bind the phosphorus, hypocalcemia and hypomagnesemia (81). Traditionally, the dosage used to treat severe hypophosphatemia has been 0.125 mmol/kg/h over a 4-h infusion (35 mmol in a 70 kg person), and a dose used to treat moderate hypophosphatemia is 0.0125 mmol/kg/h over 6 h (5.25 mmol in a 70 kg person) (84). A prospective study of eleven ICU patients with moderate hypophosphatemia and initial serum phosphorus levels of 1.6–1.9 mg/dL (0.51–0.61 mmol/L) used 15 mmol of sodium phosphate intravenously over 2 h, to be repeated every 6 h as needed. The protocol was well tolerated (85).

11.7. Summary

Electrolyte disturbances in the ICU are extremely common. The electrolyte disorder most commonly associated with seizure is hyponatremia, although extremely low Mg^{2+}, phosphate and both very low and very high Ca^{2+} values can cause seizures. Critical care physicians must be vigilant to suspect and identify electrolyte disturbances in their patients, as a growing amount of information suggests that they are a marker, and potentially a cause, of poor prognosis. Electrolyte disturbance should never be accepted as the etiology of a seizure until a thorough investigation has been undertaken.

References

1. Somjen GG (2002) Ion regulation in the brain: implications for pathophysiology. Neuroscientist 8:254–267
2. Somjen GG (2001) Mechanisms of spreading depression and hypoxic spreading depression-like depolarization. Physiol Rev 81:1065–1096
3. Rosen AS, Andrew RD (1990) Osmotic effects upon excitability in rat neocortical slices. Neuroscience 38:579–590
4. Somjen GG (1999) Low external NaCl concentration and low osmolarity enhance voltage-gated Ca currents but depress K currents in freshly isolated rat hippocampal neurons. Brain Res 851:189–197
5. Wijdicks EF, Sharbrough FW (1993) New-onset seizures in critically ill patients. Neurology 43:1042–1044
6. Sterns RH, Thomas DJ, Herndon RM (1989) Brain dehydration and neurologic deterioration after rapid correction of hyponatremia. Kidney Int 35:69–75
7. Gobbi G, Bertani G, Pini A (1997) Electrolyte, sporadic, metabolic and endocrine disorders. In: Engel J, Pedley TA (eds) Epilepsy: a comprehensive textbook. Lippincott-Raven Publishers, Philadelphia
8. Dudek FE, Obenaus A, Tasker JG (1990) Osmolality-induced changes in extracellular volume alter epileptiform bursts independent of chemical synapses in the rat: importance of non-synaptic mechanisms in hippocampal epileptogenesis. Neurosci Lett 120:267–270
9. Cluitmans FH, Meinders AE (1990) Management of severe hyponatremia: rapid or slow correction? Am J Med 88:161–166
10. Gross P, Reimann D, Henschkowski J, Damian M (2001) Treatment of severe hyponatremia: conventional and novel aspects. J Am Soc Nephrol 12(Suppl 17): S10–S14
11. Ayus JC, Olivero JJ, Frommer JP (1982) Rapid correction of severe hyponatremia with intravenous hypertonic saline solution. Am J Med 72:43–48
12. Soupart A, Decaux G (1996) Therapeutic recommendations for management of severe hyponatremia: current concepts on pathogenesis and prevention of neurologic complications. Clin Nephrol 46:149–169
13. Ellis SJ (1995) Severe hyponatraemia: complications and treatment. QJM 88:905–909
14. Leens C, Mukendi R, Foret F, Hacourt A, Devuyst O, Colin IM (2001) Central and extrapontine myelinolysis in a patient in spite of a careful correction of hyponatremia. Clin Nephrol 55:248–253
15. Oo TN, Smith CL, Swan SK (2003) Does uremia protect against the demyelination associated with correction of hyponatremia during hemodialysis? A case report and literature review. Semin Dial 16:68–71
16. Baker EA, Tian Y, Adler S, Verbalis JG (2000) Blood-brain barrier disruption and complement activation in the brain following rapid correction of chronic hyponatremia. Exp Neurol 165:221–230
17. Sterns RH, Cappuccio JD, Silver SM, Cohen EP (1994) Neurologic sequelae after treatment of severe hyponatremia: a multicenter perspective. J Am Soc Nephrol 4:1522–1530
18. Norenberg MD, Leslie KO, Robertson AS (1982) Association between rise in serum sodium and central pontine myelinolysis. Ann Neurol 11:128–135
19. Soupart A, Stenuit A, Perier O, Decaux G (1991) Limits of brain tolerance to daily increments in serum sodium in chronically hyponatraemic rats treated with hypertonic saline or urea: advantages of urea. Clin Sci (Lond) 80:77–84
20. Soupart A, Ngassa M, Decaux G (1999) Therapeutic relowering of the serum sodium in a patient after excessive correction of hyponatremia. Clin Nephrol 51:383–386
21. Soupart A, Penninckx R, Stenuit A, Perier O, Decaux G (1996) Reinduction of hyponatremia improves survival in rats with myelinolysis-related neurologic symptoms. J Neuropathol Exp Neurol 55:594–601

22. Chung HM, Kluge R, Schrier RW, Anderson RJ (1986) Postoperative hyponatremia. A prospective study. Arch Intern Med 146:333–336

23. Arieff AI (1986) Hyponatremia, convulsions, respiratory arrest, and permanent brain damage after elective surgery in healthy women. N Engl J Med 314:1529–1535

24. Cochrane JP, Forsling ML, Gow NM, Le Quesne LP (1981) Arginine vasopressin release following surgical operations. Br J Surg 68:209–213

25. Cort J (1954) Cerebral salt wasting. Lancet 1:752–754

26. Wise BL (1978) Syndrome of inappropriate antidiuretic hormone secretion after spontaneous subarachnoid hemorrhage: a reversible cause of clinical deterioration. Neurosurgery 3:412–414

27. Wijdicks EF, Vermeulen M, Hijdra A, van Gijn J (1985) Hyponatremia and cerebral infarction in patients with ruptured intracranial aneurysms: is fluid restriction harmful? Ann Neurol 17:137–140

28. Wijdicks EF, Vermeulen M, ten Haaf JA, Hijdra A, Bakker WH, van Gijn J (1985) Volume depletion and natriuresis in patients with a ruptured intracranial aneurysm. Ann Neurol 18:211–216

29. Weinand ME, O'Boynick PL, Goetz KL (1989) A study of serum antidiuretic hormone and atrial natriuretic peptide levels in a series of patients with intracranial disease and hyponatremia. Neurosurgery 25:781–785

30. Diringer M, Ladenson PW, Stern BJ, Schleimer J, Hanley DF (1988) Plasma atrial natriuretic factor and subarachnoid hemorrhage. Stroke 19:1119–1124

31. Berendes E, Walter M, Cullen P, Prien T, Van Aken H, Horsthemke J et al (1997) Secretion of brain natriuretic peptide in patients with aneurysmal subarachnoid haemorrhage. Lancet 349:245–249

32. Suarez JI, Qureshi AI, Parekh PD, Razumovsky A, Tamargo RJ, Bhardwaj A et al (1999) Administration of hypertonic (3%) sodium chloride/acetate in hyponatremic patients with symptomatic vasospasm following subarachnoid hemorrhage. J Neurosurg Anesthesiol 11:178–184

33. Qureshi AI, Suri MF, Sung GY, Straw RN, Yahia AM, Saad M et al (2002) Prognostic significance of hypernatremia and hyponatremia among patients with aneurysmal subarachnoid hemorrhage. Neurosurgery 50:749–755

34. Tanzin-Fin P, Sanz L (1992) Prostate transurethral resection syndrome. Ann Fr Anesth Reanim 11:168–177

35. Ayus JC, Arieff AI (1997) Glycine-induced hypo-osmolar hyponatremia. Ann Intern Med 157:223–226

36. Dawkins GP, Miller RA (1999) Sorbitol-mannitol solution for urological electro-surgical resection – a safer fluid than glycine 1.5%. Eur Urol 36:99–102

37. Radziwill AJ, Vuadens P, Borruat FX, Bogousslavsky J (1997) Visual ditur-bances and transurethral resection of the prostate: the TURP syndrome. Eur Neurol 38:7–9

38. Cheng JC, Zikos D, Skopicki HA, Peterson DR, Fisher KA (1990) Long-term neurologic outcome in psychogenic water drinkers with severe symptomatic hyponatremia: the effect of rapid correction. Am J Med 88:561–566

39. Tanneau RS, Henry A, Rouhart F, Bourbigot B, Garo B, Mocquard Y et al (1994) High incidence of neurologic complications following rapid correction of severe hyponatremia in polydipsic patients. J Clin Psychiatry 55:349–354

40. Morris-Jones PH, Houston IB, Evans RC (1967) Prognosis of the neurological complications of acute hypernatraemia. Lancet 2:1385–1389

41. Gall DG, Haddow JE (1969) Effects of acute hypernatraemia. Lancet 1:783

42. Palevsky PM (1998) Hypernatremia. Semin Nephrol 18:20–30

43. Polderman KH, Schreuder WO, Strack van Schijndel RJ, Thijs LG (1999) Hypernatremia in the intensive care unit: an indicator of quality of care? Crit Care Med 27:1105–1108

44. Reinhart RA, Desbiens NA (1985) Hypomagnesemia in patients entering the ICU. Crit Care Med 13:506–507

45. Ryzen E, Wagers PW, Singer FR, Rude RK (1985) Magnesium deficiency in a medical ICU population. Crit Care Med 13:19–21

46. Rubeiz GJ, Thill-Baharozian M, Hardie D, Carlson RW (1993) Association of hypomagnesemia and mortality in acutely ill medical patients. Crit Care Med 21:203–209

47. Guerin C, Cousin C, Mignot F, Manchon M, Fournier G (1996) Serum and erythrocyte magnesium in critically ill patients. Intensive Care Med 22:724–727

48. Soliman HM, Mercan D, Lobo SS, Melot C, Vincent JL (2003) Development of ionized hypomagnesemia is associated with higher mortality rates. Crit Care Med 31:1082–1087

49. Dacey MJ (2001) Hypomagnesemic disorders. Crit Care Clin 17:155–173, viii

50. Whang R (1987) Magnesium deficiency: pathogenesis, prevalence, and clinical implications. Am J Med 82:24–29

51. Ryzen E, Servis KL, Rude RK (1990) Effect of intravenous epinephrine on serum magnesium and free intracellular red blood cell magnesium concentrations measured by nuclear magnetic resonance. J Am Coll Nutr 9:1114–1119

52. Wacker W, Moore F, Ulmer D (1962) Normocalcemic magnesium deficiency. JAMA 180:161–163

53. Kingston ME, Al-Siba'i MB, Skooge WC (1986) Clinical manifestations of hypomagnesemia. Crit Care Med 14:950–954

54. Nuytten D, Van Hees J, Meulemans A, Carton H (1991) Magnesium deficiency as a cause of acute intractable seizures. J Neurol 238:262–264

55. Unachak K, Louthrenoo O, Katanyuwong K (2002) Primary hypomagnesemia in Thai infants: a case report with 7 years follow-up and review of literature. J Med Assoc Thai 85:1226–1231

56. Shalev H, Phillip M, Galil A, Carmi R, Landau D (1998) Clinical presentation and outcome in primary familial hypomagnesaemia. Arch Dis Child 78:127–130

57. Hallak M (1998) Effect of parenteral magnesium sulfate administration on excitatory amino acid receptors in the rat brain. Magnes Res 11:117–131

58. Zhang CL, Dreier JP, Heinemann U (1995) Paroxysmal epileptiform discharges in temporal lobe slices after prolonged exposure to low magnesium are resistant to clinically used anticonvulsants. Epilepsy Res 20:105–111

59. Nakamura M, Abe S, Goto Y, Chishaki A, Akazawa K, Kato M (1994) In vivo assessment of prevention of white-noise-induced seizure in magnesium-deficient rats by N-methyl-d-aspartate receptor blockers. Epilepsy Res 17:249–256

60. Schuchmann S, Buchheim K, Meierkord H, Heinemann U (1999) A relative energy failure is associated with low-Mg2+ but not with 4-aminopyridine induced seizure-like events in entorhinal cortex. J Neurophysiol 81:399–403

61. Bac P, Tran G, Paris M, Binet P (1993) Characterisitics of the audiogenic convulsive crisis in mice made sensitive by magnesium deficiency. CR Acad Sci III 316:676–681

62. Bac P, Maurois P, Dupont C, Pages N, Stables JP, Gressens P et al (1998) Magnesium deficiency-dependent audiogenic seizures (MDDASs) in adult mice: a nutritional model for discriminatory screening of anticonvulsant drugs and original assessment of neuroprotection properties. J Neurosci 18:4363–4373

63. Dreier JP, Heinemann U (1990) Late low magnesium-induced epileptiform activity in rat entorhinal cortex slices becomes insensitive to the anticonvulsant valproic acid. Neurosci Lett 119:68–70

64. Keen JH (1969) Significance of hypocalcaemia in neonatal convulsions. Arch Dis Child 44:356–361

65. Lynch BJ, Rust RS (1994) Natural history and outcome of neonatal hypocalcemic and hypomagnesemic seizures. Pediatr Neurol 11:23–27

66. Tonner DR, Schlechte JA (1993) Neurologic complications of thyroid and parathyroid disease. Med Clin North Am 77:251–263

67. Maclsaac RJ, Seeman E, Jerums G (2002) Seizures after alendronate. J R Soc Med 95:615–616

68. Leschinger A, Stabel J, Igelmund P, Heinemann U (1993) Pharmacological and electrographic properties of epileptiform activity induced by elevated K+ and lowered Ca2+ and Mg2+ concentration in rat hippocampal slices. Exp Brain Res 96:230–240

69. Bauermeister DE, Jennings ER, Cruse DR, Sedgwick VD (1967) Hypercalcemia with seizures – a clinical paradox. JAMA 201:132–133

70. Cherry TA, Kauffman RP, Myles TD (2002) Primary hyperparathyroidism, hypercalcemic crisis and subsequent seizures occurring during pregnancy: a case report. J Matern Fetal Neonatal Med 12:349–352

71. Krimsky WS, Behrens RJ, Kerkvliet GJ (2002) Oncologic emergencies for the internist. Cleve Clin J Med 69:209–210, 213–204, 216–207 passim

72. Komatsu M, Shimizu H, Tsuruta T et al (1995) Effect of lithium on serum calcium level and parathyroid function in manic-depressive patients. Endocr J 42:691–695

73. Kastrup O, Maschke M, Wanke I, Diener HC (2002) Posterior reversible encephalopathy syndrome due to severe hypercalcemia. J Neurol 249:1563–1566

74. Kaplan PW (1998) Reversible hypercalcemic cerebral vasoconstriction with seizures and blindness: a paradigm for eclampsia? Clin Electroencephalogr 29:120–123

75. Stringer JL, Lothman EW (1988) In vitro effects of extracellular calcium concentrations on hippocampal pyramidal cell responses. Exp Neurol 101:132–146

76. Swash M, Rowan AJ (1972) Electroencephalographic criteria of hypocalcemia and hypercalcemia. Arch Neurol 26:218–228

77. Brown GR, Greenwood JK (1994) Drug- and nutrition-induced hypophosphatemia: mechanisms and relevance in the critically ill. Ann Pharmacother 28:626–632

78. Zazzo JF, Troche G, Ruel P, Maintenant J (1995) High incidence of hypophosphatemia in surgical intensive care patients: efficacy of phosphorus therapy on myocardial function. Intensive Care Med 21:826–831

79. Polderman KH, Bloemers FW, Peerdeman SM, Girbes AR (2000) Hypomagnesemia and hypophosphatemia at admission in patients with severe head injury. Crit Care Med 28:2022–2025

80. Marik PE, Bedigian MK (1996) Refeeding hypophosphatemia in critically ill patients in an intensive care unit. A prospective study. Arch Surg 131:1043–1047

81. Lloyd CW, Johnson CE (1988) Management of hypophosphatemia. Clin Pharm 7:123–128

82. Kumar D, McAlister FA (1999) Rhabdomyolysis complicating unrecognized hypophosphatemia in an alcoholic patient. Can J Gastroenterol 13:165–167

83. Lee JL, Sibbald WJ, Holliday RL, Linton AL (1978) Hypophosphatemia associated with coma. Can Med Assoc J 119:143–145

84. Lentz RD, Brown DM, Kjellstrand CM (1978) Treatment of severe hypophosphatemia. Ann Intern Med 89:941–944

85. Rosen GH, Boullata JI, O'Rangers EA, Enow NB, Shin B (1995) Intravenous phosphate repletion regimen for critically ill patients with moderate hypophosphatemia. Crit Care Med 23:1204–1210

86. Johnson JE, Wright LF (1983) Thiazide-induced hyponatremia. South Med J 76:1363–1367

87. Steinhoff BJ, Stoll KD, Stodieck SR, Paulus W (1992) Hyponatremic coma under oxcarbazepine therapy. Epilepsy Res 11:67–70

88. Wakem CJ, Bennett JM (1975) Inappropiate ADH secretion associated with massive vincristine overdosage. Aust N Z J Med 5:266–269

89. Bellin SL, Selim M (1988) Cisplatin-induced hypomagnesemia with seizures: a case report and review of the literature. Gynecol Oncol 30:104–113

90. Subramanian D, Ayus JC (1992) Case report: severe symptomatic hyponatremia associated with lisinopril therapy. Am J Med Sci 303:177–179

91. Holmes SB, Banerjee AK, Alexander WD (1999) Hyponatraemia and seizures after ecstasy use. Postgrad Med J 75:32–33

92. Cherney DZ, Davids MR, Halperin ML (2002) Acute hyponatraemia and 'ecstasy': insights from a quantitative and integrative analysis. QJM 95:475–483

93. Koivikko MJ, Valikangas SL (1983) Hyponatraemia during carbamazepine therapy in children. Neuropediatrics 14:93–96

94. Cilli AS, Algun E (2002) Oxcarbazepine-induced syndrome of inappropriate secretion of antidiuretic hormone. J Clin Psychiatry 63:742

95. Mewasingh L, Aylett S, Kirkham F, Stanhope R (2000) Hyponatraemia associated with lamotrigine in cranial diabetes insipidus. Lancet 356:656

96. Rosenstein DL, Nelson JC, Jacobs SC (1993) Seizures associated with antidepressants: a review. J Clin Psychiatry 54:289–299

97. Hwang AS, Magraw RM (1989) Syndrome of inappropriate secretion of antidiuretic hormone due to fluoxetine. Am J Psychiatry 146:399

98. Goldstein L, Barker M, Segall F, Asihene R, Balser S, Lautenbach D et al (1996) Seizure and transient SIADH associated with sertraline. Am J Psychiatry 153:732

99. Vanpee D, Laloyaux P, Gillet JB (1999) Seizure and hyponatraemia after overdose of trazadone. Am J Emerg Med 17:430–431

100. Balestrieri G, Cerudelli B, Ciaccio S, Rizzoni D (1992) Hyponatraemia and seizure due to overdose of trazodone. BMJ 304:686

101. Pruthi RS, Kang J, Vick R (2002) Desmopressin induced hyponatremia and seizures after laparoscopic radical nephrectomy. J Urol 168:187

Chapter 12

Alcohol-Related Seizures in the Intensive Care Unit

Zachary Webb and Panayiotis Varelas

Abstract Alcohol abuse is a common cause of seizures resulting in admission to the intensive care unit. The cause of the alcohol-related seizures (ARS) is usually abstinence in a chronic alcoholic, although some patients may still have detectable levels of alcohol in their blood. ARS generally occur between 7 and 48 h after abstinence. Approximately half the patients presenting with ARS will have recurrent seizures (usually 2–4) within a vulnerable 6 h period following the initial ARS. Although patients with ARS rarely enter status epilepticus, alcohol withdrawal is a common contributing factor in many cases of status epilepticus. Evaluation involves searching for a focal cause of the seizure as well as looking for comorbid conditions which may complicate the management of chronic alcohol abusers, including delirium tremens. Treatment of ARS is similar to general management of alcohol withdrawal, with benzodiazepines being the mainstay of treatment. Treatment of alcohol-related status epilepticus is similar to that of other causes of status epilepticus. Phenytoin is not indicated for treatment of ARS unless the patient enters status epilepticus.

Keywords Seizure, Withdrawal, Alcohol, Status epilepticus, Intensive care, ICU, Delirium tremens, Antiepileptic, Phenytoin

12.1. Introduction

Alcohol-related seizures (ARS) are a common cause of adult onset seizures (1). Management of these patients involves careful evaluation to assess for life-threatening illness as well as causes of seizures other than alcohol. The hospital course may be complicated by status epilepticus, polysubstance abuse, intracranial pathology, delirium tremens, and other comorbid conditions.

From: *Seizures in Critical Care*: *A Guide to Diagnosis and Therapeutics*: Current Clinical Neurology, Second Edition, Edited by: P. Varelas, DOI 10.1007/978-1-60327-532-3_12, © Humana Press, a part of Springer Science+Business Media, LLC 2005, 2010

12.2. Alcohol Withdrawal Syndrome

The alcohol withdrawal syndrome is a spectrum of signs and symptoms following cessation or reduction in the intake of alcohol. In general, mild symptoms occur early and the more serious symptoms such as seizures and delirium tremens occur later in the course of withdrawal.

12.2.1. Minor Alcohol Withdrawal

Symptoms of minor alcohol withdrawal may begin within hours of the last drink, peak within 1–2 days, and generally disappear in 5–7 days (2–4). Symptoms can occur before the blood alcohol levels have reached zero (4). The patient may develop anxiety, tremor, malaise, weakness, irritability, insomnia, vivid dreams, headache, and autonomic disturbances such as tachycardia, hypertension, diaphoresis, orthostatic hypotension, and nausea. The tremor in alcohol withdrawal is a tremor of the hand and tongue and is worse when outstretched. The tremor lasts a few days and the inner shakiness and uneasiness may remain 10–14 days. After this, the patient is able to sleep throughout the night without sedation (5). Symptom severity generally relates to the duration and intensity of the alcohol intake (4).

12.2.2. Alcohol Hallucinosis

Alcohol hallucinosis is a condition that occurs in about 25% of long-term heavy drinkers (6). The patient experiences visual, auditory, tactile, or olfactory hallucinations (7). They usually begin within 12–24 h after the last drink and stop in another 24–48 h (6), although there are reports of patients developing a chronic paranoid delusional state (2). The EEG is generally normal (7) and the presence of a grossly normal sensorium helps distinguish it from delirium tremens (6).

12.2.3. Delirium Tremens

Delirium tremens is the most severe form of alcohol withdrawal. It occurs in less than 5% of patients hospitalized for alcohol withdrawal and is characterized by delirium, vivid hallucinations, and autonomic hyperactivity such as systolic hypertension, tachycardia, diaphoresis, mild hyperthermia (100.5° or less), and dilated but reactive pupils (2, 6–8). Although the range of onset may be large (6), the syndrome usually begins on the second or third day of abstinence and in most cases resolves within 5 days (5). If seizures occur in the course of alcohol withdrawal, they nearly always occur before the onset of delirium tremens. If they occur after the onset of delirium tremens, an organic cause is likely (2). The transient EEG changes that may be seen during the peak incidence of alcohol withdrawal seizures resolve before the onset of delirium tremens (9, 10). The EEG during delirium tremens is generally normal or there is an increase in fast frequencies. This fact may help in differentiating delirium tremens from other causes of altered sensorium.

Patients at risk for delirium tremens are generally older than 30 years old and have a long-standing history of alcoholism (6). The risk for delirium tremens begins at a daily consumption rate of 80 g of ethanol but becomes appreciable only at 120 g a day upwards, i.e., one half of a 750 mL bottle per day (8).

Only about 1–10% of patients with minor withdrawal symptoms will go on to develop delirium tremens (2). Medical illness or a prior history of major withdrawal also increases the risk of withdrawal delirium (2, 7).

Concurrent medical conditions are often seen and may mask the delirium tremens. Therefore one must be aware that unexplained hypertension, tachycardia, fever, or sweating may be signs of delirium tremens in a patient who is not exhibiting the usual signs and symptoms (6). Before assigning a diagnosis of delirium tremens, other causes of delirium in the alcoholic should be considered, such as pneumonia, sepsis, meningitis, hypoxia, hypercapnia, electrolyte disorders, cardiac ischemia or arrhythmia, hypertension or hypotension, hypoglycemia, hepatic disease, renal disease, thiamine deficiency, the postictal state, dehydration, medications or illicit drugs, ketoacidosis, trauma, subdural hemorrhage, intracerebral bleeding, subarachnoid hemorrhage, and acute ischemic stroke (6, 11–13).

With improved understanding and treatment, death rates have dropped from about 20% 40 years ago to just about 1% in recent years (2). Death is usually due to complications of medical illness such as pneumonia, sepsis, and arrhythmia.

12.3. Alcohol-Related Seizures

Alcohol-related seizures (ARS) are a common cause of new onset of seizures in adults (1, 9, 12). One study detected alcohol intoxication in the immediate histories of half of the patients seen in the ER for seizures (12). ARS can generally be thought of as a withdrawal phenomenon, occurring after several hours of abstinence. In some cases, however, the patient may still be intoxicated or have detectable levels of alcohol when the seizure occurs (9, 12, 14, 15).

The seizures generally occur between 7 and 48 h after cessation of alcohol (9). Seizures occurring after 72 h are likely to be associated with concurrent drug abuse or intracranial pathology (16). About half of the patients presenting with an ARS will have recurrent seizures (usually 2–4) within a vulnerable 6 h period following the initial ARS (9). Since ARS almost never occur during delirium tremens, seizures occurring after the onset of delirium are likely due to an organic cause, even if the patient has a prior history of ARS (2).

During the peak incidence of ARS, the EEG is often abnormal, showing sharp waves, spikes, paroxysmal changes and a photomyoclonic response (9, 10). This phase is very transient and usually quickly returns to normal. If the EEG is obtained after peak incidence of ARS but within the first few days of the ARS, the EEG may show increased beta activity, reduced alpha activity, or a low voltage EEG pattern (17).

Although binge drinking has been shown to cause ARS (12), the risk of having an ARS is greatest in alcoholics with a prior history of detoxification, many years of alcohol abuse, prior ARS, and a score greater than 15 on the Clinical Institute Withdrawal Assessment for Alcohol (CIWA-A) scale, a validated scale for the assessment of alcohol withdrawal severity (18–21). The typical patient is generally male, between the age of 30 and 60, experiencing a period of abstinence following a period of chronic intoxication (9).

In patients with a predisposition to seizures, such as idiopathic and post-traumatic epilepsy, much shorter periods of intoxication are required to experience ARS. In some cases, even a single evening of drinking is sufficient.

These seizures are similar to ARS in patients without epilepsy, in that they generally occur after a discrete period of abstinence and not during the period of intoxication (9).

Although ARS are usually generalized, focal seizures may occur as well. In their study of 472 adults, Ernest and Yarnell (1) found that focal seizures occurred in 24% of ARS. Of these cases, a focal lesion was found in only 15%, compared to the 47% of nonalcoholic focal seizures. Other authors have also reported a low prevalence of focal lesions in patients with focal ARS (22). These studies were during the pre-CT scan era and therefore may have underestimated the frequency of focal lesions, especially traumatic lesions (12).

It is very difficult to predict which patients will have recurrent seizures (i.e., seizures within one alcohol withdrawal episode) during the vulnerable 6 h period following an ARS. Rathlev et al. (23) conducted a retrospective analysis of the placebo arms of two prospective randomized trials of drug treatments for the prevention of recurrent alcohol-related seizures. They found that the following clinical characteristics were not predictors of recurrent seizures within 6 h following an ARS: age, gender, systolic blood pressure, diastolic blood pressure, temperature, respiratory rate, heart rate, history of ARS, history of non-alcohol-related seizures, daily ethanol intake, and duration of alcohol abuse. They did find that patients with an initial alcohol level greater than 100 mg/dL had a significantly lower risk (0%) for recurrent ARS within the study period compared to patients with blood alcohol concentration <100 mg/dL (36%, $p < 0.01$). The reason for this unexpected finding is a matter of speculation and it is possible that recurrent seizures would have been observed in some of these patients if the study period had been extended beyond 6 h. Data from a 48 h follow-up period were available from only one of the two studies. These data showed that 14% of patients developed recurrent seizures after discharge from the hospital and all of these patients except one had an alcohol level below zero on the first visit. The exception had a level of 22 mg/dL.

12.3.1. Differential Diagnosis

There are many causes for seizures in the intensive care unit (24). One must not immediately assume that alcohol is the only cause of seizure in the alcohol-dependent patient. With the help of CT or MRI scans in many of their patients, Rathlev et al. (25) conducted a chart review of emergency department patients who presented with alcohol-related seizures and found that 54% of ARS have identifiable etiologic factors other than alcohol. In reducing order of frequency, these included: past head trauma (26%), idiopathic epilepsy (16%), cerebrovascular accident (6%), non-traumatic intracranial lesions (4%), toxic/metabolic causes (3%). Hillbom reported similar findings in an older study from Finland (12). Table 12-1 provides a list of differential diagnoses to consider in ARS.

Preexisting epilepsy may be exacerbated by alcohol abuse. Chronic alcoholism results in enhanced clearance of antiepileptic medications as well as erratic compliance and a lowering of seizure threshold during periods of partial or complete abstinence. Repeated episodes of alcohol withdrawal may lead to kindling of seizures (26, 27). Alcohol abusers have an increased risk for epilepsy. However, epileptic patients overall have a lower prevalence of

Table 12-1. Differential Diagnosis of Alcohol-Related Seizures.

Alcohol or sedative drug withdrawal

Noncompliance or inconsistent use of antiepileptic medications

Head trauma (acute or remote)

Idiopathic or cryptogenic epilepsy

Illicit drug toxicity (cocaine, amphetamines, opioids, phencyclidine, MDMA, etc.)

Medication toxicity (antidepressants, antipsychotics, anticholinergics, antimicrobials, isoniazid, propranolol, opioids, theophylline, lithium, lindane, etc.)

Cerebrovascular disease

Intracranial neoplasm

CNS infection (meningitis, encephalitis, abscess, HIV, neurosyphilis)

Metabolic disorders (hypoglycemia, electrolyte disturbances)

Table 12-2. Early Postictal (Within 72 h) Signs and Symptoms Associated with Epileptic Seizures and Alcohol Withdrawal Seizures (Modified from Ref (74)).

Symptoms or signs	Epileptic seizures	Alcohol withdrawal seizures
Level of consciousness	Postictal drowsiness-sleep	Agitation-delirium
Mood	Calm	Restlessness, hallucinations
Tremor	No	Yes
Sweating	No	Yes
Blood pressure	Normal	$\uparrow$
Heart rate	Normal	$\uparrow$
Temperature	Normal or slightly $\uparrow$	Fever
Arterial blood gasses	Normal or resolving metabolic acidosis	Respiratory alkalosis or mixed (with resolving metabolic acidosis)
EEG	Postictal slowing, in 50% with interictal epileptiform discharges	Normal, low amplitude
Alcohol withdrawal scales	Normal scores	Normal or $\uparrow$ scores

alcohol abuse, possibly due to warnings from doctors and pharmacists about the increased risk for seizures and medication toxicity (28). After a seizure, within the first 24–72 h, some characteristics of the patient may help the intensivist to differentiate between epileptic seizures vs. ARS (Table 12-2).

Noncompliance or irregular use of antiepileptic medications has been shown to be a common cause of seizures including status epilepticus in alcohol abusers (22, 29). It is therefore good practice in most cases not to prescribe chronic antiepileptic drugs to alcoholics, even if there is a known seizure focus. This will be discussed in more detail later.

Recreational drug use as well as the use of certain medications have also been associated with seizures and should be considered in the differential diagnosis in ARS. Alldredge et al. (30) identified 49 illicit drug induced seizures in 47 patients from 1975 to 1987. Cocaine was the most commonly implicated drug (32 cases), followed by amphetamine (11 cases), heroin (7 cases), and phencyclidine (4 cases). Most cases resulted in a single generalized tonic clonic seizure during acute intoxication, but 7 had multiple seizures and 2 entered status epilepticus. In more recent years, MDMA (ecstasy), gamma-hydroxybutyrate (GHB), GHB prodrugs, and ketamine have become popular drugs of abuse, particular at "rave" parties. MDMA and ketamine can cause seizures, whereas it is debated if GHB and its prodrugs cause true seizures in humans (31).

Iatrogenic seizures from prescribed medication use should also be considered in alcoholics. An exhaustive list of medications that may potentially cause seizures is not the scope of this chapter, as more complete lists may be found elsewhere [see Chap. Drugs and Critical Care Seizures of ref. (32)]. Some of the medications that should be considered in the differential diagnosis of seizures in the alcohol abuser are listed in Table 12-1. Too rapid a weaning of narcotics and sedative-hypnotics in patients with long-term (>7 days) ICU care can also result in withdrawal seizures (11, 33).

Alcohol abusers are at risk for cerebrovascular structural abnormalities that may result in epilepsy such as subarachnoid hemorrhage (34), intracerebral hemorrhage (35), and ischemic stroke (36). Although there are no randomized control trials of alcohol consumption and stroke, Reynolds et al. (37) recently conducted a meta-analysis of observational studies addressing this topic. They found that moderate alcohol consumption resulted in a reduced risk of ischemic stroke but heavy intake was associated with an elevated risk of ischemic and hemorrhagic (intracerebral and subarachnoid) stroke. They looked at habitual but not binge drinking. Other studies addressing the risk of binge drinking have also found an increased incidence of ischemic and hemorrhagic stroke (34–36). There are several pathophysiological mechanisms that may contribute to alcohol-related cerebrovascular accidents. Alcohol induced cerebral vasospasm and hypertension, erythrocyte and platelet aggregation, as well as changes in fibrinolytic activity, coagulation, and bleeding time have been implicated (34, 37, 38).

Head injury, whether remote or acute, is a common cofactor causing seizures in the alcoholic patient. In addition, alcohol withdrawal symptoms may mask symptoms of head trauma (9, 12). Cerebral atrophy frequently seen in chronic alcoholics predisposes them to intracranial hemorrhage (39). One must therefore evaluate the patient with ARS for signs of cranial trauma.

Alcohol-dependent patients may also be at increased risk for seizures due to concomitant CNS infections such as meningitis, abscesses, HIV and AIDS, and neurosyphilis (3, 40). Seizures, including status epilepticus are common in patients with HIV. This is caused by a direct effect of the virus on the CNS or due to focal lesions such as toxoplasmosis, lymphoma, cryptococcal meningitis, or infarction (41). Metabolic derangements, such as hypomagnesemia and renal dysfunction, seem to increase the risk of status epilepticus in HIV infected patients (42).

Although metabolic alterations are not common causes of seizures in the alcohol-dependent patient, they should be considered and treated. Hypoglycemia may cause seizures. However, alcohol associated hypoglycemia is rarely reported in alcoholics (43). Causes of hypoglycemia in the alcoholic patient include poor nutrition, hypothermia, inhibition of gluconeogenesis, and reduced cortisol levels (3). Hypomagnesemia can cause seizures but usually only at levels less than 0.8 mEq/L (32). Although chronic alcoholism is a common cause of hypomagnesemia (44), a randomized controlled trial of parenteral magnesium showed no significant difference in withdrawal symptoms, including ARS (45).

Profound hypophosphatemia may also accompany alcohol withdrawal and at levels less than 1 mg/dL may result in antiepileptic resistant generalized seizures (32). Hyponatremia may accompany alcoholism and should be corrected to levels greater than 120 mEq/L (32). Hyperventilation with associated respiratory alkalosis may also lower seizure threshold in alcoholics (46). Wernicke disease and the Korsakoff amnestic state, which are encountered almost exclusively in alcoholics in western countries, do not include seizures in the clinical presentation. They may, however, be associated with autonomic neuropathy and syncopal episodes that may be confused with seizures. In addition, the confusional state that ensues has to be differentiated from postictal confusional states.

12.3.1.1. Sample Case

A 60-year-old widow was brought to the emergency room after being found unresponsive by her daughter. En route to the ER she had three generalized tonic-clonic seizures, each lasting about 30 s. While in the ER she received intravenous lorazepam, a loading dose of fosphenytoin, and was admitted to the intensive care unit. Phenytoin was continued and lorazepam was used as needed for withdrawal symptoms.

Further history obtained from her daughter revealed that the patient had an extensive history of alcohol abuse, including prior admissions for alcohol-related seizures. The patient would spend what little money she had on alcohol and cigarettes, until she ran out. It was estimated that the patient stopped drinking 2–3 days prior to onset of her seizures due to lack of funds for buying alcohol. She also had a known AVM in the left frontal operculum and had been prescribed phenytoin for prior alcohol-related seizures but proved to be poorly compliant with her medications.

General examination was normal except for sinus tachycardia of 136 beats per minute. Neurologic examination found her to be unresponsive to voice and pain but without focal deficits on coma examination. Complete blood count, blood chemistries, hepatic panel, arterial blood gas, and urinalysis were obtained and were significant for an elevated MCV (104), hypokalemia (2.7), hypomagnesemia (1.4), and a urinary tract infection.

The patient had no more seizures during her hospital stay but on the second day of admission developed intermittent myoclonic jerking of the right upper and lower extremities. An urgent EEG was obtained and showed no electroencephalographic correlation to the movements. The EEG did show an absence of alpha rhythm and the presence of low amplitude fast activity throughout the recording (Fig. 12-1). The myoclonic activity was attributed to her alcohol withdrawal and urinary tract infection and she responded to valproic acid and low-dose clonazepam, as well as to the treatment of her infection. An MRI of the brain showed no change in her AVM. The patient had a slow return of her normal mental status over the following few days, with waxing and waning of confusion and disorientation. Neuropsychological evaluation determined that the patient was non-decisional and she was discharged in the care of her daughter.

12.3.2. Alcohol-Related Status Epilepticus

Although patients with ARS rarely enter status epilepticus (7, 12), alcohol withdrawal is a common contributing factor in many cases of status epilepticus (22, 29, 47). From 11 to 28% of cases of status epilepticus involve

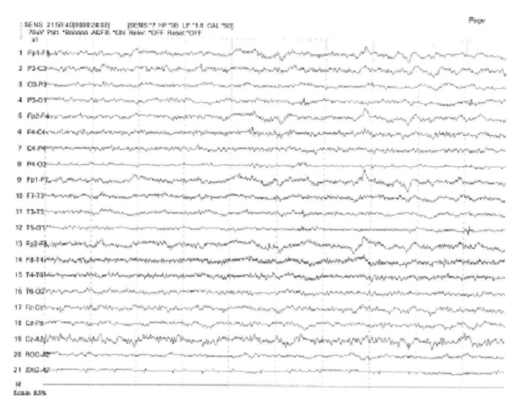

Fig. 12-1. An EEG of a 60 year old female alcoholic 1 day after a flurry of ARS and 3–4 days after her last drink. Note the absence of alpha rhythm and presence of low amplitude fast activity. The patient had a left frontal AVM but the EEG does not show evidence for this

alcohol abuse (22, 29, 47, 48). Indeed, in adult patients with no prior history of seizures, alcohol abuse was the single most common cause of status epilepticus in a study by Lowenstein and Alldredge (48). Alcohol is also occasionally implicated in nonconvulsive status epilepticus (49). Since about half of the cases of alcohol-related status epilepticus are multifactorial, a search for comorbid etiologies is necessary (22, 29). The comorbid conditions to consider in the differential diagnosis of status epilepticus in the chronic alcohol abuser are the same as those for ARS without status epilepticus (Table 12-1). Among all cases of status epilepticus in adults, discontinuation or irregular use of antiepileptics appears to be the most common etiologic factor (22, 48). Since alcoholics usually have erratic compliance with prescribed medications, antiepileptic withdrawal is a common comorbid factor in alcohol-related status epilepticus (29). Therefore, prescribing antiepileptic medications for chronic use in alcoholics may be undesirable, even if there is a seizure focus, unless the patient has proven himself to be compliant (50).

Alldredge et al. (47) found that the history of alcohol abuse in patients with alcohol-related status epilepticus did not differ from the histories of patients experiencing ARS without status epilepticus. The typical patient in each group was male, over 30 years old, with many years of heavy drinking (over 300 g ethanol daily). The status epilepticus group tended to be older and had fewer previous ARS. They also noted that alcohol-related status epilepticus was often the first presentation of ARS, occurring de novo in 44% of cases. Focal signs were noticed in 40% of alcohol-related status epilepticus cases, but they were not associated with focal CT scan or EEG findings. A lack of structural abnormalities in many cases of focal ARS has been reported by other authors (1, 22).

Treatment of alcohol-related status epilepticus is similar to that of other causes of status epilepticus. Detailed treatment of status epilepticus is covered elsewhere in this volume (see chapter Treatment of ICU Seizures and Status Epilepticus). Although phenytoin has been shown to be ineffective in preventing recurrent seizures within the vulnerable 6 h window following a common ARS *without* status epilepticus (51), it has been shown to be quite effective in treating ARS *with* status epilepticus. Alldredge et al. (47) controlled alcohol-related status epilepticus in about 67% of patients using phenytoin with or without diazepam. This was similar to their 60% response rate using phenytoin with or without diazepam to treat status epilepticus caused by other etiologies (48). Phenytoin and benzodiazepines are therefore part of the standard algorithm for treatment of alcohol-related status epilepticus (50, 52).

Some alcoholics may be taking isoniazid for tuberculosis prophylaxis or treatment. Isoniazid toxicity may cause seizures and status epilepticus by indirectly depleting GABA. Isoniazid binds with pyridoxine, which is needed in the synthesis of GABA. Seizures caused by isoniazid toxicity are resistant to phenytoin. If an alcohol-dependent patient who is known to also be taking isoniazid is experiencing refractory seizures, intravenous pyridoxine at an equivalent dose to the ingested isoniazid is given. If the dose of isoniazid is unknown, 5 g of pyridoxine is given (53, 54).

The prognosis in alcohol-related status epilepticus is generally favorable when compared to other causes of status epilepticus such as acute structural problems or metabolic disorders (48, 55). In one study (48), 90% of patients with alcohol-related status epilepticus had mild or no new neurologic deficits on discharge. These patients, however, tend to return to baseline slower than nonalcoholics, whether or not sedating medications were used, especially if there are abnormalities seen on the CT scan. About 89% of patients in one study had not returned to baseline consciousness 12 h after termination of alcohol-related status epilepticus (47). In general, a longer duration of status epilepticus results in a worse neurologic outcome (48).

12.4. Pathophysiology of Alcohol-Related Seizures

The precise pathophysiology of ARS has not been fully elucidated. It is generally accepted that abstinence or a partial reduction in alcohol intake is a key factor in the pathogenesis of ARS. Two separate research groups report that about one third of visits to the ER for ARS are on Monday. This pattern was not seen in patients who seize for reasons unrelated to alcohol. These observations support the assertion that ARS are due to withdrawal from alcohol, seizures being more frequent on Monday due to the relatively reduced availability and consumption on Sundays (12, 25). Although seizures may occur during intoxication and before alcohol levels reach zero (9, 12, 14, 15), most authors agree that ARS are primarily a withdrawal phenomenon (1, 9, 12, 22, 25, 29, 47, 48).

Although there is no known receptor for alcohol, it acts as a CNS depressant by affecting lipids and proteins in the neural membranes. Alcohol potentiates the postsynaptic effects on the GABA-A receptors in the brain, allowing chloride ion influx, resulting in a hyperpolarization of the membrane. This reduces the firing rate of the neuron, resulting in CNS sedation. The action on the excitatory NMDA receptor is just the opposite, thus causing an inhibitory effect on this receptor and further sedating the CNS (56). Ethanol also acts on non-NMDA calcium involved systems and well as serotonergic, dopaminergic, noradrenergic, opioid, and adenosinergic neural pathways (57, 58).

The genetics of ARS have only recently drawn attention. Several studies have tried to elucidate any genetic susceptibility for AES. The expression and alternative splicing of the obligatory NR1 subunit of the NMDA receptors is altered by alcohol exposure, emphasizing the involvement of the NR1 subunit, which is coded by the GRIN1 gene, in alcohol-mediated effects. In a recent study, the 2108A allele and A-containing genotypes of GRIN1 locus were over-represented in patients with a history of withdrawal-induced seizures when compared to healthy volunteers (59). Another study that examined the apolipoprotein E gene polymorphism reported a significant positive association between the ApoE3 allele group (as well as a significant negative association between the ApoE2 allele group) and a history of withdrawal seizures (60). More recently, French researchers genotyped the variable nucleotide tandem repeat of the gene and 7 single nucleotide polymorphisms encompassing the dopamine transporter (DAT1/SLC6A3) gene in a sample of 250 alcohol-dependent subjects, of whom 24% exhibited withdrawal seizures, taking into account the severity of alcohol dependence. They reported a significant role played by the 3' part of the DAT1 gene in alcohol withdrawal seizures of these alcohol-dependent patients (61).

In animal models a crucial role of the inferior colliculus has been demonstated in the initiation of audiogenic seizures (one of the models for evoking ARS in rodents). The role that this structure may play in humans is suggested by the absence of epileptiform activity in the EEG interictally (supporting the notion that these seizures are not generated in the neocortex) and the presence of abnormalities in auditory – evoked potentials (including increased latency of wave V, generated mainly by the inferior colliculus). It has also been shown that ethanol can modulate the activity of $GABA_A$ receptors, especially those containing the δ subunit. These are mostly located in the brain areas affected by alcohol intoxication (like the cerebellum, thalamic relay nuclei and the brainstem) and at the synaptic level, peri- or extrasynaptically. It has been postulated that during intense synaptic activity (such as during seizures), GABA spillover may activate these extrasynaptic receptors and induce a negative feedback to the neurons, which may explain the underlying anticonvulsant mechanism of ethanol (through potentiation of these receptors) (62). Additionally, chronic exposure to alcohol results in down regulation of the GABA-A receptors (as a result of decreases in the surface expression of α1 or γ2 subunits) (62), causing tolerance to alcohol-induced chloride ion influx (56). The NMDA receptor, on the other hand, undergoes up regulation due to chronic alcohol exposure (63). Certain areas of the brain appear to be more sensitive to the effects of chronic alcoholism (56). The increase in NMDA binding sites has been shown to occur experimentally in the hippocampus of rats (64). These changes presumably act as a compensatory mechanism for alcohol's sedating effect on the CNS. The relative excess of NMDA receptors and deficiency of GABA receptors in chronic alcoholism may result in enhanced neuroexcitation and reduced neuroinhibition. When the sedating influence of alcohol is lifted during abstinence, the result may be the rapid increase of the $\alpha4$ GABA$_A$ receptor subunits (which lead to decreased inhibitory function of the receptors) (62) and the onset of signs and symptoms of alcohol withdrawal, including ARS (63). Since benzodiazepines and barbiturates are also potentiating to the GABA-A receptor effects, they have cross-tolerance to alcohol and may alleviate the alcohol withdrawal signs and symptoms. The hypomagnesemia and zinc deficiency associated with chronic alcoholism may exacerbate the NMDA receptor mediated neurotoxicity because both magnesium and zinc are negative modulators of NMDA receptor function (63). However, magnesium supplementation does not reduce withdrawal severity or the likelihood of seizures or delirium (45). The clinical relevance of the deranged zinc metabolism is uncertain (65).

It is also hypothesized that ethanol withdrawal leads to permanent changes in the neurons, resulting in a process of kindling in which seizures become more frequent and severe with each subsequent episode of withdrawal (26, 27).

Elevated homocysteine and prolactin levels have been reported in alcoholics and may also play a role in alcohol withdrawal symptoms (66). In a recent study, 117 male patients suffering from alcohol dependency had homocysteine measured directly at admission and prolactin the morning following admission for detoxification treatment. There was a significant association for the combined assessment of both parameters and ARS, in both univariate and multivariate logistic regression analysis. The authors concluded that the combination of both, homocysteine and prolactin, may help to assess the individual risk of alcohol withdrawal seizures in clinical practice (67). Homocysteine may be metabolized into excitatory amino acids. These amino acids, as well as homocysteine itself, can act as agonists at the NMDA receptor, resulting in increased excitatory postsynaptic potentials (68, 69). The hyperhomocysteinemia may therefore lead to a relative excess of excitatory neurotransmitters compared to neuroinhibitory transmitters in the hippocampus (70), resulting in homocysteine-induced ARS.

12.5. Comorbid Medical Conditions

It is not the goal of this chapter to provide a comprehensive discussion of the many complicating medical problems that may occur in a withdrawing patient. It is useful however to mention some of the more common as well as dangerous conditions seen in these patients in the ICU. An estimated 71% of detoxifying patients have physical morbidity, primarily hepatic abnormalities, trauma, and infections (4). Gastrointestinal disease, anemia, and malnutrition are also well known complications (71). Additional drug use is common in alcohol abusers, particularly benzodiazepines. In one study, more than 41% of alcohol-dependent patients were abusing other drugs (16). As mentioned earlier in this chapter, polysubstance abuse may delay the onset of ARS. Trauma is also common in alcoholism. An estimated 50–60% of trauma patients are chronic alcoholics, and withdrawal may cause significant morbidity following trauma or surgery (72). Thiamine deficiency is relatively common, occurring in 30%

of chronic alcoholics, although the Wernicke–Korsakoff syndrome occurs in only 3–10% (7). Fluid and electrolyte abnormalities as well as hypoglycemia may also occur in the alcoholic and are discussed elsewhere in this chapter. Coma in the alcohol-dependent ICU patient may be caused by several conditions, including acute alcohol poisoning, concomitant drug overdose, head trauma, hepatic failure, intracranial hemorrhage, hypoxic encephalopathy, hypoglycemia, meningitis, hypothermia, alcoholic ketoacidosis, nonconvulsive status epilepticus, and methanol or ethylene glycol poisoning (6, 49).

12.6. Evaluation

When evaluating an alcohol-dependent patient who presents with a seizure, the physician should search for causes other than alcohol that may result in seizure activity. In particular, one must be careful not to overlook life-threatening conditions such as intracranial hemorrhage, hypoglycemia, CNS infection, and metabolic derangements. Differential diagnoses to consider are listed in Table 12-1. The management of new onset ARS consists of history, repeated physical examinations, CT scan or MRI, laboratory testing, and EEG.

A history should be obtained, if possible, from the patient, family, friends or emergency personnel. Details should include past medical history, any history of prior seizures, drinking history including any episodes of delirium tremens, when and why drinking was stopped, recent or remote serious head trauma, medications, and any medication compliance problems.

Physical examination should include a careful assessment for focal signs, level of consciousness, head trauma, signs of intracranial hypertension or herniation, signs of delirium tremens, as well general physical examination to evaluate for hepatic failure, coagulopathy, needle tracks, and other comorbid conditions (Table 12-3). Repeated neurologic examinations may help reveal

Table 12-3. Comorbid Medical Conditions in the Alcohol-Dependent Patient.[a]

Cardiovascular

Hypertension, hypotension, dilated cardiomyopathy, atrial and ventricular arrhythmias

Gastrointestinal

Pancreatitis, gastritis, esophageal varices, GI bleeding, alcoholic hepatitis, cirrhosis, liver failure

Neurologic

Wernicke–Korsakoff syndrome, epilepsy, meningitis, head trauma, meningitis, ischemic or hemorrhagic stroke, peripheral neuropathy, cerebellar degeneration

Hematologic

Anemia, leukopenia, thrombocytopenia, coagulopathy

Infectious

Meningitis, pneumonia, cellulitis, spontaneous bacterial peritonitis, HIV

Metabolic

Hypoglycemia, electrolyte disturbances, concurrent drug ingestion or withdrawal, nutritional deficiencies, alcoholic ketoacidosis, acute alcohol poisoning, methanol or ethylene glycol poisoning

Miscellaneous

Rhabdomyolysis (due to alcohol toxicity, hypokalemia, hypophosphatemia), trauma, hypothermia, poor wound healing, cancer

[a]Adapted from ref. (6, 13, 74).

declining mental status or the development of focal signs which would necessitate an urgent CT scan.

The selection of laboratory tests will depend on individual indications. The intensivist should consider obtaining a complete blood count, glucose, electrolytes, BUN, creatinine, prothrombin time, anticonvulsant levels, calcium, magnesium, phosphorus, serum or urine toxicology, alcohol level, and blood gas (3). Carbohydrate-deficient transferrin and gammaglutamyl transferase have been used as sensitive markers for alcohol overuse, but alone or in combination show poor accuracy in screening for ARS (73). Cervical spine precautions (Aspen or Philadelphia collars) and films should be considered if there is suspicion for a fall or head injury. A chest X-ray should be ordered in the patient with fever or pulmonary symptoms or signs. A lumbar puncture should be performed after the CT scan if there is any suspicion for meningitis. Evaluation for other comorbid conditions seen in the alcoholic should also be considered, depending on the clinical scenario (Table 12-3).

All new onset ARS patients require an emergent non-contrasted CT scan, regardless of whether the seizure was focal or generalized. Alcohol-related seizures may be focal or generalized and the focal seizures may or may not be related to underlying focal pathology (1, 12). Ernest et al. (75) found that in patients with a first time ARS but no other signs of major intracranial pathology, the CT scan disclosed a clinically significant intracranial process in 6.2% of patients. Of these CT-positive patients, 44% were alert, had no focal signs, and no signs of trauma. They concluded that history or signs of minor head trauma, headache, level of consciousness, or minor focal neurologic signs were not significantly associated with intracranial lesions (positive CT) when tested statistically. In slight contrast, Feussner et al. (76) studied the value of CT scan in ARS and concluded that a careful neurologic examination adequately determines which patients need a prompt CT scan. An emergent CT scan is not necessary in the patient with a documented history of focal ARS, provided the prior workup included brain imaging, the seizure had identical presentation, there are no new focal neurologic findings, there is no indication of recent head injury, and there is prompt return to baseline (50).

An EEG should also be obtained on all patients with new onset ARS. It may be ordered non-urgently, perhaps at follow-up. The aim is to identify those patients with an underlying seizure focus, which may necessitate long-term treatment with antiepileptic medications, provided they can be compliant. An abnormal interictal EEG suggests underlying epilepsy or a symptomatic focus unrelated to ARS (17). For the patient admitted to the intensive care unit, an EEG may be necessary in the management of convulsive or nonconvulsive status epilepticus, or to help differentiate delirium tremens from other causes of clouded sensorium (6, 9).

12.7. Treatment

The treatment of single or recurrent ARS is essentially the same as the treatment of the alcohol withdrawal syndrome itself (77). The pharmaceutical management of alcohol withdrawal requires the use of benzodiazepines, often with the addition of other classes of medications. Although most of these adjunctive medications don't prevent or treat seizures, they help relieve many of the other manifestations of the syndrome. This combined approach allows

Table 12.4. Criteria for Hospital Admission.[a]

New onset seizure in the chronic alcohol abuser

Recurrent seizures[b]

Moderate to severe alcohol withdrawal[b]

Comorbid illness requiring treatment (infection, arrhythmia, liver failure, dehydration, etc.) [b]

History of severe alcohol withdrawal

Fever >38.5

Wernicke's encephalopathy

Recent head injury with loss of consciousness[b]

Concurrent sedative ingestion[b]

[a] Adapted from ref. (50, 77, 78).
[b] Relative reasons for ICU admission.

lower overall doses of individual medications. The physician must also keep in mind that alcohol ingestion alters the clearance of hepatically metabolized medications, including certain antiepileptic medications. Short-term ingestion causes a reduction in clearance of many drugs, while alcohol is in the body, whereas there is increased clearance of drugs when alcohol is eliminated from the body in a chronic alcoholic. This potential effect on drug metabolism is important in drugs with a narrow therapeutic range such as phenytoin, and less important in medications with a wide therapeutic range, such as diazepam (7). Comorbid medical conditions are not infrequent in the alcohol-dependent patient and should also be considered (Table 12-3). The decision to admit a patient to the hospital for an ARS depends on several factors (Table 12-4). If it is the patient's first ARS, he should be admitted to facilitate the workup of new onset seizures. Alcohol-dependent patients often fail to comply with outpatient follow-up.

Recently, guidelines for treating ARS have been published by the European Federation of Neurological Societies Task Force (73).

12.7.1. Supportive Care

Management of the seizing alcohol-dependent patient involves stabilizing the patient with attention to airway, breathing, and circulation. A quiet, non-stimulating environment is ideal and the use of physical restraint should be kept to a minimum to help prevent worsening the agitation. It may be necessary to intubate the patient in the ICU and monitor with continuous EKG and pulse oximetry. An IV line should be established and the patient given thiamine 100 mg to reverse or prevent Wernicke's syndrome. This should be given prior to any therapy that involves glucose, to prevent further depletion of thiamine with resultant precipitation of Wernicke's syndrome. Duration of thiamine therapy is controversial, but some clinicians continue this dose for 3 days (2). Finger-stick glucose levels should be determined and IV glucose given if necessary. However, one should avoid excess glucose unnecessarily, as hyperglycemia may worsen neurologic injury in cerebral ischemia (79, 80). Intravenous glucose therapy may also cause substantial falls in serum potassium and phosphate levels (65).

The role of magnesium in seizures is controversial (44). It is a common practice to replace the magnesium deficit in chronic alcoholic patients. Magnesium sulfate given in a dose of 1 gram im or iv every 6–12 h for 48 h is one protocol. Alternatively, magnesium oxide may be given orally in a dose of 250–500 mg four times daily for 48 h, although diarrhea may occur (6). Hypocalcemia, hypokalemia, and hypophosphatemia may be associated with hypomagnesemia. Correction of the magnesium deficit helps in their resolution (44, 65). As discussed above, however, magnesium supplementation does not appear to alter withdrawal symptoms (45). Magnesium administration in patients with renal failure should be undertaken cautiously.

Hypokalemia in the alcoholic may be due to inadequate intake, diarrhea, vomiting, secondary hyperaldosteronism, magnesium depletion, or shifting of the potassium into the cells as a result of alkalosis or intravenous glucose therapy. The serum potassium concentration corresponds poorly to total potassium balance and potassium requirements may be massive (65). Hypokalemia has been suggested as a factor in the genesis of delirium tremens. However, potassium supplementation alone will not reverse delirium (6).

Withdrawing patients may also have hyponatremia as well as overhydration or dehydration. Each should be gently corrected. The patient's need for fluid and electrolytes depends on losses. Without significant gastrointestinal fluid losses, one should not assume the withdrawing patient is dehydrated. However, patients in severe withdrawal may have extensive fluid replacement needs due to hyperthermia, diaphoresis, and vomiting. If renal function is normal, a urine specific gravity of 1.025 and a urine sodium concentration of less than 10 mEq/L is an indication of volume depletion. Daily weights, and orthostatic blood pressure and pulse can also help determine fluid status. If serum sodium is normal, volume deficits are best corrected with 5% dextrose in normal saline. Hyponatremia may be due to overhydration from excessive ADH secretion or due to volume contraction from fluid losses, so replacement fluid type should be selected accordingly. In most cases, normal saline is the appropriate treatment instead of fluid restriction because these patients tend to have volume contraction. Sodium level should be corrected at least to 120 mEq/L but the rate of correction is controversial. Central pontine myelinolysis has been reported with rapid correction (2, 4, 6, 7, 32, 81).

As mentioned earlier, hypophosphatemia may occur in alcohol abusers and is a possible cause for seizures (32). Other problems that may occur with very low levels include bone pain, stiffness, weakness, loss of appetite, intention tremors, rhabdomyolysis, acute hemolysis, acute respiratory failure, and cardiac failure (2, 6). Therapy should be initiated if the serum phosphate concentration is <2.5 mg/dL. Supplementation may be by mouth or IV, starting at 20–40 mmol sodium or potassium phosphate. Caution must be exercised in renal failure and phosphate should not be given if renal failure is due to rhabdomyolysis because the damaged muscle will release phosphorus. Other contraindications to phosphate use are hypercalcemia and hypoparathyroidism (65).

Hypocalcemia in the alcoholic is usually the result of a metabolic disturbance such as hyperphosphatemia, hypomagnesemia, or some other cause of functional hypoparathyroidism. Calcium replacement is not recommended except in the treatment of hyperkalemic or hypocalcemic arrhythmias, tetany, hypocalcemic convulsions, or magnesium therapy overdose (44, 65). The metabolic disturbance causing the hypocalcemia must be treated (65).

The withdrawing alcoholic should be evaluated for acid–base derangements and managed appropriately. Acute alcohol ingestion produces a rise in urinary excretion of ammonium and titratable acid but the immediate effects are clinically inconsequential. Chronic alcohol abuse produces various acid-base abnormalities that are secondary effects of alcohol and not directly caused by the alcohol itself. Respiratory acidosis may be seen due to the respiratory depressant effects of alcohol. Metabolic acidosis in the alcoholic may be due to alcoholic ketoacidosis, methanol, or ethylene glycol poisoning. Severe lactic acidosis (lactate level 31 mmol/L, pH 6.82) has also been reported and may be due to muscle relative hypoxia during convulsions (type A) or impaired liver or renal clearance (Type B) due to thiamine deficiency (82). It may also be the result of bicarbonate loss in the stool due to the use of lactulose. Type 1, type 2, or a mixed form of renal tubular acidosis may also occur due to protein or phosphate deficiencies, or the development of cirrhosis. Patients often hyperventilate during alcohol withdrawal. This leads to respiratory alkalosis, hypokalemia, hypomagnesemia, hypophosphatemia and compensatory secondary hyperchloremic acidosis. Metabolic alkalosis may occur due to emesis (6, 65).

If meningitis is suspected, blood cultures should be obtained and empiric antibiotics given without delay. If a lumbar puncture is performed within 1–2 h after giving the antibiotics, the CSF cultures will remain positive in the majority of patients (83).

12.7.2. Benzodiazepines

The mainstay of treatment of alcohol withdrawal and ARS is benzodiazepines. Since it is not possible to predict which patients will have recurrent seizures, benzodiazepines should be administered to all patients presenting with ARS (23, 25). They have largely replaced other sedative medications such as chloral hydrate, paraldehyde, and barbiturates. Benzodiazepines act on the GABA receptors and are cross-tolerant to alcohol, effectively relieving the signs and symptoms of alcohol withdrawal. They have less respiratory and cardiac depressant effects than other CNS depressants (50). They are widely used in the neurological intensive care unit for their anxiolytic, amnestic, and anticonvulsive properties and have the potential advantage of decreasing cerebral metabolism and ICP (84). However, based on the fact that abrupt stop of alcohol consumption can lead to up-regulation of $GABA_A$ receptors with the $\alpha4$ subunit (which are benzodiazepine-insensitive, see above), benzodiazepines are expected to have only a modest effectiveness in ARS. Other medications, such as chlormethiazole (not available in the US), with more effect in $GABA_A$ receptors with the $\alpha4$ subunit, may be a better choice (62).

Several types of benzodiazepines have been used successfully in alcohol withdrawal. All are effective in controlling the signs and symptoms of alcohol withdrawal, but the longer acting ones appear better at controlling seizures (85). Although there does not appear to be one benzodiazepine with clear superiority in the treatment of alcohol withdrawal, lorazepam has some advantages in that it has an intermediate half-life, hepatic metabolism with non-active metabolites, and can be administered by mouth, IM, or IV (50). The low lipophilic properties of lorazepam allow it to remain in the serum longer, providing an anticonvulsant effect of 6–12 h, making it an ideal medication in the treatment of ARS (86).

The goal of using benzodiazepines is to give enough to keep the patient calm but awake. One protocol is to use lorazepam IV in a dose of 0.5–4.0 mg, depending on the severity of withdrawal. The dose can be repeated at 15–30 min intervals for patients in severe withdrawal, who should be observed in the ICU (2, 50). For moderate withdrawal, an oral dosing schedule may be used, giving lorazepam 6–7 mg/day in 3 divided doses, tapering to 1–2 mg/day over 4 days (50). Another approach is to give diazepam 5 mg IV every 5 min until the patient is calm (6). Short acting midazolam at an infusion rate of 20–75 mg/h has also been used and may be considered for critically ill patients (50, 87, 88). Abrupt discontinuation of benzodiazepines should be avoided to prevent benzodiazepine withdrawal seizures.

Although fixed-schedule dosing of benzodiazepines is safe and effective in the treatment of alcohol withdrawal, symptom-triggered therapy has been shown to as effective but require less medication and shorter hospital stays (85). This requires the use of a structural assessment scale, such as the Clinical Institute Withdrawal Assessment for Alcohol, revised (CIWA-Ar) scale for the monitoring of signs and symptoms. Although it is possible that symptom-triggered therapy alone may be adequate to prevent ARS (85), it is still recommended to treat all patients presenting with an ARS with benzodiazepines as soon as possible to prevent recurrence (78).

If the patient enters delirium tremens, massive amounts of benzodiazepines may be required in the ICU. Diazepam in doses of 2,640 mg in the first 48 h of treatment has been reported (89). Trauma patients experiencing withdrawal often require much larger doses than non-trauma patients to control signs and symptoms of withdrawal (72). When very large doses of benzodiazepines are used, the patient must be watched closely for respiratory depression. Likewise, if the patient has high levels of serum alcohol, the addition of a benzodiazepine may result in respiratory depression (78).

12.7.3. Antiepileptic Medications

Carbamazepine has been used successfully to treat mild to moderate alcohol withdrawal symptoms and has been used widely in Europe for this purpose (85, 90). Valproate is available in IV formulation, can be used in status epilepticus and in mice has been shown to confer protection against ARS. Data about its use either as treatment or prophylactically in ARS in humans are limited (62). Gabapentin may also show some benefit in mild to moderate withdrawal (91). In a study from Austria, gabapentin was administered in 3 doses of 300 mg daily in 30 patients with ARS for up 30 days with good results (92). The same group also used topiramate (50 mg twice/day for up to 30 days) with good results in 12 patients with ARS (93). Pregabalin, a novel lipophilic analog of GABA, was shown to reduced severity of handling-induced convulsions (a sensitive and reliable index of CNS hyperexcitability associated with ethanol withdrawal) in comparison to vehicle-treated mice. Similarly, pregabalin reduced the frequency in which EEG activity was interrupted by trains of high-voltage synchronous activity in a dose-related fashion and was effective in blocking the development of withdrawal sensitization observed in these mice. Although its use has not been reported in humans with ARS and its mechanism of action is not clear (not through GABA, but through binding to the alpha-2-delta regulatory subunit of voltage-gated calcium channels), it has a potential, because of its lack of hepatic metabolism and protein plasma binding (which may be impaired in alcoholics) (94). There is less data supporting the use of antiepileptic medications in the treatment of ARS or delirium (85). A placebo controlled, double-blinded study by Hillbom et al. did not find carbamazepine or valproic acid to be useful in treating alcohol withdrawal seizures (95).

Prophylactic antiepileptic treatment with phenytoin has not been effective in reducing primary ARS. In a randomized study of 831 patients who were admitted to a detoxification unit, phenytoin treated patients had more seizures (3%) than clorazepate treated patients (0.7%) and fewer than placebo treated patients (6.2%) during the first 96 h period (96). Although phenytoin has been shown to be effective in alcohol-related status epilepticus (47), it has been shown to be ineffective at preventing recurrent ARS within the vulnerable 6 h period following the initial ARS (51, 97, 98). In addition, IV phenytoin administration carries the risk of hypotension, arrhythmia, and cardiac arrest, and chronic oral phenytoin has several long-term consequences (99). Prescribing antiepileptic medications for chronic use in an alcoholic may have adverse consequences. Poor compliance with erratic use of antiepileptic medication results in an increase in seizure frequency due to withdrawal and possibly a kindling effect (100). In addition, antiepileptic withdrawal is a common cause of status epilepticus (22, 48). Therefore prescribing phenytoin to a patient with a known seizure focus but erratic compliance should be discouraged (50).

On the other hand, phenytoin may be used in ARS if the patient with a known seizure focus, who is normally compliant, presents with a subtherapeutic level. An intravenous loading dose of phenytoin may be administered in such cases. An oral loading dose of phenytoin can be given but would not reach a therapeutic level until the vulnerable 6 h period has passed, so iv loading is preferred (50). For those epilepsy patients who are on antiepileptic medication and abuse alcohol, abstinence or tapering of alcohol intake may result in an increased risk of seizures due to increased antiepileptic drug metabolism because of a relative lack of competing substrate (28). Therefore antiepileptic drug levels must be monitored when the patient stops drinking.

Phenytoin may also be used to treat suspected trauma induced seizures in an intoxicated or withdrawing patient during the acute phase of injury (50). Temkin et al. demonstrated that phenytoin significantly reduces seizures during the first week following head injury but did not reduce late seizures (101).

Finally, phenytoin is indicated in alcohol-related status epilepticus, as discussed above (47). Fosphenytoin, the intravenous water soluble phosphate ester of phenytoin, is safer and can be used in place of phenytoin IV. Unlike phenytoin, it may also be given intramuscularly (99).

12.7.4. Antihypertensive Agents

Antihypertensive medications can be used to treat the hyperadrenergic manifestations of alcohol withdrawal such as hypertension, tachycardia, and tremors. Clonidine has been shown to be effective in treating mild alcohol withdrawal signs and symptoms but not ARS (85, 102). Clonidine may also alleviate anxiety, diaphoresis, and insomnia associated with withdrawal (7, 102). Beta-blockers such as propranolol and atenolol may also be considered as adjunctive medications in alcohol withdrawal, but similar to clonidine, they cannot be expected to treat or prevent seizures, limiting their role in ARS. Furthermore, beta-blockers may cause delirium or mask the diagnosis of delirium tremens and have other contraindications such as hypotension, congestive heart failure, insulin dependent diabetes, and asthma or bronchospasm (50, 103).

12.7.5. Haloperidol

Haloperidol, which can be given IV, IM, and orally, is a useful adjunct in patients requiring large doses of benzodiazepines for the treatment of major alcohol withdrawal or delirium tremens in the ICU. Very high doses have been used safely in patients with serious underlying disease such as 240 mg haloperidol and 480 mg of lorazepam in 24 h (104). Haloperidol, unlike the phenothiazines, does not appear to cause seizures in humans (50, 85). No randomized studies of its use in ARS are available. Its use should be limited to an ICU setting because of the risk for respiratory depression and hypotension. Those patients treated with high IV doses of haloperidol need daily electrocardiograms and continuous EKG monitoring in an ICU to avoid widening of the QRS complex and the risk of torsades. Magnesium level should be monitored and kept at the high normal range.

12.7.6. Propofol

Propofol interacts at the GABA mediated receptor but not through the benzodiazepine site (105). It has been used to control refractory delirium tremens (106) as well as refractory status epilepticus (52). It has been reported to rarely cause seizures in high doses by an unknown mechanism (106).

12.7.7. Barbiturates

Phenobarbital is cross-tolerant with alcohol, is an extremely effective anticonvulsant, and is effective in controlling alcohol withdrawal. However, disadvantages such as hepatic enzyme induction and risk of respiratory suppression, make its use in the United States uncommon (13). However, in an ICU setting, it can be a useful adjunct to refractory seizures or status epilepticus.

12.7.8. Intravenous Alcohol

There are no controlled trials evaluating the use of ethanol in alcohol withdrawal. It is expensive to prepare, requires frequent monitoring, has a narrow therapeutic index, and has multiple medical side effects. Routine use cannot be recommended (7, 13).

12.7.9. Alcohol-Related Status Epilepticus

As mentioned above, although phenytoin is not useful in preventing recurrent ARS, it has been shown to be useful in treating alcohol-related status epilepticus (47). Alcohol-related status epilepticus is treated like other forms of status epilepticus (benzodiazepines and phenytoin, etc.) and generally responds well to standard treatments (47, 48, 77, 107). See above for further discussion, and the chapter on Treatment of ICU Seizures and Status Epilepticus.

12.7.10. Outpatient Treatment

Outpatient treatment of ARS may be considered if the patient meets several criteria. The patient must have a known history of prior ARS, and after a 6 h observation period he must be fully awake and ambulatory, without recurrent seizures or signs of moderate to severe withdrawal, have normal vital signs, and normal laboratory values (78). Other causes of seizure must ruled out by history, physical examination, and/or diagnostic tests. Patients with concomitant sedative abuse should be considered for admission since withdrawal seizures are delayed in these individuals (77). Further criteria precluding outpatient treatment are listed in Table 12.4. During the observation period, a test dose of 1–2 mg of lorazepam, 10–20 mg of diazepam, or 50–100 mg of chlordiazepoxide can be given orally. The outpatient dosing schedule depends on the severity of symptoms. One outpatient protocol consists of Lorazepam 1–2 mg three times per day, tapering over 3–6 days. This is just a guideline and the treatment should be individualized (50). Close follow-up should be arranged. Ideally the patient will be discharged home with a close family member or nonalcoholic friend to help the patient abstain, take his medications properly, eat properly, and attend follow-up appointments. Admission to a detoxification or rehabilitation unit should be considered if a safe disposition is not otherwise possible.

References

1. Earnest MP, Yarnell PR (1976) Seizure admissions to a city hospital: the role of alcohol. Epilepsia 17(4):387–393
2. Holloway HC, Hales RE, Watanabe HK (1984) Recognition and treatment of acute alcohol withdrawal syndromes. Psychiatr Clin North Am 7(4):729–743
3. Freedland ES, McMicken DB (1993) Alcohol-related seizures, Part I: Pathophysiology, differential diagnosis and evaluation. J Emerg Med 11(4):463–473
4. Yost DA (1996) Alcohol withdrawal syndrome. Am Fam Physician 54(2): 657–664, 669. Erratum in: Am Fam Physician 54(8):2377
5. Victor M, Adams RD (1953) The effect of alcohol on the nervous system. Res Publ Assoc Nerv Ment Dis 32:526–573
6. Turner RC, Lichstein PR, Peden JG Jr, Busher JT, Waivers LE (1989) Alcohol withdrawal syndromes: a review of pathophysiology, clinical presentation, and treatment. J Gen Intern Med 4(5):432–444
7. Guthrie SK (1989) The treatment of alcohol withdrawal. Pharmacotherapy 9(3):131–143
8. Chick J (1989) Delirium tremens. BMJ 298:3–4
9. Victor M, Brausch C (1967) The role of abstinence in the genesis of alcoholic epilepsy. Epilepsia 8(1):1–20
10. Wikler A, Pescor FT, Fraser HF, Isbell H (1956) Electroencephalographic changes associated with chronic alcoholic intoxication and the alcohol abstinence syndrome. Am J Psychiatry 113(2):106–114
11. Jenkins DH (2000) Substance abuse and withdrawal in the intensive care unit. Contemporary issues. Surg Clin North Am 80(3):1033–1053
12. Hillbom ME (1980) Occurrence of cerebral seizures provoked by alcohol abuse. Epilepsia 21(5):459–466
13. Chang PH, Steinberg MB (2001) Alcohol withdrawal. Med Clin North Am 85(5):1191–1212
14. Hauser WA, Ng SK, Brust JC (1988) Alcohol, seizures, and epilepsy. Epilepsia 29(Suppl 2):S66–S78
15. Yamane H, Katoh N (1981) Alcoholic epilepsy. A definition and a description of other convulsions related to alcoholism. Eur Neurol 20(1):17–24

16. Soyka M, Lutz W, Kauert G, Schwartz A (1989) Epileptic seizures and alcohol withdrawal: significance of additional use (and abuse). J Epilepsy 2(2):109–113

17. Sand T, Brathen G, Michler R, Brodtkorb E, Helde G, Bovim G (2002) Clinical utility of EEG in alcohol-related seizures. Acta Neurol Scand 105(1):18–24

18. Lechtenberg R, Worner TM (1990) Seizure risk with recurrent alcohol detoxification. Arch Neurol 47(5):535–538

19. Morton WA, Laird LK, Crane DF, Partovi N, Frye LH (1994) A prediction model for identifying alcohol withdrawal seizures. Am J Drug Alcohol Abuse 20(1):75–86

20. Essardas Daryanani H, Santolaria FJ, Gonzalez Reimers E, Jorge JA, Batista Lopez N, Martin Hernandez F, Martinez Riera A, Rodriguez Rodriguez E (1994) Alcoholic withdrawal syndrome and seizures. Alcohol Alcohol 29(3):323–328. Erratum in: 29(5):323–328

21. Foy A, March S, Drinkwater V (1988) Use of an objective clinical scale in the assessment and management of alcohol withdrawal in a large general hospital. Alcohol Clin Exp Res 12(3):360–364

22. Aminoff MJ, Simon RP (1980) Status epilepticus. Causes, clinical features and consequences in 98 patients. Am J Med 69(5):657–666

23. Rathlev NK, Ulrich A, Fish SS, D'Onofrio G (2000) Clinical characteristics as predictors of recurrent alcohol-related seizures. Acad Emerg Med 7(8):886–891

24. Varelas PN, Mirski MA (2001) Seizures in the adult intensive care unit. J Neurosurg Anesthesiol 13(2):163–175

25. Rathlev NK, Ulrich A, Shieh TC, Callum MG, Bernstein E, D'Onofrio G (2002) Etiology and weekly occurrence of alcohol-related seizures. Acad Emerg Med 9(8):824–828

26. Ballenger JC, Post RM (1978) Kindling as a model for alcohol withdrawal syndromes. Br J Psychiatry 133:1–14

27. Booth BM, Blow FC (1993) The kindling hypothesis: further evidence from a U.S. national study of alcoholic men. Alcohol Alcohol 28(5):593–598

28. Gordon E, Devinsky O (2001) Alcohol and marijuana: effects on epilepsy and use by patients with epilepsy. Epilepsia 42(10):1266–1272

29. Pilke A, Partinen M, Kovanen J (1984) Status epilepticus and alcohol abuse: an analysis of 82 status epilepticus admissions. Acta Neurol Scand 70(6):443–450

30. Alldredge BK, Lowenstein DH, Simon RP (1989) Seizures associated with recreational drug abuse. Neurology 39(8):1037–1039

31. Graeme KA (2000) New drugs of abuse. Emerg Med Clin North Am 18(4):625–636

32. Eisenschenk S, Gilmore R (2001) Seizures associated with non-neurological medical conditions. In: Wyllie E (ed) The treatment of epilepsy: principals and Practice, 3rd edn. Lippincott Williams and Wilkins, Philadelphia, pp 657–669

33. Wijdicks EF, Sharbrough FW (1993) New-onset seizures in critically ill patients. Neurology 43(5):1042–1044

34. Hillbom M, Kaste M, Rasi V (1983) Can ethanol intoxication affect hemocoagulation to increase the risk of brain infarction in young adults? Neurology 33(3):381–384

35. Juvela S, Hillbom M, Palomaki H (1995) Risk factors for spontaneous intracerebral hemorrhage. Stroke 26(9):1558–1564

36. Hillbom M, Numminen H, Juvela S (1999) Recent heavy drinking of alcohol and embolic stroke. Stroke 30(11):2307–2312

37. Reynolds K, Lewis B, Nolen JD, Kinney GL, Sathya B, He J (2003) Alcohol consumption and risk of stroke: a meta-analysis. JAMA 289(5):579–588. Erratum in: 289(21):2798

38. Larkin EC, Watson-Williams EJ (1984) Alcohol and the blood. Med Clin North Am 68(1):105–120

39. Pfefferbaum A, Rosenbloom M, Crusan K, Jernigan TL (1988) Brain CT changes in alcoholics: effects of age and alcohol consumption. Alcohol Clin Exp Res 12(1):81–87

40. Hegde A, Veis JH, Seidman A, Khan S, Moore J Jr (2000) High prevalence of alcoholism in dialysis patients. Am J Kidney Dis 35(6):1039–1043

41. Wong MC, Suite ND, Labar DR (1990) Seizures in human immunodeficiency virus infection. Arch Neurol 47(6):640–642

42. Van Paesschen W, Bodian C, Maker H (1995) Metabolic abnormalities and new-onset seizures in human immunodeficiency virus-seropositive patients. Epilepsia 36(2):146–150

43. Sucov A, Woolard RH (1995) Ethanol-associated hypoglycemia is uncommon. Acad Emerg Med 2(3):185–189

44. Graber TW, Yee AS, Baker FJ (1981) Magnesium: physiology, clinical disorders, and therapy. Ann Emerg Med 10(1):49–57

45. Wilson A, Vulcano B (1984) A double-blind, placebo-controlled trial of magnesium sulfate in the ethanol withdrawal syndrome. Alcohol Clin Exp Res 8(6):542–545

46. Victor M (1973) The role of hypomagnesemia and respiratory alkalosis in the genesis of alcohol-withdrawal symptoms. Ann N Y Acad Sci 215:235–248

47. Alldredge BK, Lowenstein DH (1993) Status epilepticus related to alcohol abuse. Epilepsia 34(6):1033–1037

48. Lowenstein DH, Alldredge BK (1993) Status epilepticus at an urban public hospital in the 1980s. Neurology 43(3 Pt 1):483–488

49. Towne AR, Waterhouse EJ, Boggs JG, Garnett LK, Brown AJ, Smith JR Jr, DeLorenzo RJ (2000) Prevalence of nonconvulsive status epilepticus in comatose patients. Neurology 54(2):340–345

50. Freedland ES, McMicken DB (1993) Alcohol-related seizures, Part II: Clinical presentation and management. J Emerg Med 11(5):605–618

51. Alldredge BK, Lowenstein DH, Simon RP (1989) Placebo-controlled trial of intravenous diphenylhydantoin for short-term treatment of alcohol withdrawal seizures. Am J Med 87(6):645–648

52. Lowenstein DH, Alldredge BK (1998) Status epilepticus. N Engl J Med 338(14):970–976

53. Delanty N, Vaughan CJ, French JA (1998) Medical causes of seizures. Lancet 352(9125):383–390

54. Wason S, Lacouture PG, Lovejoy FH Jr (1981) Single high-dose pyridoxine treatment for isoniazid overdose. JAMA 246(10):1102–1104

55. Towne AR, Pellock JM, Ko D, DeLorenzo RJ (1994) Determinants of mortality in status epilepticus. Epilepsia 35(1):27–34

56. Olmedo R, Hoffman RS (2000) Withdrawal syndromes. Emerg Med Clin North Am 18(2):273–288

57. Veatch LM, Gonzalez LP (2000) Nifedipine alleviates alterations in hippocampal kindling after repeated ethanol withdrawal. Alcohol Clin Exp Res 24(4):484–491

58. Nutt DJ, Peters TJ (1994) Alcohol: the drug. Br Med Bull 50(1):5–17

59. Rujescu D, Soyka M, Dahmen N, Preuss U, Hartmann AM, Giegling I, Koller G, Bondy B, Möller HJ, Szegedi A (2005) GRIN1 locus may modify the susceptibility to seizures during alcohol withdrawal. Am J Med Genet B Neuropsychiatr Genet 133B(1):85–87

60. Wilhelm J, von Ahsen N, Hillemacher T, Bayerlein K, Frieling H, Kornhuber J, Bleich S (2007) Apolipoprotein E gene polymorphism and previous alcohol withdrawal seizures. J Psychiatr Res 41(10):871–875

61. Le Strat Y, Ramoz N, Pickering P, Burger V, Boni C, Aubin HJ, Adès J, Batel P, Gorwood P (2008) The 3¢ part of the dopamine transporter gene DAT1/SLC6A3 is associated with withdrawal seizures in patients with alcohol dependence. Alcohol Clin Exp Res 32(1):27–35

62. Rogawski MA (2005) Update on the neurobiology of alcohol withdrawal seizures. Epilepsy Curr 5(6):225–230

63. Tsai G, Coyle JT (1998) The role of glutamatergic neurotransmission in the pathophysiology of alcoholism. Annu Rev Med 49:173–184

64. Snell LD, Tabakoff B, Hoffman PL (1993) Radioligand binding to the N-methyl-D-aspartate receptor/ionophore complex: alterations by ethanol in vitro and by chronic in vivo ethanol ingestion. Brain Res 602(1):91–98

65. Kaysen G, Noth RH (1984) The effects of alcohol on blood pressure and electrolytes. Med Clin North Am 68(1):221–246

66. Bleich S, Degner D, Kornhuber J (2000) Repeated ethanol withdrawal delays development of focal seizures in hippocampal kindling. Alcohol Clin Exp Res 24(2):244–245

67. Hillemacher T, Frieling H, Bayerlein K, Wilhelm J, Kornhuber J, Bleich S (2007) Biological markers to predict previous alcohol withdrawal seizures: a risk assessment. J Neural Transm 114(2):151–154

68. Cuenod M, Do KQ, Grandes P, Morino P, Streit P (1990) Localization and release of homocysteic acid, an excitatory sulfur-containing amino acid. J Histochem Cytochem 38(12):1713–1715

69. Lipton SA, Kim WK, Choi YB, Kumar S, D'Emilia DM, Rayudu PV, Arnelle DR, Stamler JS (1997) Neurotoxicity associated with dual actions of homocysteine at the N-methyl-D-aspartate receptor. Proc Natl Acad Sci USA 94(11):5923–5928

70. Butcher SP, Cameron D, Kendall L, Griffiths R (1992) Homocysteine-induced alterations in extracellular amino acids in rat hippocampus. Neurochem Int 20(1):75–80

71. McRae AL, Brady KT, Sonne SC (2001) Alcohol and substance abuse. Med Clin North Am 85(3):779–801

72. Spies CD, Dubisz N, Neumann T, Blum S, Muller C, Rommelspacher H, Brummer G, Specht M, Sanft C, Hannemann L, Striebel HW, Schaffartzik W (1996) Therapy of alcohol withdrawal syndrome in intensive care unit patients following trauma: results of a prospective, randomized trial. Crit Care Med 24(3):414–422

73. Bråthen G, Ben-Menachem E, Brodtkorb E, Galvin R, Garcia-Monco JC, Halasz P, Hillbom M, Leone MA, Young AB (2005) The EFNS task force on diagnosis and treatment of alcohol-related seizures. EFNS guideline on the diagnosis and management of alcohol-related seizures: report of an EFNS task force. Eur J Neurol 12(10):816

74. Tonnesen H, Kehlet H (1999) Preoperative alcoholism and postoperative morbidity. Br J Surg 86(7):869–874

75. Earnest MP, Feldman H, Marx JA, Harris JA, Biletch M, Sullivan LP (1988) Intracranial lesions shown by CT scans in 259 cases of first alcohol-related seizures. Neurology 38(10):1561–1565

76. Feussner JR, Linfors EW, Blessing CL, Starmer CF (1981) Computed tomography brain scanning in alcohol withdrawal seizures. Value of the neurologic examination. Ann Intern Med 94(4 pt 1):519–522

77. Roth HL, Drislane FW (1998) Seizures. Neurol Clin 16(2):257–284

78. D'Onofrio G, Ulrich A, Rathlev N (2002) Alcohol and seizures. In: Delanty N (ed) Seizures: medical causes and management. Humana Press, Totowa, NJ, pp 167–182

79. Browning RG, Olson DW, Stueven HA, Mateer JR (1990) 50% dextrose: antidote or toxin? Ann Emerg Med 19(6):683–687

80. Sieber FE, Traystman RJ (1992) Special issues: glucose and the brain. Crit Care Med 20(1):104–114

81. Erstad BL, Cotugno CL (1995) Management of alcohol withdrawal. Am J Health Syst Pharm 52(7):697–709

82. Hulme J, Sherwood N (2004) Severe lactic acidosis following alcohol related generalised seizures. Anaesthesia 59(12):1228–1230

83. Talan DA, Hoffman JR, Yoshikawa TT, Overturf GD (1988) Role of empiric parenteral antibiotics prior to lumbar puncture in suspected bacterial meningitis: state of the art. Rev Infect Dis 10(2):365–376

84. Mirski MA, Muffelman B, Ulatowski JA, Hanley DF (1995) Sedation for the critically ill neurologic patient. Crit Care Med 23(12):2038–2053

85. Mayo-Smith MF (1997) Pharmacological management of alcohol withdrawal. A meta-analysis and evidence-based practice guideline. American Society of Addiction Medicine Working Group on Pharmacological Management of Alcohol Withdrawal. JAMA 278(2):144–151

86. Mattson RH (1996) Parenteral antiepileptic/anticonvulsant drugs. Neurology 46(6 Suppl 1):S8–S13

87. Lineaweaver WC, Anderson K, Hing DN (1988) Massive doses of midazolam infusion for delirium tremens without respiratory depression. Crit Care Med 16(3):294–295

88. Rosenbloom A (1988) Emerging treatment options in the alcohol withdrawal syndrome. J Clin Psychiatry 49(Suppl):28–32

89. Nolop KB, Natow A (1985) Unprecedented sedative requirements during delirium tremens. Crit Care Med 13(4):246–247

90. Bjorkqvist SE, Isohanni M, Makela R, Malinen L (1976) Ambulant treatment of alcohol withdrawal symptoms with carbamazepine: a formal multicentre double-blind comparison with placebo. Acta Psychiatr Scand 53(5):333–342

91. Voris J, Smith NL, Rao SM, Thorne DL, Flowers QJ (2003) Gabapentin for the treatment of ethanol withdrawal. Subst Abus 24(2):129–132

92. Rustembegovic A, Sofic E, Tahirović I, Kundurović Z (2004) A study of gabapentin in the treatment of tonic-clonic seizures of alcohol withdrawal syndrome. Med Arh 58(1):5–6

93. Rustembegovic A, Sofic E, Kroyer G (2002) A pilot study of Topiramate (Topamax) in the treatment of tonic-clonic seizures of alcohol withdrawal syndromes. Med Arh 56(4):211–212

94. Becker HC, Myrick H, Veatch LM (2006) Pregabalin is effective against behavioral and electrographic seizures during alcohol withdrawal. Alcohol Alcohol 41(4):399–406

95. Hillbom M, Tokola R, Kuusela V, Karkkainen P, Kalli-Lemma L, Pilke A, Kaste M (1989) Prevention of alcohol withdrawal seizures with carbamazepine and valproic acid. Alcohol 6(3):223–226

96. Marx JA, Berner J,Bar-Or D et al (1986) Prophylaxis of alcohol withdrawal seizures: a prospective study. Ann Emerg Med 15:637 (abstract)

97. Chance JF (1991) Emergency department treatment of alcohol withdrawal seizures with phenytoin. Ann Emerg Med 20(5):520–522

98. Rathlev NK, D'Onofrio G, Fish SS, Harrison PM, Bernstein E, Hossack RW, Pickens L (1994) The lack of efficacy of phenytoin in the prevention of recurrent alcohol-related seizures. Ann Emerg Med 23(3):513–518

99. Holland KD (2001) Efficacy, pharmacology, and adverse effects of antiepileptic drugs. Neurol Clin 19(2):313–345

100. Hillbom ME, Hjelm-Jager M (1984) Should alcohol withdrawal seizures be treated with anti-epileptic drugs? Acta Neurol Scand 69(1):39–42

101. Temkin NR, Dikmen SS, Wilensky AJ, Keihm J, Chabal S, Winn HR (1990) A randomized, double-blind study of phenytoin for the prevention of post-traumatic seizures. N Engl J Med 323(8):497–502

102. Baumgartner GR, Rowen RC (1991) Transdermal clonidine versus chlordiazepoxide in alcohol withdrawal: a randomized, controlled clinical trial. South Med J 84(3):312–321

103. Zechnich RJ (1982) Beta blockers can obscure diagnosis of delirium tremens. Lancet 1(8280):1071–1072

104. Adams F, Fernandez F, Andersson BS (1986) Emergency pharmacotherapy of delirium in the critically ill cancer patient. Psychosomatics 27(1 Suppl):33–38

105. Jones MV, Harrison NL, Pritchett DB, Hales TG (1995) Modulation of the GABAA receptor by propofol is independent of the gamma subunit. J Pharmacol Exp Ther 274(2):962–968

106. Coomes TR, Smith SW (1997) Successful use of propofol in refractory delirium tremens. Ann Emerg Med 30(6):825–828

107. Smith BJ (2001) Treatment of status epilepticus. Neurol Clin 19(2):347–369

Chapter 13

Drug-Induced Seizures in Critically Ill Patients

Denise H. Rhoney and Panayiotis N. Varelas

Abstract Critically ill patients are prescribed numerous medications during their ICU stay. Some of them have epileptogenic potentials. The most common pathophysiologic mechanism is through GABA receptor blockade and the most commonly used family of ICU drugs, reducing the seizure threshold, is antibiotics. The exact role that these medications play in inducing a clinical or subclinical seizure, in the context of cerebral injury or other multi-organ failure, is in many cases unclear. The best treatment for drug-induced seizures is increased vigilance and prevention. Cautious measures should be used to minimize or eliminate any unwanted drug side effects by attempting to start and keep the patient on the lowest effective dose for the desired therapeutic effect. When upward dosage titration is necessary it is best to increase slowly while keeping a watchful eye on all laboratory and clinical indicators of success or failure. Free levels of antiepileptic or other medications should be considered in the critically ill, due to numerous factors affecting their final action on the pharmacologic target. If a seizure occurs clinicians should always seek a medication as the cause of the witnessed seizure and should consider replacing it with another agent that has less epileptogenic potential. Lastly, a GABAergic receptor agonist antiepileptic drug should be used as first-line antidote in most of the cases.

Keywords Seizures, Drug, Critical care

13.1. Introduction

Detection and prevention of drug-related problems during hospitalization are a focus area for many clinicians. Adverse drug events, many of which are preventable, account for more than 100,000 deaths annually in hospitalized patients (1). In addition, it is estimated that adverse drug events extend the hospital length of stay by 2 days, subsequently resulting in increased costs ranging from $2,500 to $5,500 per patient (2–4). The intensive care unit (ICU) has the highest incidence of adverse drug events and the greatest severity risk compared to other areas of

From: *Seizures in Critical Care: A Guide to Diagnosis and Therapeutics*: Current Clinical Neurology, Second Edition, Edited by: P. Varelas, DOI 10.1007/978-1-60327-532-3_13,
© Humana Press, a part of Springer Science+Business Media, LLC 2005, 2010

the hospital (5, 6). Drug-induced seizures represent a potentially serious adverse drug event. Critically ill patients with and without neurologic disease may develop seizures during their hospitalization. Bleck et al. (7) reported that over a 2-year observation period of patients without neurologic problems admitted to large university medical center intensive care units (ICUs), 12.3% experienced neurologic complications during their stay. Of the patients who developed these complications, 28% experienced seizures. Importantly patients who developed these neurologic complications demonstrated increased risk of in-hospital mortality and experienced twofold longer lengths of stay compared to those patients who did not develop these complications (7). Many complications may arise as a result of drug-related seizures including hypoxemia, shock, hyperthermia, rhabdomyolysis, metabolic acidosis, and other drug-specific complications. Therefore it is essential that all clinicians have increased vigilance towards recognition of iatrogenic seizures and associated causes.

13.1.1. Epidemiology

The true incidence of drug-induced seizures is currently unknown. The Food and Drug Administration relies upon voluntary reporting of adverse drug events, including drug-related seizures, which impacts the ability to acquire true estimates. Additionally, many patients are receiving polypharmacy, complicating the ability to make an accurate association to the offending agent. Therefore, most of the information that is available is based upon data from experimental studies and case reports/case series.

The recent Drug Abuse Warning Network (DAWN) estimated that of the total 108 million ED visits in 2005, 14% were a result of drug misuse and abuse (31% illicit drugs and 27% prescription drugs) (8). Seizures appear to be a rare effect associated with drug administration although the DAWN estimates do not report data on specific complications such as seizures. The Boston Collaborative Drug Surveillance Program evaluated over 32,000 inpatient records and found that drug-related seizures occurred in 0.08% of the group (9). More recent studies have estimated that 6.1–9% of new onset seizures and status epilepticus is drug-related (10, 11). Thundiyil et al. (12) recently assessed 386 cases of drug-related seizures reported to a poison control center and found the leading causes of seizures to be bupropion (23%), diphenhydramine (8.3%), tricyclic antidepressants (7.7%), tramadol (7.5%), amphetamines (6.9%), isoniazid (5.9%), and venlafaxine (5.9%). In the majority of these patients (68.6%) only one seizure was reported while 3.6% experienced status epilepticus as a result. When compared to data published 10 years earlier, there was a statistically significant increase in newer antidepressant-related seizures (bupropion and venlafaxine) but a decrease in tricyclic antidepressant (TCA) and cocaine-associated seizures (13). Other older reports in hospitalized patients found that the most common drugs associated with seizures were penicillins, isoniazid, insulin, lidocaine, and psychotropic agents (including TCAs and antipsychotic agents) (9, 14). Wijdicks and Sharbrough (15) found that 15% of their cohort of new onset seizures in the ICU was related to drug toxicity (antibiotics and antiarrhythmics). Drug-induced seizures are associated with poor outcome and increased risk of aspiration pneumonitis (16) along with 15% of drug-associated seizures presenting as status epilepticus (14).

13.1.2. Risk Factors

Patients with a pre-existing seizure disorder have an increased propensity to develop seizures during critical illness; however, all critically ill patients have the ability to experience seizures while hospitalized. Outside of neurological causes, other risk factors that may lower seizure threshold in critically ill patients include: electrolyte imbalance, medications, medication withdrawal, medication overdose, organ failure, glucose abnormalities, infections, alterations in volume of distribution due to post-operative fluid shifts or dialysis/continuous veno-venous hemofiltration, and ischemic-hypoxic encephalopathy (17). Many medications used routinely in critically ill patients have been associated with drug-induced seizures at both therapeutic and toxic concentrations (18, 19). Patients with critical illness have several factors that may increase their vulnerability to drug-induced seizures including altered pharmacokinetics and the use of multiple-drug regimens that could result in drug interactions. Most drug-induced seizures are concentration-dependent; therefore, anything that could result in increased central nervous system (CNS) concentrations of the drug would place the patient at risk. There is a wide spectrum of drug-related risk factors for induction of seizures including the intrinsic epileptogenicity of the agent, factors that increase serum concentrations (dose, route schedule, route of elimination, drug interactions), and factors enhancing CNS concentrations (lipid solubility, molecular weight, ionization, protein binding, transport by endogenous systems) (20). Due to the complex nature of medication regimens in critically ill patients, drug interactions especially with the cytochrome P450 (CYP450) drug-metabolizing enzymes may represent a significant risk for patients in the ICU. The CYP3A4 isoenzyme subfamily accounts for metabolism of approximately 60% of all drugs used today. In addition there are patient-related risk factors including the presence of a seizure disorder, neurologic abnormality, reduced drug elimination, and conditions that disrupt the blood–brain barrier (20).

When clinicians suspect a drug-related seizure in patients who are critically ill, important questions require to be evaluated:

Is there a temporal relationship between the initiation of the drug or dosage titration and seizure?
What was the dose prescribed compared to recommended doses?
Was the dose appropriately adjusted for organ function?
Was there an administration error?
Are there any possible drug interactions?
Does the patient have any other possible cause for a seizure-like electrolyte disturbance?

13.1.3. Prevention

The best treatment for drug-induced seizures is prevention. Increased awareness and monitoring will often identify potential problems before they occur. General principles of drug use – particularly those that have been associated with increased seizure risk – should be to use the minimally effective dose, avoid polypharmacy, and avoid abrupt discontinuation. To assist in prevention the clinician should consider the following points, especially in patients who are considered to be at increased risk for seizures, as described previously:

What is the patient age? Is there a need to adjust the dose or use smaller doses?

Is there a need for the prescribed agent?

Is there an alternative agent that may have lower potential for seizures?

Is the smallest, effective dose being used?

Is there a need to taper an agent to avoid withdrawal?

What is the appropriate titration schedule?

Is there a possibility of drug interactions with the medication regimen?

13.2. Causative Agents

There have been many agents that critically ill patients are exposed to that have been reported to cause seizures. Table 13-1 contains a list of these agents along with possible mechanisms for seizures in addition to a previously published mnemonic 21 (Otis Campbell – from the Andy Griffith TV show) that has to be adapted to apply more specifically to critically ill patients. Overall the primary mechanism by which drugs induce seizures is related to some interference with neurotransmitters in the CNS.

Table 13-1. Drug-Related Seizures in Critically Ill Patients and Associated Mechanisms.

Agent	Proposed mechanism
High-risk agents	
Antipsychotics[a]	D1 agonists and D2 antagonists are proconvulsant. Antagonism of α_1-receptors, agonism of α_2-receptors, and inhibition of histamine-1 receptors may promote seizure activity
Flumazenil[a]	Not a direct effect of the drug, rather the resultant effects of benzodiazepine reversal
Meperidine[a]	Mediated through normeperidine, a toxic metabolite that is proconvulsant
Theophylline[b]	Lower seizure threshold by elevating cyclic GMP levels in brain & antagonizes the depressant effects of adenosine on cerebral cortex (other actions include pyridoxine depletion & inhibition of GABA)
Penicillins[b]	GABA antagonists by blocking $GABA_A$ Cl$^-$ channels & prevent GABA binding to $GABA_A$ receptors
Carbapenems[b]	Prevent GABA binding to $GABA_A$ receptors
Medium-risk agents	
Bupropion	Inhibition of dopamine reuptake
Fluoroquinolones	Prevent GABA binding to $GABA_A$ receptors
Cephalosporins[b]	Prevent GABA binding to $GABA_A$ receptors
Isoniazid[b]	brain levels of GABA via inhibitory action of glutamic acid decarboxylase
Tramadol	Inhibition of monoamine (serotonin, norepinephrine) reuptake rather than to opioid effects
Tricyclic antidepressants	Inhibition of reuptake of norepinephrine or serotonin in the brain
	Overdose produces anticholinergic toxidrome (hypotension, QRS interval prolongations, ventricular arrhythmias, & seizures)

(continued)

Table 13-1.   (continued)

Agent	Proposed mechanism
Withdrawal	Disinhibition syndrome (loss of inhibitory control leading to excess stimulation and release of glutamate, NMDA, norepinephrine, and serotonin)
Alcohol	
Benzodiazepines	Opioids may possess mu-receptor anticonvulsant properties that can precipitate seizures upon withdrawal
Barbiturates	
Opioids	
Low-risk agents	
Other antidepressants	Inhibition of reuptake of norepinephrine or serotonin in the brain
Local anesthetics	Antagonism of Na+ channel
Volatile general anesthetics[b]	Activation of NMDA receptors (enflurane and sevoflurane)
Other opioids	Unknown; likely mediated by selective stimulation of opioid receptors
Antihistamines	Histamine may be anticonvulsive via central H_1 receptors
Metronidazole	Unknown
Baclofen	Inhibition of presynaptic or postsynaptic inhibitory neurons
Beta blockers	Nonspecific action on centrally located neurons (membrane-stabilizing effects)
Cyclosporine	Structural damage to central nervous system
Cocaine	Augments the effects of catecholamines by blocking the reuptake at the synaptic junction and lowers seizure threshold
Stimulants	Augment the effects of catecholamines by blocking the reuptake at the synaptic junction
Antivirals	May be the result of inhibition of mitochondrial DNA polymerase and altered mitochondrial cell function
Antiepileptic drugs	AED in high concentrations may have depressant effect on inhibitory interneurons resulting in disinhibition of excitatory neurons and facilitation of epileptic discharges
	Absence seizures may be induced by facilitating synchronization of the firing neurons in the thalamocortical network
Aspirin	Depletion of brain glucose

Mnemonic for drug-related seizures in critically ill (OTIS CAMPBELL) – Modified from reference (21).
[a]Seizures commonly occur at therapeutic doses.
[b]Seizures occasionally occur at therapeutic doses.
GABA gamma aminobutyric acid.
O – Opioid withdrawal, oral hypoglycemics; T – Tricyclic antidepressants, theophylline; I – Isoniazid, insulin; S – Sympathomimetics, salicylates; C – Cocaine, carbapenems, cyclosporine; A – Amphetamines, antibiotics, antidepressants, antipsychotics, anesthetics; M – Meperidine, Methyl xanthines; P – PCP. Propoxyphene; B – Benzodiazepine withdrawal; E – Ethanol withdrawal; L – Lithium; L – Lidocaine.

13.2.1. Analgesics

13.2.1.1. Opioids

In animals opioids are associated with electroencephalogram (EEG) proven seizure activity; however the dose required to replicate this in the clinical setting is far greater that what is administered with either analgesia or anesthesia. Therefore, outside of opioid withdrawal the three most recognized opioids that have been associated with seizures are propoxyphene, meperidine, and tramadol.

Propoxyphene is associated with seizures primarily in overdose cases where seizures have been observed in 10% of patients (22). Propoxyphene is metabolized to a toxic metabolite, norpropoxyphene, which can accumulate in overdose or with repetitive dosing (23). Patients with chronic pain syndromes may be at increased risk due to the development of tolerance to the opioids and the need for increased, repetitive doses. Toxicity with propoxyphene is similar to that observed with TCAs with a clinical presentation of both seizures and cardiotoxicity, with widening of the QRS interval observed in 20% of cases (22).

Meperidine is metabolized via N-demethylation to an active metabolite normeperidine, which is then renally excreted. Accumulation of this metabolite is associated with seizure activity and patients with renal impairment or receiving large doses are at risk (24, 25). Oral administration of meperidine will result in increased concentrations of normeperidine due to extensive first-pass metabolism, thus resulting in increased risk of seizures at therapeutic dosing (26). The elimination half-life is approximately five times as long as the parent compound (3–6 h vs. 15–40 h); thus the toxic metabolite can quickly accumulate. Typically normeperidine toxicity develops at concentrations greater than 0.8 mg/dL. EEG changes associated with normeperidine include slow wave activity and epileptiform discharges that will resolve once normeperidine is eliminated (27). Normeperidine induced seizures often begin after the onset of other clinical sequelae such as delirium, tremors, or myoclonus. Seizures that develop are usually generalized tonic-clonic. Naloxone does not reverse the toxicity and could exacerbate seizure activity. Treatment includes supportive measures and withdrawal of meperidine. Treatment with traditional antiepileptic drugs (AEDs) should be avoided as they have been shown to accelerate the conversion of meperidine to normeperidine potentially worsening the seizures (28). Return to baseline neurologic functioning is dependent upon removal of the parent compound and the toxic metabolite; so it cannot be anticipated until a few days after meperidine discontinuation.

Morphine can induce seizures at high doses in neonates with immature blood brain barriers but have never been shown to be associated with seizures in adults (29). There have been some reports of seizure activity with fentanyl, alfentanil, and sufentanil (30–34), which have not been confirmed with EEG signs of seizure activity (35, 36). Surface EEG recordings are characterized by high-voltage slow delta waves following administration of these agents (28). It has been postulated that the tonic-clonic movements originally reported is somatic muscle rigidity or subcortical seizure activity and not true seizure activity.

Tramadol is a weak mu-receptor agonist with other pharmacological properties including inhibition of serotonin and norepinephrine reuptake. Tramadol has been reported to cause seizures following overdose and also with therapeutic dosing (primarily with chronic dosing) (37). The lowest dose associated with seizures was 200 mg with the seizure occurring within 6 h of administration (38). The incidence of seizures following overdose has been reported to be around 8% (39). Subsequently, during the second year the agent was on the market, a warning letter was issued by the Food and Drug Administration to all healthcare practitioners based upon the increased number of reports of seizures they had received. In most of the cases, patients were receiving other agents that were known to increase the risk of seizures and many were overdoses (40). In a post-marketing surveillance case-controlled study in over 10,000 patients the risk of seizures with tramadol was similar to other analgesic agents (41).

Seizures can also be the result of opioid withdrawal. Interestingly, Wijdicks and Sharbrough (15) attributed one-third of new onset seizures in the critically ill patients in their cohort to opioid withdrawal. In this cohort, all patients who experienced new-onset seizures received at least 7 days of repeated intramuscular injections. Seizures related to drug withdrawal typically occur 2–4 days after last ingestion depending on the pharmacokinetic profile of the offending agent. Gradual tapering of agents that are associated with drug withdrawal, including opioids, is optimal in preventing seizures.

13.2.1.2. Salicylates

Salicylate toxicity primarily mediated through salicylic acid clinically presents with neurologic abnormalities including seizures. Most seizures are generalized and related to the depletion of brain glucose and increased CNS oxygen consumption even with normal blood glucose. First line treatment for salicylate induced seizures is benzodiazepines followed by barbiturates as second-line agents. Since seizure is the most important symptom of severe salicylate toxicity other treatments should include gastrointestinal decontamination, urine alkalinization, and hemodialysis (18).

13.2.2. Anesthetics

13.2.2.1. General Anesthetics

Seizure activity associated with general anesthetic agents is largely thought to be an uncommon event. Nonetheless seizure activity has been reported with both volatile and nonvolatile agents. These agents are commonly used in the operating or procedure rooms and rarely in the ICUs. Therefore, their potential epileptogenic effects may be encountered in critically ill patients only in cases of immediate post-op transfer to an ICU bed without passing through the recovery room.

The most widely reported volatile anesthetic agent associated with seizures is enflurane (42). This agent produces high amplitude spikes and periods of electrical silence on the EEG with the hyperexcitability originating in the limbic system and then spreading to other areas (43). Most seizures reportedly occur during recovery from anesthesia (44, 45). Interestingly, delayed seizures have also been reported up to 8 postoperative days even with an initial normal EEG (46–48). The occurrence of seizures can be minimized by using lower concentrations (less than 1.5 minimum alveolar concentrations) and avoiding hypocapnia (49). However, others have reported seizure activity with enflurane even with normocapnia in patients with seizure disorders (50). No specific recommendations are available regarding the use of these agents. However, with the availability of other volatile agents that have less seizure risk, it is best to avoid enflurane in patients with a preexisting seizure disorder or who are at risk of seizures.

There have also been a couple of reports of isoflurane-associated seizures (51, 52). In these reports, myoclonic seizures occurred 2 h after induction and progressed to generalized seizures with sustained myoclonus during recovery. However, the bulk of information in humans suggests that isoflurane has anticonvulsant properties (53, 54).

Sevoflurane has a reported incidence of seizures up to 12% in clinical trials conducted in children, healthy adults, and elective gynecological surgery (55–61). Most of the seizures were reported within 90 min of sevoflurane administration and epileptiform EEG activity was seen in over 70% of the cases. A recent case report also described seizure activity with emergence from sevoflurane anesthesia 60. When compared to isoflurane, sevoflurane has stronger epileptogenic property. Recently postulated risk factors for epileptiform activity include high alveolar sevoflurane concentration (greater than 2.0 MAC), rapid anesthetic induction, hyperventilation, history of epilepsy, and female gender (62). The concomitant use of nitrous oxide, benzodiazepine, or opioid seems to counteract the epileptogenic property of sevoflurane (59, 63). The postulated mechanism is via NMDA receptor activation, similar to that observed with enflurane, since both agents have similar molecular structure with seven fluoride atoms (64).

The seizure potential of the nonvolatile agents appears to be negligible. Some of the agents have been used intraoperatively, however, to activate epileptogenic foci during epilepsy surgery. There have been some reports of seizures associated with ketamine anesthesia (65, 66) although EEG recordings have not revealed seizure activity in patients without a seizure disorder. However, it is well described that ketamine can activate epileptogenic foci, primarily subcortical seizure activity originating in the thalamic and limbic areas, in patients with a known seizure disorder (67, 68). There is no evidence of seizure activity in cortical regions. Ketamine does posses anticonvulsant properties and has received attention as an intervention for patients with refractory status epilepticus (69).

During induction and maintenance of anesthesia, etomidate is associated with involuntary myoclonic movements, which may simulate a tonic seizure but not correlated with any epileptogenic activity (70, 71). It is also possible that this represents subcortical seizure activity (72). In patients with a history of seizure disorders, surface EEG recordings have documented proconvulsant activity of etomidate at lower concentrations (73, 74). Further studies are necessary to further evaluate the proconvulsant nature of these agents.

There have been several types of CNS reactions to propofol including twitching, hypertonia, myoclonus, and seizure activity (75). Propofol has been used in the treatment of status epilepticus; however, there are some reports correlating propofol to seizure activity in patients without a seizure disorder history (76). The seizure activity described in these reports primarily occurred during induction and emergence of anesthesia with induction doses of 0.5–5.2 mg/kg with 34% of the patients having associated EEG abnormal tracings (76). The Committee on the Safety of Medicines in the United Kingdom estimated the seizure incidence as 1 in 47,000 (77). However it is uncertain if the reports are simply "abnormal movements" or seizure activity since there is very little EEG epileptiform activity reported.

13.2.2.2. Local Anesthetics
Local anesthetics are known to be associated with both neurotoxicity and cardiotoxicity, especially following overdose in patients with and without a seizure disorder. The most commonly cited local anesthetic agents associated with seizures are lidocaine and bupivacaine.

Lidocaine can be administered to critically ill patients by different dosing routes, including topical, subcutaneous, intravenous, and intraspinal/epidural and seizures (clonic and tonic/clonic) following each route of administration has been reported. The greatest risk for neurotoxicity is following intravenous administration and when the drug is inadvertently injected directly into the blood vessel. Lidocaine is metabolized to monoethylglycinexylidide (MEGX), which can also contribute to its toxicity by lowering the seizure threshold (78).

The risk of seizures is correlated to serum concentration with seizures commonly reported with lidocaine concentrations of 8–12 mg/dL. Seizures are usually short lived ranging from a few seconds to a few minutes. At concentrations between 0.5 and 5 mg/dL, lidocaine can suppress the clinical and EEG manifestations of seizures in experimental models and has been used to treat status epilepticus in the clinical setting (79, 80). Several factors can affect serum concentrations of local anesthetics including site and rate of injection, concentration, total dose administered, use of a concomitant vasoconstrictor, degree of ionization, degree of plasma and tissue binding, age, weight, and rate of metabolism and excretion (81). Bupivacaine is similar to lidocaine in epileptogenic potential. This agent is approximately 7 times more potent than lidocaine; so toxicity can develop at doses as low as 2–3 mg/kg (82).

Patients who are at the greatest risk of local anesthetic induced seizures are those with a history of renal or hepatic failure, older age, congestive heart failure, and/or septic shock (19). In addition toxicity has been reported as a result of drug interactions with cimetidine and propranolol (83, 84). Clinicians should utilize the lowest effective dose, follow serum concentrations, and avoid long-term infusions. Treatment for seizures associated with local anesthetics should include benzodiazepines and supportive care.

13.2.3. Antiepileptic Agents

The concept of antiepileptic drugs (AED) inducing seizures is controversial and many times overlooked by clinicians. The difficulty lies in differentiating between drug effect and natural course of the disease. Seizure disorders, by themselves, are usually infrequent and unpredictable with swings between periods of seizure control success and failure. There are several conditions that have been identified that are associated with increased risk of seizures from these agents. These conditions include: (1) paradoxical reaction of the drug; (2) toxic concentrations of the AED; (3) result of AED-induced encephalopathy; (4) incorrect choice of AED in treatment of an epileptic syndrome or seizure type; (5) patients with mixed seizure types; and (6) AED withdrawal or regimen change (85). Before concluding that an increase in seizures after the introduction of a new AED is associated with that agent, alternative explanations should be explored. These include spontaneous fluctuation of seizure frequency, the presence of known seizure aggravators (such as sleep deprivation, alcohol, and electrolyte abnormality), drug interactions, concurrent use of other epileptogenic inducing drugs, progression of epilepsy, and the development of drug resistance (86).

Even when AED drugs are chosen correctly for a clinical seizure type, they may provoke an increase in seizures. This usually occurs early after a patient is started on the AED and serum concentrations are within the normal range. Paradoxical seizures appear to be more common in children than in adults. Both carbamazepine and phenytoin have been shown to provoke complex partial seizures (85). Tonic-clonic seizures have been exacerbated by carbamazepine, gabapentin, lamotrigine, and benzodiazepines, while absence or absence status has been provoked by phenobarbital, oxcarbazepine, valproate, clonazepam with valproate, and myoclonic seizures are increased with lamotrigine or oxcarbazepine (85–87).

Increased seizures may occur as a result of toxic AED serum concentrations. A neurotoxicity syndrome associated with AED overdose has been described and includes seizure exacerbation and coma (85, 86). The AEDs, which are best described to cause seizures with intoxication, include phenytoin, carbamazepine, and valproate (85). Carbamazepine has been associated with seizures following overdose or in the setting of increased carbamazepine-10,11-epoxide (active metabolite) concentrations (88, 89). Therefore drug interactions that can increase the concentration of this active metabolite, increases the risk of seizure exacerbation.

Several AEDS have been associated with development of encephalopathy. Encephalopathy presents clinically as coma, asterixis, fever, aggravation of pre-existing neurological deficits, and seizures. Agents that have been reported to cause encephalopathy include valproate, carbamazepine, and phenytoin (86). Encephalopathy due to phenytoin is not commonly associated with an increase in seizure activity. On the other hand, an increase in seizure frequency due to valproate-induced encephalopathy is common. This is generally seen within the first week of treatment but can develop within the first nine months of initiation (86). Benzodiazepines are usually ineffective in treating these seizures; therefore the best treatment is to remove the offending agent (85, 86).

Incorrect selection of AED for a given seizure type may not only be ineffective but may provoke a seizure. For example, phenytoin, gabapentin, and carbamazepine may increase the frequency of absence seizures, when incorrectly prescribed for this seizure type (19). Carbamazepine and phenytoin have been shown to provoke or intensify generalized spike and wave discharges on EEG (90, 91). In addition, myoclonic and atonic seizures are provoked by carbamazepine, lamotrigine, and gabapentin (85).

Seizure syndromes, such as West syndrome or Lennox Gastaut syndrome, consist of heterogenous seizure types, with the EEG showing continuous abnormal patterns of diffuse slowing and generalized spike and wave activity (85). Seizure exacerbation from AED is frequently reported, especially in children. The application of an AED to treat a seizure may actually unmask a second seizure component of an epilepsy syndrome, leading to an apparent increase in seizure frequency, when in fact the second seizure had been present all along. Agents that have increased seizure frequency in Lennox-Gastaut syndrome include phenytoin, carbamazepine, and benzodiazepines, while provocation of tonic seizures in West syndrome has been reported with benzodiazepines (85, 86).

In epileptic patients on antiepileptic polytherapy, seizure worsening is not easy to appreciate since worsening may be due to the withdrawal of an AED that was beneficial, rather than the introduction of a new one. An increase in seizures associated with withdrawal of the AED is expected by the decrease of seizure control resulting from the falling AED serum level. One must be watchful not only for the obvious actual removal of the medication, but also for the more insidious effective removal of the AED through the addition or withdrawal of an interacting medication. It appears that the rate of withdrawal of the AED influences the patient's susceptibility to the subsequent onset of seizures. In patients in whom the drug is quickly discontinued, there appears to be an increase in post-withdrawal seizures, as compared to the cohort of patients in whom a gradual decrease in AED dose is administered (92).

Just as the addition or deletion of medications must be carefully monitored to prevent AED toxicity, vigilance must also be maintained with respect to

Table 13-2. Effect on Present AED Plasma Levels with Addition of New AED – Adapted from (82, 216).

Added AED	Present AED							
	PHT	TPM	PHB	CBZ	VPA	LEV	BDZ	LAM
Phenytoin (PHT)	…	↓	↔	↓	↓	↔	↔	↓
Phenobarbital (PHB)	↑ then ↓	↔	…	↔	↓	↔	↓	↓
Carbamazepine (CBZ)	↔	↓	↔	…	↓	↔	↓	↑
Valproic acid (VPA)	↓/*	↓	↑	↔/+	…	↔	↑	↔
Levetiracetam (LEV)	↔	↔	↔	↔	↔	…	↔	↔
Benzodiazepines (BZD)	↓	↔	↔	↔	↔	↔	…	↔
Lamotrigine (LAM)	↔	↑	↔	+	↔	↔	↔	…
Topiramate (TPM)	↑	…	↔	↔	↓	↔	↔	↔!

* increases free PHT levels.
+ increases active epoxide metabolite.
! no change at doses up to 400 mg/day.

lowering therapeutic AED levels by new pharmacologic therapies, a common situation in the ICU. The addition of an enzyme inducing medication may speed the metabolism of an AED, causing an iatrogenic AED withdrawal when, in fact, the AED dose has remained constant. The addition of a second or third AED may have this property and can cause this effect on the first AED's level. Table 13-2 presents common interactions between AEDs.

Finally, one must consider the protein binding of several ICU drugs. Many AEDs are heavily protein bound and free drug is the active moiety and is associated with toxicity. Not uncommonly, ICU patients have low serum albumin and protein levels, leading to higher or even toxic-free AED levels; this may pass unnoticed, if not specifically checked. In addition, competition for protein binding between the various highly bound ICU medications (AEDs or others) may also lead to higher than expected active free levels of individual drugs accounting for signs of toxicity. Therefore, it is imperative in critical care that the clinician measure both total and free levels of drugs whenever possible. Table 13-3 illustrates the wide variety of protein binding that may occur with several common medications, and emphasizes the need to look at more discreet pharmacologic interactions in these medically complex patients.

13.2.4. Antimicrobial Agents

Antibiotics, especially beta-lactams, have often been linked to seizures in critically ill patients. The critically ill patient typically develops severe infections often requiring aggressive antibiotic dosing. In addition when a seizure

Table 13-3. Relative Protein-Binding Affinities for Commonly used ICU Drugs and AEDs. Adapted from (82).

Drug	% Bound
Amiodarone	96
Digoxin	20–30
Nitroglycerin	60
Atracurium	82
Vecuronium	60–90
Propofol	>95
Phenytoin	90
Valproic acid	90
Carbamazepine	75–90
Phenobarbital	20–45
Lamotrigine	55
Felbamate	25
Oxcarbazepine (MHD)	38
Topiramate	15
Zonisamide	40
Tiagabine	95
Leviracetam	<10
Vigabatrin	–
Gabapentin	–

occurs in an infected patient, additional work-up is required to exclude the co-existence of a CNS infection as a cause of the seizure. Many of the antibiotics act by antagonizing the action of GABA by various different mechanisms (*see* Table 13-1). Renal insufficiency is a well-documented risk factor for antibiotic, particularly b-lactam toxicity. The most appropriate therapy for most antibiotic-associated seizures is withdrawal of the agent and administration of benzodiazepines.

13.2.4.1. Beta-Lactams

Seizure activity has been most commonly described with the penicillin class dating back to 1945 where myoclonic twitching was described in a toddler following intraventricular administration of benzylpenicillin (93). Since that time, beta-lactams have been associated with neurotoxicity to varying degrees (*see* Table 13-4). Penicillin consistently produces seizures via any route of administration, although more common after intrathecal administration (94, 95). The most frequently reported seizure types are myoclonus and generalized tonic-clonic seizures occurring 23 to 72 h after initiation of antibiotic therapy (96, 97). Risk factors for seizures are those associated with increasing CNS concentrations and include, older age, infants, renal impairment, history of meningitis, past history of CNS abnormality, administration of intraventricular antibiotics, continuous infusion administration, and history of seizures (98).

Table 13-4. Beta Lactams Associated with Seizures.

Penicillins	Cephalosporins
Piperacillin	Cefonicid
Ticarcillin	Cephalothin
Cloxacillin	Cephalexin
Amoxicillin	Cefamandole
Ampicillin	Cefotaxime
Nafcillin	Ceftazidime
Oxacillin	Cefmetazole
Benzylpenicillin (Penicliin G)	Cefazolin

Listed in order of least seizurogenic to most seizurogenic in both classes.

Penicillin brain toxicity is also due to a decrease in active transport out of CNS, when co-administered with other drugs, including anesthetics and probenecid, leading to an accumulation in the CNS at a higher concentration than in the blood (99). Neurotoxicity has not been shown to correlate to CSF or serum concentrations of the antibiotic, while brain tissue concentration is a better indicator (99). The convulsive activity following semisynthetic penicillins has been described; however, their proconvulsant potency is lower than what is observed for benzylpenicillin (100).

Cephalosporins have a similar risk of inducing seizures in experimental models; yet in clinical practice cephalosporins rarely produce seizures unless given in high doses or in patients with renal impairment (101). Cefazolin, one of the first generation cephalosporins, in large daily doses appears to be the most epileptogenic of the class (100, 102). This is relative, of course; doses necessary to induce seizure have been reported as 50 mg of intraventricular cefazolin or 20 g of intravenous cefazolin per 24 h, which are much larger than the typically utilized dose in the ICU (99). Renal failure remains a major patient-related risk factor; doses of cefazolin must be adjusted downward, based on the patient's estimated creatinine clearance. Treatment of beta lactam-associated seizures includes benzodiazepines or barbiturates.

13.2.4.2. Carbapenems

Carbapenems are synthetic beta-lactam agents that are typically used for treating serious infections in hospitalized patients. The postulated mechanism of seizure induction is via binding to the GABAA receptor (103). The traditional carbapenem, imipenem/cilastatin, has been associated with seizures at lower concentrations than other antibiotic agents and has a reported incidence of seizures ranging from 1.8 to 6% (99, 103). Experimental studies suggest that imipenem is 10 times more neurotoxic than benzylpenicillin (104). The toxicity associated with imipenem is due to accumulation of an open lactam metabolite of imipenem with cilastatin having no role (103). The only possible role of cilastatin in increasing the risk of seizures is by the reduction in clearance of imipenem from the cerebrospinal fluid leading to CNS concentrations that may exceed serum concentrations. Risk factors for seizures associated with imipenem include high dose, renal impairment, advanced age, pre-existing neurologic abnormality, and *Pseudomonas aeruginosa* infection (105). Seizures typically occur within 3 to 7 days of treatment initiation and are generalized or focal (105, 106). The average daily dose of imipenem-cilastatin in those patients who experienced seizures ranged between 13 mg/kg and 4 g of imipenem (106). As with other beta lactam agents the treatment of choice for seizure activity is removal of the agent and administration of benzodiazepines. Phenytoin and other sodium channel blockers should be avoided. The newer carbapenems (e.g., meropenem) have lower affinity for $GABA_A$ receptor and have reduced incidence of seizures (0.8%) (107). Patients whose medical course is complicated by hydrocephalus show a marked decrease in the elimination rate of meropenem from the CSF as compared to that from the serum (103).

13.2.4.3. Fluoroquinolones

Fluoroquinolone agents are associated with seizures in animals; however in the clinical setting seizures are rare and generally associated with overdoses or in patients who are susceptible to seizures (108). The mechanism of seizures is similar to that of beta-lactams. Receptor binding affinity is likely secondary to the similarities between the chemical structures of GABA and the antibiotics (109). The incidence of CNS toxicity of fluoroquinolones was originally thought to be associated with lipophilicity of the agent although that theory has since been disproven (108). There does appear to be varying degrees of binding to the GABA receptor, which may result in inhibiting or displacing GABA from the receptors. Animal studies also suggest that these agents have an agonist effect on the glutamate receptor NMDA (110). The most epileptogenic agent is trovafloxacin followed by enoxacin, moxifloxacin, ciprofloxacin, ofloxacin, and gatifloxacin, which is equivalent in epileptogenicity to levofloxacin (108, 111). The estimated incidence in humans of seizure activity is 1% or less (112). The seizures that have been described include tonic-clonic and generalized myoclonic activity occurring anywhere from 8 h to 12 days after initiation of therapy, although seizures have been reported up to a week following discontinuation of therapy (113–115). Additionally seizures have been reported when fluoroquinolones are co-administered with theophylline and nonsteroidal anti-inflammatory drugs (19).

13.2.4.4. Isoniazid

Isoniazid (INH) remains one of the most common agents for drug-induced seizures in the United States (13). INH has a 1% to 3% risk for development of seizures. The epileptogenic potential results from INH being metabolized to hydrazines, resulting in a pyridoxine (vitamin B6) deficiency via inhibition of pyridoxine phosphokinase (the enzyme transforming pyridoxine to pyridoxal phosphate). Pyridoxal phosphate (activated B6) is required by glutamic acid decarboxylase to convert glutamic acid to GABA thus leading to decreased levels of GABA (116) Mortality associated with INH is reported as high as 19%, particularly after ingestion of 10–15 g of INH (116). An overdose of INH is frequently associated with seizures, although therapeutic doses have also been linked to seizure activity primarily in elderly patients (117, 118). Serum INH concentrations greater than 10 mg/L on presentation, greater than 3.2 mg/L 2 h after ingestion, or greater than 0.2 mg/L 6 h after ingestion are associated with severe toxicity (119). Seizures associated with INH may occur without warning usually 1–3 h after ingestion, frequently as generalized tonic-clonic seizures, which are prolonged and difficult to treat (120). Other symptoms that accompany seizures include coma and metabolic acidosis. Phenytoin is ineffective in treating seizures associated with INH. Benzodiazepines are considered first-line agents; however, patients may be refractory since the agents require the presence of GABA for their therapeutic effects. Therefore, primary treatment includes intravenous administration of pyridoxine in amounts equivalent to ingested INH dose (1 g IV pyridoxine for each gram of INH ingested (121, 122). If unknown quantities are ingested then the dose of pyridoxine should be 5 g IV. This dose may be repeated at 5–20 min intervals until control of seizures has been obtained (19, 99).

Isoniazid remains less likely than other antibiotics to cause seizures within the hospital or the ICU, as most cases of INH-induced seizure result from acute, accidental, or intentional overdose. In this case, the presence of an unexplained anion-gap metabolic acidosis with high lactate level in the presence of no seizures or after a brief seizure should alert the intensivist to the possibility of INH overdose. Damaging neurologic sequelae have resulted from exposures as low as 20 mg/kg (99). This is striking, as the recommended dosage for children requiring therapy ranges from 10 to 15 mg/kg (99). Clear understanding of dosage regimens must be carefully communicated, not only to the health care team, but also to patients or parents of patients on INH.

13.2.4.5. Metronidazole

Experimental evidence and scattered case reports suggest that metronidazole has proconvulsant activity (123–126). The mechanism of action by which metronidazole induces epileptogenicity is largely unknown (99). It is known that seizures seem to develop approximately 7–10 days following the initiation of high dose therapy (5–6 g/day) in susceptible patients (99). Patients witnessed to have seizures on metronidazole therapy were also afflicted with metastatic cancers (metronidazole was used as a radiation sensitizer) and were also treated with other medications with known pro-convulsant actions (e.g., phenothiazines, cefamandole, ciprofloxacin, and theophylline) (99). Based on these rare human reports and some limited evidence from animal experiments, metronidazole use should be considered safe, if not used in high doses or in combination with other epileptogenic drugs.

13.2.5. Antiviral Agents

Antiviral agents rarely produce seizures except when given at high doses or to patients with a seizure disorder. Ganciclovir, foscarnet, and zidovudine have been reported to cause seizures in human immunodeficiency virus (HIV)-infected patients; however, these patients have multiple reasons for seizures so it is hard to establish the causal relationship (19). Risk factors for foscarnet-related seizures include the presence of toxoplasmosis with CNS involvement and a decrease in creatinine clearance (127). Without the presence of these risk factors and in the absence of any electrolyte abnormalities, there have been no reported seizures in the foscarnet-treated population (127).

Neurologic sequelae (vomiting, hallucinations, and confusion or coma, rarely seizures) as a result of acyclovir dosing have been reported in the literature, although mostly through case reports (128). Often, this comes as a consequence of intravenous administration, but it has also been found to occur in patients receiving oral therapy. While patients with pre-existing renal dysfunction, the elderly or those patients with overdose may be most susceptible to adverse neurological events (128), seizures cannot be entirely attributed to the drug, but instead to the primary CNS insult by herpes simplex virus or varicella zoster virus. Nevertheless, acyclovir neurotoxicity is distinguished from viral encephalitis by its sudden onset, absence of fever or headache, lack of focal neurologic findings, and normal cerebrospinal fluid (129). Discontinuation of the drug and hemodialysis should be considered in case of suspicion of neurotoxicity leading to seizures from this drug.

Ganciclovir administration has been associated with seizures after the first month of administration in patients infected with the HIV. Seizures worsened with increased dosing and the seizures did not respond to phenytoin administration and stopped when ganciclovir was discontinued (130).

The incidence of seizures occurring in patients infected with HIV are higher than in the general population (131, 132) The question yet to be definitively answered is if this increased seizure risk is secondary to the disease progression itself, complicated by the many medications required to prolong life, especially in advanced disease, or if it is a manifestation of the anti-viral medications required for the prevention of this progression. In a study that followed 550 patients for one year and monitored for seizure incidence, only one patient (0.018%) had a seizure attributed to the toxic effects of anti-retroviral (zidovudine) therapy when taken in overdose with sulfonamides (131). Because of the difficulty in assessing the cause-effect relationship with these agents and seizure activity, it is accepted that AED therapy should be initiated in patients infected with HIV after their initial seizure (132). Selection of AED agent is crucial in this population, as many drug interactions and disease interactions exist. Valproate, for example, can increase viral reproduction of both the HIV virus in addition to cytomegalovirus, while phenytoin, phenobarbital, and carbamazepine may increase the metabolism of protease inhibitors via the CYP450 system (132). For more information on these interactions the interested reader should refer to the Chapter Seizures and Infection in the ICU.

13.2.6. Bronchodilators

Seizures are a frequent adverse sequela of theophylline and aminophylline toxicity mediated primarily through the antagonism of adenosine receptors, the inhibition of phosphodiesterase and the increase in cAMP; however, some have suggested other mechanisms including depletion of pyridoxine and inhibition of GABA (21). The incidence of theophylline-associated seizures is 8–14% with mortality reported as high as 50% (133). The associated EEG findings include periodic lateralized epileptiform discharges, generalized epileptiform discharges, and generalized slowing and focal status epilepticus (134). Generalized seizures occur in 33% and secondarily generalized seizures occur in 30% of patients. Almost half of patients have [3] seizures with status epilepticus occurring in 29% of them, usually without permanent neurologic sequelae (92).

Serum theophylline concentrations do not always correlate well to the risk of seizures, particularly in chronic toxicity since serum and CNS theophylline concentrations are poorly correlated (135, 136), although many reports suggest that seizures less likely occur with serum concentrations of less than 60 mg/dL (137). Some authors suggest that patients who are at increased risk of seizures be maintained with theophylline concentrations at 10–15 mg/dL (134). Seurm concentrations of >21 mg/dL are commonly associated with drug-induced seizures in acute toxicity and in one study seizures were seen in two out of three cases reaching this concentration (92). Serum concentrations do not correlate with the number of seizures a patient may develop. Nonetheless, clinicians should be aware of the risk, as other reports have also seen seizure activity in therapeutic or mildly elevated concentrations (134).

Several risk factors for seizures have been reported in patients on long-term treatment including, advanced age, previous seizure history, encephalitis, cerebral vascular insufficiency, alcohol withdrawal, and other brain anomalies (138). In addition, the potential for drug interactions may increase risk of toxicity as seizures with theophylline have been described in patients concurrently receiving theophylline along with metronidazole, ciprofloxacin, gatifloxacin, moxifloxacin, or imipenem (126). The addition of quinolone can increase theophylline serum concentrations through inhibition of theophylline metabolism. Also, theophylline has been shown to increase the antagonism of the GABAA receptor achieved by the fluoroquinolones, thus increasing the epileptogenicity of the antibiotic (99).

Seizures due to theophylline are known to be prolonged and difficult to treat. The general principle in management is to stop the seizure as soon as possible (within 5–6 h of ingestion) as a correlation exists between morbidity and mortality and the duration of seizures. Barbiturates and benzodiazepines are the cornerstone of management (phenytoin is ineffective), although many cases may require general anesthesia and aggressive gastrointestinal decontamination and hemodialysis (139). Hemodialysis and hemoperfusion is commonly used when serum theophylline concentrations are greater than 100 mg/dL following acute toxicity and greater than 60 mg/dL with chronic toxicity (140). Midazolam has been reported to be effective against refractory seizures caused by theophylline toxicity (141).

13.2.7. Immunosuppressive Agents

Seizure etiology in the post transplant patient population may be the most difficult to assess, given the level of medical complexity that these patients possess. Metabolic abnormalities, including non-ketotic hyperosmolar hyperglycemia, weakened immune systems, polypharmacy, and potential coagulopathies all pose as possible instigators of neurologic toxicity. Before the intensivist attributes seizures to a metabolic or drug cause, an extensive work-up to exclude infectious agents invading the CNS should be completed.

The most common immunosuppressive agent associated with seizures is cyclosporine. The overall incidence of CNS toxicity with cyclosporin is 10% and includes cerebellar disorders, neuropathies, and seizures (142). The incidence of seizures is approximately 3% in bone marrow transplant patients and around 1% in solid-organ transplants (142). Of solid organ transplants, cyclosporine induced seizures are more commonly reported after liver transplant compared to renal transplant. Patients with the highest risk of seizure during cyclosporine therapy include those on simultaneous high-dose steroids, children, and those with hypertension, hypomagnesemia, and/or hypoalbuminemia (143). The onset of seizures ranges from 2 to 180 days of treatment initiation (usually early during aggressive dose escalation) even in patients without risk factors for seizures. The highest risk of seizures was in patients with cyclosporine concentrations above 250 mcg/mL. Cyclosporin produces structural injury to the CNS (144). White matter is particularly susceptible to toxicity, manifested by characteristic focal lesions on magnetic resonance imaging. The brain contains high concentrations of the cytosolic-binding protein cyclophilin, which suggests increased cellular uptake of cyclosporin (142). Calcineurin inhibitors may also exacerbate an underlying seizure focus by enhancing neuronal excitability. The EEG in patients with cyclosporine neurotoxicity consists of diffuse slowing (142).

Cyclosporine's metabolic pathway may be induced by phenytoin, phenobarbital, and carbamazepine (143). Careful monitoring of cyclosporine serum concentrations is imperative in the patient who must be maintained on one of these AEDs. Valproic acid is one AED, which has failed to show any impact on the metabolism of cyclosporine (143). For that reason it may be recommended as a possible therapeutic option, although its use should be avoided in patients less than two years old who have undergone liver transplantation, as it has had reported deleterious effects on the liver itself (143). Newer AEDs, which are non-hepatic enzyme inducers, like gabapentin, oxcarbazepine, or levetiracetam may also be considered to control seizures (145). Calcineurin inhibitor-sparing regimens with mycophenolate mofetil and corticosteroids may be useful in reducing the incidence of neurotoxicity (146). Calcineurin inhibitors can then be started when encephalopathy and electrolyte shifts have resolved, usually within 48 h. Please refer to the ICU Seizures in Organ Transplantation Recipients Chapter for more information.

Other immunosuppressing agents used after organ transplantation which increase the risk of seizures include tacrolimus (FK506) and OKT3. Since tacrolimus is also a calcineurin inhibitor it has a risk of neurotoxicity similar to cyclosporine. Sirolimus is a newer agent related to tacrolimus, but its mechanism of action differs in that it does not inhibit calcineurin. No evidence of neurotoxicity with sirolimus therapy for up to 18 months has been found (147). In renal transplant patients, OKT3 caused seizures in 6% (8/122) of cases, all with non-functioning grafts, due to tubular necrosis (148).

13.2.8. Chemotherapeutic Agents

Chemotherapeutic agents may also be associated with seizures, including alkylating agents (chlorambucil and busulfan) cisplatinum, 5-flurouracil, high dose methotrexate, vincristine, etoposide, and ifosfamide (19, 149–151). The greatest risk of seizures from chemotherapeutic agents is after excessive doses such as the regimens used for myeloablative treatment in preparation for bone marrow transplant. Children also seem to be susceptible to seizures especially with chlorambucil and vincristine. Seizures occur within hours or days of drug administration, but can be delayed in patients with impaired renal or hepatic clearance.

13.2.9. Psychotropic Agents

Psychotropic drugs have been implicated in drug-induced seizures for many years. The San Francisco General Study noted that psychotropic drugs accounted for 34% of all witnessed drug-induced seizures occurring in hospitals (14). This is not surprising given the potential of these agents to lower the seizure threshold through their pharmacologic activity and through drug interactions with other medications to either result in toxicity or result in lowering of concurrent AEDs. Most of these agents utilize the CYP450 hepatic enzyme system for elimination. Thus co-administration with other agents that inhibit this system may inadvertently lead to toxicity and increased risk of seizures. The epileptogenic potential of the agents varies and data are limited regarding the impact of these agents on seizure threshold in epileptic vs. non-epileptic brains. In general, it is recommended that less epileptogenic agent is used at the lowest effective dose in patients with a history of seizures. The intensivist should be aware of the seizure potential and maintain a conservative approach to managing critically ill patients, balancing the risk and benefit in each individual patient.

13.2.9.1. Antipsychotic Agents

Seizures associated with psychotropic agents are often the cause for ICU admission, particularly as a result of overdose. Even though all patients receiving antipsychotic agents are at risk of drug-induced seizures, seizures develop most commonly upon initiation or during dosage titration, particularly rapid titration schedules. The epileptogenic potential of antipsychotics depends somewhat on the ratio of dopamine-1 (D1) to dopamine-2 (D2) blockade, as well as on the balance of glutamate and GABA activity. D1 agonists and D2 antagonists are proconvulsant. Also antagonism of α_1-receptors, agonism of α_2-receptors, and inhibition of histamine-1 receptors may promote seizure activity. Another potential mechanism is via the influence of neurosteroid sex hormones produced in the brain (152). Traditionally low potency agents were thought to possess the highest risk of seizure activity (*see* Table 13-5).

The literature suggests that chlorpromazine and other aliphatic phenothiazines (promazine and trifluoperazine) are commonly associated with seizures (1.2% overall incidence) (153, 154), while piperazine phenothiazines (fluphenazine, perphenazine, prochlorperazine, trifluoperazine) are less associated with seizures (0.3–0.9% overall incidence with therapeutic dosing) (153–155). Doses exceeding 1,000 mg per day of chlorpromazine have a 9% incidence of seizures. Seizures most commonly occur at the onset of treatment or after a rapid dose increase with other associated risk factors including an abnormal EEG tracing or evidence of a brain abnormality. Phenothiazines induce diffuse, paroxysmal EEG changes (19). In addition the phenothhiazines can interact with phenytoin and phenobarbital resulting in reduced concentrations of these AEDs placing patients at increased risk of seizures (19). Butyrophenones have been associated with seizures although haloperidol may carry a lower risk than other antipsychotic agents (155).

The atypical antipsychotic, clozapine, has a 2.8% risk of seizures with higher risk in patients receiving doses >600 mg/day (risk = 4.4–14%) or with the use of a rapid titration schedule (156, 157). Status epilepticus following clozap-

Table 13-5. Risk of Seizures Associated with Antipsychotics.

Low-risk agents	Medium-risk agents	High-risk agents
Fluphenazine	Olanzapine	Clozapine
Haloperidol	Quetiapine	Chlorpromazine
Molindone	Thioridazine	
Risperidone		
Trifluoperazine		

Adapted from (152).

ine administration has also been reported (158). Seizures occurring during clozapine therapy do not necessarily lead to discontinuation of therapy, especially since clozapine is held for refractory patients. Administration of seizure prophylaxis with valproic aid, phenytoin, or topiramate is often considered (159, 160). The risk of seizures for the remainder of newer, atypical antipsychotic agents is not well defined and appears to be low. Outside of olanzapine, none of the other second-generation antipsychotics induce EEG changes (161). Olanzapine is associated with EEG slowing and epileptiform abnormalities (161, 162). The consensus is that risperidone (0.34% incidence), olanzapine (0.9% incidence), ziprasidone (0.4% incidence), aripiprazole (0.1% incidence), quetiapine (0.8% incidence) are not associated with an increased risk of seizures (163–167). The agent causing most concern is olanzapine since it is structurally related to clozapine and isolated cases of seizures and status epilepticus have been reported at therapeutic doses (161, 168–170). The case reports of the other agents were in patients receiving polytherapy with agents which are associated with seizure activity. All patients who are predisposed to seizures should be considered at increased risk when prescribed any antipsychotic agent. When using these agents, it is best to use the lowest effective dose with slow dosage titration and avoid using them with other agents that may lower the seizure threshold.

If patients experience an antipsychotic-associated seizure and there is a need to continue therapy, then agents with the lowest potential to lower seizure threshold should be used (e.g., risperidone, haloperidol, fluphenazine, pimozide, molindone, trifluoperazine, thioridazine) (171). Phenothiazines are more likely to lower seizure threshold than butyrophenones. Therefore, haloperidol would be the agent of choice for treating delirium in the intensive care unit in patients at risk of seizures. The agents with the highest risk potential for seizures are clozapine and chlorpromazine (169, 172, 173) and in this case, should be avoided in the ICU.

13.2.9.2. Antidepressants

Antidepressant drugs have both convulsant and anticonvulsant properties. The convulsant properties are more prominent at higher concentrations. The propensity of antidepressant agents to cause seizures varies from 0.1 to 20% (*see* Table 13-6) (174–176). Since these agents are used for a variety of clinical indications ranging from depression to smoking cessation, the exposure to

Table 13-6. Risk of Seizures Associated with Antidepressants.

Minimal-risk agents	Low-risk agents	Medium-risk agents	High-risk agents
Phenelzine	SSRI	Amitriptyline	Maprotiline
Tranylcypromine	Trazodone	Imipramine	Amoxapine
	Mirtazapine	Desipramine	Clomipramine
	Nefazodone	Nortriptyline	Bupropion
		Protriptyline	
		Doxepin	
		Venlafaxine	

SSRI selective serotonin reuptake inhibitors.
Adapted from (152, 217).

these agents has increased, so it is essential to understand their seizure risk profile. It is important for the intensivist to evaluate these data (*see* Table 13-6) and then extrapolate to decision-making on initiating or continuing these agents in the ICU patient.

TRICYCLIC ANTIDEPRESSANTS

The first report of seizures associated with TCAs occurred not long after the introduction of the first agent to the market (imipramine) (177). Since that time, the overall incidence of TCA-induced seizure ranged from 4 to 20%, primarily in acute overdose (175, 176). Not all the TCAs share the same potential for seizures at therapeutic doses. Agents which have been reported to be most commonly associated with seizures are amoxapine, amitriptyline, imipramine, nortriptyline, desipramine, doxepin, and protriptyline. Clomipramine is associated with increased risk of seizures at doses greater than 300 mg/day (178). Seizures generally occur within three to 6 h post ingestion and are uncommon after 24 h (152). It has been suggested that the risk of seizures could be reduced by monitoring plasma concentrations since the isoenzymes responsible for TCA metabolism are known to be subject to genetic polymorphisms that could result in toxic concentrations in the small percentage of patients who may be lacking this isoenzyme (179). However, there is a lack of consensus on the utility of serum concentration monitoring, since the incidence of seizures in patients treated with "low dose" TCA does not differ significantly from that of the general population, implying that it is not the medication itself, but rather the brain insult that is causing the seizure (152).

Maprotiline is a semi-TCA but has a higher risk of seizures compared to other TCA, potentially related to a toxic metabolite. The risk of seizures is increased at doses above 225 mg/day. The pharmacologic action of these agents includes inhibition of serotonin and norepinephrine reuptake, histamine (H1) antagonism, and alpha-1 receptor antagonism. The exact mechanism by which these agents induce seizures has not been elucidated since many studies have found varying effects of these agents on the seizure threshold. Seizures generally occur within a few days of initiation of therapy or when changing to higher doses.

In overdose, tricyclic antidepresents (TCA) produce an anticholinergic toxidrome that includes hypotension, QRS interval prolongation, ventricular arrhythmias, and seizures. Mortality is significantly increased with the presence of seizures (180). TCA-induced seizures, with the exception of amoxapine, are generally accompanied by a widened QRS duration on electrocardiogram (181). A QRS duration of 0.10 s or longer was moderately predictive of seizures while durations of 0.16 s or longer was highly predictive of seizures (182). Seizures associated with TCA are more likely to be prolonged and multiple and associated with increased risk of medical complications (hypotension, coma, other cardiovascular complications) and death (13, 183). Treatment of TCA overdose includes supportive care, benzodiazepines for seizures, and sodium bicarbonate for cardiac toxicity.

SELECTIVE SEROTONIN REUPTAKE INHIBITORS

The selective serotonin reuptake inhibitors (SSRI) administered alone have been reported to have anticonvulsant effects (184). In overdosage situations, however, fluoxetine, sertraline, citalopram, and fluvoxamine have been reported to cause seizures (152, 185, 186). Accumulating data suggest that at therapeutic doses the incidence of seizures with fluoxetine is 0.2%; however, these agents appear to be less epileptogenic than TCA (172). Another important consideration is possible drug interactions through CYP450 since SSRI are both inhibitors and substrates for this enzyme system. It is important that clinicians carefully review all medication regimens in patients in the ICU to assess for potentially serious drug interactions. When these agents are co-administered with other agents that mimic serotonin or with monoamine oxidase inhibitors, "serotonin syndrome" may develop. This syndrome is associated with seizures, delirium, myoclonus, and autonomic instability (187, 188).

Monoamine Oxidase Inhibitors

Monoamine oxidase inhibitors are occasionally associated with seizure activity in patients suffering from hypertensive crisis as part of tyramine ingestion (189). In general, when these agents are used in the recommended doses and without external interacting factors, there is little risk of drug-induced seizures.

Bupropion

Bupropion is a unique agent that works pharmacologically by inhibiting the reuptake of dopamine, norepinephrine, and serotonin. Bupropion displays similar characteristics to TCA in overdose, although they are not structurally similar, with conduction delays on ECG reported in 2–3% of overdose cases (190). Initially the maximum recommended doses were 450–900 mg/day and the overall incidence of seizures was 2–5.4% leading to the drug being withdrawn from the market in 1986 (191). It was later re-introduced in the market with a maximum recommended dose of 450 mg/day. The incidence of seizures at doses greater than 450 mg/day has been reported to be as high as 2.2% compared to maximal doses less than 450 mg/day, which conferred a 0.44% seizure incidence (191). Bupropion was also reported to be an important cause of drug-related new-onset generalized seizures presenting to the emergency department (11). The sustained release formulation is hypothesized to have a lower epileptogenic potential since it produces lower peak concentrations compared to the immediate release product; however, there has been reports of tonic clonic seizures associated with the use of the sustained release product (191, 192). In general, bupropion is thought to have a higher risk of seizures compared to other antidepressant agents and should be used with caution in patients with seizure disorders (193, 194).

Miscellaneous Antidepressants

Both trazodone and nefazodone have very low risk of new-onset seizures and are probably safe in patients with seizure disorders. Venlafaxine is another agent pharmacologically similar to bupropion, but with lesser effect on dopamine reuptake inhibition. Cardiotoxicity with QRS interval widening and arrhythmias have been reported with venlafaxine overdose, but to a lesser extent than that experienced with TCA, although the reported incidence of seizures is also high and ranges from 8 to 14% (195).

13.2.9.3. Lithium

Lithium is well known to be associated with serious neurological side effects, especially seizures. There is limited information describing lithium's pharmacologic effects, but these are likely mediated through effects on neuronal ion transport and inhibition of norepinephrine and serotonin reuptake. The EEG changes seen after lithium administration are generalized slowing and paroxysmal diffuse alpha activity, which typically develop within one to two weeks of therapy onset and are reversible with elimination of the drug (196). Seizures associated with lithium generally occur with supratherapeutic concentrations (>3 mEq/L); however seizures have been reported in patients with therapeutic concentrations and upon drug withdrawal. Therefore it is imperative that the clinical presentation of the patient is treated instead of treating a laboratory value. Except in chronic overdosing, serum concentration correlates with severity of toxicity symptoms (197, 198). Risk factors of lithium-associated seizures include pre-existing EEG abnormality, clinical seizure disorder (including childhood febrile seizures), decreased renal function, and acute psychotic symptoms (19). Because the combination of lithium and carbamazepine has been implicated in acute neurotoxicity even with "therapeutic" concentrations of both agents, the intensivist should be aware and use alternative AED or mood stabilizing agents (199, 200). Treatment of lithium toxicity includes supportive care, gastrointestinal decontamination, enhanced elimination with hemodialysis and benzodiazepines.

13.2.10. Stimulants

Psychostimulants such as caffeine, amphetamines, methylphenidate, and modafinil are gaining increasing popularity in the treatment of diseases such as attention deficit – hyperactivity disorder (ADHD), narcolepsy, and obesity (201). Due to their diffuse action within the CNS, one would imagine the risk for seizures induced by this class of medications to be high. Studies have shown, however, that the relative epileptogenicity of these medications is quite low (202). There are no data available regarding seizure risk with their anecdotal use in ICU comatose patients.

While caffeine is certainly the most widely used medication in this class, methylphenidate remains the most widely prescribed for the aforementioned disease states. Overall, this stimulant has proven to be quite safe with regard to seizure induction. In fact, methylphenidate has actually been shown to decrease the incidence of seizure in patients with acute brain trauma (203). When this stimulant is used in patients with seizure disorders that are well controlled on AEDs, there is minimal risk of seizure exacerbation or prolongation (204). In fact, methylphenidate may increase the serum concentrations of some AEDs, including phenobarbital and primidone (202). Again, the importance of careful monitoring of serum concentrations of medications with the addition or removal of any medical therapy cannot be understated.

For patients without a previous history of seizures, if the luxury of a pre-treatment EEG is available, it may well prove beneficial in determining a patient's potential risk for developing seizures while on stimulant therapy. In one study of pediatric patients started on stimulants for ADHD, the risk of seizure in patients with a normal EEG prior to therapy was 0.6%, while for patients presenting with epileptiform abnormalities on the EEG prior to the beginning of therapy the risk was 10% ($P < 0.003$). In both groups seizures occurred during treatment with methylphenidate, except for one patient with previous history of seizures, who had one event after discontinuing the drug (204).

Modafinil is an alerting agent approved for the treatment of narcolepsy in adults. It has also been used in children with excessive daytime somnolence.

In a small case series of children with these disorders, exacerbation of seizures and psychotic symptoms was reported with modafinil therapy in 2/13 children (205).

13.2.11. Drug Withdrawal

Literature has suggested that 45% of seizures in the hospital or ICU are the result of alcohol or drug toxicity and drug withdrawal (82). Drug withdrawal may occur at several different times during the patient's hospitalization. Early withdrawal related to agents the patient ingested prior to admission might occur as patients are moved from the emergency department to the ward or the ICU or when medications are changed or abruptly stopped. Early withdrawal seizures can be attributed to many agents and may be predictable and preventable by assessment of the admission toxicology screen. More information regarding ICU seizures related to withdrawal from legal or illegal drugs can be obtained in a separate chapter.

13.2.12. Miscellaneous Agents

Baclofen is a centrally acting muscle relaxant administered either orally or intrathecally. Withdrawal from baclofen, a $GABA_B$ agonist, has been reported to be similar to ethanol and sedative withdrawal and may include seizures. Both abrupt discontinuation of oral therapy and intrathecal pump failure has been associated with seizures (206–208). The treatment of these seizures includes benzodiazepines and the readministration of oral therapy. However oral therapy may not reach sufficient CSF concentrations to be effective in patients with intrathecal pump failure (208).

Diphenhydramine is the most common antihistamine agent associated with seizures and was recently reported as the second most common agent associated with drug-induced seizures reported to a poison control center (12). Seizures associated with diphenhydramine appear to be most common in overdose situations (~5% of cases) and are generally brief and self-limited within 2–3 h of ingestion (209). Children have increased susceptibility to the convulsive effects of these agents with fatality being reported after ingesting less than 150 mg (210).

Intravenous contrast media have been associated with tonic-clonic and partial seizures within 10 min of administration. The risk is generally low (0.2–0.5%) except in patients with metastatic cancer to the brain where the incidence increased to 15% (211, 212). In animal models, the use of iodinated contrast triggered seizures when given by various routes of administration including intravenous, intra-arterial, intracerebral, and subarachnoid. Seizures are usually self-limiting occurring within 30 min of infusion with status epilepticus rarely occurring. The risk factors include dose administered, speed of administration, use of ionic agents, osmolarity, history of seizure disorder, and structural brain abnormality (211).

Beta-adrenergic blocking agents can cause seizures in overdose with the majority of cases involving propranolol (213). The cardioselective agents seem to be less epileptogenic but can still result in seizures (214).

Other agents that have been associated with seizures include exogenous administration of thyroid hormone, hypoglycemic agents, and electrolyte derangements. These areas are specifically covered in individual chapters in this book.

13.3. Treatment

The general approach for managing drug-related seizures is covered in another chapter of this text. For a detailed review of managing seizures in the intensive care unit please refer to a previously published comprehensive review by Mirski et al. (215).

13.3.1. Summary

While the overall incidence of drug-induced seizures appears to be relatively low, critically ill patients may be more vulnerable to the epileptogenicity of drugs. Unfortunately, the occurrence of drug-related seizures in critically ill patients is often difficult to assess and is dependent upon certain patient and drug attributes that would place the patients at increased risk. The complexity of the illness and delivery of care in critically ill patients certainly contribute to the risk. Numerous drugs have been implicated as a cause for seizures, but to varying degrees. The true incidence and causality is difficult to assess as most of the data is from published case reports or post-marketing surveillance programs. Therefore, clinicians should report any drug-related seizures to appropriate formulary committees or databases in order to further clarify any relationships between the drug and this adverse consequence. Prevention is the key treatment for drug-induced seizures with the first step being familiarity with the agents that may cause seizures followed by prospective assessment of drug regimens. Critically ill patients possess many of the risk factors for drug-related adverse events so recognition and vigilance is essential by all clinicians. In addition since most drug induced seizures are dose-related, it is important to use the lowest effective dose adjusted for end organ function in an effort to minimize this potentially serious adverse effect. Treatment of seizures is usually symptomatic and includes, when possible, discontinuing the offending agent. In general the first line agents for treating drug-induced seizures are benzodiazepines, which should be initiated promptly in an effort to minimize the morbidity and mortality associated with this adverse effect of drugs.

References

1. Lazarou J, Pomeranz BH, Corey PN (1998) Incidence of adverse drug reactions in hospitalized patients: a meta-analysis of prospective studies. JAMA 279(15): 1200–1205
2. Suh DC, Woodall BS, Shin SK, Hermes-De Santis ER (2000) Clinical and economic impact of adverse drug reactions in hospitalized patients. Ann Pharmacother 34(12):1373–1379
3. Classen DC, Pestotnik SL, Evans RS, Lloyd JF, Burke JP (1997) Adverse drug events in hospitalized patients. Excess length of stay, extra costs, and attributable mortality. JAMA 277(4):301–306
4. Bates DW, Spell N, Cullen DJ et al (1997) The costs of adverse drug events in hospitalized patients. Adverse Drug Events Prevention Study Group. JAMA 277(4):307–311

5. Cullen DJ, Sweitzer BJ, Bates DW et al (1997) Preventable adverse drug events in hospitalized patients: a comparative study of intensive care and general care units. Crit Care Med 25(8):1289–1297

6. Smith KM, Jeske CS, Young B, Hatton J (2006) Prevalence and characteristics of adverse drug reactions in neurosurgical intensive care patients. Neurosurgery 58(3):426–433, discussion 426–433

7. Bleck TP, Smith MC, Pierre-Louis SJ et al (1993) Neurologic complications of critical medical illnesses. Crit Care Med 21(1):98–103

8. Drug Abuse Warning Network (2005) National Estimates of Drug-Related Emergency Department Visits (2007) Substance Abuse and Mental Health Services Administration. (Accessed July 28, 2008)

9. Drug-induced convulsions (1972) Report from Boston Collaborative Drug Surveillance Program. Lancet 2(7779):677–679

10. Lowenstein DH, Alldredge BK (1993) Status epilepticus at an urban public hospital in the 1980s. Neurology 43(3 Pt 1):483–488

11. Pesola GR, Avasarala J (2002) Bupropion seizure proportion among new-onset generalized seizures and drug related seizures presenting to an emergency department. J Emerg Med 22(3):235–239

12. Thundiyil JG, Kearney TE, Olson KR (2007) Evolving epidemiology of drug-induced seizures reported to a Poison Control Center System. J Med Toxicol 3(1):15–19

13. Olson KR, Kearney TE, Dyer JE, Benowitz NL, Blanc PD (1994) Seizures associated with poisoning and drug overdose. Am J Emerg Med 12(3):392–395

14. Messing RO, Closson RG, Simon RP (1984) Drug-induced seizures: a 10-year experience. Neurology 34(12):1582–1586

15. Wijdicks EF, Sharbrough FW (1993) New-onset seizures in critically ill patients. Neurology 43(5):1042–1044

16. Isbister GK, Downes F, Sibbritt D, Dawson AH, Whyte IM (2004) Aspiration pneumonitis in an overdose population: frequency, predictors, and outcomes. Crit Care Med 32(1):88–93

17. Delanty N, Vaughan CJ, French JA (1998) Medical causes of seizures. Lancet 352(9125):383–390

18. Kunisaki TA, Augenstein WL (1994) Drug- and toxin-induced seizures. Emerg Med Clin North Am 12(4):1027–1056

19. Garcia PA, Alldredge BK (1994) Drug-induced seizures. Neurol Clin 12(1):85–99

20. Alldredge BK (1997) Drug-induced seizures: controversies in their identification and management. Pharmacotherapy 17(5):857–860

21. Wills B, Erickson T (2006) Chemically induced seizures. Clin Lab Med 26(1):185–209, ix

22. Sloth Madsen P, Strom J, Reiz S, Bredgaard Sorensen M (1984) Acute propoxyphene self-poisoning in 222 consecutive patients. Acta Anaesthesiologica Scand 28(6):661–665

23. Young RJ (1983) Dextropropoxyphene overdosage. Pharmacological considerations and clinical management. Drugs 26(1):70–79

24. Armstrong PJ, Bersten A (1986) Normeperidine toxicity. Anesth Analg 65(5):536–538

25. Knight B, Thomson N, Perry G (2000) Seizures due to norpethidine toxicity. Aust N Z J Med 30(4):513

26. Mather LE, Tucker GT (1976) Systemic availability of orally administered meperidine. Clin Pharmacol Therap 20(5):535–540

27. Kaiko RF, Foley KM, Grabinski PY et al (1983) Central nervous system excitatory effects of meperidine in cancer patients. Ann Neurol 13(2):180–185

28. Modica PA, Tempelhoff R, White PF (1990) Pro- and anticonvulsant effects of anesthetics (Part I). Anesth Analg 70(3):303–315

29. Koren G, Butt W, Chinyanga H et al (1985) Postoperative morphine infusion in newborn infants: assessment of disposition characteristics and safety. J Ped 107(6):963–967

30. Brian JE Jr, Seifen AB (1987) Tonic-clonic activity after sufentanil. Anesth Analg 66(5):481

31. Katz RI, Eide TR, Hartman A, Poppers PJ (1988) Two instances of seizure-like activity in the same patient associated with two different narcotics. Anesth Analg 67(3):289–290

32. Rao TL, Mummaneni N, El-Etr AA (1982) Convulsions: an unusual response to intravenous fentanyl administration. Anesth Analg 61(12):1020–1021

33. Safwat AM, Daniel D (1983) Grand mal seizure after fentanyl administration. Anesthesiology 59(1):78

34. Strong WE, Matson M (1989) Probable seizure after alfentanil. Anesth Analg 68(5):692–693

35. Murkin JM, Moldenhauer CC, Hug CC Jr, Epstein CM (1984) Absence of seizures during induction of anesthesia with high-dose fentanyl. Anesth Analg 63(5):489–494

36. Sebel PS, Bovill JG, Wauquier A, Rog P (1981) Effects of high-dose fentanyl anesthesia on the electroencephalogram. Anesthesiology 55(3):203–211

37. Gardner JS, Blough D, Drinkard CR et al (2000) Tramadol and seizures: a surveillance study in a managed care population. Pharmacotherapy 20(12):1423–1431

38. Marquardt KA, Alsop JA, Albertson TE (2005) Tramadol exposures reported to statewide poison control system. Ann Pharmacother 39(6):1039–1044

39. Spiller HA, Gorman SE, Villalobos D et al (1997) Prospective multicenter evaluation of tramadol exposure. J Tox 35(4):361–364

40. Kahn LH, Alderfer RJ, Graham DJ (1997) Seizures reported with tramadol. JAMA 278(20):1661

41. Gasse C, Derby L, Vasilakis-Scaramozza C, Jick H (2000) Incidence of first-time idiopathic seizures in users of tramadol. Pharmacotherapy 20(6):629–634

42. Quail AW (1989) Modern inhalational anaesthetic agents. A review of halothane, isoflurane and enflurane. Med J Aust 150(2):95–102

43. Julien RM, Kavan EM, Elliott HW (1972) Effects of volatile anaesthetic agents on EEG activity recorded in limbic and sensory systems. Can Anaesth Soc J 19(3):263–269

44. Jenkins J, Milne AC (1984) Convulsive reaction following enflurane anaesthesia. Anaesthesia 39(1):44–45

45. Rosen I, Soderberg M (1975) Electroencephalographic activity in children under enflurane anesthesia. Acta Anaesthesiologica Scand 19(5):361–369

46. Ohm WW, Cullen BF, Amory DW, Kennedy RD (1975) Delayed seizure activity following enflurane anesthesia. Anesthesiology 42(3):367–368

47. Kruczek M, Albin MS, Wolf S, Bertoni JM (1980) Postoperative seizure activity following enflurane anesthesia. Anesthesiology 53(2):175–176

48. Burchiel KJ, Stockard JJ, Calverley RK, Smith NT (1977) Relationship of pre- and postanesthetic EEG abnormalities to enflurane-induced seizure activity. Anesth Analg 56(4):509–514

49. Michenfelder JD, Cucchiara RF (1974) Canine cerebral oxygen consumption during enflurane anesthesia and its modification during induced seizures. Anesthesiology 40(6):575–580

50. Yamashiro M, Sumitomo M, Furuya H (1985) Paroxysmal electroencephalographic discharges during enflurane anaesthesia in patients with a history of cerebral convulsions. Br J Anaesth 57(10):1029–1037

51. Hymes JA (1985) Seizure activity during isoflurane anesthesia. Anesth Analg 64(3):367–368

52. Harrison JL (1986) Postoperative seizures after isoflurane anesthesia. Anesth Analg 65(11):1235–1236

53. Kofke WA, Young RS, Davis P et al (1989) Isoflurane for refractory status epilepticus: a clinical series. Anesthesiology 71(5):653–659

54. Kofke WA, Snider MT, Young RS, Ramer JC (1985) Prolonged low flow isoflurane anesthesia for status epilepticus. Anesthesiology 62(5):653–656

55. Yli-Hankala A, Vakkuri A, Sarkela M et al (1999) Epileptiform electroencephalogram during mask induction of anesthesia with sevoflurane. Anesthesiology 91(6):1596–1603

56. Jantti V, Yli-Hankala A, Vakkuri A (2001) The epileptogenic property of sevoflurane and in patients without epilepsy. Anesth Analg 92(5):1359

57. Vakkuri A, Yli-Hankala A, Sarkela M et al (2001) Sevoflurane mask induction of anaesthesia is associated with epileptiform EEG in children. Acta Anaesthesiologica Scand 45(7):805–811

58. Jaaskelainen SK, Kaisti K, Suni L, Hinkka S, Scheinin H (2003) Sevoflurane is epileptogenic in healthy subjects at surgical levels of anesthesia. Neurology 61(8):1073–1078

59. Constant I, Seeman R, Murat I (2005) Sevoflurane and epileptiform EEG changes. Paediatr Anaesth 15(4):266–274

60. Mohanram A, Kumar V, Iqbal Z, Markan S, Pagel PS (2007) Repetitive generalized seizure-like activity during emergence from sevoflurane anesthesia. Can J Anaesth 54(8):657–661

61. Woodforth IJ, Hicks RG, Crawford MR, Stephen JP, Burke DJ (1997) Electroencephalographic evidence of seizure activity under deep sevoflurane anesthesia in a nonepileptic patient. Anesthesiology 87(6):1579–1582

62. Julliac B, Guehl D, Chopin F et al (2007) Risk factors for the occurrence of electroencephalogram abnormalities during induction of anesthesia with sevoflurane in nonepileptic patients. Anesthesiology 106(2):243–251

63. Iijima T, Nakamura Z, Iwao Y, Sankawa H (2000) The epileptogenic properties of the volatile anesthetics sevoflurane and isoflurane in patients with epilepsy. Anesth Analg 91(4):989–995

64. Rudo FG, Krantz JC Jr (1974) Anaesthetic molecules. Br J Anaesth 46(3):181–189

65. Corssen G, Little SC, Tavakoli M (1974) Ketamine and epilepsy. Anesth Analg 53(2):319–335

66. Steen PA, Michenfelder JD (1979) Neurotoxicity of anesthetics. Anesthesiology 50(5):437–453

67. Ferrer-Allado T, Brechner VL, Dymond A, Cozen H, Crandall P (1973) Ketamine-induced electroconvulsive phenomena in the human limbic and thalamic regions. Anesthesiology 38(4):333–344

68. Bennett DR, Madsen JA, Jordan WS, Wiser WC (1973) Ketamine anesthesia in brain-damaged epileptics. Electroencephalographic and clinical observations. Neurology 23(5):449–460

69. Sheth RD, Gidal BE (1998) Refractory status epilepticus: response to ketamine. Neurology 51(6):1765–1766

70. Laughlin TP, Newberg LA (1985) Prolonged myoclonus after etomidate anesthesia. Anesth Analg 64(1):80–82

71. Ghoneim MM, Yamada T (1977) Etomidate: a clinical and electroencephalographic comparison with thiopental. Anesth Analg 56(4):479–485

72. Modica PA, Tempelhoff R, White PF (1990) Pro- and anticonvulsant effects of anesthetics (Part II). Anesth Analg 70(4):433–444

73. Krieger W, Copperman J, Laxer KD (1985) Seizures with etomidate anesthesia. Anesth Analg 64(12):1226–1227

74. Ebrahim ZY, DeBoer GE, Luders H, Hahn JF, Lesser RP (1986) Effect of etomidate on the electroencephalogram of patients with epilepsy. Anesth Analg 65(10):1004–1006

75. Sutherland MJ, Burt P (1994) Propofol and seizures. Anaesth Intens Care 22(6):733–737

76. Walder B, Tramer MR, Seeck M (2002) Seizure-like phenomena and propofol: a systematic review. Neurology 58(9):1327–1332

77. Bevan JC (1993) Propofol-related convulsions. Can J Anaesth 40(9):805–809

78. Blumer J, Strong JM, Atkinson AJ Jr (1973) The convulsant potency of lidocaine and its N-dealkylated metabolites. J Pharmacol Exp Ther 186(1):31–36

79. Lemmen LJ, Klassen M, Duiser B (1978) Intravenous lidocaine in the treatment of convulsions. JAMA 239(19):2025

80. Bernhard CG, Bohm E (1954) On the effects of xylocain on the central nervous system with special reference to its influence on epileptic phenomena. Experientia 10(11):474–476

81. Reynolds F (1987) Adverse effects of local anaesthetics. Br J Anaesth 59(1):78–95

82. Varelas PN, Mirski MA (2001) Seizures in the adult intensive care unit. J Neurosurg Anesth 13(2):163–175

83. Ochs HR, Carstens G, Greenblatt DJ (1980) Reduction in lidocaine clearance during continuous infusion and by coadministration of propranolol. N Engl J Med 303(7):373–377

84. Feely J, Wilkinson GR, McAllister CB, Wood AJ (1982) Increased toxicity and reduced clearance of lidocaine by cimetidine. Ann Intern Med 96(5):592–594

85. Bauer J (1996) Seizure-inducing effects of antiepileptic drugs: a review. Acta Neurolog Scand 94(6):367–377

86. Gayatri NA, Livingston JH (2006) Aggravation of epilepsy by anti-epileptic drugs. Develop Med Child Neurol 48(5):394–398

87. Gelisse P, Genton P, Kuate C et al (2004) Worsening of seizures by oxcarbazepine in juvenile idiopathic generalized epilepsies. Epilepsia 45(10):1282–1286

88. So EL, Ruggles KH, Cascino GD, Ahmann PA, Weatherford KW (1994) Seizure exacerbation and status epilepticus related to carbamazepine-10, 11-epoxide. Ann Neurol 35(6):743–746

89. Weaver DF, Camfield P, Fraser A (1988) Massive carbamazepine overdose: clinical and pharmacologic observations in five episodes. Neurology 38(5):755–759

90. Wilkus RJ, Dodrill CB, Troupin AS (1978) Carbamazepine and the electroencephalogram of epileptics: a double blind study in comparison to phenytoin. Epilepsia 19(3):283–291

91. Milligan N, Oxley J, Richens A (1983) Acute effects of intravenous phenytoin on the frequency of inter-ictal spikes in man. Br J Clin Pharmacolog 16(3):285–289

92. Schachter SC (1998) Iatrogenic seizures. Neurologic clinics 16(1):157–170

93. Walker AE, Johnson HC (1945) Convulsive factor in commercial penicillin. Arch Surg 50:69–73

94. Porter J, Jick H (1977) Drug-induced anaphylaxis, convulsions, deafness, and extrapyramidal symptoms. Lancet 1(8011):587–588

95. Gutnick MJ, Van Duijn H, Citri N (1976) Relative convulsant potencies of structural analogues of penicillin. Brain Res 114(1):139–143

96. Fossieck B, Jr., Parker RH (1974) Neurotoxicity during intravenous infusion of penicillin. A review. J Clin Pharmacol 14(10):504–512

97. Nicholls PJ (1980) Neurotoxicity of penicillin. J Antimicrobial Chemother 6(2):161–165

98. Barrons RW, Murray KM, Richey RM (1992) Populations at risk for penicillin-induced seizures. Ann Pharmacother 26(1):26–29

99. Wallace KL (1997) Antibiotic-induced convulsions. Crit Care Clin 13(4):741–762

100. De Sarro A, De Sarro GB, Ascioti C, Nistico G (1989) Epileptogenic activity of some beta-lactam derivatives: structure-activity relationship. Neuropharmacology 28(4):359–365

101. Bechtel TP, Slaughter RL, Moore TD (1980) Seizures associated with high cerebrospinal fluid concentrations of cefazolin. Am J Hosp Pharm 37(2):271–273

102. Kamei C, Sunami A, Tasaka K (1983) Epileptogenic activity of cephalosporins in rats and their structure-activity relationship. Epilepsia 24(4):431–439
103. Norrby SR (1996) Neurotoxicity of carbapenem antibacterials. Drug Saf 15(2): 87–90
104. Schliamser SE, Broholm KA, Liljedahl AL, Norrby SR (1988) Comparative neurotoxicity of benzylpenicillin, imipenem/cilastatin and FCE 22101, a new injectible penem. J Antimicro Chemother 22(5):687–695
105. Calandra G, Lydick E, Carrigan J, Weiss L, Guess H (1988) Factors predisposing to seizures in seriously ill infected patients receiving antibiotics: experience with imipenem/cilastatin. Am J Med 84(5):911–918
106. Pestotnik SL, Classen DC, Evans RS, Stevens LE, Burke JP (1993) Prospective surveillance of imipenem/cilastatin use and associated seizures using a hospital information system. Ann Pharmacother 27(4):497–501
107. Norrby SR, Gildon KM (1999) Safety profile of meropenem: a review of nearly 5,000 patients treated with meropenem. Scand J Infect Dis 31(1):3–10
108. Christ W (1990) Central nervous system toxicity of quinolones: human and animal findings. Antimicrob Agents Chemother 26(Suppl B)219–225
109. Akahane K, Sekiguchi M, Une T, Osada Y (1989) Structure-epileptogenicity relationship of quinolones with special reference to their interaction with gamma-aminobutyric acid receptor sites. Antimicrobial Agents Chemother 33(10): 1704–1708
110. Christie MJ, Wong K, Ting RH, Tam PY, Sikaneta TG (2005) Generalized seizure and toxic epidermal necrolysis following levofloxacin exposure. Ann Pharmacother 39(5):953–955
111. O'Donnell JA, Gelone SP (2000) Fluoroquinolones. Infect Dis Clin North Am 14(2):489–513, xi
112. Lietman PS (1995) Fluoroquinolone toxicities. An update. Drugs 49(Suppl 2) 159–163
113. Schwartz MT, Calvert JF (1990) Potential neurologic toxicity related to ciprofloxacin. DICP 24(2):138–140
114. Slavich IL, Gleffe RF, Haas EJ (1989) Grand mal epileptic seizures during ciprofloxacin therapy. JAMA 261(4):558–559
115. Fink MP, Snydman DR, Niederman MS et al (1994) Treatment of severe pneumonia in hospitalized patients: results of a multicenter, randomized, double-blind trial comparing intravenous ciprofloxacin with imipenem-cilastatin. The Severe Pneumonia Study Group. Antimicrob Agents Chemother 38(3):547–557
116. Coyer JR, Nicholson DP (1976) Isoniazid-induced convulsions. South Med J 69(3):294–297
117. Devadatta S (1965) Isoniazid-induced encephalopathy. Lancet 2(7409):440
118. Mahler ME (1987) Seizures: common causes and treatment in the elderly. Geriatrics 42(7):73–78
119. Orlowski JP, Paganini EP, Pippenger CE (1988) Treatment of a potentially lethal dose isoniazid ingestion. Ann Emerg Med 17(1):73–76
120. Nelson LG (1965) Grand mal seizures following overdose of isoniazid. A report of four cases. Am Rev Respir Dis 91:600–604
121. Alvarez FG, Guntupalli KK (1995) Isoniazid overdose: four case reports and review of the literature. Intensive Care Med 21(8):641–644
122. Wason S, Lacouture PG, Lovejoy FH Jr (1981) Single high-dose pyridoxine treatment for isoniazid overdose. JAMA 246(10):1102–1104
123. Frytak S, Moertel CH, Childs DS (1978) Neurologic toxicity associated with high-dose metronidazole therapy. Ann Intern Med 88(3):361–362
124. Kusumi RK, Plouffe JF, Wyatt RH, Fass RJ (1980) Central nervous system toxicity associated with metronidazole therapy. Ann Intern Med 93(1):59–60
125. Bailes J, Willis J, Priebe C, Strub R (1983) Encephalopathy with metronidazole in a child. Am J Dis Child 137(3):290–291

126. Semel JD, Allen N (1991) Seizures in patients simultaneously receiving theophylline and imipenem or ciprofloxacin or metronidazole. South Med J 84(4):465–468

127. Jayaweera DT (1997) Minimising the dosage-limiting toxicities of foscarnet induction therapy. Drug Saf 16(4):258–266

128. Kitching AR, Fagg D, Hay NM, Hatfield PJ, Macdonald A (1997) Neurotoxicity associated with acyclovir in end stage renal failure. N Z Med J 110(1043):167–169

129. Rashiq S, Briewa L, Mooney M et al (1993) Distinguishing acyclovir neurotoxicity from encephalomyelitis. J Intern Med 234(5):507–511

130. Barton TL, Roush MK, Dever LL (1992) Seizures associated with ganciclovir therapy. Pharmacotherapy 12(5):413–415

131. Pascual-Sedano B, Iranzo A, Marti-Fabregas J et al (1999) Prospective study of new-onset seizures in patients with human immunodeficiency virus infection: etiologic and clinical aspects. Arch Neurol 56(5):609–612

132. Romanelli F, Jennings HR, Nath A, Ryan M, Berger J (2000) Therapeutic dilemma: the use of anticonvulsants in HIV-positive individuals. Neurology 54(7):1404–1407

133. Zwillich CW, Sutton FD, Neff TA et al (1975) Theophylline-induced seizures in adults. Correlation with serum concentrations. Ann Intern Med 82(6):784–787

134. Bahls FH, Ma KK, Bird TD (1991) Theophylline-associated seizures with "therapeutic" or low toxic serum concentrations: risk factors for serious outcome in adults. Neurology 41(8):1309–1312

135. Gaudreault P, Guay J (1986) Theophylline poisoning. Pharmacological considerations and clinical management. Med Toxicol 1(3):169–191

136. Aitken ML, Martin TR (1987) Life-threatening theophylline toxicity is not predictable by serum levels. Chest 91(1):10–14

137. Paloucek FP, Rodvold KA (1988) Evaluation of theophylline overdoses and toxicities. Ann Emerg Med 17(2):135–144

138. Zaccara G, Muscas GC, Messori A (1990) Clinical features, pathogenesis and management of drug-induced seizures. Drug Saf 5(2):109–151

139. Henderson A, Wright DM, Pond SM (1992) Management of theophylline overdose patients in the intensive care unit. Anaesth Intensive Care 20(1):56–62

140. Olson KR, Benowitz NL, Woo OF, Pond SM (1985) Theophylline overdose: acute single ingestion versus chronic repeated overmedication. Am J Emerg Med 3(5):386–394

141. Kumar A, Bleck TP (1992) Intravenous midazolam for the treatment of refractory status epilepticus. Crit Care Med 20(4):483–488

142. Scott JP, Higenbottam TW (1988) Adverse reactions and interactions of cyclosporin. Med Toxicol Adverse Drug Exp 3(2):107–127

143. Gilmore RL (1988) Seizures and antiepileptic drug use in transplant patients. Neurol Clin 6(2):279–296

144. Truwit CL, Denaro CP, Lake JR, DeMarco T (1991) MR imaging of reversible cyclosporin A-induced neurotoxicity. AJNR 12(4):651–659

145. Glass GA, Stankiewicz J, Mithoefer A, Freeman R, Bergethon PR (2005) Levetiracetam for seizures after liver transplantation. Neurology 64(6):1084–1085

146. Ekberg H, Grinyo J, Nashan B et al (2007) Cyclosporine sparing with mycophenolate mofetil, daclizumab and corticosteroids in renal allograft recipients: The CAESAR Study. Am J Transplant 7(3):560–570

147. Maramattom BV, Wijdicks EF (2004) Sirolimus may not cause neurotoxicity in kidney and liver transplant recipients. Neurology 63(10):1958–1959

148. Thistlethwaite JR Jr, Stuart JK, Mayes JT et al (1988) Complications and monitoring of OKT3 therapy. Am J Kidney Dis 11(2):112–119

149. Kay HE, Knapton PJ, O'Sullivan JP et al (1972) Encephalopathy in acute leukaemia associated with methotrexate therapy. Arch Dis Child 47(253):344–354

150. Johnson FL, Bernstein ID, Hartmann JR, Chard RL Jr (1973) Seizures associated with vincristine sulfate therapy. J Pediatr 82(4):699–702

151. Singh G, Rees JH, Sander JW (2007) Seizures and epilepsy in oncological practice: causes, course, mechanisms and treatment. J Neurol Neurosurg Psychiatry 78(4):342–349

152. Alldredge BK (1999) Seizure risk associated with psychotropic drugs: clinical and pharmacokinetic considerations. Neurology 53(5 Suppl 2):S68–S75

153. Logothetis J (1967) Spontaneous epileptic seizures and electroencephalographic changes in the course of phenothiazine therapy. Neurology 17(9):869–877

154. Cold JA, Wells BG, Froemming JH (1990) Seizure activity associated with antipsychotic therapy. DICP 24(6):601–606

155. Remick RA, Fine SH (1979) Antipsychotic drugs and seizures. J Clin Psychiatry 40(2):78–80

156. Devinsky O, Honigfeld G, Patin J (1991) Clozapine-related seizures. Neurology 41(3):369–371

157. Ereshefsky L, Watanabe MD, Tran-Johnson TK (1989) Clozapine: an atypical antipsychotic agent. Clin Pharm 8(10):691–709

158. Wilson WH, Claussen AM (1994) Seizures associated with clozapine treatment in a state hospital. J Clin Psychiatry 55(5):184–188

159. Toth P, Frankenburg FR (1994) Clozapine and seizures: A review. Can J Psychiatry 39(4):236–238

160. Navarro V, Pons A, Romero A, Bernardo M (2001) Topiramate for clozapine-induced seizures. Am J Psychiatry 158(6):968–969

161. Centorrino F, Price BH, Tuttle M et al (2002) EEG abnormalities during treatment with typical and atypical antipsychotics. Am J Psychiatry 159(1):109–115

162. Amann BL, Pogarell O, Mergl R et al (2003) EEG abnormalities associated with antipsychotics: a comparison of quetiapine, olanzapine, haloperidol and healthy subjects. Hum Psychopharmacol 18(8):641–646

163. Barnes TR, McPhillips MA (1999) Critical analysis and comparison of the side-effect and safety profiles of the new antipsychotics. Br J Psychiatry (38):34–43

164. Citrome L (1997) New antipsychotic medications: what advantages do they offer? Postgrad Med 101(2):207–210, 213–204

165. Casey DE (1997) The relationship of pharmacology to side effects. H Clin Psychiatry 58(Suppl 10):55–62

166. Hedges D, Jeppson K, Whitehead P (2003) Antipsychotic medication and seizures: a review. Drugs Today (Barc) 39(7):551–557

167. Alper K, Schwartz KA, Kolts RL, Khan A (2007) Seizure incidence in psychopharmacological clinical trials: an analysis of Food and Drug Administration (FDA) summary basis of approval reports. Biolog Psychiatry 62(4):345–354

168. Wyderski RJ, Starrett WG, Abou-Saif A (1999) Fatal status epilepticus associated with olanzapine therapy. Ann Pharmacother 33(7–8):787–789

169. Lee JW, Crismon ML, Dorson PG (1999) Seizure associated with olanzapine. Ann Pharmacother 33(5):554–556

170. Pillmann F, Schlote K, Broich K, Marneros A (2000) Electroencephalogram alterations during treatment with olanzapine. Psychopharmacology 150(2):216–219

171. Pisani F, Oteri G, Costa C, Di Raimondo G, Di Perri R (2002) Effects of psychotropic drugs on seizure threshold. Drug Saf 25(2):91–110

172. Lee KC, Finley PR, Alldredge BK (2003) Risk of seizures associated with psychotropic medications: emphasis on new drugs and new findings. Exp Opin Drug Safety 2(3):233–247

173. Woolley J, Smith S (2001) Lowered seizure threshold on olanzapine. Br J Psychiatry 178(1):85–86

174. Rosenstein DL, Nelson JC, Jacobs SC (1993) Seizures associated with antide-pressants: a review. J Clin Psychiatry 54(8):289–299

175. Wedin GP, Oderda GM, Klein-Schwartz W, Gorman RL (1986) Relative toxicity of cyclic antidepressants. Ann Emerg Med 15(7):797–804

176. Starkey IR, Lawson AA (1980) Poisoning with tricyclic and related antidepres-sants – a ten-year review. Quart J Med 49(193):33–49

177. Brooke G, Weatherly JR (1959) Imipramine. Lancet 2:568–569

178. DeVeaugh-Geiss J, Landau P, Katz R (1989) Preliminary results from a multi-center trial of clomipramine in obsessive-compulsive disorder. Psychopharmacol Bull 25(1):36–40

179. Preskorn SH, Fast GA (1992) Tricyclic antidepressant-induced seizures and plasma drug concentration. J Clin Psychiatry 53(5):160–162

180. Lowry MR, Dunner FJ (1980) Seizures during tricyclic therapy. Am J Psychiatry 137(11):1461–1462

181. Kulig K, Rumack BH, Sullivan JB, Jr., et al (1982) Amoxapine overdose. Coma and seizures without cardiotoxic effects. JAMA 248(9):1092–1094

182. Boehnert MT, Lovejoy FH Jr (1985) Value of the QRS duration versus the serum drug level in predicting seizures and ventricular arrhythmias after an acute over-dose of tricyclic antidepressants. N Eng J Med 313(8):474–479

183. Ellison DW, Pentel PR (1989) Clinical features and consequences of seizures due to cyclic antidepressant overdose. Am J Emerg Med 7(1):5–10

184. Favale E, Rubino V, Mainardi P, Lunardi G, Albano C (1995) Anticonvulsant effect of fluoxetine in humans. Neurology 45(10):1926–1927

185. Braitberg G, Curry SC (1995) Seizure after isolated fluoxetine overdose. Ann Emerg Med 26(2):234–237

186. Kelly CA, Dhaun N, Laing WJ et al (2004) Comparative toxicity of citalopram and the newer antidepressants after overdose. J Toxicol 42(1):67–71

187. Bodner RA, Lynch T, Lewis L, Kahn D (1995) Serotonin syndrome. Neurology 45(2):219–223

188. Carbone JR (2000) The neuroleptic malignant and serotonin syndromes. Emerg Med Clin North Am 18(2):317–325, x

189. Lieberman JA, Kane JM, Reife R (1985) Neuromuscular effects of monoamine oxidase inhibitors. J Clin Psychopharmacol 5(4):221–228

190. Belson MG, Kelley TR (2002) Bupropion exposures: clinical manifestations and medical outcome. J Emerg Med 23(3):223–230

191. Davidson J (1989) Seizures and bupropion: a review. J Clin Psychiatry 50(7):256–261

192. Rissmiller DJ, Campo T (2007) Extended-release bupropion induced grand mal seizures. J Am Osteopath Assoc 107(10):441–442

193. Nierenberg AA, Cole JO (1991) Antidepressant adverse drug reactions. J Clin Psychiatry 52(Suppl):40–47

194. Johnston JA, Lineberry CG, Ascher JA et al (1991) A 102-center prospective study of seizure in association with bupropion. J Clin Psychiatry 52(11):450–456

195. Whyte IM, Dawson AH, Buckley NA (2003) Relative toxicity of venlafaxine and selective serotonin reuptake inhibitors in overdose compared to tricyclic antide-pressants. QJM 96(5):369–374

196. Struve FA (1987) Lithium-specific pathological electroencephalographic changes: a successful replication of earlier investigative results. Clin EEG 18(2):46–53

197. Hansen HE, Amdisen A (1978) Lithium intoxication. (Report of 23 cases and review of 100 cases from the literature). Quart J Med 47(186):123–144

198. Okusa MD, Crystal LJ (1994) Clinical manifestations and management of acute lithium intoxication. Am J Med 97(4):383–389

199. Mayan H, Golubev N, Dinour D, Farfel Z (2001) Lithium intoxication due to carbamazepine-induced renal failure. Ann Pharmacother 35(5):560–562

200. Shukla S, Godwin CD, Long LE, Miller MG (1984) Lithium-carbamazepine neurotoxicity and risk factors. Am J Psychiatry 141(12):1604–1606
201. Happe S (2003) Excessive daytime sleepiness and sleep disturbances in patients with neurological diseases: epidemiology and management. Drugs 63(24):2725–2737
202. Zagnoni PG, Albano C (2002) Psychostimulants and epilepsy. Epilepsia 43(Suppl 2): 28–31
203. Thomas S, Upadhyaya H (2002) Adderall and seizures. J Am Acad Child Adolesc Psychiatry 41(4):365
204. Hemmer SA, Pasternak JF, Zecker SG, Trommer BL (2001) Stimulant therapy and seizure risk in children with ADHD. Ped Neurol 24(2):99–102
205. Ivanenko A, Tauman R, Gozal D (2003) Modafinil in the treatment of excessive daytime sleepiness in children. Sleep Med 4(6):579–582
206. Green LB, Nelson VS (1999) Death after acute withdrawal of intrathecal baclofen: case report and literature review. Arch Phys Medi Rehab 80(12):1600–1604
207. Kofler M, Arturo Leis A (1992) Prolonged seizure activity after baclofen withdrawal. Neurology 42(3 Pt 1):697–698
208. Greenberg MI, Hendrickson RG (2003) Baclofen withdrawal following removal of an intrathecal baclofen pump despite oral baclofen replacement. J Tox 41(1): 83–85
209. Koppel C, Ibe K, Tenczer J (1987) Clinical symptomatology of diphenhydramine overdose: an evaluation of 136 cases in 1982 to 1985. J Tox 25(1–2):53–70
210. Magera BE, Betlach CJ, Sweatt AP, Derrick CW Jr (1981) Hydroxyzine intoxication in a 13-month-old child. Pediatrics 67(2):280–283
211. Nelson M, Bartlett RJ, Lamb JT (1989) Seizures after intravenous contrast media for cranial computed tomography. J Neurol Neurosurg Psychiatry 52(10):1170–1175
212. Avrahami E, Weiss-Peretz J, Cohn DF (1987) Focal epileptic activity following intravenous contrast material injection in patients with metastatic brain disease. J Neurol Neurosurg Psychiatry 50(2):221–223
213. Weinstein RS (1984) Recognition and management of poisoning with beta-adrenergic blocking agents. Ann Emerg Med 13(12):1123–1131
214. Das G, Ferris JC (1988) Generalized convulsions in a patient receiving ultrashort-acting beta-blocker infusion. DICP 22(6):484–485
215. Mirski MA, Varelas PN (2008) Seizures and status epilepticus in the critically ill. Crit Care Clin 24(1):115–147, ix
216. Sabers A, Gram L (2000) Newer anticonvulsants: comparative review of drug interactions and adverse effects. Drugs 60(1):23–33
217. Franson KL, Hay DP, Neppe V et al (1995) Drug-induced seizures in the elderly. Causative agents and optimal management. Drugs Aging 7(1):38–48

Chapter 14

Critical Care Seizures Related to Illicit Drugs and Toxins

Andreas R. Luft

Abstract Seizures caused by ingestion of drugs and toxins do require specific treatment aiming to terminate epileptiform activity and to eliminate the toxin. Withdrawal from regularly ingested drugs can also be accompanied by seizures requiring ICU care. This chapter discusses diagnostic and therapeutic particularities of seizures induced by illicit drugs of abuse, environmental toxins, and heavy metals.

Keywords Illicit drugs, Opiates, Sedatives, Stimulants, Solvents, Toxins, Heavy metals, Lead, Mercury, Tin, Seizures

14.1. Introduction

A variety of drugs and toxins cause seizures and status epilepticus requiring ICU admission. If intoxication is suspected, identification of the causative agent is mandatory as specific therapies aimed at toxin elimination need to be initiated in parallel to anticonvulsant treatment and supportive measures. Seizures may also occur as a result of withdrawal of recreational drugs while a patient is in the ICU for other reasons. Seizures then complicate the case and may interfere with treatment of the primary disease. Timely identification of the seizure's origin and of the drug or the toxin involved is mandatory. Companion symptoms (e.g. delirium), the patient's history, and drug screens in blood and urine must be taken into consideration.

14.2. Illicit Drugs

Chronic use, overdose (intoxication), and withdrawal are potential causes of seizures in illicit drugs users. A retrospective analysis identified 49 cases of recreational drug-induced seizures admitted to the San Francisco General Hospital between 1975 and 1987. While the great majority had one single focal or generalized seizure, seven patients had multiple convulsions and two developed status epilepticus requiring ICU admission [1]. Identified drugs were cocaine

From: *Seizures in Critical Care*: *A Guide to Diagnosis and Therapeutics*: Current Clinical Neurology, Second Edition, Edited by: P. Varelas, DOI 10.1007/978-1-60327-532-3_14, © Humana Press, a part of Springer Science+Business Media, LLC 2005, 2010

(32 cases), amphetamine (11 cases), heroin (7 cases), and phencyclidine (4 cases). All except one patient had complete recovery. A retrospective review of the California Poison Control in 2003 evaluated the causes of all drug-related seizures in 2003 [2]: Of 386 cases, 7.5 and 6.9% were related to tramadol and amphetamine use, while 37% were related to antidepressants (tricyclics, bupropione, venlafaxine), 8% to sedatives (diphenhydramine), and 6% to isoniazid.

These analyses demonstrate that hospital admissions for recreational drug-induced seizures are infrequent. Routine screening for recreational drugs in patients admitted to the hospital because of a seizure has a low yield and should only be considered if the patient's history raises suspicion for drug abuse [3]. However, if illicit drugs are suspected and seizure activity is prolonged, ICU care is necessary because management of drug-related seizures may be extremely difficult (especially in cases of cocaine abuse).

14.2.1. Opiates

Opiates include natural (endogenous: e.g., endorphin; exogenous: e.g. morphine, a constituent of the milky extract of opium poppy, *Papaver somniferum*) or synthetic (e.g. fentanyl) compounds acting on central opiate receptors and producing psychological and physical dependence. Heroin (diacetylmorphin, a lipophilic morphin analog with faster blood–brain-barrier passage) is the most commonly used recreational opiate leading to abuse and addiction. Intoxication usually caused by intravenous administration of an overdose presents with coma, respiratory depression, pinpoint but reactive pupils, and vomiting. Seizures are uncommon, which is expected given the inhibitory actions of opiates on the brain: opiate receptors (M, Δ, K) inhibit the adenylate cyclase and close Ca^{2+} channels via G-protein-mediated pathways and thereby reduce neuronal excitability. Proseizure effects of morphine have been reported in an in vitro murine hippocampus preparation precipitated by selective stimulation of mu and kappa opiate receptors [4]. In humans, seizures have been reported in 2% of heroin-overdosed patients [5], which may be attributed to heroin itself [6] or to adulterants. Inadvertent intrathecal application of morphine led to seizure in one reported case [7].

Because seizures related to opiates themselves are uncommon, other causes should be explored. These can be direct toxic effects of adulterant drugs or the other results of diseases frequently observed in the addicted population (stroke, infection, neoplasms, metabolic derangement). Adulterant drugs should be sought in laboratory analysis [8]. Acute opiate intoxication can be treated with the antagonist naloxone (2 mg iv, repeated as needed up to 20 mg). No specific recommendations exist for the use of anticonvulsants.

In contrast to acute overdose, chronic heroin abuse is an independent risk factor for seizures with an adjusted odds ratio of 2.8 ($p < 0.05$) that was increased to 3.6 when concomitant brain pathology was present [9]. Seizures sometimes accompany opiate withdrawal which in adults typically presents with flu-like symptoms. A study by Wijdicks and Sharbrough evaluating patients with new onset seizures admitted to the medical or surgical ICU at the Mayo Clinic identified sudden withdrawal of narcotics as a cause of tonic-clonic seizures [10]. Among all admissions with first-ever seizure of identifiable cause, patients in opioid withdrawal constituted the largest group. However, they represented only a small fraction of all ICU admissions during the 10-year study period (0.066%). Therefore, opioid withdrawal seizure remains a rare cause of ICU admission. General withdrawal symptoms are usually well handled with methadone (20 mg once or twice daily). Withdrawal in the neonate (neonatal abstinence syndrome, NAS) who was exposed to opiates taken by the mother is more severe and more frequently associated with seizures. Its treatment should be based on substitution of opiates. If sedatives are required, phenobarbital is preferred to diazepam [11].

The opiate oxycodone has been reported to lower seizure threshold in patients with a history of seizures or acute renal failure. One epileptic patient seized several times after ingestion of oxycodone. Seizures were controlled with carbamazepine and the opiate could be continued [12]. Seizures were also reported as a symptom of Tramadol intoxication [13] (see more details in Chap. 13).

14.2.2. Sedatives and Hypnotics

Sedative agents used for recreational purposes include benzodiazepines, barbiturates, and others (e.g., glutethimide, methaqualone). Especially barbiturates have an addictive potential of psychological and physical dependence which is between stimulants (see below) and opiates. Benzodiazepines with a lower abusive potential may also lead to withdrawal symptoms. Seizures, however, are not as common as with barbiturates. In a study in which patients were withdrawn from therapeutic doses of benzodiazepines taken for several months, withdrawal seizures were not reported [14]. As benzodiazepines and barbiturates are powerful antiepileptics, seizures have not been observed with overdose – mostly administered on suicidal purpose. However, flumazenil used as a benzodiazepine antidote, has reportedly led to partial seizures [15] and fatal status epilepticus [16].

Withdrawal from benzodiazepines and barbiturates may be complicated by seizures along with delirium tremens (in many aspects similar to alcohol withdrawal) and often requires ICU care. Seizure susceptibility is explained in part by the downregulation of GABA receptors by long-term use of these sedatives [17, 18]. Additionally, a role of the glutamatergic system is suspected because reduced susceptibility was observed after treating benzodiazepine-dependent mice with an NMDA antagonist [19].

Seizures are observed in 3% of patients going through benzodiazepine withdrawal [20]. They typically occur within 1–10 days after stopping the benzodiazepine or barbiturate, depending on the specific agent's half-life and the previously ingested dose [21]. For example, with short acting barbiturates like secobarbital, pentobarbital, or amobarbital, seizures are expected within the first 2–3 days after abrupt withdrawal of the drug and, as with alcohol, are followed occasionally by delirium tremens. Withdrawal from long-term use of pentobarbital is associated with seizures in 10% of subjects taking 600 mg per day and in 75% taking 900 mg. With lower daily doses of 400 mg, electroencephalographic changes consistent with epileptiform discharges can be found in up to one-third of patients [22]. Sedative withdrawal seizures should be treated with titrated doses of benzodiazepine or barbiturate (determination of a "stabilization dose," usually 200 mg pentobarbital every 6 h, followed by gradual tapering over 2–3 weeks). Most other anticonvulsants are ineffective.

Other sedatives, such as chloral hydrate and meprobamate, can also cause seizures during withdrawal. In contrast, glutethimide [23] and pentazocine/tripelennamine (T's and blues) can produce seizures on ingestion [24].

14.2.3. Stimulants

Psychostimulants are amphetamines, ephedrine, and methylphenidate (Ritalin). These agents release monoamines at the synaptic nerve terminals. Clinical use of amphetamines is established for treatment of narcolepsy, hyperactivity in children, and the control of obesity. Because of their widespread use, amphetamines are easy to procure. After cannabis, amphetamines are therefore the most common drugs of abuse. Use of methylenedioxymethamphetamine (MDMA, "ecstasy"), an amphetamine with stimulant and hallucinogenic properties, has quadrupled over the past decade [25]. Another psychostimulant with properties similar to MDMA is cocaine. In contrast to amphetamines, cocaine blocks the reuptake of monoamines at synaptic nerve endings.

Seizures can occur with psychostimulant overdose but also after intentional administration of high doses. Reported frequencies of cocaine-induced seizures vary between 1 and 40% [26]. In one study women were more likely to present with seizures than men (18% vs. 6%) [27]. Seizures occur with amphetamines, especially MDMA, even at intentional doses [28], but are less frequent than with cocaine [1]. Frequent acute adverse reactions of MDMA are hypothermia and hyponatremia [29]. An association exists between MDMA or cocaine use and acute catastrophic neurovascular events, such as subarachnoid hemorrhage and stroke. These events can on their own produce seizures [30, 31]. These seizures are commonly focal, whereas the typical cocaine-induced seizure is generalized. Brain imaging studies should therefore be considered in stimulant users with focal seizures. Convulsions induced by cocaine are usually of short duration and occur immediately or within a few hours. MDMA produces a secondary clonic phase after the initial ictal event [32]. Rarely status epilepticus develops requiring ICU care. Complex partial status epilepticus, i.e. nonconvulsive has been reported with alkaloid "crack" cocaine abuse (smoked) in a patient who presented with bizarre behavior thought to be "cocaine psychosis" [10]. Seizures during stimulant withdrawal have not been reported.

Responsiveness to treatment depends on the drugs: metamphetamine seizures respond to diazepam and valproate but are refractory to phenytoin. Phenytoin is more effective for cocaine-induced seizures. However, rare status epilepticus after cocaine and also after MDMA is notoriously refractory to conventional treatment and requires ICU management [27, 33–35]. 4-Methylaminorex related seizures can be treated with the calcium channel blocker flunarizine [30].

14.2.4. Solvents

Solvents include hydrocarbons, ketones, esters, and ethers and are commonly consumed by inhalation of glues, cleaning fluids, paint thinners, or anesthetics. Addictive effects resemble those of ethanol. Chronic abuse can lead to focal neurological deficits (e.g., cranial nerve palsies, internuclear ophtalmoplegia, and peripheral neuropathy) [36] and CNS demyelination [37]. Severe intoxication or oral administration can be accompanied by seizures [38, 39]. Seizures may be partial or generalized [40, 41]. Chronic solvent exposure may also lead to temporal lobe epilepsy as demonstrated by a case of occupational intoxication [42]. Seizures were fully controlled after stopping the exposure to cyclohexanone and isopropanol.

1,4-Butanediol is a solvent that is metabolized to gammahydroxybutyric acid (GHB) that acts through GABA receptors. GHB and its derivative gammabutyrolactone (GBL) have gained popularity as illicit drugs because of their sedative, anxiolytic, and euphoria-inducing effects. Poisoning leads to states of confusion, aggression, and combative behavior, and later to coma, respiratory depression, and death. Withdrawal is characterized by tremor, hallucinations, tachycardia, insomnia, and in a few reported cases by epileptic seizures [43]. In Sweden high dissemination of GHB and mortality rates comparable to those of heroin were reported [44].

14.2.5. Hallucinogens

Marijuana is the illicit drug most frequently used for recreational purposes. It is derived from the hemp plant *Cannabis sativa*. Its major hallucinogenic ingredient is Δ9-tetrahydrocannabinol (THC). THC acts via a specific receptor (CB1) expressed widely throughout the brain; certain brain lipids (anandamide) are endogenous activators of CB1 and operate as retrograde synaptic transmitters [45]. Cannabinoids have anticonvulsant properties [9, 46], which are described as being similar to those of phenytoin [47], despite different mechanisms of action [48]. Proconvulsant activity was also reported for THC in a rat model [49]; this discrepancy is likely related to species and seizure model. Cannabis withdrawal can produce a mild withdrawal syndrome consisting of anxiety, nausea, increased body temperature, and tremors. Seizures are not part of this syndrome.

Other natural (mescaline, psilocybin) and synthetic hallucinogens (lysergic acid diethylamide, LSD) are not considered epileptogenic. However, one case of grand mal seizure after an LSD overdose has been reported [50].

Phencyclidine ("Angel dust"), a hallucinogenic anesthetic, has anticonvulsant properties [51]. Intoxication, however, can lead to a severe clinical syndrome characterized by agitation, violence, psychosis, and catatonia, which can be complicated by rhabdomyolysis, hyperthermia, and seizures [52]. Fatal status epilepticus has been reported in this setting [53].

14.3. Epileptogenic Environmental Toxins

14.3.1. Marine Toxins

Among various toxins produced by marine animals or plants, domoic acid and ciguatera toxins are most relevant in view of epileptogenicity. Domoic acid (DA) is a potent excitotoxin that is produced by aglae (*Nitzschia pungens*). Humans are intoxicated via the food chain by eating mussels containing the poison. Domoic acid is an analog of kainic acid and binds to NMDA glutamate receptors [54]. Administered to rats, DA produces seizures resulting from unspecific neuronal activation throughout many brain areas. Excitotoxic brain damage ensues within certain brain regions, hippocampus and cerebellum being more vulnerable than others [55].

An epidemic DA intoxication was first identified in Canada in late 1987 [56]. After eating poisoned mussels, 107 patients developed acute gastrointestinal symptoms (76%), incapacitating headache (43%), and loss of short-term memory (25%). Twelve patients (11%) required intensive care because of seizures, coma, respiratory, or circulatory problems. One fourth of those patients died. Hippocampal and amygdaloid damage was the leading neuropathological finding [57]. Hippocampal damage, also demonstrated in survivors by reduced glucose uptake in PET imaging [57], is likely responsible for persisting seizure activity until 4 months after intoxication and for delayed onset temporal lobe epilepsy after 1 year [58]. Acute DA-induced seizure activity was resistant to phenytoin but controlled by diazepam and phenobarbital [57].

Although less epileptogenic, ciguatera fish intoxication is the most common nonbacterial marine food poisoning syndrome in humans. Ciguatoxins are heat stable polyether toxins which act by increasing the permeability of excitable membranes to sodium ions [59]. Produced by the benthic (bottom dwelling) dinoflagellate *Gambierdiscus toxicus* they enter the food chain via carnivore fish (mackarel, barracuda, rabbitfish) and reach humans. Ciguatera is endemic in tropical countries but has been observed in North America and Europe, where the diagnosis is often missed or the condition is misdiagnosed for multiple sclerosis [60]. This confusion stems from the typical ciguatera symptomatology being paraesthesiae, especially of thermo- and nociception with hot–cold inversion, occurring several hours after ingestion. Paraesthesiae usually begin periorally and then spread centrifugally. Complete restitution is common [61] but can take as long as several months and in some cases symptoms persist. Severe intoxication can lead to coma, flaccid paralysis, respiratory paralysis, and generalized tonic-clonic seizures [59, 62, 63]. Deaths have been reported [64]. Confirmation of diagnosis can be achieved by detecting the toxin in human blood using available bioassays [65, 61]. Treatment with intravenous mannitol (10 ml/kg of 20% solution infused slowly over 30–45 min) after initial fluid replacement reduces Schwann cell edema and completely reverses symptoms in up to 60% of patients [66, 59]. In a double-blind randomized study of mannitol versus normal saline treatment over 24 h, mannitol was not found superior and had more side effects [14]. Additional supportive therapy may be necessary.

14.3.2. Mushroom and Plant Toxins

The most poisonous mushrooms are of the *Amanita* species. These produce a variety of toxins (amatoxins) [67]. *Amanita phalloides* produces the cytotoxic amanitin, which can lead to acute hepatic and renal failure within days of ingestion [68]. Seizures can occur as part of fulminant hepatic failure (FHF) and are likely related to ammonia toxicity, which increases synaptic glutamate release [69]. Besides anticonvulsant and supportive therapy, specific treatments for *A. phalloides* poisoning include gastric decontamination, oral activated charcoal and lactulose, high doses of penicillin, ceftazidime, thioctic acid, or silibinin, and combined hemodialysis and hemoperfusion [70, 71]. Positive effects of acetylcysteine were also reported [72]. Benzodiazepines, as the first-line drug for agitation and seizures, have been used in the past.

Other *Amanita* species, especially *Inocybe, Clitocybe, Amanita pantherina, Amanita muscaria*, and *Psilocybe*, produce neurotoxins [73]. Examples of these toxins are ibotenic acid, stizolobic acid, and muscimol. Intoxication occurs most commonly in children (unintentional ingestion) and produces a distinctive syndrome consisting of alternating phases of drowsiness, agitation plus hallucinations, and seizures occurring within 2–3 h after ingestion [74]. In a study of nine cases of *A. pantherina* or muscarina poisoning, seizures were observed in four [75]. All seizures were controlled by standard anticonvulsant agents. In contrast to *A. phalloides* poisoning, intoxication from neurotoxic *Amanita* species is usually time limited and followed by complete recovery. However, mushroom identification should be sought, because syndromes differ in their course and treatment. Identification may be achieved from the remains of a meal [76].

Besides mushrooms, ingestion of certain plants can induce seizures. Water hemlock or other members of the *Cicuta* genus and their toxin, cicutoxin, are mostly involved. Water hemlock grows along rivers in North America. Intoxication conveys an overall mortality rate of 70% [77]. Typical symptomatology includes nausea followed by loss of consciousness and generalized seizures. In one report a patient was successfully treated with hemodialysis and hemoperfusion, forced diuresis, and artificial ventilation [78]. Other toxic plants that can sometimes induce seizures (with severe intoxication) include members of the belladonna alkaloid family (jimsonweed, nightshade), azalea, and Christmas rose [79].

Besides direct toxicity, plant ingestion can lead to intoxication by insecticides or herbicides. Amitraz is a widely used insecticide that often leads to intoxication in children. Symptoms include loss of consciousness, vomiting, hypotension, hypothermia, and generalized seizures and evolve within 2 h after ingestion [80, 81]. Benzodiazepine treatment is effective against convulsions [80]. The outcome is usually good.

14.3.3. Carbon Monoxide

Carbon monoxide (CO) is a colorless and odorless gas that is contained in exhaust fumes of motor vehicles, smoke from fires, and fumes of faulty heating systems. Intoxication results from acute inhalation or from chronic exposure to low concentrations. Seizures can occur with either acute or chronic poisoning. CO has a higher affinity for hemoglobin (forming carboxyhemoglobin) than oxygen. It therefore competitively removes oxygen from hemoglobin, thereby producing tissue hypoxia. The brain is the organ most vulnerable to hypoxia which leads to neurological symptoms ranging from dizziness to coma. CO intoxication is more common during the winter when heating systems are being used. Because initial symptoms are nonspecific, the diagnosis is often missed unless direct spectroscopic measurement of the whole blood COHb level is performed. In a prospective study COHb levels were measured in 753 unselected patients admitted to the emergency department. Those with suspected diagnosis of CO intoxication were excluded. Two patients from the entire cohort (0.3%) and 1 of 20 (5%) admitted with seizures had COHb levels of greater than 10% [82]. In several case reports mild-to-moderate CO poisoning (mild: 10–20% COHb, moderate: 20–40% COHb) presented as an isolated focal or generalized seizure [83–85]. Other symptoms of mild to moderate poisoning included headache (90%), dizziness (82%), visual disturbances, and fatigue [86]. The classic cherry-red discoloration of the skin (color of carboxyhemoglobin) is mostly seen with severe intoxication (40–60% COHb), which also leads to coma, generalized convulsions, and respiratory impairment. Global brain swelling and signs of hypoxia (hypodensities in white matter or basal ganglia) are seen on computed tomography. In one report the EEG was characterized by lateralized sharp waves and a focal electrographic seizure discharge within hours of the CO exposure associated with coma and focal motor seizures [87]. One case of CO-related nonconvulsive status epilepticus in a 70-year-old female patient has also been reported [88]. Long-term sequelae of severe intoxication range from memory deficits or extrapyramidal disorders to persistent vegetative state [89].

The therapy of choice for acute CO intoxication is hyperbaric oxygen therapy [90], which significantly reduces late sequelae [91]. Oxygen itself has neurotoxic properties: especially, when applied under high pressure, oxygen can induce seizures. In one study, seizures occurred in 0.3% of cases at 2.45 atm abs and in 2% at 2.80 atm abs [92]. Mortality remains at the 30% level if the patient is not treated with hyperbaric oxygen, but drops to less than 10% if this treatment is offered early [90, 79].

14.3.4. Heavy Metals

14.3.4.1. Introduction

Heavy metal poisoning stems from environmental pollution (e.g., herbicides, pesticides), occupational exposure (e.g., mining), and iatrogenic (e.g., antimicrobials) or intentional ingestion of recreational drugs (e.g., gasoline sniffing). Heavy metals can bind to various reactive groups (ligands) to inhibit their physiological function. Drugs designed to limit the toxic effects of heavy metals (chelators) compete with these endogenous ligands for heavy metal binding. Chelators have a greater affinity for heavy metals and form complexes which are easily eliminated from the body. Most heavy metal poisoning is secondary to chronic exposure.

14.3.4.2. Lead

Lead intoxication is common since Ancient Roman ages, when lead was ingested via water delivered through lead pipe systems. Today, most cases of lead poisoning are the result of occupational exposure. Large-scale prevention programs have been introduced to eliminate this health hazard [93]. Other cases of lead intoxication occur in children who accidentally ingest lead-containing paint or soil. Chronic lead poisoning is therefore more common in adults, whereas acute intoxication more often occurs in children. The symptoms differ: chronic exposure leads to gastrointestinal, hematological, and renal symptoms. CNS and neuromuscular symptoms predominate with acute intoxication. The neurological syndrome of lead poisoning includes vertigo, clumsiness, ataxia, headache, insomnia, restlessness, and convulsions [94, 95]. Seizures are often repetitive and tonic-clonic and are followed by somnolence with visual disturbances or coma [96, 97]. Lead binding to GABA, thereby reducing inhibition in cortical circuits, has been suggested as a possible pathophysiological mechanism for lead-induced seizures [98]. Anticonvulsants that increase GABA-mediated inhibition (sodium valproate, barbiturates, and benzodiazepines) are therefore preferred in lead-induced seizures [98]. Chronic lead exposure can also produce thiamine deficiency which lowers seizure threshold [99]. In these cases thiamine should be substituted. Other treatments for lead intoxication include chelating agents – edetate calcium disodium (CaNa^2 EDTA), dimercaprol, d-penicillamine, or succimer (2,3-dimercaptosuccinic acid). Anemia with basophilic stippling of red cells and lead lines at the metaphyses of long bones are other diagnostic findings. Blood zinc protoporphyrin (ZPP) levels can be used to assess lead exposure over the prior 3 months [100]. Excretion of lead in the urine should be assessed before and after initiation of therapy with chelating agents. Asymptomatic patients with blood lead levels greater than 80 µg/dl or symptomatic patients with blood lead concentration greater than 50 µg/dl should be treated with sodium CaNa^2 EDTA i.v., followed by oral administration of succimer for 19 days. Asymptomatic patients with blood lead concentration greater than 50 μg/dl can be treated with succimer alone. CaNa^{2+} EDTA should be combined with dimercaprol in cases with CNS symptoms [100]. Dexamethasone and mannitol should be considered in cases of cerebral edema.

14.3.4.3. Mercury

Mercury poisoning used to be a common side effect of various drugs such as antimicrobials, laxatives, and antiseptics. While these drugs have been replaced with nontoxic and more effective agents, chronic mercury exposure from cosmetics distributed in developing countries (e.g., skin whitening cream [101]) still occurs. Other sources of mercury are occupational exposure [102] and environmental pollution, especially fish containing organic mercury compounds. The FDA therefore recommends avoiding consumption of shark, swordfish, mackerel, and tilefish by pregnant women or women of childbearing age and young children [103]. Mercury intoxication causes a variety of symptoms, including gastrointestinal, renal, pulmonary, hepatic, and neurological ones. Neurotoxicity may result from excitotoxic neuronal damage due to defective glutamate reuptake by astrocytes [104].

The symptomatology of mercury intoxication depends upon the route of ingestion and on whether the exposure was acute or chronic. Acute inhalation of vapors containing high doses of elementary mercury is the most hazardous form of intoxication. Clinical signs occur within hours, consisting of gastrointestinal and respiratory symptoms, visual impairment, and generalized tonic-clonic seizures [105, 106]. Intensive care is mandatory as respiratory, renal, and hepatic failure may be fatal. In contrast, intravenous injection of doses of metallic mercury as high as 8 g are not life-threatening: In a case of suicidal injection, gastroenteritis, stomatitis mercuralis, neuropsychological symptoms, and tremor mercuralis occurred without respiratory, hepatic, or renal abnormalities [107]. The patient was successfully treated with 2,3-dimercaptopropane-1-sulfonate (DMPS), a chelating agent, and surgical removal of mercury deposits. Chronic exposure to mercury, in metallic or organic form (methylmercury) causes a neuropsychological syndrome (erethism) characterized by irritability, personality change, depression, delirium, insomnia, apathy, memory disturbances, headaches, general pain, and tremors. Hypertension, renal disturbances, allergies, and immunological conditions occur [102]. Recurrent seizures and EEG abnormalities may also be present [108]. Standard anticonvulsant therapy can be used for mercury-related seizures and epilepsy. The chelating agent DMPS should be given repetitively to remove approximately 1 mg of mercury per day of treatment [107].

14.3.4.4. Tin

Tin has neurotoxic properties as an organic compound (triethyltin, trimethyltin). These organotins are used as preservatives for textiles or wood and in the production of silicone rubber. Intoxication often occurs during occupational exposure. Symptoms include hearing loss, confusion, memory deficits, ataxia, sensory neuropathy, aggressiveness, and disturbed sexual behavior, as well as complex partial and tonic-clonic seizures. Long-term effects include epilepsy, likely because trimethyltin intoxication produces damage in amygdala, piriform cortex, and hippocampus, requiring antiepileptic treatment.

References

1. Alldredge BK, Lowenstein DH, Simon RP (1989) Seizures associated with recreational drug abuse. Neurology 39:1037
2. Thundiyil JG, Kearney TE, Olson KR (2007) Evolving epidemiology of drug-induced seizures reported to a Poison Control Center System. J Med Toxicol 3(1):15–19
3. Steele MT, Westdorp EJ, Garza AG, Ma OJ, Roberts DK, Watson WA (2000) Screening for stimulant use in adult emergency department seizure patients. J Toxicol Clin Toxicol 38:609
4. Saboory E, Derchansky M, Ismaili M, Jahromi SS, Brull R, Carlen PL, El Beheiry H (2007) Mechanisms of morphine enhancement of spontaneous seizure activity. Anesth Analg 105(6):1729–1735
5. Warner-Smith M, Darke S, Day C (2002) Morbidity associated with non-fatal heroin overdose. Addiction 97:963
6. Volavka J, Zaks A, Roubicek J, Fink M (1970) Electrographic effects of diacetyl-morphine (heroin) and naloxone in man. Neuropharmacology 9:587
7. Landow L (1985) An apparent seizure following inadvertent intrathecal morphine. Anesthesiology 62:545
8. Chiarotti M, Fucci N (1999) Comparative analysis of heroin and cocaine seizures. J Chromatogr B Biomed Sci Appl 733:127
9. Ng SK, Brust JC, Hauser WA, Susser M (1990) Illicit drug use and the risk of new-onset seizures. Am J Epidemiol 132:47
10. Ogunyemi AO, Locke GE, Kramer LD, Nelson L (1989) Complex partial status epilepticus provoked by "crack" cocaine. Ann Neurol 26:785
11. Osborn DA, Jeffery HE, Cole MJ (2002). Sedatives for opiate withdrawal in new-born infants. Cochrane Database Syst Rev (3):CD002053
12. Klein M, Rudich Z, Gurevich B, Lifshitz M, Brill S, Lottan M, Weksler N (2005) Controlled-release oxycodone-induced seizures. Clin Ther 27(11):1815–1818
13. Shadnia S, Soltaninejad K, Heydari K, Sasanian G, Abdollahi M (2008) Tramadol intoxication: a review of 114 cases. Hum Exp Toxicol. 27(3):201–205
14. Schnorf H, Taurarii M, Cundy T (2002) Ciguatera fish poisoning: a double-blind randomized trial of mannitol therapy. Neurology 58:873
15. Schulze-Bonhage A, Elger CE (2000) Induction of partial epileptic seizures by flumazenil. Epilepsia 41:186
16. Haverkos GP, DiSalvo RP, Imhoff TE (1994) Fatal seizures after flumazenil administration in a patient with mixed overdose. Ann Pharmacother 28:1347
17. Sandoval MR, Palermo-Neto J (1986) GABAergic influences on barbital withdrawal induced convulsions. Gen Pharmacol 17:431
18. Tseng YT, Wellman SE, Ho IK (1994) In situ hybridization evidence of differential modulation by pentobarbital of GABAA receptor alpha 1- and beta 3-subunit mRNAs. J Neurochem 63:301
19. Koff JM, Pritchard GA, Greenblatt DJ, Miller LG (1997) The NMDA receptor competitive antagonist CPP modulates benzodiazepine tolerance and discontinuation. Pharmacology 55:217
20. Martinez-Cano H, Vela-Bueno A, de Iceta M, Pomalima R, Martinez-Gras I (1995) Benzodiazepine withdrawal syndrome seizures. Pharmacopsychiatry 28:257
21. Committee on the review of Medicines (1980) Systematic review of the benzodiazepines. Guidelines for data sheets on diazepam, chlordiazepoxide, medazepam, clorazepate, lorazepam, oxazepam, temazepam, triazolam, nitrazepam, and flurazepam. Br Med J 280:910
22. Fraser H, Ikler A, Essig E, Isbell H (1958) Degree of physical dependence induced by secobarbital or pentobarbital. JAMA 166:126
23. Bauer MS, Fus AF, Hanich RF, Ross RJ (1988) Glutethimide intoxication and withdrawal. Am J Psychiatry 145:530
24. Caplan LR, Thomas C, Banks G (1982) Central nervous system complications of addiction to "T's and Blues". Neurology 32:623

25. Landry MJ (2002) MDMA: a review of epidemiologic data. J Psychoactive Drugs 34:163

26. Zagnoni PG, Albano C (2002) Psychostimulants and epilepsy. Epilepsia 43 (Suppl 2):28

27. Dhuna A, Pascual-Leone A, Langendorf F, Anderson DC (1991) Epileptogenic properties of cocaine in humans. Neurotoxicology 12:621

28. Burgess C, O'Donohoe A, Gill M (2000) Agony and ecstasy: a review of MDMA effects and toxicity. Eur Psychiatry 15:287

29. Gowing LR, Henry-Edwards SM, Irvine RJ, Ali RL (2002) The health effects of ecstasy: a literature review. Drug Alcohol Rev 21:53

30. Auer J, Berent R, Weber T, Lassnig E, Eber B (2002) Subarachnoid haemorrhage with "Ecstasy" abuse in a young adult. Neurol Sci 23:199

31. Klausner HA, Lewandowski C (2002) Infrequent causes of stroke. Emerg Med Clin North Am 20:657

32. Hanson GR, Jensen M, Johnson M, White HS (1999) Distinct features of seizures induced by cocaine and amphetamine analogs. Eur J Pharmacol 377:167

33. Schwartz RH, Estroff T, Hoffmann NG (1988) Seizures and syncope in adolescent cocaine abusers. Am J Med 85:462

34. Holmes SB, Banerjee AK, Alexander WD (1999) Hyponatraemia and seizures after ecstasy use. Postgrad Med J 75:32

35. Sue YM, Lee YL, Huang JJ (2002) Acute hyponatremia, seizure, and rhabdomyolysis after ecstasy use. J Toxicol Clin Toxicol 40:931

36. Szlatenyi CS, Wang RY (1996) Encephalopathy and cranial nerve palsies caused by intentional trichloroethylene inhalation. Am J Emerg Med 14:464

37. Aydin K, Sencer S, Demir T, Ogel K, Tunaci A, Minareci O (2002) Cranial MR findings in chronic toluene abuse by inhalation. AJNR Am J Neuroradiol 23:1173

38. Meredith TJ, Ruprah M, Liddle A, Flanagan RJ (1989) Diagnosis and treatment of acute poisoning with volatile substances. Hum Toxicol 8:277

39. Wells JC (1982) Abuse of trichloroethylene by oral self-administration. Anaesthesia 37:440

40. Littorin ME, Fehling C, Attewell RG, Skerfving S (1988) Focal epilepsy and exposure to organic solvents: a case-referent study. J Occup Med 30:805

41. Silva-Filho AR, Pires ML, Shiotsuki N (1992) Anticonvulsant and convulsant effects of organic solvents. Pharmacol Biochem Behav 41:79

42. Jacobsen M, Baelum J, Bonde JP (1994) Temporal epileptic seizures and occupational exposure to solvents. Occup Environ Med 51:429

43. Wojtowicz JM, Yarema MC, Wax PM (2008) Withdrawal from gamma-hydroxybutyrate, 1, 4-butanediol and gamma-butyrolactone: a case report and systematic review. CJEM 10(1):69–74

44. Knudsen K, Greter J, Verdicchio M (2008) High mortality rates among GHB abusers in Western Sweden. Clin Toxicol (Phila) 46(3):187–192

45. Wilson RI, Nicoll RA (2002) Endocannabinoid signaling in the brain. Science 296:678

46. Mechoulam R, Parker LA, Gallily R (2002) Cannabidiol: an overview of some pharmacological aspects. J Clin Pharmacol 42:11S

47. Sofia RD, Solomon TA, Barry H III (1976) Anticonvulsant activity of delta9-tetrahydrocannabinol compared with three other drugs. Eur J Pharmacol 35:7

48. Karler R, Turkanis SA (1981) The cannabinoids as potential antiepileptics. J Clin Pharmacol 21:437S

49. Turkanis SA, Karler R (1982) Central excitatory properties of delta 9-tetrahydrocannabinol and its metabolites in iron-induced epileptic rats. Neuropharmacology 21:7

50. Fisher DD, Ungerleider JT (1967) Grand mal seizures following ingestion of LSD. Calif Med 106:210

51. Leander JD, Rathbun RC, Zimmerman DM (1988) Anticonvulsant effects of phencyclidine-like drugs: relation to N-methyl-D-aspartic acid antagonism. Brain Res 454:368

52. Baldridge EB, Bessen HA (1990) Phencyclidine. Emerg Med Clin North Am 8:541
53. Kessler GF Jr, Demers LM, Berlin C, Brennan RW (1974) Letter: Phencyclidine and fatal status epilepticus. N Engl J Med 291:979
54. Stewart GR, Zorumski CF, Price MT, Olney JW (1990) Domoic acid: a dementia-inducing excitotoxic food poison with kainic acid receptor specificity. Exp Neurol 110:127
55. Cervos-Navarro J, Diemer NH (1991) Selective vulnerability in brain hypoxia. Crit Rev Neurobiol 6:149
56. Perl TM, Bedard L, Kosatsky T, Hockin JC, Todd EC, Remis RS (1990) An outbreak of toxic encephalopathy caused by eating mussels contaminated with domoic acid. N Engl J Med 322:1775
57. Teitelbaum JS, Zatorre RJ, Carpenter S, Gendron D, Evans AC, Gjedde A, Cashman NR (1990) Neurologic sequelae of domoic acid intoxication due to the ingestion of contaminated mussels. N Engl J Med 322:1781
58. Cendes F, Andermann F, Carpenter S, Zatorre RJ, Cashman NR (1995) Temporal lobe epilepsy caused by domoic acid intoxication: evidence for glutamate receptor-mediated excitotoxicity in humans. Ann Neurol 37:123
59. Pearn J (2001) Neurology of ciguatera. J Neurol Neurosurg Psychiatry 70:4
60. Ting JY, Brown AF (2001) Ciguatera poisoning: a global issue with common management problems. Eur J Emerg Med 8:295
61. Hashmi MA, Sorokin JJ, Levine SM (1989) Ciguatera fish poisoning. N J Med 86:469
62. Lange WR (1987) Ciguatera toxicity. Am Fam Physician 35:177
63. Bagnis R, Kuberski T, Laugier S (1979) Clinical observations on 3, 009 cases of ciguatera (fish poisoning) in the South Pacific. Am J Trop Med Hyg 28:1067
64. Alcala AC, Alcala LC, Garth JS, Yasumura D, Yasumoto T (1988) Human fatality due to ingestion of the crab Demania reynaudii that contained a palytoxin-like toxin. Toxicon 26:105
65. Matta J, Navas J, Milad M, Manger R, Hupka A, Frazer T (2002) A pilot study for the detection of acute ciguatera intoxication in human blood. J Toxicol Clin Toxicol 40:49
66. Palafox NA, Jain LG, Pinano AZ, Gulick TM, Williams RK, Schatz IJ (1988) Successful treatment of ciguatera fish poisoning with intravenous mannitol. JAMA 259:2740
67. Chilton WS, Ott J (1976) Toxic metabolites of *Amanita pantherina*, *A. cothurnata*, *A. muscaria* and other *Amanita* species. Lloydia 39:150
68. McPartland JM, Vilgalys RJ, Cubeta MA (1997) Mushroom poisoning. Am Fam Physician 55:1797
69. Albrecht J, Jones EA (1999) Hepatic encephalopathy: molecular mechanisms underlying the clinical syndrome. J Neurol Sci 170:138
70. Sabeel AI, Kurkus J, Lindholm T (1995) Intensive hemodialysis and hemoperfusion treatment of Amanita mushroom poisoning. Mycopathologia 131:107
71. Beer JH (1993) [The wrong mushroom. Diagnosis and therapy of mushroom poisoning, especially of Amanita phalloides poisoning]. Schweiz Med Wochenschr 123:892
72. Montanini S, Sinardi D, Pratico C, Sinardi AU, Trimarchi G (1999) Use of acetyl-cysteine as the life-saving antidote in Amanita phalloides (death cap) poisoning. Case report on 11 patients. Arzneimittelforschung 49:1044
73. Kohn R, Mot'ovska Z (1997) Mushroom poisoning–classification, symptoms and therapy. Vnitr Lek 43:230
74. Tupalska-Wilczynska K, Ignatowicz R, Poziemski A, Wojcik H, Wilczynski G (1997) Amanita pantherina and Amanita muscaria poisonings–pathogenesis, symptoms and treatment. Pol Merkuriusz Lek 3:30
75. Benjamin DR (1992) Mushroom poisoning in infants and children: the Amanita pantherina/muscaria group. J Toxicol Clin Toxicol 30:13

76. Elonen E, Tarssanen L, Harkonen M (1979) Poisoning with brown fly agaric, Amanita regalis. Acta Med Scand 205:121

77. Anonymous (1994) From the Centers for Disease Control and Prevention. Water hemlock poisoning—Maine, 1992. JAMA 271:1475

78. Knutsen OH, Paszkowski P (1984) New aspects in the treatment of water hemlock poisoning. J Toxicol Clin Toxicol 22:157

79. Kunisaki TA, Augenstein WL (1994) Drug- and toxin-induced seizures. Emerg Med Clin North Am 12:1027

80. Ertekin V, Alp H, Selimoglu MA, Karacan M (2002) Amitraz poisoning in children: retrospective analysis of 21 cases. J Int Med Res 30:203

81. Yilmaz HL, Yildizdas DR (2003) Amitraz poisoning, an emerging problem: epidemiology, clinical features, management, and preventive strategies. Arch Dis Child 88:130

82. Heckerling PS, Leikin JB, Maturen A, Terzian CG, Segarra DP (1990) Screening hospital admissions from the emergency department for occult carbon monoxide poisoning. Am J Emerg Med 8:301

83. Herman LY (1998) Carbon monoxide poisoning presenting as an isolated seizure. J Emerg Med 16:429

84. Mori T, Nagai K (2000) Carbon-monoxide poisoning presenting as an afebrile seizure. Pediatr Neurol 22:330

85. Durnin C (1987) Carbon monoxide poisoning presenting with focal epileptiform seizures. Lancet 1:1319

86. Kales SN (1993) Carbon monoxide intoxication. Am Fam Physician 48:1100

87. Neufeld MY, Swanson JW, Klass DW (1981) Localized EEG abnormalities in acute carbon monoxide poisoning. Arch Neurol 38:524

88. Brown KL, Wilson RF, White MT (2007) Carbon monoxide-induced status epilepticus in an adult. J Burn Care Res. 28(3):533–536

89. Mathieu D, Nolf M, Durocher A, Saulnier F, Frimat P, Furon D, Wattel F (1985) Acute carbon monoxide poisoning. Risk of late sequelae and treatment by hyperbaric oxygen. J Toxicol Clin Toxicol 23:315

90. Hawkins M, Harrison J, Charters P (2000) Severe carbon monoxide poisoning: outcome after hyperbaric oxygen therapy. Br J Anaesth 84:584

91. Weaver LK, Hopkins RO, Chan KJ, Churchill S, Elliott CG, Clemmer TP, Orme JF Jr, Thomas FO, Morris AH (2002) Hyperbaric oxygen for acute carbon monoxide poisoning. N Engl J Med 347:1057

92. Hampson NB, Simonson SG, Kramer CC, Piantadosi CA (1996) Central nervous system oxygen toxicity during hyperbaric treatment of patients with carbon monoxide poisoning. Undersea Hyperb Med 23:215

93. Roscoe RJ, Ball W, Curran JJ, DeLaurier C, Falken MC, Fitchett R, Fleissner ML, Fletcher AE, Garman SJ, Gergely RM, Gerwel BT, Gostin JE, Keyvan-Larijani E, Leiker RD, Lofgren JP, Nelson DR et al (2002) Adult blood lead epidemiology and surveillance—United States, 1998–2001. MMWR Surveill Summ 51:1

94. Shannon M (2003) Severe lead poisoning in pregnancy. Ambul Pediatr 3:37

95. Wedeen RP, Mallik DK, Batuman V, Bogden JD (1978) Geophagic lead nephropathy: case report. Environ Res 17:409

96. Kumar A, Dey PK, Singla PN, Ambasht RS, Upadhyay SK (1998) Blood lead levels in children with neurological disorders. J Trop Pediatr 44:320

97. Yu EC, Yeung CY (1987) Lead encephalopathy due to herbal medicine. Chin Med J (Engl) 100:915

98. Healy MA, Aslam M, Harrison PG, Fernando NP (1984) Lead-induced convulsions in young infants–a case history and the role of GABA and sodium valproate in the pathogenesis and treatment. J Clin Hosp Pharm 9:199

99. Cheong JH, Seo DO, Ryu JR, Shin CY, Kim YT, Kim HC, Kim WK, Ko KH (1999) Lead induced thiamine deficiency in the brain decreased the threshold of electroshock seizure in rat. Toxicology 133:105

100. Gordon JN, Taylor A, Bennett PN (2002) Lead poisoning: case studies. Br J Clin Pharmacol 53:451

101. Pelclova D, Lukas E, Urban P, Preiss J, Rysava R, Lebenhart P, Okrouhlik B, Fenclova Z, Lebedova J, Stejskalova A, Ridzon P (2002) Mercury intoxication from skin ointment containing mercuric ammonium chloride. Int Arch Occup Environ Health 75(Suppl):S54

102. Faria MMA (2003) Chronic occupational metallic mercurialism. Rev Saude Publica 37:116

103. Evans EC (2002) The FDA recommendations on fish intake during pregnancy. J Obstet Gynecol Neonatal Nurs 31:715

104. Juarez BI, Martinez ML, Montante M, Dufour L, Garcia E, Jimenez-Capdeville ME (2002) Methylmercury increases glutamate extracellular levels in frontal cortex of awake rats. Neurotoxicol Teratol 24:767

105. Jaffe KM, Shurtleff DB, Robertson WO (1983) Survival after acute mercury vapor poisoning. Am J Dis Child 137:749

106. Abbaslou P, Zaman T (2006) A Child with elemental mercury poisoning and unusual brain MRI findings. Clin Toxicol (Phila) 44(1):85–88

107. Winker R, Schaffer AW, Konnaris C, Barth A, Giovanoli P, Osterode W, Rudiger HW, Wolf C (2002) Health consequences of an intravenous injection of metallic mercury. Int Arch Occup Environ Health 75:581

108. Brenner RP, Snyder RD (1980) Late EEG findings and clinical status after organic mercury poisoning. Arch Neurol 37:282

Chapter 15

Management of Status Epilepticus and Critical Care Seizures

Panayiotis N. Varelas and Marianna V. Spanaki

Abstract The treatment of ICU seizures and status epilepticus may differ in the approach taken. With only one seizure, the focus should be more on defining the etiology than on treating the patient with antiepileptics, but with more prolonged or recurrent seizures, both should be pursued in parallel. Status epilepticus, if delayed or untreated, carries a grave prognosis and every ICU should have a protocol for rapid response to this neurological emergency. Continuous EEG monitoring should become mandatory, when treating status, because of the late dissociation between clinical convulsions and electrographic seizures and the inability to use the clinical examination as guide to the treatment. Focal and non-convulsive statuses have a different etiology and prognosis than generalized convulsive status epilepticus, and the treatment also differs. Several medications are available for treating seizures, but only few are available for parenteral, fast administration when treating status. The experience from using the newer antiepileptics in case of resistant status is therefore limited. Interactions between antiepileptics and common ICU medications may be significant and concurrent multi-organ failure may alter their metabolism.

Keywords Status epilepticus, Nonconvulsive status epilepticus, Antiepileptic medications, Seizures, Intensive care unit

15.1. Introduction

Status epilepticus (SE) is a true medical emergency that requires aggressive and prompt therapeutic intervention preferably in an ICU. The physician may encounter a patient with SE in the ICU, either because the patient was admitted for management of the SE or because the patient developed SE during the course of his admission for another medical reason. In our NICU some patients, who are admitted for continuous electroencephalogram (EEG) monitoring after intracranial electrode placement, may develop frank SE (after the anti-epileptic medications are withdrawn) and constitute a third category of "semi-intentional" iatrogenic SE.

From: *Seizures in Critical Care: A Guide to Diagnosis and Therapeutics*: Current Clinical Neurology, Second Edition, Edited by: P. Varelas, DOI 10.1007/978-1-60327-532-3_15, © Humana Press, a part of Springer Science+Business Media, LLC 2005, 2010

Persistent convulsive activity not responding to the usual first-line treatment requires admission to an ICU (1). This condition carries a significant mortality and morbidity and needs immediate and proper intervention. The indication for admission becomes more obscure in patients with non-convulsive SE (NCSE). This condition has a still evolving definition, unclear pathophysiology, and, most importantly, controversial prognosis. Aggressive treatment of NCSE, especially with IV administration of anti-epileptic medications, could be only justified if such intervention could clearly alter the prognosis for the better (2). As there is not enough evidence that such treatment improves the prognosis in NCSE and, actually, may cause complications (mainly hypotension and respiratory depression), the physician should individualize the admission and management to an ICU on the basis of other co-morbidities.

There are not many studies specifically reporting on admission of SE patients in an ICU. An older survey of members of the Intensive Care Society in the UK, questioned about SE resistant to initial therapy with intravenous (IV) diazepam and phenytoin, revealed that only 12% of the 408 respondents were aware of a protocol for SE in their ICUs. At that time, the authors concluded that the therapeutic and monitoring strategies used in the management of refractory SE in the UK were insufficient and needed re-evaluation (3). The same group published their experience with 26 patients admitted to a neurological ICU (NICU) with a diagnosis of SE. On transfer to the NICU only 14 (54%) were in SE; six were in drug-induced coma or were encephalopathic, and six had pseudo-SE, of whom four had been intubated. Prior to transfer most patients were treated with benzodiazepines, chlomethiazole, and phenytoin; phenytoin load was adequate in at least 7/16 cases. All those in SE on transfer had their seizures successfully controlled, but 10 patients required general anesthesia with thiopentone, propofol, ketamine, or midazolam (4). In a recent study from San Francisco, CA, patients treated with out-of-hospital benzodiazepines, and who were still in SE on arrival at the emergency department, were more likely to be admitted to the ICU, compared to those whose seizures were terminated before the arrival at the hospital (73% vs. 32%, likelihood ratio chi-square <0.001). When these groups were compared according to the cause of SE, no difference was found, suggesting that the very fact of the ongoing seizure activity, and not the underlying etiology, was the reason for ICU admission (5).

15.2. Definition

Over the last decades, the definition of SE has evolved, especially as new data regarding prognosis emerge. The International Classification of Epileptic Seizures has defined SE as any seizure lasting ≥ 30 min or intermittent seizures lasting for >30 min without recovery of consciousness interictally (6, 7).

In 1991, Bleck proposed that seizures persisting for 20 min should be defined as SE (8) and, in 1993, Ramsay suggested that a better definition should include any seizure that persists for more than twice its normal duration, even though most seizures normally last less than 5 min (9).

In 1998, Treiman et al. defined as SE the presence of two or more discrete seizures with incomplete recovery of consciousness between the seizures or continuous convulsive activity for more than 10 min (10).

More recently, Lowenstein proposed a new operational definition of SE according to which SE refers to at least 5 min of (a) continuous seizures or (b) two or more discrete seizures between which there is incomplete recovery of consciousness. In the clinical setting the need to treat continuous seizure activity promptly has been recognized and many practitioners intervene before 20 min have elapsed (11).

More controversial is the definition of NCSE. This is a condition that necessitates EEG confirmation and different criteria have been proposed by several experts. Most of them agree on the presence of altered consciousness or behavior for ≥30 min, the absence of overt clinical signs of convulsive activity during that period and the EEG presence of (1) unequivocal seizure activity or (2) periodic epileptiform discharges or rhythmic discharges with subtle clinical seizure activity or (3) rhythmic slow discharges with either clinical or EEG response to treatment (12–15).

15.3. Classification

Depending on the presence or not of convulsive activity, SE can be further defined as (a) *overt status epilepticus* with recurrent convulsions manifested as generalized motor activity [generalized convulsive SE (CSE)] or focal motor activity (partial convulsive SE) (b) *non-convulsive SE* (NCSE). NCSE can be subdivided into (a) generalized non-convulsive SE (absence NCSE) with altered consciousness associated with generalized spike and wave activity on EEG (b) complex partial NCSE, with either discrete complex partial seizures and no return of normal consciousness or a continuous state of impaired consciousness (c) myoclonic SE or generalized status myoclonicus, with more overt myoclonic activity (shock-like irregular jerks), easily distinguished from tonic-clonic convulsions (usually after global anoxic or ischemic insult or associated with myoclonic encephalopathies) lasting for at least 30 min (16) and (d) subtle generalized SE (or electrographic SE or SE in comatose patients), characterized by subtle, often unnoticed motor activity (rhythmic twitching of the arms, legs, trunk, or facial muscles, tonic eye deviation or nystagmoid eye jerking) associated with generalized epileptiform activity on the EEG (17). Diagnosis of NCSE still represents a difficult diagnosis that requires high index of clinical suspicion.

Thus, accurate diagnosis of SE is made on the basis of electro-clinical features (Table 15-1).

Table 15-1. Classification of SE.

	Convulsive SE	Non-Convulsive SE
Primary generalized SE	Tonic-clonic	Absence attacks
	Tonic	Atypical absence
	Myoclonic	Atonic seizures
Partial SE	Partial motor seizures (epilepsia partialis continua)	Aphasic
		Simple partial non-motor
		Complex partial
Secondary generalized SE	Partial seizure with secondary generalization	Subtle or in coma

15.4. Incidence and Clinical Presentation

Numerous studies confirm that SE is a common condition. It accounts for 3–5% of all emergency room admissions for seizure disorders and occurs in 2–16% of all epilepsy patients (18, 19). De Lorenzo and his colleagues in a prospective population-based epidemiological study in Richmond, VA, found that the incidence of SE was 41–61 per 100,000 patients per year. Projecting the Richmond data to the US population it was determined that 125,000–195,000 episodes per year of SE are occurring in the USA. The highest incidence of SE occurs during the first year of life and during the decades >60 years. Approximately 13% of patients have recurrence of SE and thus, the expected prevalence in the USA is higher. In this important study, partial SE of various types occurred in 25% of cases and NCSE represented approximately 4% of SE (20)

The most common type of SE encountered in ICU setting is the one presenting with generalized tonic-clonic convulsions (including secondary generalization) and diagnosis is rarely a diagnostic dilemma (21). Not all patients admitted for SE have a previous history of epilepsy; indeed, 44% of them do not have such history (22). A new insult to an epileptic brain increases the risk for SE: if there is history of epilepsy and a new acute brain insult, up to 25% of patients may develop SE (23).

The incidence of NCSE is not as well known. Overall, NCSE may account from 4% (20) to up 25% of all SE cases, depending on whether the study was population or hospital based (24, 25). Among those patients with NCSE, the incidence for complex partial SE (3.5/100,000/year) is lower than that of other types of NCSE (15/100,000/year) (19). In a large study from Richmond, VA, 164 patients were prospectively evaluated with continuous EEG monitoring for a minimum of 24 h after clinical control of CSE. After CSE was controlled, continuous EEG monitoring demonstrated that 52% of the patients did not have after-SE ictal discharges. The remaining 48% demonstrated persistent electrographic seizures and more than 14% of them manifested NCSE, predominantly of the complex partial seizure type. Because of absence of overt clinical signs of convulsive activity, the clinical detection of NCSE in these patients would not have been possible with routine neurological evaluations without the use of EEG monitoring (26). Other hospital-based studies examined the incidence of NCSE. A group from Cincinnati, OH, prospectively evaluated hospitalized patients (emergency department, wards, and ICUs) with mental status changes but no clinical convulsions for the presence of NCSE. Out of 198 cases with altered consciousness, 74 (37%) showed EEG and clinical evidence of definite or probable non-tonic-clonic SE. Of those, 42 episodes (57%) were probable or definite complex partial SE, 29 (39%) were probable or definite subtle generalized SE, and three (4%) were myoclonic SE. In 23 SE cases altered consciousness was the only clinical sign at the time of diagnosis and in 36 cases subtle motor activity was present. Neither clinical signs nor prior history predicted which patients showed SE on EEG. Non-tonic-clonic SE was associated with previous seizures in 18 cases and followed a cerebral infarction in 16 cases. Contrary to other reports, the authors did not find any relationship between duration of SE and EEG pattern. Thus, this study demonstrated that non-tonic-clonic SE is a common finding in patients with unexplained altered consciousness in the hospital and EEG is a necessary tool in the evaluation of these patients (17, 27).

There are scanty data regarding SE incidence in the ICU. Bleck et al. prospectively evaluated 1,850 patients admitted to a general medical ICU. Four patients were admitted with primary refractory status epilepticus (4.3% of primary neurological ICU admissions). Two hundred and seventeen patients with non-neurological admissions developed neurological complications and of those, 61 (28.1%) developed seizures. Six of these patients were in SE and required at least 2 antiepileptic agents in order to terminate it. Thus, 10 (0.5%) of medical ICU admissions were primary or secondary SE (21).

In another retrospective study from the Mayo Clinic, Wijdicks and Sharbrough, reported 55 patients with new onset seizures among 27,723 patients admitted in the medical or surgical ICU (0.8%). Only four (7.3%) patients with new onset seizures in these series developed SE (28).

In another study, conducted in the ICU, 236 patients (children and adults) with coma and no overt clinical seizure activity were monitored with at least 30 min continuous EEG as part of their coma evaluation. Only cases that were found to have no clinical signs of SE were included. EEG demonstrated that 19 patients (8%) met the criteria for the diagnosis of NCSE. The most common etiology was hypoxia-anoxia (42% of patients with NCSE), with second most common stroke (22%). This large-scale EEG evaluation of comatose patients without clinical signs of seizure activity found that NCSE is an under-recognized cause of coma and concluded that EEG should be included in the routine evaluation of comatose ICU patients, even if clinical seizure activity is not apparent (29).

In a more recent study, Drislane et al. retrospectively reviewed all EEGs obtained in the ICUs over a 20-year period at Beth Israel Deaconess Hospital in Boston, MA (30). By clinical and EEG evidence, 91 ICU patients with SE were identified, all with abnormal mental status: 74 were comatose. Vascular disease (in 24) and anoxia (22) were the most common causes; most had multiple medical problems. Although 76 patients had clinically evident seizures earlier (and 56, clinical SE) only 20 were thought to be in SE at the time of the diagnostic EEG. There was a median delay of 48 h from clinical deterioration until diagnosis in patients with earlier clinical seizures and 72 h without seizures. Among the 68 nonanoxic patients treated with AEDs, 38 (56%) seemed to improve in alertness, including 25 who were comatose.

Because of the type of patient population admitted, increasing availability of continuous EEG and familiarity of the NICU staff with NCSE, its reported incidence in the NICU may be higher. Using continuous EEG monitoring in 124 NICU patients, Jordan reported 34% incidence of non-convulsive seizures. Thirty-three patients (27%) were in NCSE (31).

In another retrospective study, Varelas et al. examined the use of emergent EEG (performed within 1 h from request) in the ICUs (129 tests performed) and specifically in the NICU (32 tests) (32). The most frequent reason for obtaining the test was in fact to rule out SE (68.2%). CSE was found more frequently in the ICUs than on the ward (10.1% vs. 2.3%), but for NCSE the difference was not significant (6.2% vs. 3%). Independent predictors were cardiopulmonary arrest for CSE and "rule out encephalopathy" for NCSE in the ICUs. The NICU ordered more frequently the test to exclude NCSE (25% of requests) than the other ICUs (2.1%), but, in the end, there was no difference in the incidence of CSE or NCSE (9.4% in the NICU vs. 10.3% in the other Units for CSE and 3.1% vs. 7.2% for NCSE, respectively).

Table 15-2 presents common clinical presentations of SE in the ICU.

Table 15-2. Common Clinical Presentations of Seizures in the ICU.

Seizure type	Clinical expression
Focal Motor	Face or limb motor seizure, may propagate from distal to proximal , no alteration of sensorium
Generalized Tonic-Clonic	Loss of consciousness, generalized convulsions with tonic phase followed by clonic phase and post-ictal altered sensorium. Urinary loss and tongue biting common
Complex-Partial	Disturbed sensorium (aura), can be followed by generalized tonic-clonic seizure
Non-Convulsive Status	Disturbed sensorium or loss of consciousness, minimal face or distal limb twitches

15.5. Etiology

The largest single identifiable risk factor for generalized CSE is epilepsy associated with low antiepileptic drug levels (42% in the Richmond study had epilepsy and 34% of adults had low antiepileptic drug levels (20)). Approximately 15–20% of patients with epilepsy have a history of at least one episode of status epilepticus and 12% present with SE (33). However, cerebrovascular accidents, especially in the elderly, represent the most common etiology for SE (34). Cerebral vascular disease and discontinuation of antiepileptic medications were the most prominent causes of SE, in another study from Richmond, VA, each accounting for approximately 22% of all patients in the series. The other principle etiologies were alcohol withdrawal, idiopathic, anoxia, metabolic disorders, hemorrhage, infection, tumor, drug overdose, and trauma (35).

Data from population or even hospital-based studies regarding the etiology of SE cannot be projected to the ICU. The same causes of seizures in the ICU are also responsible for SE (see Chap. 1). In a retrospective study from a tertiary referral center in London, UK, the etiology of 19 patients who were admitted to a NICU in status was unknown in six and status was due to drug reduction or withdrawal in five. Other causes included encephalitis, neurosarcoidosis, theophylline toxicity, neurocytoma, progressive myoclonic epilepsy, excess alcohol, lymphoma, and cortical dysplasia (4).

The same cerebral or systemic processes leading to CSE can also induce NCSE. In addition, prolonged CSE may evolve to NCSE (see below) and use of continuous EEG monitoring is critical for the diagnosis. Among ICUs, utilization, familiarity with the test, and patient population lead to significant differences in the etiologies assigned to NCSE. In 124 NICU patients monitored with continuous EEG, the highest percentage of non-convulsive seizures was found in those patients with metabolic coma (60%), followed by those with epilepsy (56%), brain tumor (54%), intracranial infection (33%), head trauma (28%), cerebral ischemia (26%), and intracranial hemorrhage (22%) (36). In comatose ICU patients the most common cause of NCSE was anoxia-hypoxia (42%), followed by stroke (22%), infection (5%), head trauma (5%), metabolic disorders (5%), withdrawal from alcohol, or antiepileptics (5%) and tumor (5%) (29). In a retrospective study of 100 inpatients with NCSE, the etiology was acute medical problems (52%), common in the ICU setting, epilepsy (31%), or cryptogenic (17%) (37). The cryptogenic category includes de novo generalized NCSE, which has been predominantly described in older women with drug withdrawal or intoxication with psychotropic medications

(38). In the recent study by Drislane et al. of ICU patients in SE, status was associated with anoxia in 22/91 (24%), with ischemic stroke or with infection in 32 (18% each), and with multiple medical problems in 14 (14%) (30).

15.6. Pathophysiology

Most seizures are self-terminating phenomena lasting from few seconds to few minutes. A single seizure is followed by a refractory period characterized by higher seizure threshold that prevents seizure recurrence. However, under certain conditions the mechanisms responsible for seizure termination fail and seizures recur, i.e., SE ensues. This may lead to CNS damage either directly or indirectly and further seizures.

Direct mechanisms include abnormal release of excitatory aminoacids and decreased release of inhibitory ones at the synapse. There is increased glutamate release with repetitive presynaptic activation (called facilitation) eventually leading to excitotoxic damage through Ca^{++} influx to the neurons via NMDA and AMPA receptors. At the same time, release of GABA from the presynaptic storage sites is decreased when the presynaptic neuron is activated repetitively (referred to as fading of inhibition) (39). Besides the transient synaptic effects, there are additional longer lasting ones affecting the expression of genes and leading to apoptosis of more vulnerable classes of cells, especially in the hippocampus. In addition, local epileptogenic processes, if repeated, can lead to dissemination of seizure propensity to other regions of the brain, a process named secondary epileptogenesis.

The effect that antiepileptic medications have in controlling SE may also vary with the duration of seizures and drug resistance may develop. As mentioned above, this drug resistance may be due to antiepileptic drug (AED) target alterations induced by SE, such as reduced membrane expression or increased trafficking of $GABA_A$ receptors (40), in addition to reduced GABA release. Apart from target alterations by receptor trafficking (i.e., from the synaptic membrane into endosomes, making them unavailable to the neurotransmitor), SE is known to increase the brain expression of drug efflux transporters such as P-glycoprotein (Pgp) at the blood–brain barrier, which might reduce concentrations of AEDs at their brain targets. In a recent study of two rat SE models, no increase of Pgp expression in brain capillary endothelial cells during SE was found, whereas significant overexpression was determined in both models 48 h after SE. These preliminary data suggest that, alterations in Pgp are not critically involved in refractory SE, at least in the first couple of days (41). If SE occurs in the context of pre-existing epilepsy, increased Pgp expression may already be present at the time of status onset. In this case, drugs such verapamil (a Pgp inhibitor) may reverse the resistance to AEDs, which are substrates to Pgp (phenytoin, phenobarbital), in long-lasting refractory SE (42).

Indirect CNS damage from SE is the result of systemic derangements that follow. The seminal animal studies by Meldrum have shed a light on this issue. After prolonged bicuculine-induced convulsive SE in baboons, neuronal damage and cell loss was evident in the neocortex, cerebellum, and hippocampus. When systemic factors were kept within normal physiological limits (paralyzed and artificially ventilated animals with adequate serum glucose levels), there was decreased but still present neocortical and hippocampal cell damage, but absent cerebellar cell injury (43, 44). These experiments suggest that the seizure activity per se is responsible for the neuronal damage and the systemic derangements play an additional role.

These derangements are especially important for the ICU patient who is in SE, because they are amenable to ICU treatment. Table 15-3 presents the

Table 15-3. Systemic Physiologic Changes Induced by Prolonged Generalized Convulsions or Generalized Convulsive SE – Adapted from (76, 105).

CNS

    Tissue hypoxia (decreased O_2 delivery and increased demand)

    Cerebral edema (angiogenic and cytotoxic)

    Increased CBF-$CMRO_2$

    Increased intracranial pressure

    CSF pleocytosis

    Hemorrhage

    Cerebral venous thrombosis

Cardiovascular

    Hypertension followed by hypotension

    Tachycardia

    Myocardial ischemia

    Arrhythmias

    Cardiac arrest

Respiratory

    Hypopnea/apnea

    Hypoventilation

    Aspiration

    Pulmonary hypertension and edema

    Pulmonary embolus

Metabolic

    Acidosis (both metabolic and respiratory)

    Dehydration

    Electrolyte changes (hyponatremia, hyperkalemia)

    Hypoglycemia

    Hyperthermia

Skeletomuscular

    Rhabdomyolysis

    Dislocations

    Fractures (bilateral humeral head, compression of the first four lumbar bodies)

Renal

    Acute tubular necrosis

Gastrointestinal

    Hepatic failure

Hematologic

    Peripheral leukocytosis

    Disseminated intravascular coagulopathy

most common changes by the system involved. Lothman divided the systemic changes after convulsive SE into two phases (39). During phase 1 (or early phase, within the first 30 min) the initial consequences of a prolonged seizure or SE are an increase in the cerebral blood flow (CBF) and a massive increase of plasma catecholamines, leading to increased blood pressure, heart rate, serum glucose, sweating, and body temperature. Cardiac arrhythmias are common. Acidosis is the result of increased serum lactate and CO_2 retention. Minute ventilation may be increased in this phase, but later, periods of hypopnea predominate and can be exacerbated with respiratory depressant antiepileptics, such as barbiturates and benzodiazepines. In a clinical study, the pH ranged between 6.28 and 7.5 in 70 spontaneously ventilating patients with SE: it was <7.35 in 59 and <7.0 in 23 patients. Thirteen patients had $PaCO_2$ >60 mm Hg and overall 30 patients had a respiratory component to the acidosis (45). Acidosis is markedly attenuated with neuromuscular blockade, indicating anaerobic muscle metabolism as a major source of lactate (44). Hypoxia, on the other hand, is usually modest. In primate models of SE, the mean PaO_2 was 58–68 mm Hg and alone did not seem to induce cerebral injury (43, 46). After approximately 30 min of seizing, the patient enters the second phase (or late phase) of SE. The systemic and cerebral protective mechanisms progressively fail, leading to multi-organ compromise: Hypotension, cardiac failure with increased pulmonary capillary leaking (leading to neurogenic pulmonary edema), loss of cerebral autoregulation (resulting in a systemic pressure dependent CBF, which together with the increased intracranial pressure exacerbates the cerebral hypoperfusion), renal failure secondary to rhabdomyolysis or acute tubular necrosis, hypoglycemia and hepatic failure, severe electrolyte abnormalities (hyperkalemia which may reach life-threatening levels), and a disseminated coagulopathy. Cardiac arrhythmias are life-threatening in up to 60% of patients with prolonged SE (47). Sinus tachycardia or supraventricular tachycardia is most common and can be complicated by the rapid infusion of antiepileptics such as phenytoin. Temperature elevation of 40° in seizing primates can be reached within 60–90 min after SE onset and, if persisting for >3 h, leads to neuropathic changes greater than those predicted from the seizure duration alone. When the baboons were paralyzed, the mean temperature increase was only 2.05 °C over a 7-h observation. A similar dangerous temperature elevation has been observed in humans. Seventy out of 90 patients with SE had hyperthermia, with maximum temperature reaching 107°F. The duration of hyperthermia outlasted the duration of SE, with most patients remaining febrile at 12 h after the cessation of the convulsions, but only 3/27 were febrile at 48 h (45).

Another important characteristic of late-phase status is an electromechanical dissociation that occurs and may lead to misinterpretation of the clinical situation: convulsions may decrease or evolve to minor twitching, although electrical cerebral seizure activity continues as NCSE (26). Table 15-4 presents a scheme of these evolving stages. It is interesting to note that SE is a dynamic state, with different characteristics, depending on when the patient is examined (48). Thus depending on the time of observation in the ICU, the patient may have obvious grand mal convulsions or only subtle twitching of the fingers, abdomen, or face or nystagmoid jerks of the eyes or no clinical activity, while being in deep coma state. Although the chances in the ICU are that the intensivist will be notified early, because of vital sign monitoring and frequent examinations by the ICU staff, this may not be the case with a patient who was

Table 15-4. Clinical and EEG Seizure Correlation During Generalized SE – Adapted From (48, 54, 105).

Time	Clinical activity	EEG activity
Onset	Discrete convulsions	Discrete seizure activity
	Continuous convulsions	Merging seizure activity
Minutes	Continuous convulsions	Continuous seizure activity
	Minimal twitching in face or distal extremities	Intermittent suppression between bursts of seizure activity
Hours	No muscular activity	Periodic epileptiform discharges on a flat background

just admitted for ongoing status. This possibility must be kept in mind and all previously seizing patients, who do not regain consciousness soon, should be monitored with a continuous EEG to exclude ongoing NCSE.

15.7. Differential Diagnosis

Although generalized tonic-clonic convulsions, associated with tongue biting, irregular respirations, froth in the mouth, urine incontinence, and postictal diminished responsiveness are quite characteristic, this is not the case with several other repetitive abnormal movements or postures which may be witnessed in the ICU. Usually, there is a false positive interpretation of various non-epileptic phenomena as seizures or, if continuous, as SE and several unnecessary tests are ordered. Convulsive SE differential diagnosis should include among others continuous or multifocal subcortical myoclonus (postanoxic syndromes, Creutzfeld –Jacob disease, metabolic encephalopathies), asterixis, tics, hemifacial spasm or myokymia, fasciculations (spontaneous or after depolarizing paralytic drug administration), rigors due to sepsis, intermittent decorticate or decerebrate posturing, and psychogenic SE following anesthesia (Table 15-5) (49, 50). A careful clinical history, an interview of the staff who witnessed the abnormal movements, and a review of ICU medications, as well as of the most recent appropriate laboratory tests, would be enough to make a sound diagnosis. It is imperative that the ICU nurses and medical staff are familiar with seizures and status and know not only what to do, but also what to look for and document. Although one would expect the opposite, it is alarming that in the recent study by Drislane et al. the level of suspicion was inadequate and the delay to diagnosis significant in the ICUs: out of 76 patients who had clinically evident seizures earlier (and 56 of them clinical SE!) only 20 were thought to be in SE at the time of the diagnostic EEG. This was translated to a median delay of 48 h from clinical deterioration until diagnosis in patients with earlier clinical seizures and 72 h in those without seizures (30). Many times, however, there is no previous history of seizures, the onset of movements was not witnessed, or the clinical presentation is atypical. In these situations of doubt, three major diagnostic steps should be taken, in parallel with the emergent treatment that should be administered to stop the seizures. Firstly, if there is no known cerebral pathology, a computerized tomography (CT) of the head should be ordered. Not every patient who has a seizure needs a CT (for example children with febrile seizures), but the very presence of the patient in the ICU is a proof of complex organ dysfunctions,

Table 15-5. Differential Diagnosis of ICU Seizures or SE.

Myoclonus
Toxic/metabolic
Infectious/inflammatory/autoimmune
Spinal cord disease
Brain stem/subcortical
Cortical
Epileptic
Tics
Tremor
Asterixis
Clonus
Posturing
Hydrocephalic opisthotonus
Shivering-rigors
Hiccoughs
Psychogenic status epilepticus after anesthesia
Narcolepsy-cataplexy
Syncope
Transient ischemic attacks
Transient global amnesia
Voluntary movement
Pseudo-seizures or psychogenic nonepileptic status epilepticus (PNESE)

which may lead to the development of cerebral pathology. Secondly, a number of biochemical and hematologic tests should be ordered, which are the same included in the treatment of SE algorithm, because they have a dual diagnostic and therapeutic significance. Thirdly, an EEG, preferably continuous and with video recording, should be ordered (see below). The sensitivity of the test may be compromised by the treatment already administered, but still it remains the cornerstone of the differential diagnosis. There are not many data regarding the usefulness of emergent EEG, but in a mixed ICU-ward population of 261 patients, Varelas et al. found that the presence of any epileptic activity on the emergent EEG was independently predicted by a history of cardiorespiratory arrest (odds ratio 2.6, 95% CI 1.12–6.25) or witnessed seizures before the test was performed (2.2, 1.2–4.1). A history of stroke on admission and a first ever ordered EEG were negative predictors for epileptic activity on the test (0.2, 0.006–0.65 and 0.38, 0.16–0.88, respectively) (51).

Without the EEG, clinical suspicion may be misleading, but there are still some characteristics of SE that may be helpful to differentiate refractory generalized CSE from a psychogenic nonepileptic SE (PNESE) variety (52). In a recent study in the emergency setting, Holtkamp et al. reported that patients with PNESE were younger, had port systems implanted more frequently, received higher doses of benzodiazepines until seizure termination or respiratory failure, and had lower serum creatine kinase levels (52).

In the next sections we will examine the data available regarding the indications and timing for ordering the test and the results of the test.

15.8. EEG

15.8.1. Indications and Timing

Almost all experts agree that EEG is a valuable test in the management of SE. When it should be ordered is more controversial. During the first 15 min, the majority of experts do not find a reason to spend valuable time and resources initiating the test (7, 9). Others, however, argue that EEG has to be started immediately (53) or when there is no improvement in the level of consciousness during the first 15 (21) or 30 min (27) after the initiation of treatment. The real onset of SE, in case is not known, may be another reason to order the test, as the presence of a specific phase according to the classification of Treiman et al. (54) in the recording may have a diagnostic and prognostic value (55). During the late phase (30–60 min after the "time zero"), an emergent EEG has a more clear indication, if the neurological examination of the patient is compromised by the treatment (sedatives, paralytics) (27) or when the depth of barbiturate coma needs to be monitored. A prolonged emergent EEG in this setting may be more useful (27, 51, 53, 55). Another reason to order the test during this late phase is when, after the cessation of the tonic-clonic activity due to appropriate treatment, the patient is slow to return to the baseline status. In that case, NCSE has to be excluded, as in any case of unexplained altered or fluctuating level of consciousness (17, 31, 56). Finally, an emergent EEG could be considered, if for any reason there is suspicion for pseudo-status (57) or to differentiate myoclonic SE from non-epileptic myoclonus (55).

If the EEG shows seizures, especially NC seizures or SE or highly suspicious interictal activity (periodic epileptiform discharges, see below), one should strongly argue that the patient needs continuous EEG monitoring, instead of just routine EEG. Many experts actually argue that the CEEG should become another monitoring tool (like the EKG), especially in specialized ICUs, such as the NICU, to "detect and protect" (58). The switch from routine to continuous can be easily done by the EEG technicians. However, analyzing the data in real time is far from optimal in the majority of hospitals, especially during after hours.

15.8.2. EEG Findings in SE

15.8.2.1. Generalized Convulsive SE

The grand mal attack is initiated by an abrupt loss of voltage of a few seconds duration [desynchronization, electro-decremental period followed by very fast activity (20–40/s)] in a generalized distribution that corresponds to the tonic phase. Muscle activity usually obscures the recording, but if there is any doubt and the ICU patient is intubated and mechanically ventilated, one should consider paralytic agents to remove it. In patients who are curarized rhythmical activity at about 10/s with rapidly increasing amplitude follows the phase of desynchronization. Approximately 10 s after the onset of a seizure, slower frequencies are seen in the theta and delta ranges. This phase is followed by repetitive bursts of poly-spike and wave complexes that correspond to the clonic phase of the seizure. The last clonic contraction is followed by postictal flatness of several seconds. In an ongoing status, EEG shows slowing and disorganization in the interval until fast low-voltage spiking with focal onset or primary generalization indicates the onset of a new attack. It is very characteristic that the postictal suppression of brain activity that is seen after a single generalized tonic clonic seizure is not usually seen in SE (59). The default of postictal flattening may indicate failure of active inhibition in the postictal stage. A reasonable hypothesis indicates that this type of inhibition that stems from cerebellar structures is weakened by hypoxia.

In the aforementioned study from the Richmond, VA group, after CSE was controlled, continuous EEG monitoring demonstrated that 52% of patients had no after-SE ictal discharges and manifested EEG patterns of generalized slowing, attenuation, periodic lateralizing epileptiform discharges (PLEDS), focal slowing, and/or burst suppression. The remaining 48% demonstrated persistent electrographic seizures. These results suggested that EEG monitoring after treatment of CSE is essential to recognition of persistent electrographic seizures and NCSE unresponsive to routine therapeutic management of CSE, despite the fact that clinically the patient may seem responding (no convulsions) (26, 34).

15.8.2.2. Generalized NCSE or Absence Status

The EEG findings in the ictal episode consist of classical continuous spike and wave activity in 41% of the cases. There is usually a history of absence of seizures in childhood with typical 3 Hz spike-and-wave discharges or a history of mental retardation, diffuse brain dysfunction, and Lennox-Gastaut syndrome with slower (<2.5 Hz) spike-and-wave discharges (38). Fragmented spike-waves occurring in repetitive bursts are also quite common (28%). Spike-wave activity shows the typical frontal midline maximum. Rhythmical slow activity in the delta or theta range of either frontal or occipital predominance was found in 15.6% (59).

15.8.2.3. Complex Partial Status

In Complex partial status, EEG findings consist of focal onset of electrographic seizures (usually in a temporal or extratemporal distribution) on a slow and disorganized background, intermixed with single or multi-spike wave complexes interictally, in the context of a confusional state. However, rapid generalization can occur and the initial focus may be obscured until treatment is given (15).

15.8.2.4. Focal Motor Status

Epilepsia Partialis Continua may be associated with a completely normal EEG. In other cases rolandic spiking can be seen in conjunction with contralateral twitching.

15.8.2.5. Tonic Status

Tonic status is associated with runs of rapid spikes or very fast poly-spikes in generalized synchrony with frontal maximum.

15.8.2.6. Myoclonic Status

A variety of EEG patterns accompany myoclonic status. The most common pattern consists of generalized periodic complexes (spikes, poly-spikes, or sharp waves) with attenuation of activity between complexes. The second most common pattern presents with burst-suppression (60).

15.8.2.7. NCSE vs. Metabolic Encephalopathy

A number of patients thought to be in NCSE display EEG characteristics of encephalopathy (14). In a study by Granner and Lee, the EEG patterns in patients with NCSE were not uniform: 26% of the 85 patients examined had rhythmic slow waves in the delta range with intermittent spikes (61). It is not clear if these rhythmic waves are the result of the underlying cerebral injury or a primary expression of NCSE. Triphasic waves (TW) have typically a small negative (upward) deflection, followed by a large positive wave, which is followed by another low-amplitude, longer negative slow wave (62). They have a generalized distribution, recur at 0.5–2 Hz, and are not considered to be epileptic in origin. TW with epileptiform characteristics (spike morphology, waxing and waning) have to be differentiated from TW due to a metabolic encephalopathy and this is not always easy in the ICU, where both conditions can coexist. The inclusion in the NCSE definition of a response to benzodiazepine is not enough, however, as even metabolic TW (for example associated with hyperammonemia) can respond to IV diazepam. Fountain and Waldman retrospectively examined the EEG response to benzodiazepines in 10 patients with definitively diagnosed metabolic encephalopathy. TW resolved persistently in four patients and intermittently in six patients. Background activity slowed in five patients and was attenuated in five patients. Unresponsive patients did not arouse and three of five drowsy patients became less responsive after the drug was given (63). If administration of benzodiazepines results in resolution of the EEG abnormality and clinical improvement, the diagnosis of NCSE is straightforward. If clinical improvement does not occur but the EEG improves, this lack of improvement may be due to the underlying encephalopathy state causing the TWs (62). However, there are cases of NCSE where the clinical response is delayed (64) (and mistakenly not associated with the drug given hours or days before) or absent: in a recent study of 100 case with NCSE, 25/64 (39%) did not have a clinical response and 10/64 (16%) not even an EEG response to benzodiazepines (37).

Another area of contention, beyond the TWs, is the relationship of NCSE or seizures with periodic epileptiform discharges (PEDs). With more frequent use of continuous video-EEG monitoring in critically ill patients, these findings of yet unclear significance and evolving nomenclature came to the limelight. There is debate over their significance, if indeed they represent ictal or interictal activity, and the aggressiveness of the treatment to be used against them (see Chap. 2). Most experts believe that they are interictal, representing "an irritative pattern found in temporal proximity to seizures proper; the footprints rather than the animal itself" as Peter Kaplan eloquently put it (62). Many times there is no clinical motor correlate, but the patient's mental status is quite impaired. On the EEG several different patterns may be encountered.

Periodic lateralized epileptiform discharges (PLEDs) are bi or polyphasic (surface negative) discharges, consisting of spikes or polyspikes with or without slow waves, that occur at 0.5–2 Hz over one hemispheric area. If PLEDs occur independently and asynchronously over both hemispheres they are referred to BiPLEDs. If they occur in synchrony over both hemispheres, they are referred to as generalized periodic epileptiform discharges (GPEDs). Over the course of the illness the vast majority of these patients will also have seizures (62). Stimulus-induced rhythmic periodic or ictal discharges (SIRPIDs) have been recently described in critically ill patients stimulated by sensory or other alerting stimuli: Hirsch et al. evaluated 150 CEEGs and reported 33 patients with SIRPIDs (22%), all but 5 admitted to an ICU (65). Clinically, all patients were stuporous or comatose on the day the EEG showed SIRPIDs and all, except one (who had consistently reproducible, irregular semirhythmic jerking of one arm during stimulation–induced GPEDs), did not have any clinical correlate with the SIRPIDs. SIRPID patterns included PEDs in 21 patients (in 9 they were lateralized, i.e., PLEDs), rhythmic patterns with evolution that fulfilled criteria for ictal discharges in 18 patients (12 unilateral), and frontal rhythmic delta activity (FRDA) in 14 patients. Regarding etiology, eight patients had prior epilepsy and 24 acute brain injury. Half the patients (17 of 33) had seizures, clinical or subclinical, during the acute illness in addition to SIRPIDs, and half (16 of 33) did not. SE occurred during the acute illness in 11 (30%) patients. No significant difference was found in the incidence of clinical seizures in patients with SIRPIDs (30%) compared with those without (45%). Clinical CSE, however, was independently associated with focal (odds ratio 8, 95% CI 2–32.5) or ictal-appearing SIRPIDs (3.2, 1–10.2).

15.9. Outcome

Many studies have documented the high morbidity and mortality of convulsive SE and emphasized the importance of prompt intervention to improve outcomes (7, 35). Mortality in convulsive SE ranges from 15 to 22% in adults, but may be lower (3%) in children (18, 20, 45, 66). In the Richmond population study it was estimated that 22,200–42,000 deaths per year from SE occur in the United States (20). Morbidity and mortality in generalized CSE are attributed to three factors: (1) brain injury caused by an acute insult that induces SE, (2) systemic metabolic and physiologic effects of CSE, and (3) neuronal damage from the abnormal electrical activity of SE. The main factors that influence mortality in CSE are (1) the underlying cause (regarded by most authorities the most important variable), (2) the duration of SE (mortality 32% if persistent for >1 h vs. 2.7% if <1 h), (3) the treatment, and (4) the age of the patient (children have better outcome than adults) (13, 35, 67).

The etiology of SE plays the most important role in mortality. In the large study of 253 adults from Richmond, VA, Towne et al. found that SE associated with anoxia (60%), tumors (36%), metabolic etiologies (31%), infection (31%), and CNS hemorrhage (38.5%) had higher mortality. Ethanol and anti-epileptic medication withdrawal were associated with decreased mortality. The mortality rate is 20% when the cause cannot be determined. In the multivariate analysis, duration >1 h, anoxia, and age were independent risk factors for mortality after SE. The mortality rates of focal (30%) and generalized (21%) SE were not significantly different in this study. Neither race nor sex did affect mortality significantly (35).

Seizure duration is also predictive of both treatment success rate and mortality. As time passes, SE becomes more refractory to treatment (22). Seizures lasting longer than 60 min are associated with higher mortality rate than status lasting 30–59 min (35). However, seizures of 10–29 min duration have a mortality rate of 4.4% (68). In another retrospective analysis from Columbia Presbyterian Hospital in New York, NY, Mayer et al. did not find a difference in mortality between patients with refractory SE (23%) and those with non-refractory SE (13%), but this may be due to the small number of patients. It was clear, though, that those patients with refractory SE stayed longer in both NICU and hospital (7.5 vs. 1 day, $P<0.001$ and 32.5 vs. 11 days, $P<0.001$) and had reduced Glasgow Outcome Scale score at discharge compared to that at admission ($P=0.02$) (69).

In NCSE, outcome is less well documented. Patients with absence SE do not have permanent neurologic deficits and do not die from their status. In contrast, complex partial status epilepticus (CPSE) can be accompanied by considerable morbidity and mortality. CPSE like generalized CSE can be precipitated by acute lesions such as stroke or encephalitis, which are responsible for subsequent morbidity. Aggressive and early antiepileptic treatment may not alter the poor outcome in those patients who present in coma. There may also be resistance to the drug treatment: in the aforementioned study, Mayer et al. found that NCSE was an independent risk factor for refractoriness to treatment (69). In the large, double-blinded study by Treiman et al. 134 patients with subtle generalized SE were randomized to receive four different IV regimens (10). No difference in the success rate among the regimens was found. However, outcomes for subtle SE were significantly worse at 30 days (50.1% of patients with overt SE were discharged from the hospitals vs. only 8.8% of those with subtle SE, $P<0.001$). Similarly, hypotension requiring treatment occurred more often in patients with subtle SE ($P<0.001$). During the first 12 h after the end of the infusions, no patient with subtle SE regained consciousness, compared to 17% of patients with overt SE (but with no significant difference among the four treatment groups).

A published retrospective analysis from the University of Virginia identified 100 consecutive patients with NCSE from an EEG database. Patients were divided into three groups on the basis of etiology: acute medical, epilepsy, and cryptogenic. Overall mortality was 18%. Subgroup analysis showed that mortality was 27% (14/52) in the acute medical group, 3% (1/31) in the epilepsy group, and 18% (3/17) in the cryptogenic group ($P<0.02$). Mortality was also different between those patients with severe mental status impairment (39%) and those with mild impairment (7%, $P<0.001$), and between those patients with acute complications (36%) and those without complications (7%, $P<0.0002$). Two additional, interesting observations from this study were (1) the absence of correlation between generalized spike-wave discharges on EEG and mortality and (2) the independent association of mental status impairment and etiology with mortality ($P<0.001$) (37). Thus, although not universally accepted, some authorities believe that it is appropriate to early diagnose and treat NCSE, as duration from 36 to 72 h may lead to serious morbidity and mortality (70).

15.10. Goals of ICU Management of Seizures and SE

Management of ICU seizures and SE should include (1) emergent medical management, (2) termination of seizures, (3) prevention of recurrence of seizures, and (4) prevention or treatment of complications. To what extent these goals are met in clinical practice is unclear. In the aforementioned survey of 408 intensivists from the UK, it was shown that following failure of initial management of resistant SE, a benzodiazepine infusion (35%), or anesthetic induction agent (32%) were the preferred second-line treatments. The majority of respondents (57%) gave anesthetic induction agents within 60 min of the start of SE. Thiopentone was administered in 82% of these cases. Clinical assessment was used to monitor the response to the treatment in almost half the cases. However, in more specialized ICUs, such as pediatric or neurological or neurosurgical units, the majority of responders used a cerebral function monitor in addition to the clinical examination, emphasizing the greater experience these physicians had (3).

15.10.1. Emergent Medical Management

Basic life support with maintenance of airway, breathing, and circulation should be provided as soon as the diagnosis of a seizure or SE is established. Tracheal intubation is important in maintaining adequate oxygenation and preventing aspiration pneumonia. However, few patients with one or more seizures, but almost all patients with SE (especially refractory) need intubation. Adequate oxygen supply with a non-rebreather facial mask and airway patency with oral or nasopharyngeal devices may be enough measures for a patient who has had one or more seizures, but has stopped having convulsions. On the other hand, most ICU physicians would intubate a patient in SE for airway protection and for anticipation of administration of respiratory depressant anti-epileptics. The goal after intubation is adequate oxygenation (initially 100% FiO_2) and ventilation with a goal of normal pH: initial hyperventilation in a paralyzed patient with metabolic acidosis is acceptable, but frequent arterial blood gases are necessary to avoid subsequent respiratory alkalosis, which may further decrease seizure threshold (71). Paralytics are almost always used for the intubation of a seizing patient, but short-acting agents, such as IV rocuronium (0.6–1.2 mg/kg) or vecuronium (0.1 mg/kg), are preferable to succinylcholine, which can induce severe hyperkalemia in neurological patients. As for sedation, thiopental can be used at 3–5 mg/kg, a drug which can also help in seizure control. At least two large IV catheters should be inserted and carefully secured for fluid, drug administration and withdrawal of blood samples. This is not easy in a convulsing patient: an alternative site, such as external jugular catheterization or an alternative route such as intramuscular or rectal administration should be sought. Continuous electrocardiogram, pulse oximetry, and temperature monitoring should be initiated. Non-invasive blood pressure measurements should be started, but the physician should be reluctant to treat elevated pressure during the convulsion phase, unless it is extreme (for example >230 mm Hg systolic) or there is suspicion that it is the primary cause of the seizures (see the Chapter 9 on Extreme Hypertension, Eclampsia and Critical Care Seizures). Usually, control of the seizures with the first- line anti-epileptic drugs would be enough to reduce the blood pressure. Continuous invasive monitoring of blood pressure should be reserved for patients in SE given anti-epileptics with strong hypotensive effect, such as barbiturates.

Routine or continuous EEG recording should be used to assess the presence or absence of ongoing seizure activity and to direct effective and rational treatment, but this should not delay or distract the rest of the urgent management (see above).

Blood samples should be obtained for blood count, glucose, electrolytes, liver enzymes, creatinine kinase, toxicology screen, arterial blood gases, and anti-epileptic drug levels if appropriate. If hypoglycaemia is confirmed, glucose 50 ml of 50% solution should be given. Hyperglycaemia may exacerbate neuronal damage caused by SE; therefore, glucose should only be administered when lab results confirm hypoglycaemia (72, 73). However, the glucose measurement can be done at the bedside rapidly and this is preferable. If this option is not available, the history of the patient is unknown, or there is a strong suspicion of hypoglycemia and the glucose measurement will take several minutes to be completed, we recommend giving 1 ampule of D/W 50%, than wait for the results. In case of history of alcoholism, 100 mg of IV thiamine is given first along with glucose to avoid precipitating Wernicke's encephalopathy. If the history of the patient is unknown, thiamine should be administered at the same dose.

Lumbar puncture is indicated, if there are no signs of increased intracranial pressure and an infectious process causing SE is highly suspected (which is uncommon). Twenty percent of patients with SE may have "benign postictal pleocytosis" (up to 70 white blood cells/mm^3) (74). This SE-induced pleocytosis is usually polymorphonucleocitic in the differential (45) and this may help identify primary viral encephalitis as the cause of SE (where the differential is mainly mononucleocytic (1)). This latter case may be resistant to treatment to the point that the term "malignant SE" has been coined (75). Eight out of 54 (15%) patients with SE may have CSF protein elevation >50 mg/100 ml, but in only one case the value exceeded 75 mg/100 ml (45).

15.10.2. Termination of Seizures and Prevention of Recurrence of Seizures

As a general rule, one brief generalized tonic-clonic seizure in the ICU is not an indication for anti-epileptic drug administration. By the time the drugs are available at the bedside the seizure is usually over. Close monitoring of the patient's vital signs, bed padding, and the initiation of a work-up for identifying the cause are usually adequate measures (Table 15-6). Sometimes the etiology is obvious, for example severe hyponatremia, and management should be focused on correcting the abnormality rather than treating the seizure. In other situations, however, where the presence of an intracranial pathology is already known (for example stroke or extra-axial hematoma), and the patient had never been loaded with anti-epileptic medications, the balance shifts towards covering the patient with an anti-epileptic drug in anticipation of new seizures (as an expression of enhanced cerebral irritability from the lesion). Most times in the ICU, because of routine venous accessibility, this is accomplished through an IV load, but per os loading is an acceptable alternative depending on the circumstances. Because of the complexity of ICU patients, the intensivist

Table 15-6. Management of Brief Single ICU Seizure (<60 s) – Adapted from (288)

Observe. Eliminate etiology
Consider chronic therapy: phenytoin 15–20 mg/kg or fosphenytoin 15–20 mg/kg phenytoin equivalents (PE) loading dose and 300–400 mg/day. Goal serum level 10–20 mcg/ml or free level 1–2 mcg/ml
Phenytoin intolerant patients: IV/PO valproic acid, 15–20 mg/kg load, maintenance 600–3,000 mg/day or PO carbamezapine 600–1,200 mg/day
Seizure precautions – padding bed rails, increased observation

should individualize the extent of the evaluation, but in most cases a CT of the head to exclude new intracranial pathology and an EEG to confirm epileptic discharges are the minimal non-metabolic work-up that should be ordered.

If the seizure is prolonged enough or recurs after few minutes, there is enough time to have the proper medications at the bedside. In this situation most intensivists would try to break the convulsion by administering benzo-diazepines IV for the short-term control of the seizing patient and loading the patient with an IV anti-epileptic, such as phenytoin or valproate for the long-term control (Table 15-7). Because at this point it may not be clear if the flurry of seizures heralds the entry of SE, some intensivists will also consider intubating the patient in anticipation of more seizures and the need for airway control during the work-up. However, this may not be necessary in most of the cases, unless the patient is obstructing the upper airway or is vomiting or the second line drugs fail to control the seizures.

If the seizures continue and the patient meets the criteria for SE a treatment algorithm should be initiated without delay (Table 15-8). The earlier the treatment is initiated, the easier the termination of seizures: 80% of patients had

Table 15-7. Management of a Prolonged Seizure or >1 Seizures in the ICU – Adapted from (288).

Check oxygen saturation, vital signs. Consider intubation, if risk of aspiration
IV benzodiazepine-lorazepam 1–2 mg, diazepam 10–20 mg or midazolam 2–5 mg with concurrent loading dose phenytoin or fosphenytoin (PE) 15–20 mg/kg and maintenance 300–400 mg/day
Phenytoin intolerant: Valproic acid IV load 15–20 mg/kg, maintenance 400–600 mg q6h
Seizure precautions – padding bed rails, increased observation

Table 15-8. Treatment of ICU Recurrent or Refractory Seizures >5 min or >2 Discrete Seizures Without Recovery of Consciousness – Adapted from (2, 7, 9, 11, 50, 53, 79, 105, 108, 158, 288).

Consider as status epilepticus
ABC. Preserve airway and oxygenation by intubation
Measure blood glucose at bedside. IV 100 mg thiamine and glucose, only if less 40–60 mg/100 dL or unable to have a fast result. At the same time draw blood for blood count, electrolytes, liver enzymes, creatinine kinase, toxicology screen, arterial blood gases, and anti-epileptic drug levels
Immediate benzodiazepines – IV lorazepam 5–10 mg, diazepam 20–40 mg, or midazolam 5–20 mg over 5 min
Phenytoin loading dose 20 mg/kg at 50 mg/min or fosphenytoin 20 mg/kg PE at 150 mg/min. Consider Valproic acid IV load 15–20 mg/kg (may be administered up to 500 mg/min IV), maintenance 400–600 mg q6h in phenytoin intolerant patients
Continuous EEG, if available
If seizures continue, phenytoin or fosphenytoin (additional 5–10 mg/kg or 5–10 mg/kg PE). Consider Valproic acid IV load 15–20 mg/kg, maintenance 400–600 mg q6h
If seizures continue for more than 60 min: diagnose Refractory Status and institute pharmacological EEG seizure suppression, 10–20 s burst-suppression, if necessary – propofol 2 mg/kg bolus IV and 100–150 mcg/kg/min infusion or thiopental 3–4 mg/kg bolus IV and 0.3–0.4 mg/kg/min. Hemodynamic support – fluids, pressors, inotropes
Once EEG suppressed, complete loading of anticonvulsant, add additional benzodiazepine if necessary, and consider weaning infusion agent several hours later (preferably 12–24 h) while optimal serum anticonvulsant levels are documented
If seizures persist, consider prolonged barbiturate or anesthetic coma with pentobarbital 12 mg/kg at 0.2–0.4 mg/kg/min followed by an infusion of 0.25–2.0 mg/kg/h for continued EEG suppression

termination of SE when treated within 30 min of onset and <40% when treated after the first 2 h from onset (22). If the seizures persist despite 2 or 3 first or second line IV antiepileptics, SE is considered refractory and special measures are taken in the ICU. In the following sections we will review the available medication options and the rationale for their use.

15.10.3. Rationale for Using Specific Anti-Epileptic Medications

Treatment of recurrent seizures and status epilepticus requires fast drug absorption and, therefore, parenteral administration is essential. Among the currently available standard antiepileptics, only phenytoin, phenobarbital, and valproate are available in injectable preparations. In addition, antianxiety drugs (such as diazepam, lorazepam) and anesthetics (such as amorbabital, pentobarbital, thiopental, midazolam, and propofol) are available in parenteral forms. In order to act rapidly, the drugs need to cross the blood–brain barrier readily. This is the case with most drugs that are effective in acute seizure management: they are highly lipid-soluble and thus cross in seconds to minutes. High lipid solubility also leads to redistribution from the central compartment (blood and extracellular fluid) to peripheral compartments (fat and organs). The redistribution leads to a drop in plasma concentrations. Therefore, repeat infusions are necessary to maintain adequate plasma levels. Continuous administration increases the concentration of the drug in the central compartment and leads to saturation of the peripheral compartment to the degree that the drug no longer redistributes. If drug administration ceases, plasma levels will be maintained by diffusion from the peripheral to the central compartment, which may result in unfavorable side effects, such as prolonged obtundation or cardiorespiratory collapse. These effects are dangerous and account for some of the morbidity and mortality associated with SE (76).

The rationale for using benzodiazepines as first-line drug was until recently based on small uncontrolled studies. The first randomized, double-blind study was conducted by Leppik et al. who compared diazepam to lorazepam in patients with SE. Both drugs were highly efficacious at controlling the seizures (see below) (77). Another randomized, non-blinded clinical trial compared a combination of diazepam and phenytoin to phenobarbital in 36 patients with generalized convulsive SE. The cumulative convulsion time had a strong trend to be shorter for the phenobarbital group than for the diazepam/phenytoin group (median 5 vs. 9 min, $P<0.06$). The response latency (elapsed time from the initiation of therapy to the end of the last convulsion) had also a tendency for being shorter for the phenobarbital group (median 5.5 vs. 15 min, $P<0.10$). The frequencies of intubation, hypotension, and arrhythmias were similar in the two groups (78). The results of this study, although not reaching statistical significance due to the small number of patients, provided evidence of the safety and efficacy of phenobarbital, but did not convince the majority of the medical community, who preferred shorter acting agents with a safer clinical profile.

Ten years later, a landmark study from the Veterans Affairs Status Epilepticus Cooperative Study Group was published (10). It was a randomized, double-blind, multicenter trial from 16 VA medical centers of four IV regimens, either for overt SE or subtle SE: diazepam (0.15 mg/kg) followed by phenytoin (18 mg/kg), lorazepam (0.1 mg/kg), phenobarbital (15 mg/kg), and phenytoin alone (18 mg/kg). Interestingly, lorazepam followed by phenytoin, the most commonly used combination today, was not included. If the first treatment had failed, an algorithm to follow with a second and third treatment regimen was also available. Treatment was considered successful when all motor and EEG seizure activity ceased within 20 min after the beginning of the drug infusion and when there was no return of seizure activity during the following 40 min. Five hundred seventy patients were enrolled. Three hundred eighty-four patients had verified overt convulsive SE and 134 subtle SE. An important finding was that SE has to be controlled with the first antiepileptic agent: the second agent was successful in only 7% of cases when the first one failed. In the convulsive SE group, lorazepam was successful in 64.9% of patients, phenobarbital in 58.2%, diazepam plus phenytoin in 55.8%, and phenytoin in 43.6% ($P=0.02$, but in the intention-to-treat analysis only with a trend). Lorazepam was significantly superior to phenytoin in a pair-wise comparison ($P=0.002$). In the subtle SE group no significant differences among the treatments were detected (17.9%, 24.2%, 8.3% and 7.7%, respectively for the four regimens, $P=0.18$, in the intention-to-treat analysis $P=0.91$). There were no differences among the treatment groups with respect to recurrence during the 12-h study period, the incidence of adverse reactions (hypoventilation, hypotension, cardiac arrhythmias), or the outcome at 30 days. However, comparing the two types of SE, outcomes for subtle SE were significantly worse at 30 days (50.1% of patients with overt SE were discharged from the hospitals vs. only 8.8% of those with subtle SE, $P<0.001$). Similarly, hypotension requiring treatment occurred more often in patients with subtle SE ($P<0.001$). During the first 12 h after the end of the infusions, no patient with subtle SE regained consciousness, compared to 17% of patients with overt SE (but with no significant difference among the four treatment groups). At 30 days, the outcome of patients who responded to the first-line drug in both the overt and subtle SE groups was better than that of those who did not respond. Mortality in the non-responders was twice as high as that in the responders. On the basis of these results, Treiman and colleagues concluded that lorazepam was more efficacious than phenytoin in overt SE treatment and overall easier to use than the other regimens. Also on the basis of these results, various treatment algorithms have been proposed which combine treatment first with lorazepam and then with phenytoin within the first 30 min after SE onset (79). After these measures fail and if the patient is in the ICU, anesthesia with midazolam or propofol is suggested. Alternatively, phenobarbital is tried first for the next 30 min, before one proceeds to general anesthesia. The current notion, however, is to individualize the treatment to the patient, than follow a strict, inflexible algorithm: for example, there are selected patients with good response to IV lorazepam, who may benefit from subsequent oral administration of the drug instead of an additional medication (80). When the first-line drugs fail to control SE, the subsequent choices have markedly reduced efficacy (10), because of either intrinsic refractoriness or delay of treatment with reduced probability for response (81). Until now we do not have a way to predict which patient will not respond to treatment and for whom the intensivist should, for example, skip treatment steps and go directly to general anesthesia. Mayer et al. examined the issue of predictive factors for refractory SE in a retrospective study of 74 patients with 83 episodes of SE. Refractory SE was defined as seizures occurring for >60 min despite treatment with benzodiazepines and an adequate loading of a second standard IV antiepileptic.

In 57 (69%) episodes seizures occurred after benzodiazepine treatment and in 26 (31%) even after a second agent was administered (i.e., fulfilling the criteria for refractory SE). NCSE and focal motor seizures at onset were independent risk factors for refractory SE in the multivariate analysis (odds ratio 11.6, 95% CI 1.3–11.1, $P=0.03$ and 3.1, 1.1–9.1, $P=0.04$, respectively) (69).

However, there is no standardized management of refractory SE even among neurologists specializing in critical care. A survey among 63 (out of 91 participants who responded) experts in this field from Austria, Germany, and Switzerland found that two thirds would apply another non-anesthetising drug (such as phenobarbital) for both convulsive and complex partial SE after the failure of first line drugs. A general anesthetic was more often used in convulsive than in complex partial SE as an alternative (35% vs. 16%, $P=0.02$). All participants would proceed to general anesthesia for ongoing seizures after these measures had failed in case of convulsive SE and, interestingly, 75% of them in case of non-convulsive SE. One third of participants would not use EEG, but only aim for clinical seizure termination. The vast majority (72%) responded that they would start weaning general anesthesia within 24–48 h (82).

In the following sections we will present the individual drugs used in the treatment of ICU seizures. Some of the most important data regarding pharmacokinetics, adverse effects, and efficacy, based on published studies pertinent to the ICU, will be presented to the interested reader. Table 15-9 presents an

Table 15-9. Doses, Half-Life, and Elimination Route for Antiepileptic Medications Used in the ICU for Prolonged Seizures or SE (2, 4, 7, 79, 105, 108, 183).

	IV Loading dose	Maximum rate	Maintenance (po-IV)	T 1/2	Elimination
Diazepam	0.15–0.25 mg/kg	5 mg/min		24–57 h	Hepatic
Lorazepam	0.05–0.1 mg/kg	2 mg/min		8–25 h	Hepatic
Midazolam	0.1–0.3 mg/kg	4 mg/min	0.08–0.4 mg/kg/h	1.5–4 h	Hepatic
Clonazepam	1 mg (repeat ×4)	2 mg/min	10 mg/day	20–40 h	Hepatic
Clomethiazole	40–100 ml	5–15 ml/min	0.5–20 ml/min	–	–
Phenytoin	15–20 mg/kg	50 mg/min	4–5 mg/kg/day	12–48 h	Hepatic
Fosphenytoin	15–20 mg PE/kg	150 mg PE/min	4–5 mg PE/kg/day	10–15 min	Hepatic, RBC, tissues
Lidocaine	1.5–2 mg/kg	50 mg/min	3–4 mg/kg/h	1.8 h	Hepatic
Lacosamide	100 mg	1–2 mg/min	50–400 mg/day	13 h	Renal
Levetiracetam	1,500 mg (up to 3 g)	Within 15 min	1–3 g/day	7 h	Renal
Valproic acid	10–25 mg/kg	1.5–3 mg/kg/min	15–50 mg/kg/day	7–18 h	Hepatic
Thiopental	2–4 mg/kg	250 mg/min	3–5 mg/kg/h	14–34 h	Hepatic
Pentobarbital	6–12 mg/kg	50 mg/min	0.5–2 mg/kg/h	20 h	Hepatic
Phenobarbital	15–20 mg/kg	100 mg/min	1–4 mg/kg/day	75–120 h	Hepatic, renal (25%)
Propofol	1–2 mg/kg	5 min	5–10 mg/kg/h initially, reduced to 1–3 mg/kg/h	0.5–1 h	Hepatic
Paraldeyde	5–10 ml rectally	Glass syringes	Repeated in 15–30 min	3 h	Hepatic, lungs
Isoflurane	0.8–2% inhaled	Anesthetic system	Titrate to burst-suppression		Lungs

PE phenytoin equivalents.

overview of these medications. A more in-depth analysis can be found in standard Epilepsy and Pharmacology textbooks.

15.10.4. Medications Used to Control ICU Seizures and SE (Table 15-9)

15.10.4.1. Benzodiazepines

INTRODUCTION

Benzodiazepines have maintained a significant role as first line IV treatment for acute seizures or SE since they were shown to be broad spectrum and potent anticonvulsant agents (83). Their effect is at the synaptic level via the benzodiazepine $GABA_A$ receptor complex. They enhance the inhibitory GABA action by increasing the Cl- channel openings and hyperpolarizing the postsynaptic neuron (84, 85). However, one must keep in mind that first line anticonvulsants like benzodiazepines and phenytoin fail to terminate convulsive SE in 31–50% of cases (11, 69).

DIAZEPAM

Diazepam is a highly lipid-soluble benzodiazepine, which has been used extensively during the last decades, but recently has lost some popularity to lorazepam. It is recommended that diazepam be administered by direct IV injection through a needle or a catheter rather than by infusion. Because of its solubility profile it rapidly enters the brain tissue. However, it redistributes to other parts of the body (fat stores and muscle) in approximately 15–20 min after it enters the brain. This results in loss of the clinical effect because of a fall in the brain levels. Its distribution half-life is 30–60 min and its elimination half-life 24–57 h (86). Nonetheless, sedative adverse effects are persistent and cumulative in particular with repeated administration, as the drug remains in the fat stores. It has been shown that 5–10 mg/min of diazepam can terminate seizures in 5–10 min in 70–80% of patients. The recommended dose is 10–20 mg (0.15–0.25 mg/kg, at a rate of ≤5 mg/min) (77).

In cases in which prolonged IV treatment is recommended for longer-term management, the use of an alternative drug is advised. The injectable solution contains 5 mg/ml diazepam in a mixture containing 40% propylene glycol and 10% ethanol and can cause local tissue irritation, venous thrombosis or phlebitis, and pain at the site of injection. Careful monitoring of vital signs is recommended to prevent systemic adverse effects such as hypotension, respiratory depression, profound sedation, and coma. Co-administration of other sedatives such as barbiturates can increase the risk of serious systemic side effects (49, 76, 87, 88).

Diazepam can also be given by rectal administration. Two controlled clinical studies were conducted to demonstrate the effectiveness of rectal diazepam in treating seizure clusters. The trials were randomized, double-blind, placebo-controlled with the first dose administered at the onset of an identified episode. Seizure frequency was measured over the course of 12 h. Both trials showed that a significantly greater percentage of diazepem–treated patients that ranged from 55% to 62% were seizure free during the observation periods compared with placebo-treated patients. Somnolence was the most commonly reported adverse effect and in over 500 patients treated with rectal diazepam not a single episode of respiratory depression was reported (89, 90). Despite this favorable drug profile, rectal diazepam administration in the

ICU should be considered only in the very few patients without immediate IV access (for example those who, during their convulsions, lose their IV access, continue to seize, and have no obvious veins for cannulation). However, newer benzodiazepines, such as IM midazolam, may be better suited for those problematic administration route cases (see below).

LORAZEPAM

Lorazepam is closely related to diazepam in terms of efficacy and adverse effects. It has become the drug of choice in the acute management of seizures as the drug is less lipid-soluble than diazepam and subject to less rapid redistribution. Its distribution half-life is <10 min and its elimination half-life 8–25 h (86). A single injection is highly effective and it has been associated with lower risk of cardiorespiratory depression and hypotension than diazepam. The anticonvulsant effect lasts approximately 6–12 h, making it preferable to diazepam (15–30 min) and particularly appropriate for the management of withdrawal seizures (7). In a randomized, double-blind trial, lorazepam was compared with diazepam in the treatment of 81 episodes of SE. Patients received one or two doses of 10 mg of diazepam or 4 mg of lorazepam IV. The onset of action did not differ significantly (mean time to end the seizures was 2 min for diazepam and 3 min for lorazepam). Seizures were controlled in 89% of the episodes treated with lorazepam and 76% treated with diazepam. Adverse effects, such as respiratory depression, occurred in 13% of the lorazepam-treated and in 12% of the diazepam-treated patients (77). This slightly superior clinical profile of the drug was also confirmed in the pediatric population. The two drugs were compared in 102 children in a prospective, open, "odd and even dates" trial. Convulsions were controlled in 76% of patients treated with a single dose of lorazepam and in 51% of those treated with a single dose of diazepam. In this study, some patients received lorazepam rectally with 100% efficacy. Significantly fewer patients treated with lorazepam required additional anticonvulsants to terminate the seizures. Respiratory depression occurred in 3% of lorazepam-treated patients and 15% of diazepam-treated patients. Interestingly, no patient who received lorazepam required admission to an ICU(91).

In another recent retrospective study, efficacy, safety, and cost of lorazepam treatment in 90 episodes of SE were compared to those of diazepam. Fewer seizure recurrences followed lorazepam administration (given either as first, second, or third dose of benzodiazepine, $P = 0.0006$). There was no difference in adverse effects or cost. The authors recommended that lorazepam be the first line therapy in preference to diazepam in adults with convulsive SE (92).

Because of the strong tendency for tolerance following lorazepam treatment, longer-term maintenance antiepileptic drugs must be given in addition. The recommended dose of lorazepam is 0.05–0.1 mg/kg (usually 4 mg), repeated after 10 min if necessary. The rate of injection should not exceed 2 mg/min.

MIDAZOLAM

Midazolam is a unique water-soluble compound, whose benzepine ring closes when in contact with serum and converts it into a highly lipophilic structure, crossing rapidly the blood–brain barrier. Its water solubility leads to rapid absorption by intramuscular injection or by intranasal or buccal administration. Midazolam is 96% protein-bound and is metabolized in the liver before renal excretion. It has an ultra-short distribution half-life of <5 min and a short elimination half-life of 1.5–4 h (86). Thus, its action is very short and seizures may recur few minutes after they have stopped. However, in the ICU the volume of distribution may be expanded and the half-life may be prolonged, especially with liver dysfunction (93). Acidosis can also reduce the lipid solubility of the drug by opening the benzepine ring structure and thus, decrease CNS entrance and seizure control. Despite these deficiencies, midazolam is probably the best benzodiazepine that can be used as a continuous infusion, because of its favorable kinetics and the lack of propylene glycol as a vehicle (which can cause cardiac arrhythmias). An IV bolus of 0.1–0.3 mg/kg, at a rate not to exceed 4 mg/min, can be repeated once after 15 min. The recommended rate for IV infusion is 0.08–0.4 mg/kg/h.

The high water solubility of midazolam and rapid absorption make it a better agent for IM injection than the other benzodiazepines, when IV administration route becomes a problem in the ICU (94). The mean half-life of IM midazolam (2 h) is slightly longer than the IV route. IM diazepam and lorazepam have a relatively slower absorption, induce local discomfort or can precipitate at the injection site, and are not recommended for the treatment of SE (7). However, IM midazolam has been successfully used to stop frequent seizures or SE within 5–10 min in children and adults (95–99). In a prospective, randomized study in the emergency department IM midazolam was compared to IV diazepam in their ability to stop seizures. Eleven patients received diazepam (0.3 mg/kg, maximum 10 mg) and 13 midazolam (0.2 mg/kg, maximum 7 mg). Midazolam was administered faster, because of no need for starting an IV line (mean time from arrival to administration of the drug was 3.3 vs. 7.8 min, $P=0.001$) and resulted in faster cessation of seizures (mean time from arrival to cessation 7.8 vs. 11.2 min, $P=0.047$) (97). The usual IM dose of midazolam is 5–10 mg (0.2 mg/kg).

More recently, Ulvi et al. prospectively evaluated midazolam infusion in 19 patients with refractory SE (not responding to initial IV administration of 0.3 mg/kg diazepam (three times at 5-min intervals), 20 mg/kg phenytoin, and 20 mg/kg phenobarbital). These patients were given an IV bolus of midazolam (200 mcg/kg) followed by a continuous infusion at 1 mcg/kg/min. The dose was increased by 1 mcg/kg/min every 15 min until seizures were controlled. In 18 (94.7%) patients, seizures were completely controlled in a mean time of 45 min, at a mean infusion rate of 8 mcg/kg/min. No significant changes in blood pressure, heart rate, oxygen saturation, or respiratory status were noticed. The mean time to full consciousness after stopping the infusion was 1.6 h and the mean infusion duration of midazolam was 14.5 h (100).

We like to use midazolam in our NICU in intubated and mechanically ventilated patients admitted with SE during after hours (when there is less expertise available reading the CEEG). In addition to other AEDs, midazolam infusion is started at 5 mg/h and if clinical or electrographic seizures are witnessed or suspected by the NICU on-call staff, the dose can be increased up to 10 mg/h. The infusion is usually discontinued early in the morning (for example at 6 am), in order to have CEEG époques before and after the infusion of the drug. This information is useful for making a final plan during morning rounds. So far, our personal experience is complete control of seizures or significant reduction during the night infusion time (101).

15.10.4.2. Phenytoin and Fosphenytoin

Phenytoin is insoluble in water, and the parenteral formulation contains 40% propylene glycol, 10% alcohol, as well as sodium hydroxide to adjust the pH to 12. This solution is highly caustic to veins and it may cause necrosis to the surrounding tissues by extravasation. The rate of administration has been limited to a maximum of 50 mg/min, although in clinical practice it is given more slowly – over 25–45 min in the adult patient – to minimize the pain at the injection site and reduce the risk of cardiovascular toxicity from the propylene glycol diluent. It should be mixed only with normal saline and other drug administration through the same line should be avoided. As a lipid-soluble compound, phenytoin readily enters the brain (it reaches peak levels within 15 min) and its redistribution out of the CNS is slower than that of the benzodiazepines, providing some evidence for binding of phenytoin to the brain (102). The drug is 96% protein bound and competes with other highly bound medications. With low albumin levels, one should consider measuring free instead of total phenytoin levels. Fast infusion of the drug carries the risk for hypotension and QT prolongation; therefore, ECG and frequent blood pressure measurements are recommended. Pain, edema, and distal to the infusion site ischemia characterize the "purple-glove" syndrome, which occurred in 9/152 (5.9%) patients who received phenytoin through a peripheral IV line (103). There may be a delay of several hours between the infusion and the clinical presentation of the syndrome, which makes the recognition difficult. Nevertheless, phenytoin is a highly effective drug in treating SE (104).

Fosphenytoin sodium is a phosphate ester prodrug of phenytoin that was developed as a replacement for parenteral phenytoin and was approved in the US market in 1996. After administration, phenytoin is cleaved from the prodrug by phosphatases found in the liver, red blood cells, and many other tissues. The conversion rate is not affected by age, hepatic status, or the presence of other drugs. Unlike phenytoin, fosphenytoin is freely soluble in aqueous solutions, including IV solutions. It is supplied as a ready-mixed solution of 50 mg/ml in water for injection and is buffered to a pH 8.6–9.0. This relatively lower pH of the vehicle for fosphenytoin is responsible for the lack of local adverse side effects at the injection site as opposed to the highly alkaline IV phenytoin solution. Fosphenytoin can be administered IV or IM and it is extensively bound (~95%) to plasma albumin. The dosage of the drug is expressed in phenytoin equivalents (PE). Seventy-five mg of fosphenytoin result in 50 mg of phenytoin in the serum after the enzymatic conversion; 75 mg of fosphenytoin is therefore labeled as 50 mg phenytoin equivalent (thus 15 mg PE of fosphenytoin is the same as 15 mg of phenytoin) (105). The drug is administered IV or IM at doses corresponding to customary phenytoin sodium loading (15–20 mg PE/kg) and consistently produces therapeutic plasma phenytoin concentrations (total 10–20 µg/ml and free 1–2 µg/ml). A maintenance dose of 4–7 mg PE/kg can be given either IV or IM. Therapeutic phenytoin concentrations are attained in most patients within 10 min of rapid IV fosphenytoin infusion (up to 150 mg PE/min) and within 30 min of slower IV infusion (<100 mg/min) or IM injection. Maximal total plasma phenytoin concentration increases with increasing fosphenytoin dose, but is less affected by increasing the infusion rate at a given dose level. It is recommended, following fosphenytoin administration, that phenytoin concentrations not be monitored until complete conversion of fosphenytoin to phenytoin is established.

As the conversion half-life is approximately 10–15 min (106), conversion is completed within 1–1.5 h; serum phenytoin peaks at 30 min following the start of IV fosphenytoin infusion and at 3 h after IM injection.

Fosphenytoin has fewer local adverse side effects (pain, itching, or burning at the site of injection) when given IV or IM compared with IV phenytoin. The most common CNS side effect incidence, such as nystagmus, somnolence, ataxia, and headache, does not differ between phenytoin and fosphenytoin (107). Fosphenytoin has been associated with hypotension in 7.7% of patients, which rarely lead to an intervention and with higher pruritus than phenytoin (108). Phenytoin, mistakenly administered at fosphenytoin rates, can lead to cardiac arrest (109); therefore, intensivists have to be very careful while prescribing the drug in the ICU during emergencies. Paresthesias of the lower abdomen, back, head, or neck have been reported with fosphenytoin in particular, when high doses and rapid infusion rate were used. They rapidly resolve without sequelae. A possible explanation is the competitive displacement of derived phenytoin from plasma protein binding sites by fosphenytoin. Earlier and higher unbound phenytoin plasma concentrations, and thus an increase in systemic adverse effects, may also occur following IV fosphenytoin loading doses in patients with a decreased ability to bind fosphenytoin and phenytoin (renal or hepatic disease, hypoalbuminaemia, the elderly). Close vital sign monitoring and reduction in the infusion rate by 25–50% are recommended for these, frequently encountered, ICU patients (110).

An issue of concern with the drug is its cost (14–18 times as expensive as generic phenytoin). In a small study comparing the cost in an emergency department, fosphenytoin (given in 39 patients) had lower overall hospital cost than phenytoin (given in 19 patients), mainly because of the associated complications with the latter (111). A subsequent larger, open label, study by Coplin et al. did not replicate the advantage of fosphenytoin (112). Whether these results can be extrapolated to the ICU remains to be seen.

15.10.4.3. Valproic Acid (VPA)

Valproate is an antiepileptic drug with broad spectrum activity against absence seizures (113), generalized tonic-clonic seizures (114), focal seizures (115, 116), and myoclonic seizures (117).

The drug has enjoyed increasing popularity in the ICU, especially after the introduction of the parenteral formulation. Although VPA is safe and generally well tolerated, there have been early reports of altered hepatic function and of several fatalities in patients taking VPA in combination with other antiepileptics (118). Careful monitoring of hepatic function is required in patients being treated with VPA, but dose reduction alone may be effective in preventing hepatic complications. In order to provide information on which patients are at risk for VPA-induced hepatotoxicity, Dreifuss et al. conducted a retrospective review of all reports of fatal hepatic dysfunction received by Abbott laboratories between 1978 and 1984. Patients found to be at the greatest risk for developing fatal hepatotoxicity were children <2 years treated with multiple antiepileptics, and who had other medical conditions, congenital abnormalities, mental retardation, developmental delay, or other neurologic diseases (119). From 1980 to 1986 the number of VPA-related hepatic fatalities had declined from eight to one, while the number of patients treated had increased nearly six-fold. Nevertheless, VPA is relatively contraindicated in cirrhosis or hepatic failure where it can accumulate and further promote liver damage (see below). Additional side effects are dose-related thrombocytopenia, platelet dysfunction and coagulopathies (4% incidence in children (120)), pancreatitis, and elevated ammonia.

Valproate sodium injection (Depacon) is approved for use when clinical factors make oral administration difficult or impossible. The pharmacokinetics of the oral and parenteral forms are similar, but if fast therapeutic levels is the goal, like in many ICU situations, the IV form has significant advantages. It can be delivered at a more physiological pH, does not require organic solvents, and has a wider range of solution compatibility compared to phenytoin. In addition, it does not cause sedation or respiratory compromise like the barbiturates or benzodiazepines and has a safer hypotension profile compared to phenytoin and the barbiturates (121). The drug has an elimination half-life between 7.2 and 17.7 h in studies given to healthy volunteers and this may be due to its 90–95% plasma protein binding (122–124). Depacon was approved for infusions up to 10–15 mg/kg at 1.5–3 mg/kg/min in the absence of other anti-epileptics and in patients who are valproate-naive. IM injection may produce muscle necrosis and should be avoided.

In a multicenter, open-label trial examining safety of IV VPA, 318 patients with previously treated epilepsy were enrolled; a need for parenteral VPA therapy for various reasons was documented. The median dose of IV VPA was 375 mg given over 1 h. Fifty-four (17%) patients experienced transient adverse effects, such as headache (2.4%), local reactions (2.2%), somnolence, and nausea without vomiting (2.2%). The side effects led 6 patients to withdraw from the study (124). However, these recommended doses generally result in sub-therapeutic levels of VPA, and they have been challenged in subsequent studies. In a small study by Venkataraman and Wheless, 24 infusions of IV valproate were carried out electively in 21 patients with epilepsy. The dose ranged from 21 to 28 mg/kg (mean 24.2 mg/kg) and was weight-adjusted. Target infusion rates were 3 or 6 mg/kg/min, i.e., over 4–8 min. No significant BP changes or EKG abnormalities were reported. On the basis of these results the authors suggested a rate of 6 mg/kg/min (125). Doses up to 40 mg/kg (126) have been given without serious side effects including significant changes in blood pressure, electrographic abnormalities, or respiratory depression. This is in contrast to other commonly used parenteral antiepileptics, such as lorazepam, phenobarbital, diazepam, and fosphenytoin, which have been variably associated with hypoventilation, cardiac arrhythmias, or hypotension (10, 127).

Intravenous VPA has not been approved for the management of status epilepticus (SE). However, the use of IV valproate in SE has been reported in the medical literature in both children and adults (38, 128–131) and recently in a rat model of SE induced by intra-hippocampal application of 4-aminopyridine (132). It has been used in both CSE and NCSE.

Price evaluated 24 neurosurgical patients with generalized CSE refractory to diazepam, treated with IV VPA, either as a bolus of 400 mg followed by infusion of 100 mg/h or 15 mg/kg load followed by 6 mg/kg/h infusion. Seizure control was achieved in 6/15 (40%) patients within 2 h in the first group and in 7/9 (78%) patients within 1 h in the second. Only one patient developed thrombocytopenia, without a clear cause-and-effect relationship ever established (133).

In one study conducted in Europe, the efficacy of IV sodium valproate was evaluated in 23 valproate-naïve adult patients with SE (8 with convulsive and 15 with non-convulsive). A loading dose of 15 mg/kg followed by 1 mg/kg/h infusion led to VPA levels of 68.5 mg/L at 1 h, which was deemed satisfactory. Disappearance of SE in <20 min was considered successful, while in >30 min was considered a failure. Use of IV valproate resulted in the resolution of SE in 19 (83%) patients (7/8 with convulsive and 12/15 with NCSE). All 4 patients who failed to respond to VPA, as well as to other anti-epileptics, had SE secondary to cerebral lesions. There were no relapses of SE within the first 24 h. All patients showed a slight reduction in systolic blood pressure and heart rate, but none required treatment for that. The serum concentrations varied most in 4 patients older than 80 years, but valproate was still well tolerated. Despite these promising results, the authors suggested that IV valproate be used cautiously in the elderly (130).

Another study assessed the safety and efficacy of IV valproate in 35 patients with SE. Twenty patients had failed treatment with benzodiazepines, and 3 patients had failed phenytoin treatment. SE was interrupted in 27/35 (77%) patients; the majority of them responded during the bolus infusion. Among the 8 patients considered treatment failures, 5 patients were also refractory to other antiepileptic drugs, 2 patients responded to an increased valproate dose, and 1 patient responded to clonazepam. Two patients developed nausea and allergic skin rash after the VPA in these series (134).

A case report of a 38-year-old man who presented with NCSE after his carbamazepine level became sub-therapeutic has been reported by Chez et al. The patient was loaded with 30 mg/kg IV VPA and responded for 6 h. Seizures recurred when the level fell to 32 mg/L and he received a second loading dose with complete success (128).

Another case of a 25-year-old woman with history of absence epilepsy in childhood and catamenial exacerbation of eye fluttering and dysphasia, successfully treated with 500 mg of IV VPA over 30 min, has been reported by Kaplan (38). A similar case of a 28-year-old woman with history of absence epilepsy in childhood and tonic-clonic seizures as an adolescent, who presented with nonrhythmic whole body myoclonic jerks while on therapeutic phenytoin, was reported by Sheth and Gilal. The patient received IV VPA 500 mg over 30 min with clinical and EEG response (135).

In a small retrospective review of hospital records, 13 patients with SE and hypotension received IV VPA therapy. Mean age of patients was 74 and the mean loading dose of VPA was 25 mg/kg (range 14.7–32.7), at a mean rate of 36.6 mg/min (range 6.3–100). There were no significant changes in blood pressure, pulse, or use of vasopressors, suggesting that VPA loading at these high rates is well tolerated, even in patients with cardiovascular instability. Seizures were controlled in 4 (31%) patients with IV VPA, but eventually all patients died as a consequence of their underlying illness (six were post-anoxic and three had stroke) (127). The same group presented their results of using IV VPA in 30 patients on a later occasion. Control of seizures was achieved in 5/11 (45%) of patients with overt convulsive SE, 2/6 (33%) of patients with subtle SE, 4/8 (50%) patients with complex partial SE, and all four (100%) patients with simple partial SE. Among patients with overt convulsive SE, the mean duration of SE prior to treatment in patients who responded was 2.6 h vs. 36 h in those who did not respond (136).

Table 15-10. Indications for Use of IV Valproic Acid in SE – Adapted from (121).

1. As adjunctive agent, after benzodiazepines and phenytoin/fosphenytoin have been properly given and while preparations are being made for third-line agents (propofol, midazolam, or barbiturates)

2. Once third-line agents have been given without complete cessation of SE

3. Instead of third-line agents in patients who do not wish to be mechanically ventilated

4. Patients allergic to one or more other antiepileptics

5. Absence SE or myoclonic SE as first or second line agent

On the basis of a review of the available literature until mid-2000, Hodges and Mazur suggested 3 clinical situations, where IV VPA could be considered as a third- or fourth-line agent for the treatment of SE (Table 15-10). We also added a use in patients who have a well documented allergic reaction to phenytoin or fosphenytoin.

This sequence of treatment options may be challenged by new data comparing phenytoin to VPA. In a retrospective study of 63 patients treated with IV VPA (average dose 31.5 mg/kg, range 10–78 mg/kg), because of allergy to phenytoin, myoclonus, or refractoriness to the other AEDs, Limdi et al. reported 63.3% efficacy, which was increasing with the order that the drug was used (higher as a fourth AED than as a first AED). The rate of administration in this study reached 500 mg/min in the majority of patients, with minimal adverse events (137). In a prospective study from India, Misra et al. evaluated 68 patients with CSE who were randomly assigned to two treatment groups, either VPA 30 mg/kg IV over 15 min or phenytoin 18 mg/kg IV at a rate of 50 mg/min. Interestingly, no benzodiazepines were used before VPA or phenytoin. If seizures failed to be controlled after this first-line treatment, the other agent was subsequently used. Seizures were aborted in 66% in the VPA group and 42% in the PHT group. As a second-line treatment in refractory patients, VPA was effective in 79% and PHT was effective in 25%. The side effects in the two groups did not differ (138).

This study is the first to demonstrate superiority of VPA over phenytoin. These results were not replicated in a subsequent randomized study, which compared 50 patients treated with IV VPA with 50 age and sex-matched patients treated with phenytoin, but after administration of benzodiazepines without success. Intravenous VA was successful in 88% and IV phenytoin in 84% of patients of SE (no significant difference), with a significantly better response in patients of SE <2 h. As in the study by Misra et al. the total number of adverse events did not differ significantly between the two treatment groups (139). Lastly, in a prospective, quasi-randomized open-label study, Gilad et al. treated patients who presented in the emergency department with SE or acute repetitive seizures with either IV VPA 30 mg/kg or IV phenytoin 18 mg/kg over 20 min in a 2:1 ratio. No benzodiazepines were initially used and in case of failure of the first drug to control seizures, the other one followed. Seventy-four adult patients participated in the study, 49 in the VPA and 25 in the phenytoin arm. In 43 (87.8%) of the VPA patients, the seizures discontinued, and no rescue medication was needed. Similar results were found in the PHT group in which seizures of 22 (88%) patients were well controlled. Side effects were found in 12% of the PHT group, and in none of the VPA group (140). In another recent prospective study from Norway, Olsen et al. treated 41 patients with SE or serial seizure attacks with 25 mg/kg of IV VPA loading dose over 30 min, followed by continuous infusion of 100 mg/h for at least 24 h. All patients had initially received diazepam as first-line unsuccessful treatment. In 76% of the cases (31 of 41), seizures stopped and anesthetic agents were not required (141).

Despite the small numbers and conflicting results, these small unblinded studies show better safety profile of VPA compared to phenytoin, at least equivalent efficacy, and tolerability of higher infusion rates (up to 6 mg/kg/min), and may begin to challenge the current treatment algorithms. In fact some European guidelines from Spain, Italy, and Belgium recommend IV VPA as an alternative to phenytoin second-line treatment for benzodiazepine resistant SE, but the European Federation of Neurological Societies guideline does not yet support that (142–147).

15.10.4.4. Barbiturates

Issues with High Barbiturate Dose Use in the ICU

These are potent antiepileptic medications and can be used either as additives to the anti-epileptic regimen for better seizure control (infrequently as first or second-line drugs due to several serious adverse effects) or as inducers of general anesthesia in case of refractory SE. A major problem with these medications is the need for complete and prolonged support of vital organs when administered in high doses that challenges and exhausts many ICU resources. The neurological examination, an important assessment tool in all cases where an intracranial pathology is associated with SE (for example hemorrhage, tumor, or trauma), is reduced to few brainstem reflexes (the last retained reflex with increasing depth of coma being the pupillary response) or complete disappearance of all indications of brain activity. This reduces our ability to differentiate between brain death, on going non-convulsive epileptic activity, and profound sedation and obviates the need for ancillary bedside tests including an EEG or a transcranial Doppler for the presence of cerebral flow. Respiratory depression with barbiturates obligates endotracheal intubation and mechanical ventilation. Frequent suctioning of the respiratory secretions is necessary because of ciliary immobility and cough suppression. Cardiovascular adverse events are equally hazardous. Hypotension due to both vasodilatation and myocardial depression occurs in almost every case. Central venous pressure (goal 6–8 mm Hg) or less often pulmonary wedge pressure (goal 12–14 mm Hg) monitoring and vasopressor and inotrope infusion (dopamine 10–20 mcg/kg/min or neosynephrine 1–8 mcg/kg/min) with continuous arterial blood pressure monitoring are standard in our ICU with prolonged administration of high dose pentobarbital or other barbiturates. A hemodynamic treatment protocol for thiopental infusion has been recently published with a goal of mean arterial pressure >65 mm Hg: all 10 patients had Swan-Ganz catheter placement. Pulmonary capillary wedge pressure was kept >10 mm Hg and if the cardiac index was <3 L/min, the patient was started on dopamine or dobutamine infusion, otherwise on norepinephrine (148). These measures will also keep adequate renal perfusion and urinary output, which are usually decreased with barbiturate coma. With deep coma, poikilothermia ensues and special care should be taken to keep the temperature to the predefined range. On the other hand, all barbiturates are potent immunosuppressives (149) and special care should be taken to avoid nosocomial infections.

All procedures should be performed under strict sterility, samples of potentially infected fluids (bronchial secretions, urine, blood) should be collected with even low suspicion level, and all infections should be aggressively treated. Enteral nutrition through nasogastric or nasojejunal tubes, although feasible (150), is usually problematic because of gastric and bowel hypomobility. Intestinal infarction can complicate ileus during high barbiturate dosage (151). Therefore, in many cases total parenteral nutrition through a dedicated central line port becomes necessary. Immobility leads to skin ulceration and deep venous thromboses, increasing the risk for pulmonary embolism. Frequent repositioning of the patient in bed and special inflatable or rotating mattresses decrease the incidence of the former. Elastic stockings, sequential compression devices, and low-molecular weight heparin administration are common measures taken in the ICU to avoid the latter.

DEPTH AND DURATION OF BARBITURATE COMA

Most authorities agree that ICU patients on barbiturate coma should be monitored with EEG, preferably on a continuous basis. However, there is no consensus regarding the depth of the EEG suppression that must be achieved. Some experts recommend a burst-suppression pattern of 5–10 s (148, 152), while others advocate for complete suppression or "flat record" (9). In a retrospective study of 35 patients treated with pentobarbital for refractory SE, persistent seizure control was achieved in 6/12 (50%) patients reaching a burst-suppression level as the greatest depth of EEG suppression and in 17/20 (85%) patients reaching a "flat" record ($P = 0.049$). Three patients with neither pattern but just slow EEG had also persistent control. Survival was non-significantly better in the more suppressed group (25% vs. 60%, $P = 0.08$). Isolated epileptiform discharges during the barbiturate infusion did not correlate with relapse of status. These results suggest that patients with deeper suppression appear to have fewer relapses and a better outcome, as well as that it is not necessary to suppress all epileptiform discharges (153). However, one has to balance the benefits of the deeper suppression level with the adverse effects such a more aggressive treatment portends. A systematic review evaluated studies describing use of midazolam or propofol or pentobarbital for refractory SE. Compared with seizure suppression, titration of treatment to EEG background suppression level was associated with a lower frequency of breakthrough seizures (4 vs. 53%; $P < 0.001$), but also a higher frequency of hypotension (76 vs. 29%; $P < 0.001$). No difference in short-term mortality was found among these three anesthetic agents (154). Another recent retrospective study of 127 episodes of SE (excluding post-anoxic cases), 49 of which were refractory to treatment, did not find any benefit regarding mortality in achieving burst suppression (via barbiturates, propofol, or combination of anesthetic agents) (155). The criticism of this study was that one third of patients were not monitored by continuous EEG and that no patient achieved complete and sustained burst suppression (156). Therefore, the majority of experts agree that the more aggressive treatment goal of burst suppression should be tried in cases of refractory SE (1).

There is also no general agreement regarding the duration of the induced barbiturate coma (157). Most authorities believe that 12–24 h are enough (1, 79), but some recommend up to 96 h (158). Krishnamurthy and Drislane conducted a retrospective analysis of 40 patients with 44 refractory SE episodes on pentobarbital coma. Patients with more prolonged treatment

(>96 h) and those receiving phenobarbital at the time of pentobarbital taper were less likely to relapse (159). Treatment is gradually tapered and the patient is closely monitored clinically and electrographically for recurrence of seizures. If seizures return, the process is reversed and the patient re-anesthetized for progressively longer periods, as needed. Therapeutic levels of additional antiepileptics should be reached (for example phenytoin level of 20–25 mcg/ml) before a new weaning trial. A load of phenobarbital sometimes is helpful. Mirski et al. described a patient with refractory generalized SE, who was treated with barbiturate-induced burst suppression coma for 53 days with good neurologic recovery (160). Initially, pentobarbital was used, with serum pentobarbital levels necessary to control EEG seizure activity ranging from 40 to 95 mg/L (177–419 μmol/L). After the first 15 days, phenobarbital was introduced and kept at levels that reached 220–290 mg/L (947–1249 μmol/L) for seizure control. In addition, phenytoin with over-therapeutic levels of 25–35 mg/L (99–139 micro mol/L; unbound phenytoin concentration 2.0–4.0 mg/L [7.9–15.9 μmol/L]) was used. Maintaining these concentrations required 2,500–3,000 mg/day of phenobarbital and 800–1,200 mg/day of phenytoin. Overall, the patient spent 79 days in the ICU. This extreme case reveals the feasibility of an aggressive treatment approach.

Thus, although some general rules are applicable, treatment should be individualized through "trial and error" attempts. The intensivist should always seek other therapeutic options such as hypothermia, resection surgery, or brain stimulation (see below).

Phenobarbital

Parenteral phenobarbital is available in preparations that are highly alkaline and may irritate the tissues. Phenobarbital's entry into the brain is more gradual than with more lipid-soluble compounds such as benzodiazepines. Therefore, peak concentrations in the brain may not occur for 15–20 min after the peak blood concentration is reached. This represents a limitation that makes phenobarbital not the best choice as a first-line drug. Phenobarbital is solely eliminated by the liver and has a prolonged half-life of 4 days (75–120 h). This pharmacokinetic property may be advantageous as it is associated with prolonged antiepileptic effect. However, if the dose is excessive, reversal of the effect will be slow. Phenobarbital can cause severe sedation and even coma, but in children paradoxical hyperkinetic reactions are not uncommon. Elderly with cerebral disease may also exhibit confusion and irritability rather than sedation. Sedation subsides with chronic therapy. Respiratory depression and hypotension can occur especially if it is given as a second- or third-line drug to a patient previously treated with benzodiazepines or other barbiturates. In most cases, intubation and maintenance of ventilation are essential if phenobarbital is administered. Dupuytren contractures and folate-deficient megaloblastic anemia, requiring supplementation are not uncommon with more chronic use. The recommended loading dose is 10–20 mg/kg at a rate of 100 mg/min (usual adult dose 600–800 mg) followed by a maintenance dose of 1–4 mg/kg/day (7, 79, 105).

Thiopental

Thiopental is a highly effective anticonvulsant medication with some potential cerebral protective action. It has rapid onset of action and reduces the intracranial pressure, cerebral blood flow, and cerebral metabolism.

Thiopental is the preferred drug for barbiturate-induced anesthesia for refractory SE in Europe (3). A recent study from Finland reported the outcomes of 10 patients treated with high-dose thiopental for refractory SE in an ICU. The median time from seizure onset to burst-suppression EEG was 11.5 (6–12) hours and from ICU admission to starting thiopental anesthesia 113 (80–132) minutes. The median dose of thiopental to achieve burst-suppression was 19 (13–21) mg/kg and the median infusion rate to maintain the burst suppression 7 (5–8) mg/kg/h. The median duration of ventilation was 8.5 days and the median ICU length of stay 10 days. Eight patients developed atelectasis and nine received antibiotics based on clinical signs of infection (148). This small study is indicative of the difficulties encountered in the ICU with such treatment. Sedation, hypotension, and respiratory depression that requires intubation and mechanical ventilation usually occur. The drug has a strong tendency to accumulate, the elimination half-life may extend to 14–36 h (157), and a prolonged recovery time of days should be expected after the anesthetic doses are used for the treatment of SE. Monitoring of the blood levels of the drug or its active metabolite pentobarbitone is advisable. Other less common adverse effects include spasm at the site of injection, hepatic dysfunction, pancreatitis, and hypersensitivity reactions. Administration of thiopental requires full cardiorespiratory support with IV fluids, pressors, and prolonged EEG monitoring to maintain a burst-suppression pattern. Hypotension below 90 mmHg is a sign that thiopental should be lowered. All these adverse effects make the drug less suitable for elderly patients or those with cardiac, hepatic, or renal disease (2). The recommended dose is 2–4 mg/kg IV bolus given over 20 s followed by 3–5 mg/kg/h infusion in 0.9% sodium chloride solution. Thiopental should be slowly withdrawn 12 h after the last seizure has ceased and when optimal levels of antiepileptic drugs are documented.

PENTOBARBITAL

Pentobarbital is an alternative to phenobarbital and thiopental (an active metabolite of the latter). It has a shorter elimination half-life than phenobarbital (approximately 24 h, range 15–60 h) (152). Because of the short action of the drug, withdrawal results in a fairly prompt recovery of consciousness. However, seizures may also recur, as with all barbiturates, during the withdrawal period. In the retrospective study by Krishnamurthy and Drislane, 40 patients were treated for refractory SE with pentobarbital coma. Eight of 9 (89%) patients with relapse of seizures after the drug was discontinued died, compared to only 9/26 (35%) with persistently controlled seizures ($P<0.005$). Etiology was the major determinant of relapse and survival, with 19/20 (95%) patients with chronic epilepsy, infections, or focal lesions having achieved good control as compared with 2/9 (22%) with multiple medical problems ($P<0.001$). In this study, treatment delay did not predict a worsened outcome. Hypotension caused dose reduction, but never required treatment discontinuation (159).

Sedation, respiratory depression, and hypotension due to both vasodilatation and myocardial depression commonly occur. Decerebrate posturing and flaccid paralysis have been reported. Flaccid paresis may persist for weeks after withholding pentobarbital. Blood level monitoring is not very helpful, as there is inconsistent relationship between serum level and seizure control. Lactic acidosis due to 40% v/v propylene glycol content in pentobarbital infusion has recently been reported in a patient receiving the infusion at a rate of 10 mg/kg/h. Twelve hours later, the patient developed an anion gap metabolic acidosis, elevated serum lactate level, hyperosmolality, and increased osmolal gap, which improved after discontinuation of the drug (161). The recommended IV dose is 6–15 mg/kg over 1 h followed by infusion of 0.25–2.0 mg/kg/h or higher until burst-suppression EEG pattern is evident. In a literature review until September 2001, Claassen et al. compared the efficacy of midazolam, propofol, and pentobarbital for the treatment of refractory SE (154). No prospective, randomized trial was found. Overall 28 studies, mainly case series, with a total of 193 patients were included. Mortality was not different between the groups. Compared to the other two medications, pentobarbital was associated with a lower frequency of short-term treatment failure (8 vs. 23%; $P<0.01$) and breakthrough seizures (12 vs. 42%; $P<0.001$), and was changed to a different continuously infused anti-epileptic (3 vs. 21%; $P<0.001$). However, a higher frequency of hypotension was reported with pentobarbital (77 vs. 34%; $P<0.001$).

15.10.4.5. Propofol

Propofol is a potent anticonvulsant non-barbiturate anesthetic, with barbiturate-like and benzodiazepine-like effects at the $GABA_A$ receptor (162). It has rapid onset of action (within 3 min) and recovery (5–10 min after the drug has been stopped). It is metabolized in the liver and thus, affected by liver disease. Usage for SE management in anesthetic doses always requires assisted ventilation. Neuroexcitatory effects possibly through subcortical disinhibition result in muscle rigidity, opisthotonos, or myoclonic jerks (2). These involuntary movements are usually not associated with EEG changes. However, not all experts agree with this thesis (163): propofol has been shown to increase the frequency of spikes during electrocorticography and to activate neocortical foci (164, 165). A systemic review of reports on seizure-like phenomena (SLP) associated with propofol was conducted by Walder et al. In 70 patients without epilepsy, SLP happened during induction in 24 (34%), during maintenance in two (3%), during emergence in 28 (40%), and were delayed in 16 (23%). Most frequent clinical presentations of SLP were generalized tonic-clonic seizures in 30 patients (43%), increased tone with twitching and rhythmic movements not perceived as generalized tonic-clonic seizures in 20 (36%), and involuntary movements in 11 (16%). EEG was performed in 24 patients, in all after the SLP had stopped. Two patients had generalized spikes and three general slowing. Out of 11 patients with epilepsy, seven (64%) had generalized tonic-clonic seizures during emergence. Only two patients had an EEG that showed generalized spikes and slowing in one patient and focal temporal spikes in the other. The time point of the SLP occurrence according to this study suggests that a change in cerebral concentration of propofol may be causative, because it is quite rare to witness these phenomena during the maintenance phase of anesthesia (163).

The recommended dose is 2 mg/kg bolus followed by continuous infusion of 5–15 mg/kg/h initially, reducing to 1–3 mg/kg/h. When seizures have been controlled for at least 12 h, the drug should be slowly tapered over 12 h. To prevent rebound seizures, a decremental rate of 5% of the maintenance infusion per hour (i.e., over approximately 24 h (2)) or 1 mg/kg or less every 2 h has been recommended. Propofol infusion may cause hypotension that can be prevented by adequate use of vasopressors and IV fluids. Bradycardia including asystole has also been reported (166). Metabolic acidosis, increased incidence of infection, rhabdomyolysis (166), and lipidemia may occur after prolonged use, but the use of 2% formulation of propofol has reduced the incidence of the latter. A propofol-infusion syndrome has been described in children and adults (167, 168). Cremer et al. reported seven adult cases with head injury in a neurosurgical ICU. Five of them died because of progressive myocardial failure and arrhythmias, rhabdomyolysis, metabolic acidosis, and hyperkalemia. All patients received propofol at rates >5 mg/kg/h for >58 h. Interestingly, the incidence was higher after the introduction of 2% propofol (5% before vs. 17% after), although it did not reach statistical significance. The authors discouraged these high doses of propofol for long periods (169). We also recently reported an association between propofol and catecholamine infusions (to support low blood pressure) in patients with traumatic head injury (170). A small retrospective study comparing propofol to midazolam for the treatment of refractory SE, found that the two agents did not differ in clinical or electrographic seizure control. Propofol-treated patients with Acute Physiology and Chronic Health Evaluation (APACHE) II score of ≥20 had higher mortality ($P=0.05$) (171).

A more recent, prospective study of 10 patients with refractory SE showed that propofol had to be titrated at high doses (median rate 9.5 mg/kg/h) to induce burst-suppression pattern for at least 12 h. Three patients had recurrence of their seizures after the propofol was tapered (172). These preliminary data suggest that midazolam may be tried before propofol, especially if used for several days.

15.10.4.6. Ketamine

Animal data suggest that during SE there is an initial response to GABAergic agonists, which is lost later in the course, at about the same time that NMDA receptor-mediated transmission becomes enhanced (173). NMDA antagonism at this late state, when SE becomes refractory (i.e., not responding to benzodiazepines, propofol, or barbiturates) seems a logical next step (174). Ketamine is an NMDA antagonist, which has been used in refractory SE in both animal models (175) and humans (176). In a recent report, for example, a 22-year-old woman with mitochondriopathy and pre-existing epilepsy developed SE not responding to benzodiazepines, phenytoin, thiopental, and propofol. SE was terminated within days after supplemental administration of continuous ketamine infusion to midazolam. The authors suggested that ketamine should be incorporated into therapeutic regimens for difficult-to-treat SE (177). In a case report of subtle SE, ketamine controlled the seizures, but 3 months later diffuse cerebellar and worsened cerebral atrophy, raising the possibility of NMDA antagonist-mediated neurotoxicity was found (178). On the basis of this report, we would caution against its use until more data are available.

15.10.4.7. Isoflurane

Isoflurane, which produces electrographic suppression and has no reported organ toxicity, is the most commonly used volatile anesthetic for treating refractory SE not responding to IV agents (179). It has minimal hepatic or renal metabolism (thus, no toxicity to the organs) and most is exhaled unchanged. Compared to other volatile anesthetics it also has less cardiac and blood pressure effects. Its major limitation for more widespread use is the lack of scavenging apparatus in most ICUs. In addition, the experience with the agent has been limited: only small case series of its use have been reported. Kofke et al. have administered isoflurane for 1–55 h, in 9 patients with 11 episodes of SE. Seizures stopped in all patients and burst-suppression patterns on EEGs were achieved. Hypotension was recorded in all patients. Seizures resumed upon discontinuation of isoflurane on eight of 11 occasions. Six of the nine patients died and the three survivors sustained cognitive deficits. This small series suggest that isoflurane is an effective, rapidly titratable anticonvulsant, but does not reverse the underlying process leading to refractory seizures (180). In another retrospective study, Mirsattari et al. reported 7 patients treated with an average of 10 AEDs in addition to isoflurane (one patient also received desflurane for 19 days). Regardless of seizure type, isoflurane and desflurane consistently stopped epileptic discharges with adequate, sustained EEG burst suppression within minutes of initiation of the inhalation therapy. Four patients had good outcomes and 3 died. Complications during the inhalation therapy included hypotension (7/7), atelectasis (7/7), infections (5/7), paralytic ileus (3/7), and deep venous thrombosis (2/7) (181).

Isoflurane has also been suggested as an anti-epileptic agent in patients with acute intermittent porphyria (108). Its dose is titrated for end-tidal concentration of 0.8–2% and burst-suppression on the EEG.

15.10.4.8. Other Less Commonly Used Medications for SE

Lidocaine can be tried as a second-line drug for the treatment of early SE (182). The drug has a cell membrane stabilizing effect that reduces ion exchange and depolarization. Its action is not prolonged and with repeated doses there is significant risk for toxicity and even exacerbation of seizures (see Chapter 13 of Drug-induced Seizures in Critically Ill Patients). It is administered as a bolus of 1.5–2 mg/kg IV over 2 min, which can be repeated only once (total dose up to 200 mg). A continuous IV infusion of 3–4 mg/kg/h should not extend for >12 h.

Paraldeyde is a cyclic polymer of acetaldehyde with foul odor that has to be administered through a glass syringe (plastic tubing systems or syringes should be avoided). It has been used in the past extensively for treating SE, but during the last decades has lost popularity with the advent of newer antiepileptics. It has to be taken from fresh preparations kept in dark containers, because, if decomposed, it can induce toxicity or thrombosis of veins and micro-embolism if given IV. The preferred route is per rectum. It is rapidly absorbed and its anti-epileptic effect is evident within few minutes and is usually long lasting. Most of the metabolism occurs in the liver, but 20–30% of the dose is exhaled through the lungs. Sedation, cardiorespiratory depression, and metabolic acidosis with increased lactate are the major adverse effects. The drug is diluted by the same volume of water (5–10 ml for adults) and given rectally in a dose of 5–10 g.

Clomethiazole is given as an IV bolus followed by a continuous infusion, but its popularity has declined because of the risk for accumulation with prolonged use. However, the drug has rapid onset of action and can be titrated to desired effect. Cardiorespiratory arrest is a real risk with higher infusion rates or prolonged use and the patient should be continuously monitored. Other adverse effects include sedation, vomiting, phlebitis, fluid overload, and electrolyte disturbances. It is administered as a bolus of 320–800 mg

(40–100 ml) at a rate of 5–15 ml/min, followed by an infusion of 1–4 ml/min and titration to response (183).

Verapamil, a Ca^{++} channel antagonist with inhibitory effects on the P-glucoprotein (an efflux transporter for several AEDs, the overexpression of which is thought to convey resistance to AEDs during prolonged SE – see above in Pathophysiology), has been successfully administered IV (0.034 mg/min) to terminate SE after 37 days in an 11-year-old boy (42).

15.10.5. Newer Antiepileptics in the Treatment of Prolonged Seizures or SE (Table 15-11)

15.10.5.1. Introduction

Several newer antiepileptics have currently found their place in the epileptologist's armamentarium (184–187). Their use in the ICU is limited by the paucity of data regarding specific indications for their use in SE and their availability in only parenteral preparations, with slower onset of action. There are situations, however, where the intensivist should seriously consider using one or more of these agents: as adjuncts to the parenteral antiepileptics when there is a failure to control the seizures or when a specific organ dysfunction or disease prohibits the use of other antiepileptics. The small case-series available show that these newer antiepileptics can be used in cases of refractory SE, but they do not address the issue of when one should switch to or add them to the treatment. The question remains: use them just when one has already tried unsuccessfully all the other options and after the patient had been seizing for hours without control or earlier, when seizures are more amenable to

Table 15-11. Newer Anti-Epileptics: Dose, Half-Life, and Elimination Route – Adapted from (88).

	Dose	Half-life (h)	Elimination	Side effects
Gabapentin	900–3,600 mg/day	5–9	Renal	Drowsiness, ataxia, headache, fatigue
Topiramate	200–600 mg/day	18–23	Renal, hepatic (40%)	Weight loss, renal stones, paresthesias
Levetiracetam	1–3 g/day IV or po	7	Renal	Somnolence, infection, headache
Lacosamide	100–200 mg IV or po q 12 h	13	Renal	Dizziness, ataxia, prolongation of PR interval and syncope, suicidal ideation
Vigabatrine	1–3 g/day	4–7	Renal	Peripheral field constriction, depression
Tiagabine	15–45 mg/day	4–5	Hepatic	Dizziness, fatigue, SE induction
Zonisamide	100–600 mg/day	27–38[a], 63	Renal, hepatic	Rash, somnolence, dizziness, anorexia
Felbamate	1,200–3,600 mg/day	13[a]–30	Hepatic, renal (40%)	Aplastic anemia, hepatitis, weight loss
Lamotrigine	200–600 mg/day	15[a]–29[b]–60[c]	Hepatic	Rash, headache, somnolence, diplopia
Carbamazepine	400–2,400 mg/day	5–25	Hepatic	SIADH, neutropenia, aplastic anemia, rash
Oxcarbazepine	900–2,400 mg/day	8–10	Hepatic, renal (MHD)	Rash, ataxia, SIADH

[a] Enzyme-inducing co-medication
[b] Monotherapy.
[c] Valproic co-medication.
SIADH syndrome of inappropriate secretion of antidiuretic hormone, *MHD* active oxcarbazepine metabolite.

treatment? Because of lack of studies or guidelines, we feel that the intensivist should individualize the use of these drugs, on the basis of the etiology of the seizures, clinical status of the patient, and the potential for adverse effects or interaction with other critical care or antiepileptic medications. In the following sections we present a synopsis of the pharmacological action of each one of them, adverse effects, and available data regarding their use in SE.

15.10.5.2. Felbamate

Felbamate (FBM) has been approved as add-on therapy and monotherapy in adults with partial epilepsy with and without generalization and as adjunctive treatment in children with Lennox-Gastaut syndrome since 1993. FBM mechanism of action is not well known. It is very likely that it blocks the NMDA receptors. It is extensively metabolized by the liver, a property that leads to a number of drug–drug interactions. General use is limited because of occurrence of aplastic anemia and hepatic failure in some patients. FBM has not been used in the treatment of SE. However, studies have shown that FBM displays a potent seizure-protective effect in animal models of self-sustaining and kainic acid -induced SE. These results suggest that FBM might be useful when standard antiepileptics fail in the treatment of refractory cases of SE (188, 189).

15.10.5.3. Gabapentin

Gabapentin (GBP) has a structural relationship to GABA, the main inhibitory neurotransmitter in the brain. Nonetheless, it has little or no action at the GABA receptor. It is very likely that it binds to a calcium channel receptor in the cerebral neocortex and hippocampus. It lacks hepatic metabolism and it is entirely excreted by the kidneys in an unchanged form. Gabapentin was approved as add-on therapy for partial and secondarily tonic-clonic seizures. It has a moderate anticonvulsant effect and it is mainly used as analgesic in certain painful neuropathy syndromes.

In one case report, a patient on high dose GBP (8,000 mg/day) for back surgery and no prior history of epilepsy developed convulsive SE following gabapentin withdrawal (190). Another patient with a family history of benign adult familial myoclonic epilepsy developed myoclonic SE after GPN administration. Although he did not respond to benzodiazepines, he improved after discontinuing the gabapentin (191). In another case, a female patient with acute intermittent porphyria was admitted to the ICU with quadriparesis and change of mental status. Later in the course, she developed face and arm twitching and was started on gabapentin 300 mg tid, with increased seizure frequency and eventually convulsive SE. The patient was started on propofol and within few days she left the ICU on gabapentin 900 mg tid (192). Recently, another case of acute intermittent porphyria and SE, successfully treated with propofol and GPN, has been reported (193). Therefore, in patients seizing during a porphyric exacerbation, GPN may be considered as a therapeutic option.

15.10.5.4. Lamotrigine

Lamotrigine (LMG) was approved as adjunctive or monotherapy in partial or generalized epilepsy and in Lennox-Gastaut syndrome. In experimental seizure models, LMG has a similar profile of action to that of phenytoin and carbamazepine. It seems that it stabilizes the neuronal membranes by blocking voltage-dependent sodium channels. It is extensively metabolized in the liver through glucuronidation. LMG levels are increased by sodium valproate and lowered by phenytoin, carbamazepine, and phenobarbital. The effect of LMG on the severity of seizures and the seizure-induced neuronal damage was studied in animal models of SE. Treatment with LMG was shown to have only a mild effect on SE-induced neuronal damage in rats (194). In another experimental study, the effect of LMG for treatment of SE in rats was compared to that of phenytoin. Doses of LMG within or higher than the "therapeutic" concentration used for chronic epilepsy failed to prevent the onset of generalized tonic-clonic seizures while phenytoin was effective (195).

Human reports of LMG use in SE also exist. In one case report, generalized CSE that presented with recurrent tonic seizures was treated with 600 mg of lamotrigine over 4 h through a nasogastric tube (200 mg for 3 administrations at 2-h intervals). Reduction in seizure frequency was observed 5 h following initial administration of LMG (196).

Interestingly, cases of NCSE and myoclonic SE treated with LMG have also been reported. In a retrospective analysis of three patients who developed NCSE after replacement of VPA with LTG, Trinka et al. reported that the episodes of NCSE presented as an acute confusional state with mild myoclonus. Ictal EEG showed generalized spike-wave or polyspike-wave activity. The clinical symptoms and the EEG responded promptly to IV benzodiazepines and patients remained well controlled with dose reduction of LTG (in one patient) or discontinuation of LTG (in two patients) (197). In another case report, myoclonic SE was developed when LMG was added to clobazam (CLB) and vigabatrin (VGB) at a dose of 20 mg/kg for treatment of Lennox-Gastaut syndrome in an 8-year-old girl. Discontinuation of LTG resulted in rapid disappearance of clinical and electrophysiological manifestations of myoclonic ME (198). There are also reports of SE induced by LTG overdose in a 29-year-old man who intentionally ingested large doses of LTG and pregabalin and who had decreased level of consciousness and seizures (199). Another patient with localization-related epilepsy ingested an overdose of lamotrigine tablets in a suicide attempt and was in prolonged CSE. He was eventually controlled with benzodiazepines (200). These reports should alarm the intensivist who would like to try the drug in ICU patients with frequent seizures or SE, that if no improvement follows LTG treatment, a re-evaluation of the situation with an EEG may be warranted.

15.10.5.5. Levetiracetam

Levetiracetam (LEV) was approved as an add-on therapy for refractory partial onset seizures with or without secondary generalization. The mechanism of action is poorly understood. It binds to the synaptic vesicle protein 2A (which regulates vesicular traffic and neurotransmitter release), inhibits the N-type high voltage-activated Ca^{++} channel currents, and suppresses the activity of negative allosteric modulators (such as zinc and beta carbolines) in the chloride influx via GABA and glycine-gated channels (therefore restoring chloride influx) (201–203). It is metabolized by plasma hydrolysis and not through the cytochrome P450 system. LEV and its inactive metabolites are excreted 60–70% renally and the remaining 30% via the fecal route. Renal elimination is proportional to the renal clearance, and the half-life increases in renal insufficiency.

A significant advantage of the drug is that it virtually has no known interaction with the majority of ICU-used drugs, including other antiepileptics.

This was explored in a retrospective study conducted in the NICU at the University of Cincinnati by Szaflarski et al. (204). These authors analyzed the data of 379 critically ill patients and reported that phenytoin used prior to the NICU admission was frequently replaced with LEV monotherapy. Patients treated with LEV monotherapy when compared to other AEDs had lower complication rates and shorter NICU stays. Older patients and patients with brain tumors or strokes were preferentially treated with LEV for prevention and/or management of seizures.

LEV has been used in the treatment of SE. Rossetti et al. retrospectively analyzed 23 patients with SE treated with enteral LEV (205). The median daily dose of LEV was 2,000 mg (range: 750–9,000 mg). Ten patients (43%) responded. Initiation of treatment and dosage were significantly different between responders and non-responders: all responders had received LEV within 4 days after the beginning of their SE episode and were administered less than 3,000 mg LEV/day. These authors concluded that LEV may be a useful alternative in SE if administered early, even in intubated patients, and that escalating the dosage beyond 3,000 mg/day will unlikely provide additional benefit.

In another study from Jena, Germany, Rupprecht et al. compared 8 patients who received LEV as a second line agent for NCSE with 11 patients treated with conventional IV medications for NCSE (206). Those patients treated with LEV showed a marked clinical improvement with final cessation of ictal EEG-activity and clinical symptoms of NCSE within 3 days (mean 1.5 days). The response to conventional treatment was similarly effective but there were severe side effects whereas no relevant side effects in the LEV-treated group were noticed. The authors report no significant differences in hospitalization time, time in intensive care unit, and outcome between the LEV group and the control group.

LEV has also been used in patients with refractory SE. Patel et al. published a small series of 6 patients with refractory SE (not responding to at least 2 antiepileptic medications), who eventually responded to enteral LEV (dose range 500–3,000 mg/day) within 12–96 h (207).

LEV became also available in a parenteral form. Although it is considered bioequivalent to the enteral form and should be administered IV at a similar to the per os dose, it will build serum levels at a much faster rates (500–1,500 mg can be given within 15 min), a potential advantage in case of SE. In fact, even higher infusion rates (up to 2,500 mg IV over 5 min) were tolerated in healthy adults, with adverse effects (dizziness, 52.8%; somnolence, 33.3%; fatigue, 11.1%; headache, 8.3%) consistent with the established safety profile for the oral formulation (208). Additionally, it may be considered an attractive alternative in critically ill patients in general, where the enteral administration may lead to delayed or erratic absorption or when swallowing or nasogastric tube placement is not deemed possible. Parenteral LEV has been used for treatment of SE in a study from Basel, Switzerland (209). In this retrospective study, Ruegg et al. used IV LEV to treat 50 critically ill patients, 24 of whom were in SE. These patients in SE received 20 mg/kg IV LEV within 15 min and in 16 (67%) of them (including 4, who received the drug as first-line treatment for simple partial or NCSE) SE ceased. Except for transient thrombocytopenia in 2/50 patients, no other serious or life-threatening side-effects were reported by the authors. These results were replicated in the study by Knake et al.

who recently reported their experience with the use of IV LEV for the treatment of 18 episodes of benzodiazepine refractory focal SE in 16 patients, including four patients with secondary generalized SE (210). SE was controlled in all patients by the given combination of drugs. Additional antiepileptic medications after the IV LEV were necessary in two episodes.

Whether or not these retrospective data from small case series support the notion that LEV can be effectively used to treat SE remains to be seen.

15.10.5.6. Zonisamide

Zonisamide (ZNS) is a sulfonamide derivative that has been used in Japan since 1989. It was approved as an add-on therapy for refractory partial epilepsy. It exerts its action by blocking sodium and calcium channels. It has hepatic metabolism through the cytochrome P450 system. In a rat model of secondarily generalized SE induced by kainic acid, Takano et al. showed that 40 min following IV administration of ZNS, seizure propagation from the primary focus was inhibited, but there was no suppression of the epileptic activity in the focus (211). When IV ZNS will be clinically available is unknown.

15.10.5.7. Topiramate

Topiramate is an antiepileptic drug with multiple mechanisms of action. It exhibits voltage-sensitive, use dependent, sodium-channel blockade and elevates brain GABA levels. It also antagonizes excitatory glutamatergic transmission. Both animal and human data suggest that topiramate may have a beneficial effect in SE and may have neuroprotective properties in animal models of focal ischemia and SE, probably via its inhibitory effect on the mitochondrial permeability transition pore (212). Administration of topiramate after experimental SE in rats can attenuate seizure-induced hippocampal neuronal injury (213). A suspension of topiramate was administered via nasogastric tube in 6 patients in SE with a duration that ranged from 23 h to 38 days. In these case-series, topiramate was effective against both generalized convulsive SE and NCSE. In some patients seizure control, achieved by topiramate, averted the need for barbiturate coma, mechanical ventilation, and ICU admission. In three patients, standard treatment with consecutive IV antiepileptic medications, consisting of loading doses of lorazepam or diazepam, fosphenytoin, phenobarbital, pentobarbital, valproate, midazolam, or propofol failed to control seizure activity. Topiramate was administered at a dose ranging from 300 mg/day to 1,600 mg/day. The time to response to topiramate ranged from several hours to 10 days. The authors concluded that the parenteral formulation, when it becomes available, would allow wide spread use of topiramate in SE (214).

In another small series, topiramate was used to treat successfully two patients with refractory generalized SE and one with complex partial SE (215). Another patient with occipital strokes post nephrectomy, who was treated with several antiepileptics for refractory complex partial SE, including clobazam, carbamazepine, paraldehyde, and general anesthesia for 38 days, eventually responded to 400 mg topiramate bid via a nasogastric tube (216). Recently, topiramate aborted refractory SE within 21 h in 3 children after being administered as a 10 mg/kg/day dose for 2 consecutive days and followed by maintenance doses of 5 mg/kg/day (217). Therefore, topiramate may be a useful adjunct to the ICU treatment of refractory SE. Although anecdotal, we have had positive personal experience with the drug in our NICU.

In a few patients with refractory SE, we administered it at doses 200 initially and then 400 mg/day via a nasogastric tube. Seizures were controlled and subsequently the dose was tapered off by 50 mg/day every 1–2 days.

15.10.5.8. Tiagabine

Tiagabine (TGB) was initially approved as adjunctive therapy or monotherapy in partial or secondarily generalized seizures. TGB is a derivative of the GABA uptake inhibitor nipecotic acid and increases the cerebral GABA concentration. Although it is metabolized by the P450, it does not affect the concentration of other adjunctive antiepileptics. There have been a number of reports of NCSE development during TGB treatment in pediatric and adult patients (218–220). The patients presented with acute intermittent or progressive chronic confusion and the diagnosis was based on the EEG findings. TGB reduction or discontinuation led to clinical and EEG improvement. In one case report, the patient developed CSE after a TGB overdose (221).

In a review article, a panel of experts attempted to determine whether an increased risk of SE and complex partial SE is associated with TGB therapy. They reviewed 13 cases in which an EEG, performed on patients with altered mental status taking TGB, showed spike-and-wave discharges (SWDs). In addition, they reviewed all cases of suspected SE from TGB clinical trials. The panel concluded that the majority of patients had had prior EEGs with similar findings and there was no overall difference in the frequency of SE or CPSE between TGB and placebo-treated patients from placebo-controlled trials. The major risk factor for the occurrence of SE and CPSE in both the TGB and placebo-treated groups was a prior episode of SE ($P<0.0001$) (222). On the basis of these results, we do not recommend TGB as an alternative antiepileptic medication for the treatment for SE in the ICU, if there is a previous history of convulsive or complex partial SE.

15.10.5.9. Carbamazepine (CBZ) and Oxcarbazepine (OXC)

CBZ is one of the most commonly used and studied antiepileptics, with a wide range of action against both partial and secondarily generalized seizures, that has yet to find its role in the ICU. CBZ, although not one of the newer antiepileptics, is mentioned here, because of the commercial lack of an IV formulation and the marketing of its 10-keto analog, OXC, which has a more favorable adverse effect profile. Both block voltage-sensitive sodium channels, NMDA receptor-activated sodium, and calcium influx, with stabilization of the cell membrane. CBZ is metabolized to 10,11-epoxide in the liver and it is this metabolite that has antiepileptic action, and also plays a significant role in the attributed side effects. OXC does not have an epoxide or auto-induction, but exerts its actions through its 10-monohydroxy metabolite (MHD). Both can cause skin rashes in up to 5% of patients (with 25% cross-reactivity), but hyponatremia, due to SIADH, is more common with OXC (20% of treated patients may have a Na+ <135 mEq/L, usually responding to lowering the dose and fluid restriction).

CBZ can be dissolved in glycofurol (a common vehicle for other antiepileptics) and other compounds and administered intravenously. This injectable CBZ has been used to control seizures in a mice model of CSE, with antiepileptic activity evident as early as 30 s and peak at 3 min (223). Despite this potential, the IV formulation has not been marketed yet. In the ICU, rectally administered CBZ at 6 mg/kg, does not offer any advantage compared to the po route (same absorption and time to achieve maximum serum concentration (224)) in the management of SE. CBZ can exacerbate the non-convulsive seizures of the Lennox-Gastaut syndrome in childhood or induce myoclonic, partial (225), or absence SE (226, 227) , which can be particularly resistant to treatment with other antiepileptics, can cause increased intracranial pressure or transient MRI abnormalities (226) and can only respond to withholding the drug (225). In adolescent patients with idiopathic generalized epilepsy use of CBZ has also been reported to induce NCSE, which may be misdiagnosed as psychiatric disorder (228). This syndrome is believed to be due to the high epoxide and low CBZ levels in patients treated with other drugs that increase the conversion (phenytoin, phenobarbital and, especially, valproate) (225). CBZ intoxication can lead to alpha coma and SE (229), that may be resistant to even barbiturates and can be lethal (230). Midazolam infusion was successful in one case of overdose (230).

There are no studies specifically addressing the use of OXC in SE. A single blind, clinical study from Finland examined the antiepileptic effect of substituting carbamazepine with OXC on 16 profoundly mentally retarded in-patients. Although the anticonvulsive efficacy of the drug was considered better than that of CBZ in half the patients, two of them developed their first episode of SE during the trial (231). Therefore, both CBZ and OXC, despite their excellent antiepileptic properties, lack the fast action needed in the ICU to treat SE and can have potential for seizure exacerbation.

15.10.5.10. Pregabalin

This newer agent has been used for treating neuropathic pain and postherpetic neuralgia, as well as an adjunct in the treatment of focal epilepsies. Its mechanism is probably via reduction of the synaptic release of neurotransmitors, because of its binding to the alpha 2-delta subunits of Ca^{++} channels. Pregabalin has been reported to induce myoclonic SE in 2 patients treated for chronic pain (232) and probably should not be used in the ICU until more data support its efficacy and safety. See also pregabalin use for alcohol related seizures in the Chap. 12.

15.10.5.11. Lacosamide

This novel agent was approved by FDA on 28 October 2008 for the adjunctive treatment of partial-onset seizures in patients 17 years of age and older with epilepsy. The mode of action is unclear, but the drug binds to the collapsin response mediator protein 2 (CRMP-2), a phosphoprotein expressed mainly in the CNS and playing a role in neuronal differentiation and control of axonal outgrowth. This drug is renally eliminated (233). Although a substrate for the CYP2C19, its metabolite is inactive. Reduction of the maximum daily dose up to 300 mg/day is recommended in patients with severe renal insufficiency and in those with mild to moderate hepatic insufficiency. After hemodialysis, an extra dose of 50% should be considered. It is available in oral and IV formulations (a potential advantage in ICU patients). In a double blind, double-dummy, randomized inpatient trial, 60 patients with partial-onset epilepsy received either IV lacosamide plus oral placebo or IV placebo plus oral lacosamide. During treatment period, patients received twice-daily doses of lacosamide equivalent to their oral dose in another open-label lacosamide trial (range 200–600 mg/day). Intravenous lacosamide showed a similar safety and tolerability profile to oral lacosamide when used as replacement therapy (234).

There is only one case report of its use in a patient with NCSE, who responded to its IV formulation (200 mg IV bolus within 3–5 min, followed by 100 mg po q12 h the next day) (235).

15.10.6. Hypothermia

Hypothermia decreases the oxygen consumption and metabolic rate of the brain. There has been growing evidence of its beneficial effects in stroke and head trauma. Even in earlier studies, hypothermia has been recognized as a useful measure to decrease seizure activity (236). There are animal data showing that hypothermia ameliorates and hyperthermia aggravates brain damage from seizures or SE (237). In a rat model of kainic acid-induced seizures and SE, ictal discharges were decreased by 50% with mild hypothermia (28°C) and nearly abolished when body temperature was further lowered to 23°C. There was no hippocampal cell loss in hypothermic rats, whereas gross cell loss in the hippocampus was observed at normal body temperature. Hyperthermia (42°C), on the other hand, markedly aggravated the seizures and hippocampal damage induced by kainic acid in all rats; all animals died of tonic seizures within 2 h (238, 239).

In addition, hypothermia may have a synergistic effect on thiopental-induced burst-suppression EEG pattern. Kim et al. compared normothermic to hypothermic (33.3°C) patients undergoing cerebral aneurysm clipping with EEG monitoring after a thiopental bolus was given: the onset time for suppression was shortened and the duration of suppression and of isoelectric EEG were prolonged in the group with mild hypothermia (240). Moderate hypothermia (30–31°C) in addition to thiopental-induced coma has been used in 3 children with refractory SE. The seizures were controlled and 48 h to 5 days later the patients were rewarmed at a rate of 1°C every 3–4 h (241).

Recently, Corry et al. treated 4 patients with refractory SE with hypothermia (goal 31–33°C) via an endovascular cooling system (242). These patients also received midazolam or pentobarbital infusions for rapid seizure control and were maintained hypothermic for 24 h. If no seizures recurred, they were rewarmed at a rate of 0.5°C every 4 h. Therapeutic hypothermia was successful in aborting seizure activity in all four patients, allowing midazolam infusions to be discontinued. In 3 patients a burst-suppression EEG was reached. After rewarming, two patients remained seizure-free, and all four demonstrated a marked reduction in seizure frequency. Thus, although there are no randomized clinical studies evaluating the effect of hypothermia on SE, we prefer to keep our ICU patients with SE normothermic or slightly hypothermic.

15.10.7. Resective Surgery

This strategy is usually reserved for cases of partial refractory SE, with an identifiable epileptic focus. This approach has been reported in a child with complex partial SE or in patients who fail to respond to 3 courses of cerebral suppressant therapy for at least 2 weeks (243, 244). Duane et al. reported a 7-year-old boy with left hemiparesis secondary to right hemispheric cortical dysplasia. Burst-suppression pattern during pentobarbital coma was not successful and he seemingly had generalized spike and waves on the EEG and scattered areas of regional hypometabolism bilaterally on the [18F]fluorodeoxyglucose positron emission tomography. When the EEG was reviewed with increased time resolution, however, spikes suggested a right hemisphere origin. The patient underwent bilateral intracarotid amobarbital spike-suppression test that showed only minimal suppression of epileptiform discharges with injection of the left carotid, but complete suppression of spike activity after right-sided carotid injection. A right hemispherectomy was performed with complete cessation of status epilepticus (245). In a recent study, Ng et al. reported a total of 5 children who presented with refractory SE, including complex partial SE, epilepsia partialis continua, and "status gelasticus." Multiple medical therapies had failed to control their seizures, and focal resection was performed. Seizures were fully controlled in four patients, and in one patient seizure frequency was reduced by more than 90% (246).

In our NICU we had the experience of two patients with persistent failure of weaning from the barbiturate coma who underwent intracranial grid placement and mapping of the epileptogenic focus and had excellent outcome after surgical resection. More recently, we reported a patient with neuro-sarcoidosis in complex partial SE, with occasional generalization, who failed barbiturate coma treatment. This patient had an epileptic focus identified through intracranial electrode placement, surgical resection, and successful outcome (101). Despite these case reports or small case series, safety and effectiveness of resective surgery has yet to be proved in a controlled study.

15.10.8. Brain Stimulation

Refractory SE has been reported to respond to various methods of brain stimulation, including low frequency cortical stimulation via subdural electrodes (0.5 Hz stimulations to the ictal onset zones in 30 min trains daily for 7 consecutive days). This 26 year-old woman, who was on two anesthetics plus high doses of 2–4 enteral AEDs responded after 1 day of stimulation and one anesthetic agent was successfully discontinued. Seizures only returned by the fourth day when the second anesthetic had been reduced by 60%. Upon returning, seizures arose from only one of the five original ictal onset zones (247).

Vagal nerve stimulation has also become one of the treatment options in epilepsy. A 30-year-old man with refractory SE was placed on pentobarbital coma in another case report. He underwent left vagal nerve stimulator placement after nearly 9 days of barbiturate coma, with stimulation initiated in the operating room. On the following day, EEG revealed resolution of previously observed periodic lateral epileptiform discharges and the patient was free of seizures (248).

Electroconvulsive therapy (3 sessions/week, 6 total) was administered in a patient who was in refractory SE, not responding to pentobarbital coma for 40 days. After the second session the barbiturate was removed and eventually the patient recovered within 1 month (249).

15.10.9. Prevention and Treatment of Complications

Complications of generalized tonic-clonic seizures can be divided into acute systemic complications due to the sympathetic overdrive and the stress of extreme motor activity and to persistent neurological complications that occur at a later stage (250). Most of these complications have been already presented under the section pathophysiology of SE.

One of the most common complications encountered with SE is hyperthermia: it is usually due to excessive muscle activity rather than infection (45), but there are few cases where a CNS infection is the cause of SE. Therefore, the intensivist should be vigilant and order the appropriate work-up in atypical cases. Hyperthermia can spontaneously resolve following seizure control. However active cooling is recommended if body temperature exceeds 40°C. Because of the aforementioned beneficial results of hypothermia from experimental animal models (238), we believe more aggressive and earlier treatment of fever should be instituted in the ICU. Pilot data of hypothermia use in SE in humans suggest some efficacy (see above).

Extreme muscle activity also leads to lactic acidosis (46). Catecholamine excess can cause hyperglycemia, which can further exacerbate acidosis through anaerobic metabolism. Lactic acidosis has also been reported with high-dose propofol and pentobarbital use (see above). Acidosis, induced by hypercarbic ventilation, attenuates neuronal injury in a rat model of SE (251).

Hyperglycemia, on the other hand, may have detrimental effects in several types of brain injury (for example ischemia), but its effects are less clear in SE. Regional brain glucose utilization during seizures is increased in the brain, especially the hippocampus (252). In a rat model of L-allylglycine-induced SE, Swan et al. studied the lactate and glucose content of hippocampal cells at increasing plasma glucose concentrations. Although brain lactate concentration was elevated in SE and maximal in the high-glucose group, it did not reach ischemia levels thought to induce cell death nor did it correlate with neuropathologic damage (253). The intracellular pH, however, decreased in hyperglycemic rabbits with pentylenetetrazole induced SE (73). Therefore, although hyperglycemia should be avoided in the management of several underlying cerebral injurious processes, which may lead to SE, this may not be the case when seizures or SE ensue. Our personal preference is to start all our ICU non-hypoglycemic patients in SE on fingerstick checks q6 h for the first 24 h and treat glucose readings >130 mg/dl with subcutaneous insulin on the basis of a "non-aggressive" sliding scale (part of a tight glucose control protocol that is used in all patients admitted to our Neuro-ICU).

Another common complication is rhabdomyolysis, which may cause acute tubular necrosis and renal failure if left untreated. Patients should be screened for myoglobinuria and serum creatinine level should be measured. If myoglobinuria is detected or creatinine levels are highly elevated, serum potassium monitoring, urinary alkalinization, and forced diuresis should be considered. Special attention to rhabdomyolysis after high-dose, prolonged propofol infusions (as part of the propofol infusion syndrome) should be paid in the Neuro-ICU, especially if catecholamine infusions are used to support the blood pressure (170).

Cardiorespiratory complications include arrhythmias, hypotension, respiratory depression, neurogenic pulmonary edema, central apnea, and pulmonary aspiration (see above). Mean arterial pressure is elevated because of elevated total peripheral resistance, which can lead to decreased cardiac output. Patients with atherosclerotic cardiovascular risk factors may have a gradual deterioration in hemodynamic parameters, whereas other patients decline acutely (47, 254–256)

15.11. Management of Focal SE

Although single or multiple focal involuntary movements are not commonly encountered in the ICU, the intensivist should be familiar with the remote possibility that sensory complaints, changes of mental status, or speech or visual disturbances represent seizures.

Focal SE encompasses a wide range of clinical manifestations lasting for >30 min, including epilepsia partialis continua (EPC or Kojewnikoff's epilepsy, defined as continuous focal jerking of a body part, usually distal limb, over hours, days, or years) (257), opercular myoclonic SE (OMASE, characterized by fluctuating cortical dysarthria without true aphasia associated with epileptic myoclonus involving bilaterally the glossopharyngeal musculature) (258), sensory SE (259), aphasic SE (260), or occipital lobe SE (presenting as visual loss, mimicking migraine) (261). These focal seizures generate a lot of questions in the ICU, regarding their nature, need for treatment and outcome, because staff is more familiar with the clinical presentation and treatment of generalized tonic-clonic SE. However, until a more diffuse process is excluded (for example hypoglycemia), their very presence indicates focal cerebral pathology that should alert the clinician. Common causes include vascular or traumatic lesions, epilepsy (benign epilepsy of childhood with rolandic spikes), tumors or Russian spring-summer, or Rasmussen's encephalitis (see Chap. 1). More diffuse processes are much less common, with non-ketotic hyperglycemic diabetes mellitus (262) and hyponatremia, mitochondrial encephalopathies (MELAS-MERRF), paraneoplastic syndromes (263), or antibiotics (penicillin, azlocillin-cefotaxime (264)) the most prominent (265). Rasmussen's encephalitis was the most common cause of EPC in patients younger than 16 and cerebrovascular disease in older patients in a British series of 36 cases (257). Acute disease was also found in most of the 41 patients described by Drislane et al. vascular disease being present in over half of them (266). More recently, inflammatory or autoimmune EPC was reported. In a case from Turkey, a patient diagnosed with neuro-Behcet disease developed EPC resistant to treatment (267). In another case report from the same country, a 37-year-old woman presented with migrating focal motor SE. She was found to have autoimmune thyroiditis and was treated successfully with IV steroids. The authors recommended anti-thyroid antibody screening for multifocal motor status epilepticus cases of unspecified cause (268). In another case report, a 19-year-old Japanese man presented with EPC. Clobazam improved the EPC, but action myoclonus developed, which responded to oral tandospirone (30 mg/day, as 5-hydroxyindole acetic acid was markedly decreased in the CSF). In this patient, the MR structural images were unremarkable, but cerebral SPECT showed decreased uptake in the left thalamus and bilateral frontal lobes. Antibodies against glutamate receptor subunit ε2 were positive in the CSF (269).

Focal SE except for the etiologic implications is also important because it may precede or follow generalized clinical seizures or SE (266). An EEG may be ordered when there is suspicion of secondary generalization or when a new focal neurologic deficit cannot be explained by neuroimaging alone. Subdural hematomas in particular are lesions in which it is important to consider the possibility of focal SE as the reason of worsening symptoms or mental status changes (266).

Although EPC is notoriously resistant to anti-epileptics, in up to one third of cases there may be improvement or complete resolution with treatment (257). Focal SE usually necessitates polypharmacy, which, in our experience as well as in others, must include phenytoin or phenobarbital, although there are no randomized studies comparing these medications to the newer anti-epileptics or placebo. The same guidelines presented in Tables 15-6, 15-7, and 15-8 can be used, but most physicians would be reluctant to reach general anesthesia to control focal seizures. In non-motor simple partial SE there is no evidence that secondary brain damage ensues. On the other hand, the outcome of focal SE with motor symptoms is more strongly related to the underlying condition. As an example, tight glucose control in a case of non-ketotic hyperglycemia resolved the EPC in two separate episodes (262). EPC following Rasmussen's has worse prognosis, because of the progressive nature of the disease (266, 270). It should be kept in mind that the longer acting anti-epileptics appear more helpful and that the response to the drugs may be quite delayed in focal SE (up to 48 h in one series (266)). Intravenous nimodipine, a calcium channel blocker, has been used to successfully treat two patients with EPC (271), but no controlled trials exist. In another study, all four patients with simple partial SE treated with IV valproate (mean loading dose of 22.9 ± 7.9 mg/kg) achieved seizure control with mean levels of 92.2 ± 50.1 mg/L (136). Repetitive transcranial magnetic stimulation (rTMS) has also been used in recent reports. Seven patients with EPC of mixed etiologies were treated with rTMS applied over the seizure. rTMS was delivered in high-frequency (20–100 Hz) bursts or as prolonged low-frequency (1 Hz) trains and resulted in a brief (20–30 min) pause in seizures in 3/7 patients and a lasting (> or = 1 day) pause in 2/7. These authors also conducted a literature search, which identified six additional reports of EPC treated with rTMS where seizures were suppressed in 3/6. Seizures were not exacerbated by rTMS in any patient. Generally mild side effects included transient head and limb pain, and limb stiffening during high-frequency rTMS trains (272).

15.12. Management of NCSE

Compared to convulsive SE, there are no widely accepted guidelines or treatment protocols and this may be due to the still evolving definition, the inclusion of different clinical syndromes under the same rubric, and the paucity of animal or human data showing significant secondary neuronal damage (14). The extent and aggressiveness of treatment are unknown, but the presumed cause and type of NCSE may be helpful stratifying it: for example, if NCSE is secondary to epilepsy, treatment with anesthetic anti-epileptics and induction of burst-suppression may rarely be necessary, because of the better response and outcome in these cases (273, 274). Supplementing low antiepileptic levels in these patients and individualizing the work-up for an additional or triggering etiology may be enough measures. If, on the other hand, the NCSE is due to acute medical causes or is cryptogenic, more aggressive treatment is warranted (37). Other factors, which may play a role in the decision to treat by the intensivist, are the age of the patient and the potential for adverse drug effects (14). Elderly ICU patients with NCSE treated with IV benzodiazepines have increased mortality that may be independent of the severity of the illness (275). Six of 16 treated patients in this small case-series required emergent endotracheal intubation, some accompanied by hypotension, after the drug was administered.

Lastly, in the large, double-blinded study by Treiman et al. 134 patients with subtle generalized SE (defined as coma with ictal EEG discharges with or without rhythmic twitching of the arms, legs, trunk, or facial muscles or tonic eye deviation or nystagmoid eye jerking), were randomized to receive four different IV regimens (10). No difference in seizure control between lorazepam, phenytoin alone, diazepam and phenytoin, or phenobarbital was found. The success rate ranged between 7.7% (phenytoin alone) and 24.2% (phenobarbital), a disappointing outcome.

Although most authorities believe that absence SE does not induce neuronal damage and thus treatment does not constitute a medical emergency, seizures have still to be terminated. The first-line drugs of choice are IV benzodiazepines: diazepam (0.2–0.3 mg/kg), lorazepam (0.1 mg/kg), or clonazepam (0.5–1 mg). As second-line drugs, IV phenytoin or valproate can be used. In children, etho-suximide or valproate (age >2 years) are recommended as maintenance drugs for typical absence; therefore, they can be tried in the status setting. Crouteau et al. have reported an 11-year-old boy with absence SE after Lennox-Gastaut syndrome treated successfully in the pediatric ICU with propofol (bolus of 50 mg followed by infusion of 3.7 mg/kg for 30 min) (276). The patient needed endotracheal intubation after propofol was administered. There was a marked improvement on the EEG and the patient was extubated in 90 min.

Complex partial SE, on the other hand, may induce neuronal injury in animals (277) and humans (13). It can be precipitated by focal lesions such as stroke or encephalitis and seems to add an extra morbidity to these disorders (70, 278). Therefore, although treatment may not need to be instituted as urgent or aggressive as in convulsive SE (because it lacks the systemic complications of the latter), it should still aim at termination of the status within the first few hours, because serious mortality and morbidity have been associated with status duration from 36 to more than 72 h (70). As diagnosis of the condition may already be delayed (in 10/23 patients in the series from the emergency department the diagnosis was delayed by >24 h (56)), treatment should be started as soon as the diagnosis is confirmed. Some patients have rapid clinical or EEG improvement, but in many it is more gradual and delayed: 10/23 (43%) patients in the series of Kaplan had rapid EEG resolution of status, but clinical improvement only after 1 day (56); only 3/24 (12.5%) elderly ICU patients with NCSE in the series of Litt et al. responded to treatment within 24 h and more than half responded after the first 2 days to treatment (275). Thus, although a fast response to the treatment confirms the diagnosis, absence of response does not exclude it (37, 56, 64). Benzodiazepines administered po are the first-line drugs for treatment of complex partial SE, followed by a longer-acting antiepileptic, such as po phenytoin or valproate. Oral clobazam (10–20 mg/day over a period of 2–3 days) has also been recommended (15). Intravenous benzodiazepines (lorazepam) followed by IV phenytoin or pheno-barbital are kept for more persistent cases of complex partial SE. Intravenous valproate (30 mg/kg) has been successfully used to control NCSE in patients with sub-therapeutic carbamazepine levels (128) and complex partial SE (136). Topiramate by nasogastric tube has also been used for refractory complex partial SE in small series of patients (214–216). Recently, IV levetiracetam was also used to treat NCSE (279). In a retrospective study of 8 patients with NCSE treated with levetiracetam and compared to 11 controls (treated with conventional antiepileptics), Rupprecht et al. reported a marked clinical improvement with final cessation of ictal EEG-activity and clinical symptoms of NCSE within 3 days of starting levetiracetam. The response to conventional treatment was similarly effective but there were severe side effects whereas no relevant side effects in the LEV-treated group were noticed. There were no significant differences in hospitalization time, time in the ICU, and outcome between the levetiracetam group and the control group (206). It is unclear whether more aggressive treatment with general anesthetics as next step is warranted for refractory complex partial SE, as there are no studies evaluating outcomes and most cases are self-terminating (15, 273, 274).

Finally, there is also no uniform approach regarding treatment of comatose patients with NCSE or comatose patients with prolonged subtle movements. If the electrographic seizures follow a convulsive SE, the treatment should be as aggressive as with convulsive status, i.e., following the same protocol. If the electrographic seizures, however, follow an anoxic brain event and are associated with subtle movements, there are little data suggesting that aggressive treatment with IV antiepileptics and general anesthesia improves outcome. Most experts believe that post-anoxic EEG patterns of burst-suppression, periodic discharges, or encephalopathic triphasic waves indicate underlying widespread cortical damage and, therefore, represent agonal events (15). Several treatments have been tried, without convincing results. The large, randomized Brain Resuscitation Clinical Trial I, conducted in comatose patients admitted to an ICU after cardiac arrest, did not find any effectiveness or improvement of outcomes by administering an additional – to the standard treatment – single intravenous loading dose of thiopental (30 mg/kg of body weight) (280). In the series of Celesia et al. only 1/13 patients with cardiorespiratory arrest and generalized status myoclonicus (GSM) responded to IV lorazepam 4 mg and recovered fully. This patient did not have an EEG. IV phenytoin failed to stop the seizures in 6/9 treated patients with GSM and IV phenobarbital or diazepam in all patients treated. IV lorazepam (4–10 mg) successfully controlled the seizures in 3 out of 4 patients (281). None of the 11 patients with post anoxic myoclonic SE in the series by Young et al. responded to treatment with IV phenytoin, phenobarbital, diazepam, lorazepam, or clonazepem (via nasogastric tube) and all patients died (16). In the prospective study by Krumholz et al. comatose patients with myoclonic SE post cardiopulmonary resuscitation were treated early and aggressively with benzodiazepines, phenytoin, and barbiturates: 7/19 (37%) of patients received 2 antiepileptics and 12/19 (63%) 3 or more. Despite therapy, seizures or myoclonic SE were often difficult to stop and, even after they were controlled, the outcome did not seem to improve significantly (282). However, the authors advocated early and aggressive treatment, as their results suggested that seizures or myoclonic SE may contribute to progressive neurologic injury. Alternative treatments, such as high dose IV magnesium (to elevate the serum levels up to 14.2 mEq/L), were not effective in one patient with myoclonic SE (283).

15.13. Management of Seizures and SE with Antiepileptics in ICU Patients with Organ Dysfunction

15.13.1. Hepatic Failure

Because of their renal clearance, low protein binding and metabolism, gabapentin, leviracetam, and vigabatrin seem excellent choices (Table 15-11). However, there are not many data regarding these newer anti-epileptic drugs. Vigabatrin may normalize plasma alanine aminotransferase levels, making impossible to use it as an index of the hepatic dysfunction (284).

Phenytoin can accumulate and its plasma protein binding capacity is reduced. Reduction of the dose and frequent determinations of free levels are required in order to continue using the drug. Phenobarbital is metabolized in the liver, but is also partially excreted unchanged in the urine (20–25% of the dose). Biliary excretion is minimal and cholestasis is not a reason to adjust the dosage. Therefore, it can be used po or IV, but one should remember that its half-life in hepatic failure may be prolonged up to 130 h. Measuring serum levels of the drug and close monitoring for respiratory depression are recommended. The same is true for the benzodiazepines: oxazepam is a short-acting drug without oxidative metabolism, but is not available in IV form. All benzodiazepine dosing, except for oxazepam, should be reduced with liver failure. Lack of active metabolites makes lorazepam a better choice than diazepam, which should be avoided. The short acting barbiturates, such as pentobarbital and thiopental are completely metabolized in the liver and should not be used because of poor elimination. In addition to hepatotoxicity, which is idiosyncratic and mainly encountered in young children (see above), and pancreatitis, valproic acid can induce elevations of ammonia. In epileptic patients without hepatic disease, this adverse effect does not require treatment, unless symptomatic (285). However, it can lead to confusion when treating patients with hepatic dysfunction and baseline hyperammonemia, who may clinically worsen; therefore, VPA is generally contraindicated in hepatic failure. If absolutely necessary to be used, the dosage should be reduced, because the half-life of the drug is increased up to 18 ± 5 h.

15.13.2. Renal Failure

Drugs hepatically metabolized should be used instead of those with renal elimination, but there are several details that are important to remember. Phenytoin has decreased half-life and the unbound fraction is increased. Free levels should be followed and doses should be smaller and more frequent (q8 h). Only the free fraction is dialyzable; therefore, there is usually no need for extra dosing post dialysis. A significant amount of phenobarbital, on the other hand, is dialyzable and has to be supplemented post dialysis with careful monitoring of the levels. Because of the potential for accumulation, the dosage of the drug should be reduced. Valproic acid is barely affected by renal failure, as it is mainly hepatically metabolized. As with phenytoin, the decreased protein binding in uremia may lead to elevated free levels, which should be followed. Dialysis does not affect its levels. An increased risk for valproic-induced pancreatitis has been reported in uremic patients (286) and amylase should be measured in case of unexplained abdominal pain. Benzodiazepines do not seem to be affected by uremia or dialysis and, generally, their dose does not need adjustment. Because diazepam's active metabolite and oxazepam are renally excreted, caution is advised with their use in severe uremia.

Among the enterally administered anti-epileptic drugs, carbamazepine together with valproic acid is a good option, as its levels are barely affected in uremia and there is no need for post dialysis supplementation. However, rare instances of idiosyncratic renal damage have been reported with this drug (287). Tiagabine, an hepatically metabolized antiepileptic can also be used without any dosage adjustment in uremia, but if the patient is in status, it should probably be avoided (see above). With gabapentin a sliding scale dosage based on creatinine clearance has been recommended:

- >60 ml/min, 400 mg tid
- 30–60 ml/min, 300 mg bid
- 15–30 ml/min, 300 mg qd
- <15 ml/min, 300 mg every other day

Because the drug is highly dialyzable, an extra dose of 200–300 mg should be also given after each dialysis session.

If levetiracetam is used in renal failure the following dosing schedule is recommended based on creatinine clearance:

- >80 ml/min, 500–1,000 mg bid
- 50–80 ml/min, 500–1,000 mg bid
- 30–50 ml/min, 250–750 bid
- <30 ml/min, 250–500 mg bid
- End stage renal disease –hemodialysis, 500–1,000 mg/day

Following dialysis, 250–500 mg extra IV or po levetiracetam can be administered.

Topiramate and zonisamide induce formation of renal calculi and should be probably avoided in case of single kidney, history of renal stones, and after kidney transplantation.

15.13.3. HematoPoetic Dysfunction

Immunosuppressed or post chemotherapy ICU patients have special needs regarding the anti-epileptic drug use. Phenytoin can lead to megaloblastic anemia, responding to folate supplementation. An idiosyncratic pseudolymphoma syndrome, with diffuse lymphadenopathy, fever, and skin rash, different than the more common hydantoin lupus-like rash, can be misdiagnosed as true lymphoma and lead to unnecessary diagnostic work-up. Thrombocytopenia is much less common with phenytoin, but is a dose-related adverse effect of valproic acid. Usually only purpura or petechiae occur and only rarely organ bleeding. However, in the ICU, in pre- or postoperative patients or those with active bleeding or coagulopathy, any drop in the platelet count should lead to a decrease of the dose of the drug or substitution with an alternative agent. Neutropenia is less common with valproic acid, but a well-known adverse effect of carbamazepine (10%, usually during the first few months of use). The drug should be stopped only in case of white cell count <2,500 or absolute neutropenia (<1,000 polymorphonuclear cells). Carbamazepine can also induce aplastic anemia. Phenobarbital when chronically administered can induce folate-deficient megaloblastic anemia, but this is rarely a problem in the ICU. The benzodiazepines have no significant hematologic adverse effects.

15.14. Drug Interaction in the ICU

Several of the interactions between antiepileptics and common medications used in the ICU have been mentioned in the other chapters of this book. The physician treating ICU seizures or SE should be familiar with the most important of them, before he assumes treatment failure or is surprised by obvious signs of toxicity. Table 15-12 presents the effects of these drugs on anti-epileptic medication levels. Aluminum hydroxide, magnesium hydroxide, and calcium antiacids can decrease the absorption of enterally administered

Table 15-12. Effects of Common ICU Medications on Anti-Epileptics – Adapted from (288–291).

| Added drug | Effect on plasma level of primary agents | | |
	Phenytoin	Carbamazepine	Valproate
Salicylates	↑		↑
Ibuprofen	↑		
Erythromycin		↑↑	↑
Chloramphenicol	↑		
Trimethoprim	↑		
Isoniazide	↑	↑	↑
Fluconazole, ketoconazole	↑↑	↑	
Propoxyphene	↑	↑↑	
Amiodarone	↑	↑	
Diltiazem, verapamil		↑	
Cimetidine	↑↑	↑	
Omeprazole	↑		
Chlorpromazine			↑
Ethanol	↓		
Folic acid	↓		
Rifampicin	↓		
Digitoxin	↓		
Cyclosporine	↓		
Warfarin	↓		
Theophylline	↓		
Glucocorticosteroids	↓		

↓ decrease, ↑ increase.

Table 15-13. Effects of Anti-Epileptics on Common ICU Medications – Adapted from (288–291).

| ICU medication | Effect of antiepileptic agents | | |
	Phenytoin	Carbamazepine	Phenobarbital
Warfarin	↓	↓↓	↓↓
Theophylline	↓↓	↓↓	↓↓
Corticosteroids	↓↓	↓↓	↓↓
Haloperidol		↓	↓
Lithium		↑	
Tricyclics	↓	↓	↓
Cyclosporine	↓↓	↓↓	↓↓
Nimodipine	↓	↓	↓
Non-depolarizing paralytics	↓	↓	

↓ decrease, ↑ increase.

phenytoin, lowering its level. Conversely, antiepileptic medications can affect the metabolism of numerous ICU drugs and few of these interactions are presented in Table 15-13. Finally, anti-epileptic medications interact with each

Table 15-14. Interaction Between Anti-Epileptic Medications – Adapted from (288).

Added drug	Effect on plasma level of primary agents								
	PHT	**PB**	**CBZ**	**OXC**	**VPA**	**TB**	**LTG**	**ZNS**	**BDZ**
PHT		~	↓	↓	↓	↓	↓	↓	
PB	↑, then ↓		~	↓	↓	↓	↓		↓
CBZ	~	~	↓	↓	↓	↓	↓	↓	↓
OXC			↑[b]				↓		
VPA	↓[a]	↑	~ or ↑[b]				↑		↑
ZNS			↑[b]						
BDZ	↓	~			~				

PHT phenytoin, *PB* phenobarbital, *CBZ* carbamazepine, *VPA* valproate, *TB* tiagabine, *OXC* oxcarbazepine, *ZNS* zonisamide, *BDZ* benzodiazepines.

↓ decrease, ↑ increase, ~ variable.

[a] Free DPH level.

[b] Epoxide.

other (Table 15-14) and the intensivist using polypharmacy in the management of epileptic seizures should consider potential changes in the free or total levels of individual medications.

References

1. Holtkamp M (2007) The anaesthetic and intensive care of status epilepticus. Curr Opin Neurol 20:188–193
2. Walker MC (2003) Status epilepticus on the intensive care unit. J Neurol 250: 401–406
3. Walker MC, Smith SJ, Shorvon SD (1995) The intensive care treatment of convulsive status epilepticus in the UK. Results of a national survey and recommendations. Anaesthesia 50:130–135
4. Walker MC, Howard RS, Smith SJ, Miller DH, Shorvon SD, Hirsch NP (1996) Diagnosis and treatment of status epilepticus on a neurological intensive care unit. QJM 89:913–920
5. Alldredge BK, Gelb AM, Isaacs SM et al (2001) A comparison of lorazepam, diazepam, and placebo for the treatment of out-of-hospital status epilepticus. N Engl J Med 345:631–637
6. Gastaut H (1983) Classification of status epilepticus. Adv Neurol 34:15–35
7. Treatment of convulsive status epilepticus (1993) Recommendations of the Epilepsy Foundation of America's Working Group on Status Epilepticus. JAMA 270:854–859
8. Bleck TP (1991) Convulsive disorders: status epilepticus. Clin Neuropharmacol 14:191–198
9. Ramsay RE (1993) Treatment of status epilepticus. Epilepsia 34:S71–S81
10. Treiman DM, Meyers PD, Walton NY et al (1998) A comparison of four treatments for generalized convulsive status epilepticus. Veterans Affairs Status Epilepticus Cooperative Study Group. N Engl J Med 339:792–798
11. Lowenstein DH (1999) Status epilepticus: an overview of the clinical problem. Epilepsia 40(Suppl 1):S3–S8 discussion S21–S22
12. Husain AM, Mebust KA, Radtke RA (1999) Generalized periodic epileptiform discharges: etiologies, relationship to status epilepticus, and prognosis. J Clin Neurophysiol 16:51–58

13. Krumholz A (1999) Epidemiology and evidence for morbidity of nonconvulsive status epilepticus. J Clin Neurophysiol 16:314–322 discussion 353

14. Kaplan PW (1999) Assessing the outcomes in patients with nonconvulsive status epilepticus: nonconvulsive status epilepticus is underdiagnosed, potentially overtreated, and confounded by comorbidity. J Clin Neurophysiol. 16:341–352

15. Walker MC (2001) Diagnosis and treatment of nonconvulsive status epilepticus. CNS Drugs 15:931–939

16. Young GB, Gilbert JJ, Zochodne DW (1990) The significance of myoclonic status epilepticus in postanoxic coma. Neurology 40:1843–1848

17. Privitera M, Hoffman M, Moore JL, Jester D (1994) EEG detection of nontonic-clonic status epilepticus in patients with altered consciousness. Epilepsy Res 18:155–166

18. Hauser WA (1990) Status epilepticus: epidemiologic considerations. Neurology 40:9–13

19. Shorvon S (1994) The outcome of tonic-clonic status epilepticus. Curr Opin Neurol 7:93–95

20. DeLorenzo RJ, Hauser WA, Towne AR et al (1996) A prospective, population-based epidemiologic study of status epilepticus in Richmond, Virginia. Neurology 46:1029–1035

21. Bleck TP, Smith MC, Pierre-Louis SJ, Jares JJ, Murray J, Hansen CA (1993) Neurologic complications of critical medical illnesses. Crit Care Med 21:98–103

22. Lowenstein DH, Alldredge BK (1993) Status epilepticus at an urban public hospital in the 1980s. Neurology 43:483–488

23. Barry E, Hauser WA (1994) Status epilepticus and antiepileptic medication levels. Neurology 44:47–50

24. Dunne JW, Summers QA, Stewart-Wynne EG (1987) Non-convulsive status epilepticus: a prospective study in an adult general hospital. Q J Med 62:117–126

25. Celesia GG (1976) Modern concepts of status epilepticus. JAMA 235:1571–1574

26. DeLorenzo RJ, Waterhouse EJ, Towne AR et al (1998) Persistent nonconvulsive status epilepticus after the control of convulsive status epilepticus. Epilepsia 39:833–840

27. Privitera MD, Strawsburg RH (1994) Electroencephalographic monitoring in the emergency department. Emerg Med Clin North Am 12:1089–1100

28. Wijdicks EF, Sharbrough FW (1993) New-onset seizures in critically ill patients. Neurology 43:1042–1044

29. Towne AR, Waterhouse EJ, Boggs JG et al (2000) Prevalence of nonconvulsive status epilepticus in comatose patients. Neurology 54:340–345

30. Drislane FW, Lopez MR, Blum AS, Schomer DL (2008) Detection and treatment of refractory status epilepticus in the intensive care unit. J Clin Neurophysiol 25:181–186

31. Jordan KG (1999) Continuous EEG monitoring in the neuroscience intensive care unit and emergency department. J Clin Neurophysiol 16:14–39

32. Varelas PN, Hacein-Bey L, Hether T, Terranova B, Spanaki MV (2004) Emergent electroencephalogram in the intensive care unit: indications and diagnostic yield. Clin EEG Neurosci 35:173–180

33. Hesdorffer DC, Logroscino G, Cascino G, Annegers JF, Hauser WA (1998) Incidence of status epilepticus in Rochester, Minnesota, 1965–1984. Neurology 50:735–741

34. Jaitly R, Sgro JA, Towne AR, Ko D, DeLorenzo RJ (1997) Prognostic value of EEG monitoring after status epilepticus: a prospective adult study. J Clin Neurophysiol 14:326–334

35. Towne AR, Pellock JM, Ko D, DeLorenzo RJ (1994) Determinants of mortality in status epilepticus. Epilepsia 35:27–34

36. Jordan KG (1999) Nonconvulsive status epilepticus in acute brain injury. J Clin Neurophysiol 16:332–340 discussion 353

37. Shneker BF, Fountain NB (2003) Assessment of acute morbidity and mortality in nonconvulsive status epilepticus. Neurology 61:1066–1073

38. Kaplan PW (1999) Intravenous valproate treatment of generalized nonconvulsive status epilepticus. Clin Electroencephalogr 30:1–4

39. Lothman EW (1998) Biological consequences of repeated seizures. In: Engel J, Pedley TA (eds) Epilepsy: a comprehensive textbook, vol 1. Lippincott-Raven, Philadelphia-New York, pp 481–497

40. Loscher W (2007) Mechanisms of drug resistance in status epilepticus. Epilepsia 48(Suppl 8):74–77

41. Bankstahl JP, Loscher W (2008) Resistance to antiepileptic drugs and expression of P-glycoprotein in two rat models of status epilepticus. Epilepsy Res 82(1):70–85

42. Iannetti P, Spalice A, Parisi P (2005) Calcium-channel blocker verapamil administration in prolonged and refractory status epilepticus. Epilepsia 46:967–969

43. Meldrum BS, Brierley JB (1973) Prolonged epileptic seizures in primates. Ischemic cell change and its relation to ictal physiological events. Arch Neurol 28:10–17

44. Meldrum BS, Vigouroux RA, Brierley JB (1973) Systemic factors and epileptic brain damage. Prolonged seizures in paralyzed, artificially ventilated baboons. Arch Neurol 29:82–87

45. Aminoff MJ, Simon RP (1980) Status epilepticus. Causes, clinical features and consequences in 98 patients. Am J Med 69:657–666

46. Meldrum BS, Horton RW (1973) Physiology of status epilepticus in primates. Arch Neurol 28:1–9

47. Boggs JG, Painter JA, DeLorenzo RJ (1993) Analysis of electrocardiographic changes in status epilepticus. Epilepsy Res 14:87–94

48. Treiman DM (1995) Electroclinical features of status epilepticus. J Clin Neurophysiol 12:343–362

49. Parry T, Hirsch N (1992) Psychogenic seizures after general anaesthesia. Anaesthesia 47:534

50. Leppik IE (1993) Status epilepticus. In: Wyllie E (ed) The treatment of epilepsy: principles and practice. Lea and Febige, Philadelphia, pp 678–685

51. Varelas PN, Spanaki MV, Hacein-Bey L, Hether T, Terranova B (2003) Emergent EEG: indications and diagnostic yield. Neurology 61:702–704

52. Holtkamp M, Othman J, Buchheim K, Meierkord H (2006) Diagnosis of psychogenic nonepileptic status epilepticus in the emergency setting. Neurology 66:1727–1729

53. Walsh GO, Delgado-Escueta AV (1993) Status epilepticus. Neurol Clin 11:835–856

54. Treiman DM, Walton NY, Kendrick C (1990) A progressive sequence of electroencephalographic changes during generalized convulsive status epilepticus. Epilepsy Res 5:49–60

55. Thomas P (1997) Status epilepticus: indications for emergency EEG. Neurophysiol Clin 27:398–405

56. Kaplan PW (1996) Nonconvulsive status epilepticus in the emergency room. Epilepsia 37:643–650

57. Pakalnis A, Drake ME Jr, Phillips B (1991) Neuropsychiatric aspects of psychogenic status epilepticus. Neurology 41:1104–1106

58. Vespa P (2005) Continuous EEG monitoring for the detection of seizures in traumatic brain injury, infarction, and intracerebral hemorrhage: "to detect and protect". J Clin Neurophysiol 22:99–106

59. Niedermeyer E, Lopes Da Silva F (eds) (1999) Electroencephalography: basic principles, clinical applications and related fields. Lippincott-Williams, Baltimore

60. Jumao-as A, Brenner RP (1990) Myoclonic status epilepticus: a clinical and electroencephalographic study. Neurology 40:1199–1202

61. Granner MA, Lee SI (1994) Nonconvulsive status epilepticus: EEG analysis in a large series. Epilepsia 35:42–47

62. Kaplan PW (2007) EEG criteria for nonconvulsive status epilepticus. Epilepsia 48(Suppl 8):39–41

63. Fountain NB, Waldman WA (2001) Effects of benzodiazepines on triphasic waves: implications for nonconvulsive status epilepticus. J Clin Neurophysiol 18:345–352

64. Fagan KJ, Lee SI (1990) Prolonged confusion following convulsions due to generalized nonconvulsive status epilepticus. Neurology 40:1689–1694

65. Hirsch LJ, Claassen J, Mayer SA, Emerson RG (2004) Stimulus-induced rhythmic, periodic, or ictal discharges (SIRPIDs): a common EEG phenomenon in the critically ill. Epilepsia 45:109–123

66. Logroscino G, Hesdorffer DC, Cascino G, Annegers JF, Hauser WA (1997) Short-term mortality after a first episode of status epilepticus. Epilepsia 38:1344–1349

67. DeLorenzo RJ, Towne AR, Pellock JM, Ko D (1992) Status epilepticus in children, adults, and the elderly. Epilepsia 33(Suppl 4):S15–S25

68. DeLorenzo RJ, Garnett LK, Towne AR et al (1999) Comparison of status epilepticus with prolonged seizure episodes lasting from 10 to 29 minutes. Epilepsia 40:164–169

69. Mayer SA, Claassen J, Lokin J, Mendelsohn F, Dennis LJ, Fitzsimmons BF (2002) Refractory status epilepticus: frequency, risk factors, and impact on outcome. Arch Neurol 59:205–210

70. Krumholz A, Sung GY, Fisher RS, Barry E, Bergey GK, Grattan LM (1995) Complex partial status epilepticus accompanied by serious morbidity and mortality. Neurology 45:1499–1504

71. Guaranha MS, Garzon E, Buchpiguel CA, Tazima S, Yacubian EM, Sakamoto AC (2005) Hyperventilation revisited: physiological effects and efficacy on focal seizure activation in the era of video-EEG monitoring. Epilepsia 46:69–75

72. Pulsinelli WA, Levy DE, Sigsbee B, Scherer P, Plum F (1983) Increased damage after ischemic stroke in patients with hyperglycemia with or without established diabetes mellitus. Am J Med 74:540–544

73. Tomlinson FH, Anderson RE, Meyer FB (1993) Effect of arterial blood pressure and serum glucose on brain intracellular pH, cerebral and cortical blood flow during status epilepticus in the white New Zealand rabbit. Epilepsy Res 14:123–137

74. Simon RP (1985) Physiologic consequences of status epilepticus. Epilepsia 26(Suppl 1):S58–S66

75. Holtkamp M, Othman J, Buchheim K, Masuhr F, Schielke E, Meierkord H (2005) A "malignant" variant of status epilepticus. Arch Neurol 62:1428–1431

76. Shorvon S (2000) Emergency treatment of epilepsy. In: Shorvon S (ed) Handbook of epilepsy treatment. Blackwell Science, Malden, MA, pp 173–194

77. Leppik IE, Derivan AT, Homan RW, Walker J, Ramsay RE, Patrick B (1983) Double-blind study of lorazepam and diazepam in status epilepticus. JAMA 249:1452–1454

78. Shaner DM, McCurdy SA, Herring MO, Gabor AJ (1988) Treatment of status epilepticus: a prospective comparison of diazepam and phenytoin versus phenobarbital and optional phenytoin. Neurology 38:202–207

79. Lowenstein DH, Alldredge BK (1998) Status epilepticus. N Engl J Med 338:970–976

80. Lowenstein DH (2003) Treatment options for status epilepticus. Curr Opin Pharmacol 3:6–11

81. Bleck TP (2002) Refractory status epilepticus in 2001. Arch Neurol 59:188–189

82. Holtkamp M, Masuhr F, Harms L, Einhaupl KM, Meierkord H, Buchheim K (2003) The management of refractory generalised convulsive and complex partial status epilepticus in three European countries: a survey among epileptologists and critical care neurologists. J Neurol Neurosurg Psychiatry 74:1095–1099

83. Zbinden G, Randall LO (1967) Pharmacology of benzodiazepines: laboratory and clinical correlations. Adv Pharmacol 5:213–291

84. Meldrum BS, Chapman AG (1986) Benzodiazepine receptors and their relationship to the treatment of epilepsy. Epilepsia 27(Suppl 1):S3–S13

85. Amrein R, Hetzel W (1991) Pharmacology of drugs frequently used in ICUs: midazolam and flumazenil. Intensive Care Med 17(Suppl 1):S1–S10

86. Reves JG, Fragen RJ, Vinik HR, Greenblatt DJ (1985) Midazolam: pharmacology and uses. Anesthesiology 62:310–324

87. Bell DS (1969) Dangers of treatment of status epilepticus with diazepam. Br Med J 1:159–161

88. Shorvon S (2000) Antiepileptic drugs. In: Shorvon S (ed) Handbook of epilepsy treatment. Blackwell Science, Oxford, UK, pp 85–172

89. Cereghino JJ, Mitchell WG, Murphy J, Kriel RL, Rosenfeld WE, Trevathan E (1998) Treating repetitive seizures with a rectal diazepam formulation: a randomized study. The North American Diastat Study Group. Neurology 51:1274–1282

90. Dreifuss FE, Rosman NP, Cloyd JC et al (1998) A comparison of rectal diazepam gel and placebo for acute repetitive seizures. N Engl J Med 338:1869–1875

91. Appleton R, Sweeney A, Choonara I, Robson J, Molyneux E (1995) Lorazepam versus diazepam in the acute treatment of epileptic seizures and status epilepticus. Dev Med Child Neurol 37:682–688

92. Cock HR, Schapira AH (2002) A comparison of lorazepam and diazepam as initial therapy in convulsive status epilepticus. QJM 95:225–231

93. Dirksen MS, Vree TB, Driessen JJ (1987) Clinical pharmacokinetics of long-term infusion of midazolam in critically ill patients–preliminary results. Anaesth Intensive Care 15:440–444

94. Towne AR, DeLorenzo RJ (1999) Use of intramuscular midazolam for status epilepticus. J Emerg Med 17:323–328

95. Wroblewski BA, Joseph AB (1992) The use of intramuscular midazolam for acute seizure cessation or behavioral emergencies in patients with traumatic brain injury. Clin Neuropharmacol 15:44–49

96. Galdames D, Aguilera M, Fabres L (1997) Midazolam in the treatment of status epilepticus and frequent seizures in adults. Epilepsia 38:12

97. Chamberlain JM, Altieri MA, Futterman C, Young GM, Ochsenschlager DW, Waisman Y (1997) A prospective, randomized study comparing intramuscular midazolam with intravenous diazepam for the treatment of seizures in children. Pediatr Emerg Care 13:92–94

98. Mayhue FE (1988) IM midazolam for status epilepticus in the emergency department. Ann Emerg Med 17:643–645

99. McDonagh TJ, Jelinek GA, Galvin GM (1992) Intramuscular midazolam rapidly terminates seizures in children and adults. Emerg Med 4:77–81

100. Ulvi H, Yoldas T, Mungen B, Yigiter R (2002) Continuous infusion of midazolam in the treatment of refractory generalized convulsive status epilepticus. Neurol Sci 23:177–182

101. Varelas PN (2008) How I treat status epilepticus in the Neuro-ICU. Neurocrit Care 9:153–157

102. Treiman DM (1989) Pharmacokinetics and clinical use of benzodiazepines in the management of status epilepticus. Epilepsia 30(Suppl 2):S4–S10

103. Jamerson BD, Dukes GE, Brouwer KL, Donn KH, Messenheimer JA, Powell JR (1994) Venous irritation related to intravenous administration of phenytoin versus fosphenytoin. Pharmacotherapy 14:47–52

104. Jones GL, Wimbish GH, McIntosh WE (1983) Phenytoin: basic and clinical pharmacology. Med Res Rev 3:383–434

105. Chapman MG, Smith M, Hirsch NP (2001) Status epilepticus. Anaesthesia 56: 648–659

106. Browne TR, Kugler AR, Eldon MA (1996) Pharmacology and pharmacokinetics of fosphenytoin. Neurology 46:S3–S7

107. Boucher BA (1996) Fosphenytoin: a novel phenytoin prodrug. Pharmacotherapy 16:777–791

108. Payne TA, Bleck TP (1997) Status epilepticus. Crit Care Clin 13:17–38
109. DeToledo JC, Lowe MR, Rabinstein A, Villaviza N (2001) Cardiac arrest after fast intravenous infusion of phenytoin mistaken for fosphenytoin. Epilepsia 42:288
110. Fischer JH, Patel TV, Fischer PA (2003) Fosphenytoin: clinical pharmacokinetics and comparative advantages in the acute treatment of seizures. Clin Pharmacokinet 42:33–58
111. Marchetti A, Magar R, Fischer J, Sloan E, Fischer P (1996) A pharmacoeconomic evaluation of intravenous fosphenytoin (Cerebyx) versus intravenous phenytoin (Dilantin) in hospital emergency departments. Clin Ther 18:953–966
112. Coplin WM, Rhoney DH, Rebuck JA, Clements EA, Cochran MS, O'Neil BJ (2002) Randomized evaluation of adverse events and length-of-stay with routine emergency department use of phenytoin or fosphenytoin. Neurol Res 24:842–848
113. Villarreal HJ, Wilder BJ, Willmore LJ, Bauman AW, Hammond EJ, Bruni J (1978) Effect of valproic acid on spike and wave discharges in patients with absence seizures. Neurology 28:886–891
114. Wilder BJ, Ramsay RE, Murphy JV, Karas BJ, Marquardt K, Hammond EJ (1983) Comparison of valproic acid and phenytoin in newly diagnosed tonic-clonic seizures. Neurology 33:1474–1476
115. Beydoun A, Sackellares JC, Shu V (1997) Safety and efficacy of divalproex sodium monotherapy in partial epilepsy: a double-blind, concentration-response design clinical trial. Depakote Monotherapy for Partial Seizures Study Group. Neurology 48:182–188
116. Penry JK, Dean JC (1988) Valproate monotherapy in partial seizures. Am J Med 84:14–16
117. Bourgeois BFD (1995) Valproic: clinical use. In: Levy RH, Mattson RH, Meldrum BS (eds) Antiepileptic drugs. Raven Press, New York
118. Willmore LJ, Wilder BJ, Bruni J, Villarreal HJ (1978) Effect of valproic acid on hepatic function. Neurology 28:961–964
119. Dreifuss FE, Santilli N, Langer DH, Sweeney KP, Moline KA, Menander KB (1987) Valproic acid hepatic fatalities: a retrospective review. Neurology 37:379–385
120. Gerstner T, Teich M, Bell N et al (2006) Valproate-associated coagulopathies are frequent and variable in children. Epilepsia 47:1136–1143
121. Hodges BM, Mazur JE (2001) Intravenous valproate in status epilepticus. Ann Pharmacother 35:1465–1470
122. Zaccara G, Messori A, Moroni F (1988) Clinical pharmacokinetics of valproic acid–1988. Clin Pharmacokinet 15:367–389
123. Ramsay RE, Uthman B, Leppik IE et al (1997) The tolerability and safety of valproate sodium injection given as an intravenous infusion. J Epilepsy 10:187–193
124. Devinsky O, Leppik I, Willmore LJ et al (1995) Safety of intravenous valproate. Ann Neurol 38:670–674
125. Venkataraman V, Wheless JW (1999) Safety of rapid intravenous infusion of valproate loading doses in epilepsy patients. Epilepsy Res 35:147–153
126. Uberall MA, Trollmann R, Wunsiedler U, Wenzel D (2000) Intravenous valproate in pediatric epilepsy patients with refractory status epilepticus. Neurology 54:2188–2189
127. Sinha S, Naritoku DK (2000) Intravenous valproate is well tolerated in unstable patients with status epilepticus. Neurology 55:722–724
128. Chez MG, Hammer MS, Loeffel M, Nowinski C, Bagan BT (1999) Clinical experience of three pediatric and one adult case of spike-and-wave status epilepticus treated with injectable valproic acid. J Child Neurol 14:239–242
129. Alehan FK, Morton LD, Pellock JM (1999) Treatment of absence status with intravenous valproate. Neurology 52:889–890
130. Giroud M, Gras D, Escousse A (1993) Use of injectable valproic in status epilepticus. Drug Invest 5:154–159

131. Yu KT, Mills S, Thompson N, Cunanan C (2003) Safety and efficacy of intra-venous valproate in pediatric status epilepticus and acute repetitive seizures. Epilepsia 44:724–726

132. Martin ED, Pozo MA (2003) Valproate suppresses status epilepticus induced by 4-aminopyridine in CA1 hippocampus region. Epilepsia 44:1375–1379

133. Price DJ (1989) Intravenous valproate: experience in neurosurgery. Royal Society of Medicine Service, International Congress and Symposium Series, vol. 152. Royal Society of Medicine Services Limited, London

134. Peters CN, Pohlmann-Eden B (1999) Efficacy and safety of intravenous valproate in status epilepticus. Epilepsia 40:149–150

135. Sheth RD, Gidal BE (2000) Intravenous valproic acid for myoclonic status epilepticus. Neurology 54:1201

136. Naritoku DK, Sinha S (2001) Outcome of status epilepticus treated with intravenous valproate. Neurology 56:A235

137. Limdi NA, Shimpi AV, Faught E, Gomez CR, Burneo JG (2005) Efficacy of rapid IV administration of valproic acid for status epilepticus. Neurology 64:353–355

138. Misra UK, Kalita J, Patel R (2006) Sodium valproate vs phenytoin in status epilepticus: a pilot study. Neurology 67:340–342

139. Agarwal P, Kumar N, Chandra R, Gupta G, Antony AR, Garg N (2007) Randomized study of intravenous valproate and phenytoin in status epilepticus. Seizure 16:527–532

140. Gilad R, Izkovitz N, Dabby R et al (2008) Treatment of status epilepticus and acute repetitive seizures with i.v. valproic acid vs phenytoin. Acta Neurol Scand 118(5):296–300

141. Olsen KB, Tauboll E, Gjerstad L (2007) Valproate is an effective, well-tolerated drug for treatment of status epilepticus/serial attacks in adults. Acta Neurol Scand Suppl 187:51–54

142. Meierkord H, Boon P, Engelsen B et al (2006) EFNS guideline on the management of status epilepticus. Eur J Neurol 13:445–450

143. Kalviainen R (2007) Status epilepticus treatment guidelines. Epilepsia 48(Suppl 8): 99–102

144. Serrano-Castro PJ, Casado-Chocan JL, Mercade-Cerda JM et al (2005) The Andalusia Epilepsy Society's Guide to Epilepsy Therapy 2005: III. Antiepileptic therapy in special situations. Rev Neurol 40:683–695

145. van Rijckevorsel K, Boon P, Hauman H et al (2006) Standards of care for non-convulsive status epilepticus: Belgian consensus recommendations. Acta Neurol Belg 106:117–124

146. van Rijckevorsel K, Boon P, Hauman H et al (2005) Standards of care for adults with convulsive status epilepticus: Belgian consensus recommendations. Acta Neurol Belg 105:111–118

147. Minicucci F, Muscas G, Perucca E, Capovilla G, Vigevano F, Tinuper P (2006) Treatment of status epilepticus in adults: guidelines of the Italian League against Epilepsy. Epilepsia 47(Suppl 5):9–15

148. Parviainen I, Uusaro A, Kalviainen R, Kaukanen E, Mervaala E, Ruokonen E (2002) High-dose thiopental in the treatment of refractory status epilepticus in intensive care unit. Neurology 59:1249–1251

149. Devlin EG, Clarke RS, Mirakhur RK, McNeill TA (1994) Effect of four i.v. induction agents on T-lymphocyte proliferations to PHA in vitro. Br J Anaesth 73:315–317

150. Magnuson B, Hatton J, Williams S, Loan T (1999) Tolerance and efficacy of enteral nutrition for neurosurgical patients on pentobarbital coma. Nutr Clin Practice 14:131–134

151. Olson KR, Pond SM, Verrier ED, Federle M (1984) Intestinal infarction complicating phenobarbital overdose. Arch Intern Med 144:407–408

152. Rashkin MC, Youngs C, Penovich P (1987) Pentobarbital treatment of refractory status epilepticus. Neurology 37:500–503

153. Krishnamurthy KB, Drislane FW (1999) Depth of EEG suppression and outcome in barbiturate anesthetic treatment for refractory status epilepticus. Epilepsia 40:759–762

154. Claassen J, Hirsch LJ, Emerson RG, Mayer SA (2002) Treatment of refractory status epilepticus with pentobarbital, propofol, or midazolam: a systematic review. Epilepsia 43:146–153

155. Rossetti AO, Logroscino G, Bromfield EB (2005) Refractory status epilepticus: effect of treatment aggressiveness on prognosis. Arch Neurol 62:1698–1702

156. Bergey GK (2006) Refractory status epilepticus: Is EEG burst suppression an appropriate treatment target during drug-induced coma? What is the Holy Grail? Epilepsy Curr 6:119–120

157. Rossetti AO (2007) Which anesthetic should be used in the treatment of refractory status epilepticus? Epilepsia 48(Suppl 8):52–55

158. Treiman DM (1999) Convulsive status epilepticus. Curr Treat Options Neurol 1:359–369

159. Krishnamurthy KB, Drislane FW (1996) Relapse and survival after barbiturate anesthetic treatment of refractory status epilepticus. Epilepsia 37:863–867

160. Mirski MA, Williams MA, Hanley DF (1995) Prolonged pentobarbital and phenobarbital coma for refractory generalized status epilepticus. Crit Care Med 23:400–404

161. Miller MA, Forni A, Yogaratnam D (2008) Propylene glycol-induced lactic acidosis in a patient receiving continuous infusion pentobarbital. Ann Pharmacother 42:1502–1506

162. Stecker MM, Kramer TH, Raps EC, O'Meeghan R, Dulaney E, Skaar DJ (1998) Treatment of refractory status epilepticus with propofol: clinical and pharmacokinetic findings. Epilepsia 39:18–26

163. Walder B, Tramer MR, Seeck M (2002) Seizure-like phenomena and propofol: a systematic review. Neurology 58:1327–1332

164. Hodkinson BP, Frith RW, Mee EW (1987) Propofol and the electroencephalogram. Lancet 2:1518

165. Hufnagel A, Elger CE, Nadstawek J, Stoeckel H, Bocker DK (1990) Specific response of the epileptic focus to anesthesia with propofol. J Epilepsy 3:37–45

166. Hanna JP, Ramundo ML (1998) Rhabdomyolysis and hypoxia associated with prolonged propofol infusion in children. Neurology 50:301–303

167. Strickland RA, Murray MJ (1995) Fatal metabolic acidosis in a pediatric patient receiving an infusion of propofol in the intensive care unit: is there a relationship? Crit Care Med 23:405–409

168. Perrier ND, Baerga-Varela Y, Murray MJ (2000) Death related to propofol use in an adult patient. Crit Care Med 28:3071–3074

169. Cremer OL, Moons KG, Bouman EA, Kruijswijk JE, de Smet AM, Kalkman CJ (2001) Long-term propofol infusion and cardiac failure in adult head-injured patients. Lancet 357:117–118

170. Smith H, Sinson G, Varelas P (2009) Vasopressors and propofol infusion syndrome in severe head trauma. Neurocrit Care 10(2):166–172

171. Prasad A, Worrall BB, Bertram EH, Bleck TP (2001) Propofol and midazolam in the treatment of refractory status epilepticus. Epilepsia 42:380–386

172. Parviainen I, Uusaro A, Kalviainen R, Mervaala E, Ruokonen E (2006) Propofol in the treatment of refractory status epilepticus. Intensive Care Med 32:1075–1079

173. Walton NY, Treiman DM (1991) Motor and electroencephalographic response of refractory experimental status epilepticus in rats to treatment with MK-801, diazepam, or MK-801 plus diazepam. Brain Res 553:97–104

174. Rice AC, DeLorenzo RJ (1999) N-methyl-D-aspartate receptor activation regulates refractoriness of status epilepticus to diazepam. Neuroscience 93:117–123

175. Borris DJ, Bertram EH, Kapur J (2000) Ketamine controls prolonged status epilepticus. Epilepsy Res 42:117–122

176. Sheth RD, Gidal BE (1998) Refractory status epilepticus: response to ketamine. Neurology 51:1765–1766

177. Pruss H, Holtkamp M (2008) Ketamine successfully terminates malignant status epilepticus. Epilepsy Res 82(2–3):219–222

178. Ubogu EE, Sagar SM, Lerner AJ, Maddux BN, Suarez JI, Werz MA (2003) Ketamine for refractory status epilepticus: a case of possible ketamine-induced neurotoxicity. Epilepsy Behav 4:70–75

179. Kofke WA, Bloom MJ, Van Cott A, Brenner RP (1997) Electrographic tachyphylaxis to etomidate and ketamine used for refractory status epilepticus controlled with isoflurane. J Neurosurg Anesthesiol 9:269–272

180. Kofke WA, Young RS, Davis P et al (1989) Isoflurane for refractory status epilepticus: a clinical series. Anesthesiology 71:653–659

181. Mirsattari SM, Sharpe MD, Young GB (2004) Treatment of refractory status epilepticus with inhalational anesthetic agents isoflurane and desflurane. Arch Neurol 61:1254–1259

182. Aggarwal P, Wali JP (1993) Lidocaine in refractory status epilepticus: a forgotten drug in the emergency department. Am J Emerg Med 11:243–244

183. Shorvon S (2001) The management of status epilepticus. J Neurol Neurosurg Psychiatry 70:II22–II27

184. Duncan JS (2002) The promise of new antiepileptic drugs. Br J Clin Pharmacol 53:123–131

185. Perucca E (1999) The clinical pharmacokinetics of the new antiepileptic drugs. Epilepsia 40(Suppl 9):S7–S13

186. Cramer JA, Fisher R, Ben-Menachem E, French J, Mattson RH (1999) New antiepileptic drugs: comparison of key clinical trials. Epilepsia 40:590–600

187. White HS (1999) Comparative anticonvulsant and mechanistic profile of the established and newer antiepileptic drugs. Epilepsia 40(Suppl 5):S2–S10

188. Mazarati AM, Baldwin RA, Sofia RD, Wasterain CG (2000) Felbamate in experimental model of status epilepticus. Epilepsia 41:123–127

189. Chronopoulos A, Stafstrom C, Thurber S, Hyde P, Mikati M, Holmes GL (1993) Neuroprotective effect of felbamate after kainic acid-induced status epilepticus. Epilepsia 34:359–366

190. Barrueto F Jr, Green J, Howland MA, Hoffman RS, Nelson LS (2002) Gabapentin withdrawal presenting as status epilepticus. J Toxicol Clin Toxicol 40:925–928

191. Striano P, Coppola A, Madia F et al (2007) Life-threatening status epilepticus following gabapentin administration in a patient with benign adult familial myoclonic epilepsy. Epilepsia 48:1995–1998

192. Pandey CK, Singh N, Bose N, Sahay S (2003) Gabapentin and propofol for treatment of status epilepticus in acute intermittent porphyria. J Postgrad Med 49:285

193. Bhatia R, Vibha D, Srivastava MV, Prasad K, Tripathi M, Bhushan Singh M (2008) Use of propofol anesthesia and adjunctive treatment with levetiracetam and gabapentin in managing status epilepticus in a patient of acute intermittent porphyria. Epilepsia 49:934–936

194. Halonen T, Nissinen J, Pitkanen A (2001) Effect of lamotrigine treatment on status epilepticus-induced neuronal damage and memory impairment in rat. Epilepsy Res 46:205–223

195. Walton NY, Jaing Q, Hyun B, Treiman DM (1996) Lamotrigine vs. phenytoin for treatment of status epilepticus: comparison in an experimental model. Epilepsy Res 24:19–28

196. Pisani F, Gallitto G, Di Perri R (1991) Could lamotrigine be useful in status epilepticus? A case report. J Neurol Neurosurg Psychiatry 54:845–846

197. Trinka E, Dilitz E, Unterberger I et al (2002) Non convulsive status epilepticus after replacement of valproate with lamotrigine. J Neurol 249:1417–1422

198. Guerrini R, Belmonte A, Parmeggiani L, Perucca E (1999) Myoclonic status epilepticus following high-dosage lamotrigine therapy. Brain Dev 21:420–424

199. Braga AJ, Chidley K (2007) Self-poisoning with lamotrigine and pregabalin. Anaesthesia 62:524–527

200. Dinnerstein E, Jobst BC, Williamson PD (2007) Lamotrigine intoxication provoking status epilepticus in an adult with localization-related epilepsy. Arch Neurol 64:1344–1346

201. Lynch BA, Lambeng N, Nocka K et al (2004) The synaptic vesicle protein SV2A is the binding site for the antiepileptic drug levetiracetam. Proc Natl Acad Sci U S A 101:9861–9866

202. Niespodziany I, Klitgaard H, Margineanu DG (2001) Levetiracetam inhibits the high-voltage-activated Ca(2+) current in pyramidal neurones of rat hippocampal slices. Neurosci Lett 306:5–8

203. Rigo JM, Hans G, Nguyen L et al (2002) The anti-epileptic drug levetiracetam reverses the inhibition by negative allosteric modulators of neuronal GABA- and glycine-gated currents. Br J Pharmacol 136:659–672

204. Szaflarski JP, Meckler JM, Szaflarski M, Shutter LA, Privitera MD, Yates SL (2007) Levetiracetam use in critically ill patients. Neurocrit Care 7:140–147

205. Rossetti AO, Bromfield EB (2006) Determinants of success in the use of oral levetiracetam in status epilepticus. Epilepsy Behav 8:651–654

206. Rupprecht S, Franke K, Fitzek S, Witte OW, Hagemann G (2007) Levetiracetam as a treatment option in non-convulsive status epilepticus. Epilepsy Res 73:238–244

207. Patel NC, Landan IR, Levin J, Szaflarski J, Wilner AN (2006) The use of levetiracetam in refractory status epilepticus. Seizure 15:137–141

208. Ramael S, Daoust A, Otoul C et al (2006) Levetiracetam intravenous infusion: a randomized, placebo-controlled safety and pharmacokinetic study. Epilepsia 47:1128–1135

209. Ruegg S, Naegelin Y, Hardmeier M, Winkler DT, Marsch S, Fuhr P (2008) Intravenous levetiracetam: treatment experience with the first 50 critically ill patients. Epilepsy Behav 12:477–480

210. Knake S, Gruener J, Hattemer K et al (2008) Intravenous levetiracetam in the treatment of benzodiazepine refractory status epilepticus. J Neurol Neurosurg Psychiatry 79:588–589

211. Takano K, Tanaka T, Fujita T, Nakai H, Yonemasu Y (1995) Zonisamide: electrophysiological and metabolic changes in kainic acid-induced limbic seizures in rats. Epilepsia 36:644–648

212. Frisch C, Kudin AP, Elger CE, Kunz WS, Helmstaedter C (2007) Amelioration of water maze performance deficits by topiramate applied during pilocarpine-induced status epilepticus is negatively dose-dependent. Epilepsy Res 73:173–180

213. Niebauer M, Gruenthal M (1999) Topiramate reduces neuronal injury after experimental status epilepticus. Brain Res 837:263–269

214. Towne AR, Garnett LK, Waterhouse EJ, Morton LD, DeLorenzo RJ (2003) The use of topiramate in refractory status epilepticus. Neurology 60:332–334

215. Bensalem MK, Fakhoury TA (2003) Topiramate and status epilepticus: report of three cases. Epilepsy Behav 4:757–760

216. Reuber M, Evans J, Bamford JM (2002) Topiramate in drug-resistant complex partial status epilepticus. Eur J Neurol 9:111–112

217. Perry MS, Holt PJ, Sladky JT (2006) Topiramate loading for refractory status epilepticus in children. Epilepsia 47:1070–1071

218. Mangano S, Cusumano L, Fontana A (2003) Non-convulsive status epilepticus associated with tiagabine in a pediatric patient. Brain Dev 25:518–521

219. Kellinghaus C, Dziewas R, Ludemann P (2002) Tiagabine-related non-convulsive status epilepticus in partial epilepsy: three case reports and a review of the literature. Seizure 11:243–249

220. Skardoutsou A, Voudris KA, Vagiakou EA (2003) Non-convulsive status epilepticus associated with tiagabine therapy in children. Seizure 12:599–601

221. Ostrovskiy D, Spanaki MV, Morris GL 3rd (2002) Tiagabine overdose can induce convulsive status epilepticus. Epilepsia 43:773–774

222. Shinnar S, Berg AT, Treiman DM et al (2001) Status epilepticus and tiagabine therapy: review of safety data and epidemiologic comparisons. Epilepsia 42: 372–379

223. Loscher W, Honack D (1997) Intravenous carbamazepine: comparison of different parenteral formulations in a mouse model of convulsive status epilepticus. Epilepsia 38:106–113

224. Graves NM, Kriel RL, Jones-Saete C, Cloyd JC (1985) Relative bioavailability of rectally administered carbamazepine suspension in humans. Epilepsia 26: 429–433

225. So EL, Ruggles KH, Cascino GD, Ahmann PA, Weatherford KW (1994) Seizure exacerbation and status epilepticus related to carbamazepine-10, 11-epoxide. Ann Neurol 35:743–746

226. Callahan DJ, Noetzel MJ (1992) Prolonged absence status epilepticus associated with carbamazepine therapy, increased intracranial pressure, and transient MRI abnormalities. Neurology 42:2198–2201

227. Osorio I, Reed RC, Peltzer JN (2000) Refractory idiopathic absence status epilepticus: a probable paradoxical effect of phenytoin and carbamazepine. Epilepsia 41:887–894

228. Marini C, Parmeggiani L, Masi G, D'Arcangelo G, Guerrini R (2005) Nonconvulsive status epilepticus precipitated by carbamazepine presenting as dissociative and affective disorders in adolescents. J Child Neurol 20:693–696

229. Ono A, Yano T, Sawaishi Y, Komatsu K, Takada G (2001) A case of carbamazepine intoxication with alpha coma and status epilepticus. No To Hattatsu 33:528–532

230. Spiller HA, Carlisle RD (2002) Status epilepticus after massive carbamazepine overdose. J Toxicol Clin Toxicol 40:81–90

231. Sillanpaa M, Pihlaja T (1988) Oxcarbazepine (GP 47 680) in the treatment of intractable seizures. Acta Paediatr Hung 29:359–364

232. Knake S, Klein KM, Hattemer K et al (2007) Pregabalin-induced generalized myoclonic status epilepticus in patients with chronic pain. Epilepsy Behav 11:471–473

233. Doty P, Rudd GD, Stoehr T, Thomas D (2007) Lacosamide. Neurotherapeutics 4:145–148

234. Biton V, Rosenfeld WE, Whitesides J, Fountain NB, Vaiciene N, Rudd GD (2008) Intravenous lacosamide as replacement for oral lacosamide in patients with partial-onset seizures. Epilepsia 49:418–424

235. Kellinghaus C, Berning S, Besselmann M (2009) Intravenous lacosamide as successful treatment for nonconvulsive status epilepticus after failure of first-line therapy. Epilepsy Behav 14(2):429–431

236. Vastola EF, Homan R, Rosen A (1969) Inhibition of focal seizures by moderate hypothermia. A clinical and experimental study. Arch Neurol 20:430–439

237. Lundgren J, Smith ML, Blennow G, Siesjo BK (1994) Hyperthermia aggravates and hypothermia ameliorates epileptic brain damage. Exp Brain Res 99:43–55

238. Liu Z, Gatt A, Mikati M, Holmes GL (1993) Effect of temperature on kainic acid-induced seizures. Brain Res 631:51–58

239. Maeda T, Hashizume K, Tanaka T (1999) Effect of hypothermia on kainic acid-induced limbic seizures: an electroencephalographic and 14C-deoxyglucose autoradiographic study. Brain Res 818:228–235

240. Kim JH, Kim SH, Yoo SK, Kim JY, Nam YT (1998) The effects of mild hypothermia on thiopental-induced electroencephalogram burst suppression. J Neurosurg Anesthesiol 10:137–141

241. Orlowski JP, Erenberg G, Lueders H, Cruse RP (1984) Hypothermia and barbiturate coma for refractory status epilepticus. Crit Care Med 12:367–372

242. Corry JJ, Dhar R, Murphy T, Diringer MN (2008) Hypothermia for refractory status epilepticus. Neurocrit Care 9:189–197

243. Ma X, Liporace J, O'Connor MJ, Sperling MR (2001) Neurosurgical treatment of medically intractable status epilepticus. Epilepsy Res 46:33–38

244. Ng YT, Kim HL, Wheless JW (2003) Successful neurosurgical treatment of childhood complex partial status epilepticus with focal resection. Epilepsia 44:468–471

245. Duane DC, Ng YT, Rekate HL, Chung S, Bodensteiner JB, Kerrigan JF (2004) Treatment of refractory status epilepticus with hemispherectomy. Epilepsia 45:1001–1004

246. Ng YT, Kerrigan JF, Rekate HL (2006) Neurosurgical treatment of status epilepticus. J Neurosurg 105:378–381

247. Schrader LM, Stern JM, Wilson CL et al (2006) Low frequency electrical stimulation through subdural electrodes in a case of refractory status epilepticus. Clin Neurophysiol 117:781–788

248. Patwardhan RV, Dellabadia J Jr, Rashidi M, Grier L, Nanda A (2005) Control of refractory status epilepticus precipitated by anticonvulsant withdrawal using left vagal nerve stimulation: a case report. Surg Neurol 64:170–173

249. Carrasco Gonzalez MD, Palomar M, Rovira R (1997) Electroconvulsive therapy for status epilepticus. Ann Intern Med 127:247–248

250. Fountain NB (2000) Status epilepticus: risk factors and complications. Epilepsia 41(Suppl 2):S23–S30

251. Sasahira M, Lowry T, Simon RP (1997) Neuronal injury in experimental status epilepticus in the rat: role of acidosis. Neurosci Lett 224:177–180

252. Evans MC, Meldrum BS (1984) Regional brain glucose metabolism in chemically-induced seizures in the rat. Brain Res 297:235–245

253. Swan JH, Meldrum BS, Simon RP (1986) Hyperglycemia does not augment neuronal damage in experimental status epilepticus. Neurology 36:1351–1354

254. Kreisman NR, Gauthier-Lewis ML, Conklin SG, Voss NF, Barbee RW (1993) Cardiac output and regional hemodynamics during recurrent seizures in rats. Brain Res 626:295–302

255. Darnell JC, Jay SJ (1982) Recurrent postictal pulmonary edema: a case report and review of the literature. Epilepsia 23:71–83

256. Terrence CF, Rao GR, Perper JA (1981) Neurogenic pulmonary edema in unexpected, unexplained death of epileptic patients. Ann Neurol 9:458–464

257. Cockerell OC, Rothwell J, Thompson PD, Marsden CD, Shorvon SD (1996) Clinical and physiological features of epilepsia partialis continua. Cases ascertained in the UK. Brain 119(Pt 2):393–407

258. Thomas P, Borg M, Suisse G, Chatel M (1995) Opercular myoclonic-anarthric status epilepticus. Epilepsia 36:281–289

259. Manford M, Shorvon SD (1992) Prolonged sensory or visceral symptoms: an under-diagnosed form of non-convulsive focal (simple partial) status epilepticus. J Neurol Neurosurg Psychiatry 55:714–716

260. Wells CR, Labar DR, Solomon GE (1992) Aphasia as the sole manifestation of simple partial status epilepticus. Epilepsia 33:84–87

261. Walker MC, Smith SJ, Sisodiya SM, Shorvon SD (1995) Case of simple partial status epilepticus in occipital lobe epilepsy misdiagnosed as migraine: clinical, electrophysiological, and magnetic resonance imaging characteristics. Epilepsia 36:1233–1236

262. Huang CW, Hsieh YJ, Pai MC, Tsai JJ, Huang CC (2005) Nonketotic hyperglycemia-related epilepsia partialis continua with ictal unilateral parietal hyperperfusion. Epilepsia 46:1843–1844

263. Mut M, Schiff D, Dalmau J (2005) Paraneoplastic recurrent multifocal encephalitis presenting with epilepsia partialis continua. J Neurooncol 72:63–66
264. Wroe SJ, Ellershaw JE, Whittaker JA, Richens A (1987) Focal motor status epilepticus following treatment with azlocillin and cefotaxime. Med Toxicol 2:233–234
265. Schomer DL (1993) Focal status epilepticus and epilepsia partialis continua in adults and children. Epilepsia 34(Suppl 1):S29–S36
266. Drislane FW, Blum AS, Schomer DL (1999) Focal status epilepticus: clinical features and significance of different EEG patterns. Epilepsia 40:1254–1260
267. Aktekin B, Dogan EA, Oguz Y, Karaali K (2006) Epilepsia partialis continua in a patient with Behcet's disease. Clin Neurol Neurosurg 108:392–395
268. Aydin-Ozemir Z, Tuzun E, Baykan B et al (2006) Autoimmune thyroid encephalopathy presenting with epilepsia partialis continua. Clin EEG Neurosci 37:204–209
269. Kato Y, Nakazato Y, Tamura N, Tomioka R, Takahashi Y, Shimazu K (2007) Autoimmune encephalitis with anti-glutamate receptor antibody presenting as epilepsia partialis continua and action myoclonus: a case report. Rinsho Shinkeigaku 47:429–433
270. Scholtes FB, Renier WO, Meinardi H (1996) Simple partial status epilepticus: causes, treatment, and outcome in 47 patients. J Neurol Neurosurg Psychiatry 61:90–92
271. Brandt L, Saveland H, Ljunggren B, Andersson KE (1988) Control of epilepsy partialis continuans with intravenous nimodipine. Report of two cases. J Neurosurg 69:949–950
272. Rotenberg A, Bae EH, Takeoka M, Tormos JM, Schachter SC, Pascual-Leone A (2009) Repetitive transcranial magnetic stimulation in the treatment of epilepsia partialis continua. Epilepsy Behav 14:253–257
273. Meierkord H, Holtkamp M (2007) Non-convulsive status epilepticus in adults: clinical forms and treatment. Lancet Neurol 6:329–339
274. Treiman DM, Walker MC (2006) Treatment of seizure emergencies: convulsive and non-convulsive status epilepticus. Epilepsy Res 68(Suppl 1):S77–S82
275. Litt B, Wityk RJ, Hertz SH et al (1998) Nonconvulsive status epilepticus in the critically ill elderly. Epilepsia 39:1194–1202
276. Crouteau D, Shevell M, Rosenblatt B, Dilenge ME, Andermann F (1998) Treatment of absence status in the Lennox-Gastaut syndrome with propofol. Neurology 51:315–316
277. Lothman EW, Bertram EH, Bekenstein JW, Perlin JB (1989) Self-sustaining limbic status epilepticus induced by 'continuous' hippocampal stimulation: electrographic and behavioral characteristics. Epilepsy Res 3:107–119
278. Scholtes FB, Renier WO, Meinardi H (1996) Non-convulsive status epilepticus: causes, treatment, and outcome in 65 patients. J Neurol Neurosurg Psychiatry 61:93–95
279. Farooq MU, Naravetla B, Majid A, Gupta R, Pysh JJ, Kassab MY (2007) IV levetiracetam in the management of non-convulsive status epilepticus. Neurocrit Care 7:36–39
280. Brain Resuscitation Clinical Trial I Study Group (1986) Randomized clinical study of thiopental loading in comatose survivors of cardiac arrest. N Engl J Med 314:397–403
281. Celesia GG, Grigg MM, Ross E (1988) Generalized status myoclonicus in acute anoxic and toxic-metabolic encephalopathies. Arch Neurol 45:781–784
282. Krumholz A, Stern BJ, Weiss HD (1988) Outcome from coma after cardiopulmonary resuscitation: relation to seizures and myoclonus. Neurology 38:401–405
283. Fisher RS, Kaplan PW, Krumholz A, Lesser RP, Rosen SA, Wolff MR (1988) Failure of high-dose intravenous magnesium sulfate to control myoclonic status epilepticus. Clin Neuropharmacol 11:537–544

284. Williams A, Sekaninova S, Coakley J (1998) Suppression of elevated alanine aminotransferase activity in liver disease by vigabatrin. J Paediatr Child Health 34:395–397

285. Zaret BS, Beckner RR, Marini AM, Wagle W, Passarelli C (1982) Sodium valproate-induced hyperammonemia without clinical hepatic dysfunction. Neurology 32:206–208

286. Moreiras Plaza M, Rodriguez Goyanes G, Cuina L, Alonso R (1999) On the toxicity of valproic-acid. Clin Nephrol 51:187–189

287. Hogg RJ, Sawyer M, Hecox K, Eigenbrodt E (1981) Carbamazepine-induced acute tubulointerstitial nephritis. J Pediatr 98:830–832

288. Varelas PN, Mirski MA (2001) Seizures in the adult intensive care unit. J Neurosurg Anesthesiol 13:163–175

289. Roberts C, French JA (2002) Anticonvulsants in acute medical illness. In: Delanty N (ed) Seizures. Medical causes and management. Humana Press, Inc, Totowa, NJ, pp 333–356

290. Shorvon S (1993) The drug treatment of epilepsy. In: Hopkins A, Shorvon S, Cascino G (eds) Epilepsy. Chapman and Hall, London, p 178

291. Leppik IE, Wolff DL (1993) Antiepileptic medication interactions. Neurol Clin 11:905–921

Index